Clinician's Manual of Pediatric Nephrology

Clinician's Manual of Pediatric Nephrology

editors

Deepa H Chand
Akron Children's Hospital, USA

Rudolph P Valentini
Children's Hospital of Michigan, USA

World Scientific

NEW JERSEY • LONDON • SINGAPORE • BEIJING • SHANGHAI • HONG KONG • TAIPEI • CHENNAI

Published by

World Scientific Publishing Co. Pte. Ltd.
5 Toh Tuck Link, Singapore 596224
USA office: 27 Warren Street, Suite 401-402, Hackensack, NJ 07601
UK office: 57 Shelton Street, Covent Garden, London WC2H 9HE

British Library Cataloguing-in-Publication Data
A catalogue record for this book is available from the British Library.

CLINICIAN'S MANUAL OF PEDIATRIC NEPHROLOGY

ISBN-13 978-981-4317-87-0
ISBN-10 981-4317-87-X

Typeset by Stallion Press
Email: enquiries@stallionpress.com

Printed in Singapore by Mainland Press Pte Ltd.

To my best friend and husband, Bipan; my proudest achievements, Sunita and Sameer; and my parents, Hasmukh and Mina; for all of their love and support over the years.

Deepa H. Chand

To my loving wife, Nancy, and my wonderful children, Alexander and Lauren.

Rudolph P. Valentini

Preface

When we set out to create this handbook, we began with our target audience in mind. We wanted to produce a manual that would provide pediatric and pediatric nephrology trainees with a handy guide to solving kidney- and bladder-related problems. We created a comprehensive outline combining both introductory and advanced renal subject matters. Next, we invited numerous experts, including nephrologists, radiologists, and urologists, to participate in this project in an effort to optimize the instructional nature of the manual. We are indebted to the efforts of our contributors who met the challenge of writing on complex pediatric nephrology related topics and did so in a concise manner, against tight deadlines, and while still tending to their "day jobs" in patient care and research. We would also like to thank our publishing company for giving us this opportunity and believing in the project from the outset.

The efforts of many have resulted in an informative handbook that will be enriching to our target audience. If successful, it will meet our goals of improving the care of children with renal disorders. In a less direct manner, we hope this manual will inspire young pediatricians to pursue a career in the exciting field of pediatric nephrology. An increase in the pediatric nephrology work force will undoubtedly improve the access of children with renal disorders to specialists, thereby leading to better outcomes for our patients. We hope you find this guide useful, and we welcome your comments.

Kind regards,
Deepa H. Chand
Rudolph P. Valentini

Contents

Contributors

Farah N. Ali, MD, MSci
Assistant Professor of Pediatrics
Feinberg School of Medicine
Northwestern University
Division of Pediatric Kidney Diseases
Children's Memorial Hospital
USA

Uri S. Alon, MD
Professor of Pediatrics
Director, Bone and Mineral Disorders Clinic
The Children's Mercy Hospital and Clinics
University of Missouri-Kansas City School of Medicine
USA

Brian Becknell, MD, PhD
Department of Pediatrics
Nationwide Children's Hospital / The Ohio State University
USA

Marcus R. Benz, MD
Division of Pediatric Nephrology
Children's Hospital
University of Munich
Germany

John J. Bissler, MD
Clark D. West Chair of Nephrology
Professor of Pediatrics
Associate Program Director for Research and Academic Careers
Division of Nephrology and Hypertension
Cincinnati Children's Hospital Medical Center
and the University of Cincinnati College of Medicine
USA

Michael C. Braun, MD, FASN
Associate Professor of Pediatrics and Molecular Medicine
Division of Pediatric Nephrology and Hypertension
Department of Pediatrics
University of Texas Medical School at Houston
USA

Patrick D. Brophy, MD
Director Pediatric Nephrology
Associate Professor
Carver College of Medicine
University of Iowa Children's Hospital
USA

Vimal Chadha, MD
Associate Professor of Pediatrics
Chair, Section of Nephrology
Virginia Commonwealth University Medical Center
USA

Deepa H. Chand, MD, MHSA, FASN
Director, Dialysis Services
Akron Children's Hospital
Assistant Professor of Pediatrics
Northeastern Ohio Universities College of Medicine
USA

Swasti Chaturvedi, MBBS, MD, FRACP
Clinical Fellow, Division of Nephrology,
The Hospital for Sick Children
Canada

Maria E. de Ferris, MD, MPH, PhD
Associate Professor
University of North Carolina at Chapel Hill
USA

William R. DeFoor, MD, MPH
Associate Professor
Division of Pediatric Urology
Cincinnati Children's Hospital
USA

Prasad Devarajan, MD
Louise M. Williams Endowed Chair
Professor of Pediatrics and Developmental Biology
Director of Nephrology and Hypertension
Director, Clinical Nephrology Laboratories
CEO, Dialysis Unit
Cincinnati Children's Hospital Medical Center
University of Cincinnati College of Medicine
USA

Azam Eghbal, MD
Director, Pediatric Radiology Fellowship
Department of Pediatric Radiology
Akron Children's Hospital
USA

Marlo A. Eldridge, CPNP
Co-Director, Pediatric Voiding Dysfunction Clinic
Johns Hopkins Hospital
USA

Daniel Feig, MD, PhD, MS
Associate Professor, Pediatrics
Chief, Pediatric Hypertension Program
Texas Children's Hospital
Baylor College of Medicine
USA

John W. Foreman, MD
Chief, Pediatric Nephrology and Professor of Pediatrics
Department of Pediatrics
Duke University Medical Center
USA

Aaron Friedman, MD
Ruben-Bentson Professor and Chair
Department of Pediatrics
University of Minnesota
USA

Rasheed A. Gbadegesin, MBBS, MD
Assistant Professor of Pediatrics
Department of Pediatrics
Duke University Medical Center
USA

Denis F. Geary, MB, MRCP, FRCPC
Professor of Paediatrics
University of Toronto
Division of Nephrology
The Hospital for Sick Children
Canada

Jens Goebel, MD
Associate Professor of Pediatrics
Clinical Director, Nephrology and Hypertension
Medical Director of Kidney Transplantation
Cincinnati Children's Hospital Medical Center
USA

Susan E. Ingraham, MD, PhD
Fellow, Pediatric Nephrology
Nationwide Children's Hospital
USA

Gaurav Kapur, MD
Assistant Professor of Pediatrics
Wayne State University School of Medicine
Division of Pediatric Nephrology
Children's Hospital of Michigan
USA

Sanjeev Kaul, MD, MCh
Urology Resident
Henry Ford Hospital
USA

David Kershaw, MD
Associate Professor
Division Director Pediatric Nephrology
Robert C. Kelsch Collegiate Professor
C.S. Mott Children's Hospital
University of Michigan
USA

Larisa G. Kovacevic, MD
Director, Voiding Dysfunction Clinic
Co-Director, Pediatric Kidney Stone Clinic
Pediatric Urology
Children's Hospital of Michigan
USA

Yegappan Lakshmanan, MD, FAAP
Chief, Pediatric Urology
Children's Hospital of Michigan
USA

Craig B. Langman, MD
Isaac A. Abt MD Professor of Pediatrics
Northwestern University's Feinberg School of Medicine
Head, Division of Pediatric Kidney Diseases
Children's Memorial Hospital
USA

Christoph Licht, MD, FASN
Assistant Professor of Paediatrics
Division of Nephrology
The Hospital for Sick Children
Canada

Natalie Lussier, MS, RD/LD
Akron Children's Hospital
USA

Shaunna Lyon, MD
Lecturer of General Pediatrics
Department of Pediatrics
University of Iowa Children's Hospital
Carver College of Medicine
University of Iowa
USA

John D Mahan, MD
Assistant Dean for Faculty Development
Professor, Department of Pediatrics
Program Director
Pediatric Residency and Pediatric Nephrology Fellowship Programs
Vice-Chair for Education, Department of Pediatrics
Director, OSU College of Medicine Center for Education and Scholarship
The Ohio State University College of Medicine
USA

Shefali Mahesh, MD
Assistant Professor of Pediatrics
Northeastern Ohio Universities College of Medicine
Division of Pediatric Nephrology
Akron Children's Hospital
USA

Eric Z Massanyi, MD
Resident, Urology, Akron General Hospital
Akron Children's Hospital
USA

Tej K. Mattoo, MD, DCH, FRCP (UK)
Professor of Pediatrics
Wayne State University School of Medicine
Chief, Pediatric Nephrology and Hypertension
Children's Hospital of Michigan
USA

Kevin D. McBryde, MD
Medical Officer
Food and Drug Administration
Center for Devices and Radiological Health
Office of Device Evaluation
Division of Reproductive, Abdominal & Radiological Devices
Gastroenterology and Renal Devices Branch
USA

Daniel R. McMahon, MD, FAAP
Akron Children's Hospital
USA

Meredith Miller, RD/LD
Digestive Disease Institute
Cleveland Clinic
USA

Mark M. Mitsnefes, MD, MS
Associate Professor of Pediatrics
Cincinnati Children's Hospital Medical Center
USA

Corina Nailescu, MD
Assistant Professor of Clinical Pediatrics, Indiana University
Pediatric Nephrology & Hypertension Section
Medical Director of Pediatric Kidney Transplantation
James Whitcomb Riley Hospital for Children
USA

Carla M. Nester, MD
Assistant Professor of Pediatric Nephrology, Dialysis & Transplantation
Department of Pediatrics
University of Iowa Children's Hospital
Carver College of Medicine
University of Iowa
USA

Christina Nguyen, MD
Clinical Fellow, Pediatric Nephrology
Children's Hospital of Pittsburgh
USA

Abiodun A. Omoloja, MD
Associate Professor, Department of Pediatrics
Boonshoft School of Medicine
Wright State University.
Pediatric Nephrologist
Dayton Children's Medical Center Dayton, Ohio
USA

Hiren P. Patel, MD
Ohio State University College of Medicine
Nationwide Children's Hospital
USA

Elahna Paul, MD, PhD
Harvard Medical School
Pediatric Nephrology
Massachusetts General Hospital
USA

Alyssa A. Riley, MD
Fellow
Texas Children's Hospital
Baylor College of Medicine
USA

Michael Rubin, MD
Chief, Department of Pediatric Radiology
Akron Children's Hospital
USA

Franz Schaefer, MD
Professor of Pediatrics
Pediatric Nephrologist, Hypertensiologist DHL
Head, Division of Pediatric Nephrology
Director, KfH Kidney Center for Children and Adolescents
Heidelberg University Center for Pediatrics and Adolescent Medicine
Germany

Scott J. Schurman, MD
Associate Professor of Pediatrics, Pediatric Nephrology
Vice-Chair, Clinical Affairs
Upstate Medical University
USA

Curtis A. Sheldon, MD, FAAP
Professor and Chair
Division of Pediatric Urology
Cincinnati Children's Hospital
USA

Laurence Shoemaker, MD
Associate Professor of Pediatrics
Division of Nephrology
University of Louisville
USA

William E. Smoyer, MD, FASN
C. Robert Kidder Chair
Vice President, Clinical and Translational Research
Director, Center for Clinical and Translational Research
The Research Institute at Nationwide Children's Hospital
Professor of Pediatrics
The Ohio State University
USA

Michael J.G. Somers, MD
Harvard Medical School
Division of Nephrology
Children's Hospital Boston
USA

Konggrapun Srisuwan, MD
Nephrology Division, Department of Pediatrics
Phramongkutklao Hospital and College of Medicine
Thailand

Heather Stewart, MD
Internal Medicine and Pediatric Nephrology Fellow
University of North Carolina at Chapel Hill
USA

C. Frederic Strife, MD
Emeritus Professor of Pediatrics
Division of Nephrology,
Cincinnati Children's Hospital and
The University of Cincinnati College of Medicine
USA

Rudolph P. Valentini, MD
Vice President of Medical Affairs
Director of Dialysis Services
Children's Hospital of Michigan
Associate Professor of Pediatrics
Wayne State University School of Medicine
USA

Rene G. Van De Voorde III, MD
Assistant Professor, Pediatrics
Division of Pediatric Nephrology and Hypertension
Medical Director, Dialysis Unit
Cincinnati Children's Hospital Medical Center
Cincinnati, OH
USA

Victoria Vitale, MS, RD/LD
Akron Children's Hospital
USA

Thomas R. Welch, MD
Professor and Chair of Pediatrics
Upstate Medical University
Medical Director
Upstate Golisano Children's Hospital
USA

Amy C. Wilson, MD, MS
Assistant Professor of Pediatrics, Indiana University
Pediatric Nephrology and Hypertension Section
James Whitcomb Riley Hospital for Children
USA

Robert P. Woroniecki, MD, MS
Assistant Professor of Pediatrics
Associate Director, Pediatric Nephrology Training Program
Albert Einstein College of Medicine
USA

Part I

Introduction

1

Anatomy and Physiology of the Nephron

Christina Nguyen, Deepa H. Chand and Rudolph P. Valentini

Renal Development

Human kidney development begins in the fifth week of gestation, with the first functioning nephron formed by week 9. Urine production commences at 12 weeks gestation. By 32–34 weeks gestation, glomerulogenesis is completed and no new nephrons are formed. Development of the kidney is derived from two components of the metanephros: the ureteric bud and metanephric mesenchyme. The ureteric bud gives rise to the collecting duct, renal calyces, renal pelvis, ureter, and trigone of the bladder, whereas the metanephric mesenchyme gives rise to all the epithelial cell types, the proximal convoluted tubule, ascending and descending loops of Henle, and the distal convoluted tubule. The development of the kidney involves four processes: outgrowth of the ureteric bud, branching of the ureteric bud, patterning of the cortical and medullary collecting duct system, and formation of the pelvicalyceal system. Glomerular capillaries appear to arise from angiogenesis from in growth of existing capillaries in the developing embryo.

Renal Anatomy

Gross anatomy

The kidneys are located retroperitoneally. The kidney is covered by a smooth, fibrous capsule. The right kidney is positioned slightly lower than the left. Each kidney is approximately 5 cm in length at birth, growing to an adult size of 11–12 cm by late adolescence. Along the medial margin of the kidney rests the hilus. This is where the renal pelvis, artery, vein, lymphatics, and nerve plexus pass into the renal sinus. The renal pelvis extends into a funnel-shaped system, the calyces, which attaches to the renal papillae.

The kidneys receive 20% of the cardiac output, approximately 1 liter/minute of blood flow. The renal artery is a direct branch of the aorta and divides into anterior and posterior branches at the hilus. These branches create lobar arteries that run toward the papillae and branch into interlobar arteries. The interlobar arteries ascend to the corticomedullary junction where they continue into the arcuate arteries that run parallel to the kidney surface. The interlobar arteries continue to ascend from the arcuate arteries, forming afferent arterioles at the level of the cortex. Efferent arterioles form a peritubular capillary network in the cortex to carry blood from the glomeruli. The blood from the capillaries drains into the interlobular, arcuate, and interlobar veins, ultimately leaving the kidney through the renal vein.

The kidney is divided into two units, the cortex and medulla. The medulla consists of 8–18 pyramids, whose bases rest at the corticomedullary junction. The apices of the pyramid form papillae. From the base of the pyramid, medullary rays extend into the cortex. These consist of collecting ducts and the straight portions of the proximal and distal tubules. The functional unit of the kidney is the nephron, consisting of the glomerulus and its associated tubule. The tubule can be divided into three subdivisions: the proximal convoluted tubule, loop of Henle, and distal convoluted tubule. Nephrons originating from the outer and mid-cortical glomeruli have short loops of Henle that reach the outer medulla where as juxtamedullary nephrons have long loops of Henle that extend into the inner medulla.

The nephron (Fig. 1)

Glomeruli are located within the cortex and are responsible for the formation of an ultrafiltrate of plasma. It is an elaborate structure consisting of capillaries, mesangial cells, and glomerular epithelial cells, both visceral (podocytes) and parietal. The fenestrated endothelium is the initial barrier to the passage of blood components. The glomerular basement membrane (GBM) is composed of type IV collagen, fibronectin, and glycosaminoglycans that are negatively charged. It is located between the endothelium and visceral epithelium. It has three layers: the *lamina densa*, *lamina rara externa* and *lamina rara interna*. The GBM serves as a size and charge-selective barrier to macromolecule passage. Podocytes are in close contact with the GBM. The spaces between adjacent foot processes, slit pores, are closed be a thin membrane known as the slit diaphragm. The podocytes

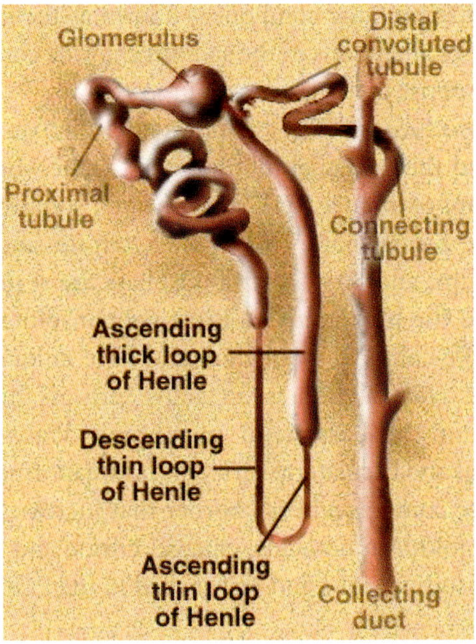

Figure 1. Diagram of the nephron [Source: http://apbio12007.blogspot.com/2007_12_01_archive.html].

have long cytoplasmic processes that divide into foot processes that are negatively charged and are essential in maintaining the normal structure and function of the filtration barrier. Mesangial cells lie in the mesangial matrix. They provide structural support for the capillary loops and contain filaments. The cells are stimulated by angiotensin II, causing the filaments to contract and thereby limiting filtration by decreasing the surface area for filtration. Mesangial cells are also phagocytic and sequester immune complexes in some forms of glomerulonephritis.

The juxtaglomerular apparatus is located at the vascular pole of the glomerulus. It contains the terminal portion of the afferent arteriole and the initial portion of the efferent arteriole. A group of cells at that vascular pole contain granules that secrete renin. Renin (*angiotensinogenase*) is an enzyme involved in the generation of angiotensin I through cleavage of angiotensinogen produced by the liver. This sets up the cascade of the renin–angiotensin–aldosterone system which is important in blood pressure regulation, as well as sodium and potassium regulation. The start of the thick ascending limb contains a specialized tubular component known as the *macula densa*. The *macula densa* senses alterations in the sodium chloride concentration, sending a feedback response that regulates renin secretion.

The kidneys produce 180 liters of filtrate per day, yet only excrete 1–2 liters of urine and the proximal tubule serves as the workhorse for reabsorption. Here, approximately 65–70% of water, sodium and potassium, 100% of glucose, bicarbonate, amino acids, citrate, and small peptides, 40–50% of calcium, and 80–95% of phosphate are reabsorbed from the tubular fluid into the blood stream. Proximal convoluted tubules (PCT) are lined by simple cuboidal epithelium and have unique surface specializations. Sodium reabsorption is an active process mediated through Na^+/K^+-ATPase on the basolateral membrane. Water moves directly through the apical and basolateral surfaces via aquaporins, water channels. The apical surface contains a brush border that increases the surface area of the cell by 36 fold. Amino acids, glucose, citrate and bicarbonate ions are coupled with sodium ions and reabsorbed in the PCT down a concentration gradient.

The thin loop of Henle extends from the proximal tubule to the start of the thick ascending limb (TAL) and has no active transport of sodium or chloride anywhere along its course. Molecule transportation occurs through the countercurrent multiplication mechanism. The descending limb is permeable to water, but not sodium and chloride whereas the ascending limb is impermeable to water and highly permeable to sodium and chloride. Therefore, water diffuses out of the descending limb through aquaporin channels and subsequently, the sodium exits the ascending limb down its concentration gradient.

The TAL is a component of the distal tubule and is subdivided into a medullary and cortical segment. The cortical TAL is the site of 60–70% of the filtered magnesium reabsorption through a passive process drive by tight junction proteins paracellin-1 and claudin-19. Both the cortical and medullary TAL are the sites of Na^+/K^+-ATPase active transport. Invaginations of the basolateral membrane hold the transporters and are therefore responsible for active reabsorption of sodium chloride which is important in urinary concentrating and diluting mechanisms. The TAL serves as the site of action of loop diuretics. It is impermeable to water and active reabsorption of sodium creates a hypertonic interstitium and ensures the delivery for a hypotonic tubular fluid to the distal convoluted tubule (DCT). The DCT is the principal site of action of thiazide diuretics.

The collecting duct is the final segment of the distal nephron. The connecting tubule bridges between the DCT and collecting duct. This is the site of critical hormonal regulation via aldosterone and vasopressin. The collecting duct changes its appearance between the cortex and papillary tip. In the cortex, there are principal and intercalated cells. The principal cells are the site of salt and water transport and intercalated cells are critical to acid–base regulation. The medullary collecting duct more closely resembles the tall cells of the transitional epithelium that lines the bladder. A number of genetic diseases involving abnormalities of tubular transport in various segments of the nephron are listed in Table 1.

Table 1. Molecular basis of genetic disorders of renal transport

Inherited disorder	Location	Protein defect
X-linked Hypophosphatemic rickets	Proximal tubule	PHEX gene
Fanconi syndrome	Proximal tubule	Many: dependent on underlying cause of Fanconi syndrome
Dent disease	Proximal tubule	Chloride channel transporter CLC–5 Cl^-/H^+ exchanger
Bartter syndrome	TAL	Type I: Na–K–2Cl cotransporter (NKCC2) Type II: Apical potassium Channel (ROMK) Type III: Basolateral chloride channel (ClC–Kb) Type IV: Barttin protein
Gitelman syndrome	DCT	Thiazide-sensitive Na–Cl cotransporter (NCCT)
Liddle syndrome Pseudohypoaldosteronism type I	Collecting duct	Epithelial sodium channel (ENaC)
Nephrogenic diabetes insipidus	Collecting duct	X-linked: Arginine vasopressin receptor (V2R), 90% of cases Autosomal: Aquaporin 2 water channel, 10% of cases

Suggested Reading

Akbar S, Moe S. (2009) Disorders of calcium and phosphorus. In: Greenberg AM. (ed.) *Primer on Kidney Diseases* (5th ed.) Saunders Elsevier. pp. 118–128.

Burns J. (2009) Disorders of magnesium homeostasis. In: Greenberg AM. (ed.) *Primer on Kidney Diseases* (5th ed.) Saunders Elsevier. pp. 129–134.

Hellman N, O'Seaghdha C. (2009) *The Renal Fellow Network.* [http://renalfellow.blogspot.com/]

Madsen K, Verlander J. (2004) Renal structure in relation to function. In: Wilcox CS, Tisher CC. (eds.) *Handbook of Nephrology and Hypertension* (5th ed.) Lippincott Williams and Wilkins. pp. 3–13.

Piscione T, Waters A. (2008) Structural and functional development of the kidney. In: Geary D, Schaefer F. (eds.) *Comprehensive Pediatric Nephrology.* Mosby Elsevier Health Sciences. pp. 91–130.

Rose B, Post T. (2009) *Glomerular Anatomy and Function.* [http://www.uptodate.com] Accessed January 2010.

2
The Urinalysis

Hiren P. Patel

Introduction

The urinalysis is one of the most commonly utilized tests in pediatrics. This is not only due to its ease of collection and testing, but also the potential usefulness of the information. Urine testing can identify a number of renal, urinary tract, and systemic disorders. A basic review of the urinalysis, urine microscopic analysis, and quantitative urine protein testing will be presented.

Technique

The urinalysis should be performed on a freshly voided specimen to limit false positive and false negative results. If urine will not be tested for more than an hour, it should be refrigerated. If refrigerated, urine should be warmed to room temperature before testing. Other measures to reduce false readings include proper handling of urine dipsticks and avoiding prolonged immersion of dipstick in urine. A midstream urine specimen will reduce contamination.

Screening Urinalysis

The merits of mass screening of asymptomatic healthy children have been debated for some time. The American Academy of Pediatrics had previously recommended a screening urinalysis at four points during childhood, but the most recent preventive health care recommendation no longer mentions obtaining a screening urinalysis in an asymptomatic child at any age. Minor abnormalities on screening urinalysis are common but often are either transient or due to a false positive reading. In the United States, mass screening of asymptomatic individuals has not been shown to be cost effective.

Urine dipstick testing

When interpreting urinalysis results, it should be kept in mind that not all abnormal results are clinically significant. In addition, false positive and false negative results are common (see Table 1).

Table 1. Causes of false positive and false negative results in urine dipstick testing

Urine Dipstick test	False positives	False negatives
Specific gravity	Contamination during collection/storage	None
pH	High pH from urease producing organisms (e.g. *Proteus mirabilis*), prolonged standing of urine	Low pH from mixing of reagents from adjacent test pads
Blood	Oxidizing contaminants (e.g. hypochlorite), microbial peroxidase associated with UTI	High ascorbic acid, large nitrites, high SG
Protein	Fever, exercise, alkaline urine, concentrated urine, presence of cells/bacteria in urine	Dilute urine, low molecular weight proteins
Glucose	Strong oxidizing agents in urine container	Ascorbic acid, high SG, exposure to humid environment
Ketones	Captopril, methyldopa	Prolonged standing of urine, moisture on test pad
Bilirubin	Rifampin, chlorpromazine	Ascorbic acid, prolonged standing in light
Urobilinogen	Alkaline urine, sulfonamides (for Multistix®)	Broad spectrum antibiotics, discolored urine, prolonged standing in light
Nitrite	Urine contamination, medications which turn urine color to red, gross hematuria	Inadequate dietary nitrate intake (vegetables), non nitrate reducing bacteria, insufficient incubation time for conversion of nitrate to nitrite, ascorbic acid, high urobilinogen
Leukocyte esterase	Contamination with vaginal fluid, oxidizing agents, Trichomonas	Ascorbic acid, high protein, high glucose, high SG, cephalosporins, tetracycline, nitrofurantoin

SG, specific gravity; UTI, urinary tract infection. [Reproduced with permission from Patel HP. (2006) The abnormal urinalysis. *Pediatr Clin N Am* **53**: 325–337.]

Color and appearance

The normal appearance of a freshly voided urine sample is clear with pale to dark yellow color depending on urine concentration. A number of medications and foods can alter urine color (Table 2). The differential diagnosis for cloudy appearing urine is listed in Table 3. If cloudy urine obtained and suspicion for urinary tract infection (UTI) is nil, urinalysis with microscopy should be repeated on a freshly voided specimen after increasing fluid intake.

Table 2. Foods and medications that may discolor urine

Urine color	Food	Medication
Bright yellow–orange	Carrots, rhubarb	Phenazopyridine, rifampin, sulfasalazine, riboflavin, thiamine, multivitamin
Red–pink	Beets, rhubarb, food coloring	Senna, deferoxamine, phenolphthalein
Brown–black	Blackberries	Metronidazole, nitrofurantoin, quinolones, chloroquine, methyldopa, levodopa
Blue–green		Methylene blue, vitamin B complex

Table 3. Differential diagnosis of cloudy urine

Urinary tract infection/bacteruria
Pyuria
Crystalluria
Calcium–phosphorous precipitation
Alkaline urine
Elevated urine calcium or phosphorous
Prostatic secretions
Elevated urine urates
Prolonged standing of urine (> 1 hour)
Concentrated urine

Specific gravity

The specific gravity (SG) reagent on the dipstick is a measure of urine concentration and should be interpreted with the clinical situation in mind. A urine SG of 1.010 approximates a urine osmolality of 300 mOsm/L. In a healthy child, the urine SG simply reflects recent fluid intake. A high urine

SG may reflect dehydration in someone who has been ill. Low urine SG in a dehydrated patient indicates inability of kidneys to appropriately concentrate urine.

pH

Urine pH is reliable only on a freshly voided specimen and ranges from 5–8 in healthy individuals. It is useful in clinical situations such as metabolic acidosis and certain types of kidney stones. A low urine pH promotes formation of uric acid and cystine stones while high urine pH promotes calcium-phosphate precipitation.

Hemoglobin

The urine dipstick is very sensitive to intact red blood cells (RBCs) and free hemoglobin. Due to the high sensitivity, transient microscopic hematuria is common. Therefore, the initial step in asymptomatic children with microscopic hematuria and no other abnormalities on urinalysis or physical exam is to obtain at least two repeat urinalyses at least one week apart. When urine dipstick is persistently positive for blood, a urine microscopic exam should be performed. The differential diagnosis of hematuria is extensive and discussed in more detail in a later chapter.

Protein

Normal urine protein excretion (see Table 4) consists mostly of Tamm-Horsfall protein, which is secreted by the tubules. The primary protein excreted in glomerular disorders is albumin. The proteinuria in tubular

Table 4. Reference values for urine protein measurements

Test	Normal	Nephrotic range
Urine dipstick	Negative–trace	$\geq 3^+$ (300 mg/dL)
Urine protein to creatinine ratio (mg/mg)	≤ 0.2 (> 2 year old) < 0.5 (6m–24m)	> 2
24-hour urine protein	< 4 mg/m^2/hr	> 40 mg/m^2/hr
Urine albumin to creatinine ratio (mg/mg)	≤ 0.03	
24-hour urine albumin	< 20 mcg/m	

disorders mostly consists of low molecular weight proteins typically reabsorbed by healthy tubules. One limitation of the urine dipstick is it primarily detects albumin, not low molecular weight proteins. Additionally, the sensitivity of this dipstick is insufficient to detect microalbuminuria (see below).

Proteinuria can be an important marker of kidney disease. Negative or trace protein on the dipstick is considered normal, while 1+ protein (30 mg/dL) or greater should be monitored. Table 1 lists causes of false positives for urine protein. If a concern for a false positive or negative reading exists, proteinuria should be quantified by urine protein/creatinine ratio on a random urine specimen. Evaluation of proteinuria is discussed in more detail in a subsequent chapter.

Glucose

The presence of glucose in the urine may reflect hyperglycemia or proximal tubular dysfunction. Typically, glycosuria does not appear until the plasma level exceeds 180 to 200 mg/dL, at which point the glucose load in the filtrate exceeds the proximal tubule's capacity to completely reabsorb glucose. If glycosuria occurs, serum glucose level should be checked. If normal, then glycosuria may reflect a proximal tubular defect in ability to reabsorb a normal filtered glucose load. This could be an isolated defect termed renal glucosuria (benign) or part of a generalized proximal tubulopathy referred to as Fanconi syndrome.

Ketones

Increased breakdown of fatty acids leads to ketogenesis, which usually occurs in setting of altered glucose metabolism. A small amount of ketones in the urine may be seen in healthy children after a brief fast. Urine ketones are expected in individuals on a high-fat/low-carbohydrate diet (e.g. ketogenic diet). More pathologic causes of ketonuria include uncontrolled diabetes mellitus, acute illnesses with limited food intake, liver disease and certain forms of glycogen storage disease.

Bilirubin and urobilinogen

Conjugated bilirubin is water soluble and appears in the urine, whereas unconjugated bilirubin remains protein-bound. Most conjugated bilirubin is eliminated by the gastrointestinal tract via bile. Detection of bilirubin in urine suggests obstruction to bile outflow or hepatitis.

Urobilinogen is a product of conjugated bilirubin metabolized by colonic bacteria. Some urobilinogen is reabsorbed and enters the portal circulation. Most of this urobilinogen is processed by the liver while a small amount is excreted in the urine. Patients with liver dysfunction may have decreased hepatic uptake of urobilinogen, leading to increased urine excretion. Increased urine urobilinogen and negative bilirubin can be seen with increased hemolysis or tissue bleeding. Decreased urine urobilinogen may be seen with severe biliary obstruction (absence of bilirubin in the intestines) and with broad-spectrum antibiotics (decreased urobilinogen formation in the colon).

Nitrite and leukocyte esterase

Positive urine nitrites are strongly suggestive of gram negative bacilli and a urine culture should be performed. Since bacteria require up to four hours to convert urinary nitrate to nitrite, a false negative can occur if urine is present in the urinary tract for insufficient time period. Leukocyte esterase in the urine suggests presence of neutrophils, which could be due to bacterial UTI or sterile pyuria from another inflammatory process (see Table 5).

Thus, nitrites have high specificity and lower sensitivity for detecting UTI while leukocyte esterase has high sensitivity and lower specificity. Combining both tests results in relatively high sensitivity and low false-positive rate. Nonetheless, UTI must be confirmed with a urine culture.

Urine Microscopy

Microscopic examination of the urine can provide useful diagnostic information, especially when urine dipstick is abnormal. To examine the urine sediment, approximately 10 ml of urine is centrifuged for five minutes at moderate speed, then the supernatant is decanted and the remaining drop is examined on a clean slide. This must be done on a freshly voided specimen.

Table 5. Differential diagnosis of sterile pyuria

Infection of the Genitourinary Tract
Viral cystitis
Renal abscess
Urethritis
Epididymitis
Balanitis
Tuberculosis
Inflammation of the Genitourinary Tract
Glomerulonephritis
Interstitial nephritis
Hemorrhagic cystitis
Tumor
Renal papillary necrosis
Kidney stones
Fever
Inflammation in Proximity of the Urinary Tract
Vulvovaginitis
Appendicitis

Cells

Red blood cells

A child with persistently positive urine dipsticks for blood should have the presence of increased RBCs confirmed with urine microscopy. In most labs, up to 3–5 RBCs per high power field is considered normal. A patient with red or brown urine with a dipstick strongly positive for blood but minimal RBCs on microscopy, rhabdomyolysis (myoglobinuria) or intravascular hemolysis (hemoglobinuria) should be excluded. Microscopic exam may underestimate RBC number in a dilute yellow urine specimen, due to RBC lysis in a hypotonic environment.

Urine microscopy can also be useful in evaluating source of hematuria. Presence of dysmorphic RBCs and RBC casts suggest a glomerular hematuria. Lack of dysmorphic RBCs and casts suggest lower urinary tract bleeding although a renal etiology cannot be ruled out. Dysmorphic RBCs may have membrane blebs, irregular surface or other membrane defects, but crenated RBCs in a concentrated urine specimen are normal.

White blood cells

Greater than 5–10 white blood cells (WBCs) per high power field is usually considered abnormal. Pyuria suggests UTI although many other causes of sterile pyuria can occur (Table 5). WBCs from the vagina can contaminate the urine and give a false positive result. Thus, urine culture should be performed to confirm UTI. Prolonged standing of hypotonic urine can result in a false negative due to lysis of WBCs.

Eosinophils

Urine eosinophilia (greater than 1% of total urine WBCs) has been proposed to be a useful marker in identifying medication-induced acute interstitial nephritis. However, urine eosinophils can be seen with other renal disorders. The false positive and false negative rate of urine eosinophils is too high to be useful for distinguishing interstitial nephritis. Urine eosinophils are not measured in a standard urinalysis; it requires a special Wright stain to assist in detection.

Epithelial cells

Renal tubular cells, urinary tract transitional cells and squamous epithelial cells may be noted on microscopic exam. All three cells types may be observed in normal urine in small amounts. Increased numbers of renal tubular cells may be observed with acute tubular necrosis and injury from nephrotoxic agents. Squamous epithelial cells line the distal third of the urethra and in females, may originate from the vagina or vulva. Large amounts of squamous epithelial cells in the urine suggest contamination.

Bacteria

Detection of bacteria on urine microscopy in asymptomatic patients is most likely due to contamination with normal flora from either the external urethral meatus or vagina. In centrifuged urine, the bacteria will clump and be more easily seen.

Casts

Urinary casts, which are formed in the distal nephron, consist of a Tamm-Horsfall mucoprotein matrix with or without additional elements. Casts can be easily missed if microscopy is not performed within 30 minutes after voiding. Several different types of casts may be seen on urine microscopy (see Table 6), but hyaline casts are most common. Hyaline casts are primarily mucoproteins and typically clinically insignificant. They may be increased with decreased urine output, concentrated urine, fever and exercise. Cellular casts are of greater significance when present.

Table 6. Differential diagnoses of urinary casts. glomerulonephritis (GN)

Cast	Differential diagnosis
Hyaline	Normal health, fever, exercise, diuretics, renal disease
Granular	Normal health, glomerular disease, tubular disease, infection
Waxy	Advanced renal failure
Fatty	Nephrotic syndrome
Red blood cell	GN, tubulointerstitial nephritis, acute tubular injury/necrosis
White blood cell	Pyelonephritis, GN, tubulointerstitial nephritis
Epithelial cell	Acute tubular injury/necrosis, tubulointerstitial nephritis, GN

Crystals

Urine crystals are commonly reported on microscopy, but usually of limited clinical significance. Crystal formation depends on numerous factors including solute concentration, ionic strength, urine pH, and presence of promoters or inhibitors. Fluid intake, dietary intake and body metabolism alter these factors. Certain medications such as sulfonamides and ampicillin may crystallize in the urine. Healthy children often possess urine that is supersaturated with calcium oxalate, calcium phosphate and sodium urate; the presence of these crystals on urine microscopy does not necessarily indicate the patient is forming stones. Cystine, tyrosine and leucine crystals, on the other hand, are always pathologic.

Quantitative Urine Protein Measurements

Twenty-four hour urine collections have traditionally been considered the gold standard for quantifying urine protein excretion. However, they are cumbersome and difficult to obtain accurately, especially in younger children. Fortunately, the urine protein/creatinine ratio and albumin/creatinine ratio from a random urine specimen can estimate the 24-hour excretion of protein and albumin with reasonable accuracy. These spot urine protein/creatinine ratios can also be used to monitor therapy. As such, the ease of use and accuracy of the spot urine protein/creatinine ratios has essentially eliminated the need for 24-hour urine collection for proteinuria in the pediatric patient.

Urine protein/creatinine ratio

The urine protein/creatinine ratio more accurately estimates the degree of proteinuria compared to urine dipstick, being much less prone to false negative and false positive results. The urine sample should ideally be a first morning void. Reference values for the urine protein/creatinine ratio are listed in Table 4.

Urine albumin/creatinine ratio

Microalbuminuria refers to a urine albumin excretion rate above the normal range (see Table 4), but below the threshold of detection by standard urine dipsticks. By definition, microalbuminuria is only detectable by a urine quantification test. As with protein, the urine albumin to creatinine ratio on a random sample (preferably first morning void) correlates reasonably well with albumin excretion in a timed urine sample. Microalbuminuria is the earliest clinical finding of diabetic nephropathy, but diabetic children with elevated urine albumin to creatinine ratios should also be evaluated for orthostatic proteinuria.

Summary

The urinalysis is an oft-employed test in pediatrics. While very useful, the urinalysis by dipstick is subject to false positive and false negative results, as well as transient findings. The interpretation of abnormal urinalysis results and need for further evaluation should be guided by the clinical situation. Further evaluation may include simply retesting the urine to check for persistence of abnormal findings or additional testing for underlying conditions. In certain situations, urine microscopic exam and quantification testing are useful follow-up studies to urine dipstick testing.

Suggested Reading

American Academy of Pediatrics Committee on Practice and Ambulatory Medicine and Bright Futures Steering Committee. (2007) Recommendations for preventive pediatric health care. *Pediatr* **120**: 1376.

American Academy of Pediatrics Committee on Quality Improvement, Subcommittee on Urinary Tract Infection. (1999) Practice parameter: the diagnosis, treatment, and evaluation of the initial urinary tract infection in febrile infants and young children. *Pediatr* **103**: 843–852.

Hogg RJ, Portman RJ, Milliner D, *et al.* (2000) Evaluation and management of proteinuria and nephrotic syndrome in children: recommendations from a pediatric nephrology panel established at the National Kidney Foundation conference on proteinuria, albuminuria, risk, assessment, detection, and elimination (PARADE). *Pediatr* **105**: 1242–1249.

Patel HP. (2006) The abnormal urinalysis. *Pediatr Clin N Am* **53**: 325–337.

Simerville JA, Maxted WC, Pahira JJ. (2005) Urinalysis: a comprehensive review. *Am Fam Phys* **71**: 1153–1162.

3

Evaluation of Renal Function in the Pediatric Patient

Susan E. Ingraham and Hiren P. Patel

Introduction

As in all patient evaluations, workup of kidney function begins with patient's history and physical examination. Blood pressure, clinical status, fluid balance, and urine output may all be important indicators of renal function. For example, "normal" urine output in a child with clinical signs of dehydration may be a sign of a renal concentrating defect. Oliguria, edema, and hypertension may signal acute kidney injury. Renal tubular disorders may present with polyuria, polydipsia, growth retardation, or failure to thrive. If history and physical examination indicate a need to further evaluate renal function, initial steps usually involve urinalysis and measurement of serum creatinine and blood urea nitrogen (BUN). Additional tests may be needed and will be discussed below.

The Basic Serum Chemistries: BUN and Creatinine

Urea is the end result of protein metabolism in the human body. It is freely filtered at the glomerulus and up to 50% is reabsorbed in the tubules. Blood urea nitrogen levels are sensitive indicators of renal disease, becoming elevated when renal function is decreased by 25–50%. However, the BUN is not specific for kidney disease, since it may be affected by nonrenal factors as well. A decreased BUN level is rarely of clinical interest, but may be due to inadequate protein intake or severe liver disease. Increased BUN or azotemia is due to either increased protein catabolism or impaired kidney function. Increased protein catabolism may result from ingestion of a high-protein diet, severe physiological stress, corticosteroid use or bleeding in the gastrointestinal (GI) tract (where blood is digested and absorbed). Impaired renal function leading to azotemia is further classified into prerenal, intrinsic, or postrenal etiologies.

Creatinine results from the enzymatic degradation of creatine and phosphocreatine during muscle catabolism, and is typically released from skeletal muscle at a steady rate. The serum creatinine level in a healthy individual correlates closely with the skeletal muscle mass. Creatinine is freely filtered by the glomerulus, and a small amount is also secreted into the filtrate in the proximal tubule. A few drugs including cimetidine, trimethoprim, triamterene, amiloride, and probenecid block tubular secretion of creatinine, and therefore may cause a modest increase in serum creatinine level despite lack of renal injury. Serum creatinine level is the most commonly used marker for "renal function," since it is fairly sensitive for changes in glomerular function, and is more specific than BUN.

Glomerular Function Tests

Glomerular Filtration Rate (GFR)

GFR is the most useful measurement of renal function. Other kidney functions (including tubular transport, vitamin D activation, and erythropoietin production) decline as GFR decreases. GFR is central to the National Kidney Foundation guidelines for the definition, classification, and management of chronic kidney disease, described in more detail elsewhere. Knowledge of a patient's GFR is essential for the appropriate prescription of fluids, solutes, and medications.

GFR is the volume of ultrafiltrate passing into the nephron tubules per unit time. GFR depends on the total number of filtering nephrons and the filtration rate of each individual nephron. The latter depends on the glomerular transcapillary hydrostatic pressure difference, plasma oncotic pressure, and glomerular plasma flow rate. The standard units for GFR are milliliters per minute (ml/min). In children, GFR is normalized to ideal adult body surface area, giving units in ml/min/1.73 m^2. This standardized approach allows GFR to follow a predictable developmental course in a normal pediatric patient (Table 1). GFR decreases when nephrons are lost to injury, disease or surgery. However, compensatory changes often occur

Table 1. Glomerular filtration rates in healthy infants, children, and young adults (adapted from Schwartz and Guignard)

Age	Normal GFR (ml/min/1.73m^2)
Preterm babies	
1–30 days	10–60
1–4 months	50–85
Term babies	
< 1 week	25–40
1– weeks	45–60
1–3 months	50–90
4–6 months	65–100
7–12 months	70–110
1–2 years	75–120
Children	
3–4 years	90–125
5–12 years	95–135
Adolescents	
12–15 years	100–135
Young adults	
16–34 years	100–125

in the remaining nephrons such that reduction in renal function is less than predicted from extent of anatomic change. This compensatory ability is often referred to as "renal reserve." GFR cannot be measured directly, but many approaches have been developed to indirectly measure or estimate GFR.

Clearance

GFR is measured indirectly using the concept of renal clearance. Clearance of a substance is the plasma volume from which a substance would be completely removed to equal the urinary excretion rate of the substance per unit time. The clearance of a substance freely filtered by the glomerulus without further renal handling (i.e. reabsorption, secretion, or metabolism in the tubules or collecting ducts) closely approximates true GFR.

Renal clearance of any substance is calculated by:

$$C = (U \times V)/P$$

C represents clearance of a substance, U is urinary concentration of the substance, V is volume of urine per given time period, and P is concurrent plasma concentration of the substance. Although 24-hour urine collection is the common standard for calculating clearance, any carefully timed urine collection (e.g. a 12-hour collection) may be sufficient. A variety of substances, both endogenous and exogenous, have been used for GFR determination by measuring clearance.

Inulin

Inulin is an exogenous marker whose clearance has long been considered the "gold standard" for GFR measurement due to absent protein binding or tubular handling. Unfortunately, clinical determination of inulin clearance is cumbersome and technically difficult; moreover, inulin is currently unavailable for clinical use in the United States and several other countries. Therefore, alternative methods for GFR measurement/estimation are currently used.

Creatinine clearance

Creatinine is most commonly used endogenous marker for formal GFR measurement. Creatinine clearance is determined by measuring creatinine concentrations of a timed urine collection and a concurrent serum sample. Creatinine clearance is calculated as follows:

$$\begin{aligned}&\text{Creatinine clearance (mL/min/1.73 m}^2\text{)}\\&= [(U_{Cr} \times V)/(P_{Cr} \times T)] \times (1.73/\text{BSA})\end{aligned}$$

Where U_{Cr} is urine creatinine concentration in mg/dL, V is total urine volume collected during the sampling period in mL, P_{Cr} is plasma/serum creatinine concentration in mg/dL, T is duration of urine sampling period in minutes (24 h = 1440 min), and BSA is the patient's body surface area in m^2. As discussed, creatinine undergoes both glomerular filtration and tubular secretion in the kidney. Therefore, creatinine clearance is not a perfect measure of GFR, because secreted creatinine plus filtered creatinine will be included in the urine concentration. When GFR is normal, the secreted portion of urine creatinine is negligible. When GFR is low (<30 ml/min/1.73m^2), tubular secretion approaches or even exceeds amount filtered at the glomerulus. Therefore, creatinine clearance overestimates GFR in advanced kidney disease. For individuals with low GFR, averaging creatinine clearance and urea clearance gives a more accurate estimate of true GFR.

Other methods to measure GFR

Many other exogenous substances have been used in clinical or research settings for GFR determination by measuring renal clearance. These include iohexol, iothalamate, diethylene triamine penta-acetic acid (DTPA), and ethylene diamine tetra-acetic acid (EDTA). A nuclear GFR test involves labeling an exogenous substance with a radioactive tracer (^{99}Tc-DTPA is most common in the United States; ^{51}Cr-EDTA in Europe), intravenous infusion, and determining GFR by either measuring renal uptake of radiotracer using a gamma camera, or plasma disappearance of tracer using serial plasma concentration measurements. The gamma camera method also allows determination of GFR of each individual kidney, but does not measure total GFR as accurately as obtaining serial plasma concentrations.

Cystatin C

Cystatin C is an endogenous protein produced by all nucleated cells at a relatively constant rate and uninfluenced by muscle mass, gender, or body composition over the age of one, up to 50 years of age. In healthy individuals greater than one year, serum cystatin C is approximately 1 mg/liter. Cystatin C is catabolized and almost completely reabsorbed in the proximal tubule, therefore, cystatin clearance is not useful. Nonetheless, serum cystatin C levels closely correlate with GFR, and may be more sensitive to subtle alterations in renal function than serum creatinine. To estimate GFR from serum cystatin C level in children:

$$\log_{10}(\text{GFR}) = 1.962 + [1.123 \times \log_{10}(1/\text{cysC})]$$

where cysC is serum cystatin C concentration (mg/L) and GFR is ml/min/1.73m^2. Factors other than renal function, including C-reactive protein levels and smoking status, may affect serum cystatin C levels.

Furthermore, cystatin C may appear in the urine during glomerular or tubular injury, raising doubts about reliability of cystatin C in estimating GFR in acute kidney injury.

Equations to estimate GFR

Close relationships between muscle mass and creatinine production, and between creatinine clearance and glomerular function, have led to the concept of estimating GFR from serum creatinine level and anthropomorphic data. In pediatrics, this is typically done using the Schwartz formula:

$$eGFR = kL/S_{Cr}$$

eGFR is ml/min/1.73m^2, L is length/height of patient in centimeters, S_{Cr} is serum creatinine in mg/dl, and k is a constant determined empirically by Schwartz and colleagues. The k value for different age groups is listed in Table 2. The Schwartz formula generates good estimates for GFR in patients with normal or mildly impaired renal function, and in many circumstances is preferable to complicated measurements of clearance. However, it becomes unreliable in situations in which height is not an accurate reflection of muscle mass (such as severe obesity, limb amputations, bodybuilding, and malnourishment), as well as situations where GFR is rapidly changing (e.g. acute kidney injury). In advanced chronic renal failure, the Schwartz formula tends to overestimate GFR.

Table 2. Values of k for GFR estimating formulas in children. The equation for both formulae is kL/S_{Cr}. GFR, glomerular filtration rate; k, constant; L, height in cm; S_{Cr}, serum creatinine (mg/dl)

Age	Schwartz	Modified bedside Schwartz*
Premature infants < 1 year	0.33	
Full term infants < 1 year	0.45	
Children 1–12 years	0.55	0.413
Females 13–20 years	0.55	0.413
Males 13–20 years	0.70	0.413

*Applies to children ages 1 to 18 with GFR < 75 ml/min/1.73m^2.

It should be noted that the original Schwartz formula was developed using creatinine values measured by Jaffe chromogen methods. This laboratory technique has largely been replaced by enzymatic (creatinase) measurements. The enzymatic methods generate serum creatinine measurements typically 10–20% lower than the Jaffe technique, so the original Schwartz formula may overestimate GFR when serum creatinine is measured by newer laboratory methods. In 2009, the Schwartz formula was re-evaluated and revised. The new Schwartz formula is based on patient height, serum creatinine, serum cystatin C, BUN and gender:

$$GFR = 39.1(L/S_{Cr})^{0.516} \times (1.8/cysC)^{0.294} \times (30/BUN)^{0.169} \times (L/1.4)^{0.188} \times (\text{gender correction})$$

GFR is ml/min/1.73 m^2, L is length/height of patient in meters, S_{cr} is serum creatinine in mg/dl, cysC is serum cystatin C in mg/L, BUN is in mg/dl, and the gender correction is 1 for females and 1.099 for males. A good approximation of the above formula was obtained with a simplified "bedside" equation:

$$eGFR = 0.413(L/S_{Cr})$$

eGFR is ml/min/1.73 m^2, L is length/height of patient in centimeters, and S_{cr} is serum creatinine in mg/dl. These equations were determined and tested in pediatric patients with varying degrees of chronic kidney disease. Additional studies are needed to validate these formulas for use in children with GFR > 75 ml/min/1.73 m^2.

The Schwartz and modified Schwartz equations were developed specifically for pediatric use. Different equations are used to estimate GFR in adults, based on serum creatinine, age, gender, race, and body weight. The Modification of Diet in Renal Disease (MDRD) and Cockcroft-Gault equations are the most commonly used in adult medicine, but are inappropriate for children.

Tubular Function Tests

In most cases where renal impairment is suspected, alteration of glomerular function is the primary concern. However, renal tubules play a critical role in fluid and electrolyte homeostasis, and tubular defects can cause significant impairment in the adaptive renal response to fluid or electrolyte changes. Tubular function includes processes specific to the proximal tubule (phosphate, glucose, bicarbonate, and amino acid handling) as well as the distal tubule (urinary acidification, and concentration) while other solutes (sodium, potassium) are processed throughout the nephron. There may be generalized proximal tubular failure (e.g. Fanconi syndrome) or disorders in specific tubular functions (e.g. nephrogenic diabetes insipidus, renal tubular acidosis [RTA], or renal glycosuria). When suspicion of tubular defects exists, detailed evaluation of renal tubular functions may be needed.

Assessment of tubular function in acute renal failure

A common clinical problem is distinguishing prerenal azotemia from intrinsic renal injury in the setting of acute azotemia, oliguria, and evidence of intravascular volume depletion (e.g. shock, dehydration, congestive heart failure). Several parameters may be assessed to evaluate the integrity of tubular function to distinguish between the two categories in such a situation (Table 3). In prerenal azotemia, tubular function is intact, and the kidneys should therefore be able to appropriately conserve salt and water in response to reduced effective circulating blood volume, whereas this response is impaired with intrinsic tubular injury. Newborns and children with preexisting tubular disorders or injury may have findings suggestive of intrinsic renal failure despite actually having superimposed prerenal azotemia, due to limited tubular function.

Table 3. Laboratory data to distinguish prerenal azotemia from intrinsic renal injury

Lab	Prerenal azotemia	Intrinsic renal injury
Serum BUN/Cr ratio	> 20	< 10
Urine osmolality (mOsm/L)	> 500	< 350
Urine specific gravity	≥ 1.025	≤ 1.015
Urine Na^+ (mmol/L)	< 15	> 40
Fe_{Na^+}	< 1%	> 2%
Fe_{urea})	< 35%	> 50%

BUN, blood urea nitrogen; Cr, creatinine; FE, fractional excretion; Na, sodium.

Water

Antidiuretic hormone (ADH) is upregulated in intravascular volume depletion. In prerenal azotemia with intact tubular function, this manifests as high urine osmolality and specific gravity compared to inappropriately iso-osmolar or even dilute urine with tubular injury.

Sodium

Sodium reabsorption is the driving force for reabsorption of water and other solutes. In response to volume depletion, sodium reabsorption is enhanced with normal tubule function in an effort to conserve sodium and water. This results in low urine sodium in prerenal azotemia compared to inappropriately higher sodium levels with acute tubular injury. Enhanced sodium reabsorption in the proximal tubule increases urea reabsorption. This results in serum BUN elevated out of proportion to the creatinine leading to elevated serum BUN/creatinine ratio.

Fractional excretion of sodium

The fractional excretion of sodium (Fe_{Na^+}) is superior to measuring urine sodium in isolation for determining the state of renal sodium handling at a given time point. The formula is:

$$Fe_{Na^+} = [(U_{Na^+} \times P_{Cr})/(U_{Cr} \times P_{Na^+})] \times 100\%$$

Fe_{Na^+} is expressed as a percentage, U_{Na^+} is urine sodium concentration, P_{Cr} is plasma creatinine, U_{Cr} is urine creatinine concentration, and P_{Na^+} is serum sodium (because the equation is a ratio, any units may be used as long as the units are consistent). The Fe_{Na^+} is unreliable if the child has received diuretics. In that case, fractional excretion of urea (calculated in the same manner as Fe_{Na^+}) may be used instead.

Assessment of urinary solutes

Potassium

Renal excretion of potassium is largely controlled by the distal nephron. Renal tubular defects may be associated with either hyperkalemia or hypokalemia. Random urine potassium testing is of limited use, although a urine potassium concentration greater than 20 mEq/L in a hypokalemic patient suggests renal potassium wasting. The fractional excretion of potassium (Fe_{K^+}) may be calculated in a manner analogous to Fe_{Na^+}; normal Fe_{K^+} is 10–30%, and a value greater than 40% suggests renal tubular potassium wasting.

Transtubular potassium concentration gradient

Aldosterone plays an important role in renal handling of potassium, and action of aldosterone-mediated sodium/potassium exchange in the distal tubule is evaluated by calculation of transtubular potassium concentration gradient (TTKG). TTKG should be calculated in the hyperkalemic patient when urine osmolality exceeds plasma osmolality, using the formula:

$$\text{TTKG} = (U_{K^+} \times P_{Osm})/(U_{Osm} \times P_{K^+})$$

U_{K^+} is urine potassium concentration, P_{K^+} is plasma potassium concentration, and P_{Osm} and U_{Osm} are osmolality of plasma and urine, respectively. TTKG > 10 indicates appropriate aldosterone-mediated response in the kidney, and the hyperkalemia is likely due to increased potassium load. A TTKG below seven in the setting of hyperkalemia suggests impaired potassium secretion due to aldosterone deficiency or resistance. A TTKG > 2.5 in a hypokalemic child is indicative of deficient aldosterone suppression. The TTKG is unreliable if urine sodium < 25 mmol/L since low urine sodium will limit potassium secretion.

Chloride

Measurement of urine chloride may be helpful in assessment of metabolic alkalosis. Metabolic alkalosis with urine chloride level > 10 mmol/L suggests a renal cause for alkalosis, whereas lower values are found with extrarenal chloride loss (e.g. pyloric stenosis or cystic fibrosis).

Calcium

Urine calcium levels may be useful in evaluation of patients with kidney stones or isolated hematuria. Traditionally, a 24-hour urine collection was performed to measure the total calcium excretion, with hypercalciuria defined as excretion of > 4 mg/kg/day in a child over six years of age. Urine calcium excretion may also be assessed on a random urine sample as a urine calcium to urine creatinine ratio. Measuring urine creatinine in infants can be challenging as the diaper or other absorptive materials may trap creatinine; therefore, urine collection by squeezing diaper or using cotton balls may underestimate urine creatinine. In older children and adults, a calcium/creatinine ratio > 0.2 mg/mg is diagnostic of hypercalciuria. The ratio in infants and younger children is typically higher (see Table 4).

Table 4. Normal urinary excretion of calcium, oxalate, uric acid and citrate in the pediatric population (partially adapted from Alon and Milliner)

Urine solute	Age	Random (Solute/ creatinine ratio)	Timed (24-hour urine collection)
Calcium	0–6 months	< 0.8 mg/mg	
	7–18 months	< 0.6 mg/mg	
	1.5–6 years	< 0.42 mg/mg	
	≥ 6 years	< 0.21 mg/mg	< 4 mg/kg/24h
Oxalate	< 1 year	< 0.3 mg/mg	
	1–5 years	< 0.15 mg/mg	
	> 5 years	< 0.05 mg/mg	
	2–18 years		< 52 mg/1.73m^2/24h
Uric acid	> 2 years		< 815 mg/1.73m^2/24h
	> 3 months	< 0.53 mg/dL GFR*	< 0.56 mg/dL GFR*
Citrate	> 6 years		> 0.180 mg/mg Cr

*calculated as (urine uric acid x serum Cr)/urine Cr, all units in mg/dL.
Cr, creatinine.

Phosphate

Phosphate balance is controlled predominantly by reabsorption of phosphate in the proximal tubule, which depends on plasma phosphate concentration and on GFR. Assessment of the proximal tubular phosphate handling may be calculated as the tubular maximum reabsorption of phosphate corrected for GFR (TmP/GFR):

$$TmP/GFR = P_P - (U_P \times P_{Cr}/U_{Cr})$$

P_P is plasma phosphate concentration, U_P is urine phosphate, P_{Cr} is plasma creatinine and U_{Cr} is urine creatinine, and all units are in mg/dl. Normal TmP/GFR is in the 2.8–4.4 mg/dL range. A value below 2.8 in the setting of hypophosphatemia indicates tubular wasting of phosphate.

Uric acid, oxalate, citrate

Elevated urinary excretion of uric acid and oxalate are risk factors for kidney stones, while high urine levels of citrate are protective against stones and nephrocalcinosis. As with urine calcium levels, these factors may be measured in 24-hour urine collection or a random urine sample as a ratio normalized to creatinine; however, the 24-hour collection is preferred (see Table 4).

Amino acids

Amino acids are filtered through the glomerulus and reabsorbed by proximal tubular cells. Urinary amino acid profiling may be diagnostic in certain inborn errors of metabolism, such as phenylketonuria, maple syrup urine disease, cystinuria, homocystinuria, Hartnup disease, arginonosuccinic aciduria, histidinemia, and citrullinuria. A generalized increase in urinary amino acid excretion is characteristic of global proximal tubule dysfunction, or Fanconi syndrome.

Glucose

Glucose is filtered by the glomerulus and reabsorbed by the proximal tubule. If filtered glucose load exceeds the capacity of glucose transport, glycosuria occurs. This occurs in setting of hyperglycemia (diabetes mellitus, insulin resistance, or iatrogenic infusion) or when proximal tubular function is impaired. The normal serum glucose threshold before urinary excretion of glucose is observed is 180 mg/dL. A crude test for proximal tubular glucose handling can therefore be performed by testing serum and urine glucose levels concurrently. The presence of glucose in the urine when the serum glucose is < 180 mg/dL suggests a proximal tubular glucose handling defect.

Renal handling of acid and base

The kidney is an active participant in acid–base homeostasis. Bicarbonate is freely filtered by the glomerulus, and is largely reclaimed by absorption in the proximal tubule. In the distal tubule and collecting ducts, acid is excreted in the form of ammonium ions to further refine acid–base balance.

Plasma anion gap

The plasma anion gap is calculated as the difference between measured anions and cations in the blood. The commonly used equation for plasma anion gap is:

$$AG_P = Na^+ - (Cl^- + HCO_3^-)$$

Na^+, Cl^-, and HCO_3^- are serum sodium, chloride, and bicarbonate concentrations, respectively. A normal anion gap is 10–12 mEq/L ± 4. A higher anion gap indicates the presence of an unmeasured anion, often an organic acid such as lactate or acetoacetate. A normal anion gap in the setting of metabolic acidosis suggests gastrointestinal losses of bicarbonate or RTA.

Urine pH

Urine pH has been used as an indicator of renal response to alterations in serum pH, particularly when evaluating metabolic acidosis. Excretion of alkaline urine in setting of metabolic acidosis suggests defective renal handling of acid–base balance, and possibly a distal RTA. However, alkaline urine can occur with urinary tract infections, hypokalemia, or a vegetarian diet. Thus, urine pH is less specific than urine anion gap in estimating renal NH_4^+ excretion.

Urine anion gap (also known as urinary net charge)

An anion gap may also be calculated on a urine sample, and can provide important information about the renal response in acidemia. The formula for urine anion gap takes into account the most prevalent measurable cations and anions:

$$AG_U = Na^+ + K^+ - Cl^-$$

Na^+, K^+ and Cl^- are urine sodium, potassium, and chloride concentrations, respectively. Normally, the urine anion gap should be positive due to unmeasured anions such as sulfates and phosphates. In metabolic acidosis, AG_U should become negative due to compensatory increase in hydrogen excretion via ammonium chloride (NH_4Cl) by the distal tubule. Patients with distal RTA show impaired renal NH_4^+ excretion and inappropriately positive or neutral urine anion gap. Urine anion gap is unreliable in neonates, high serum anion gap metabolic acidosis, low urine sodium, or absence of acidosis.

Urine osmolal gap

The urine ammonium concentration can be estimated from calculation of the urine osmolal gap. This calculation requires the measurement of urine osmolality as well as urine sodium, potassium, urea nitrogen, and glucose concentrations. The calculated urine osmolality is estimated from:

$$(2 \times [Na^+ + K^+]) + [\text{urea nitrogen}]/2.8 + [\text{glucose}]/18$$

Na^+ is urine sodium concentration in mEq/L, K^+ is urine potassium in mEq/L, urea nitrogen is urine urea nitrogen in mg/dL, and glucose is urine glucose in mg/dL.

The gap between measured and calculated urine osmolality represents ammonium salts present in urine, and the approximate ammonium concentration of urine (in mEq/L) is one half of the difference between measured and calculated urine osmolality. A urine osmolal gap below 40 mEq/L (corresponding to a urine ammonium concentration of < 20 mEq/L) in the setting of metabolic acidosis indicates a distal RTA.

Fractional excretion of bicarbonate

Bicarbonate is a useful indicator of renal handling of acid–base balance, particularly the proximal tubular function of bicarbonate reabsorption. A normally functioning proximal tubule reabsorbs more than 95% of the bicarbonate filtered by the glomerulus. This function may be assessed by calculating the fractional excretion of bicarbonate:

$$FE_{HCO_3^-} = (U_{HCO_3^-} \times P_{Cr})/(U_{Cr} \times P_{HCO_3^-}) \times 100\%$$

$Fe_{HCO_3^-}$ is expressed as a percentage, $U_{HCO_3^-}$ is urine bicarbonate concentration, P_{Cr} is plasma creatinine, U_{Cr} is the urine creatinine concentration, and $P_{HCO_3^-}$ is serum bicarbonate (as equation is a ratio, any units may be used as long as they are consistent). The blood should be adequately alkalinized (serum bicarbonate above 24) prior to performing this test. A $Fe_{HCO_3^-}$ greater than 15% indicates a proximal RTA. The $Fe_{HCO_3^-}$ is <5% in normal individuals and distal RTA. An intermediate value (5–15%) is found in hyperkalemic (Type IV) RTA.

Urinary concentrating ability

The concentration of urine may be measured by specific gravity or osmolality. Urine specific gravity may range from <1.005 to >1.035 for maximally dilute and concentrated urine, respectively. Urine osmolality ranges from 50–1400 mOsm/L. For most individuals, the first morning urine (i.e. after an overnight fast) is more concentrated than urine produced later in the day. In a child with a suspected urinary concentrating defect, first morning urine samples should be tested for osmolality or specific gravity. A urine osmolality > 800 mOsm/L or specific gravity > 1.015 effectively rules out a significant urine concentrating defect. If repeated first morning samples are consistently more dilute than these cutoff values, a water deprivation test may be considered.

Water deprivation test

In a water deprivation test, a patient being evaluated for polyuria, polydipsia, and/or a suspected urinary concentrating defect undergoes serial testing of blood and urine electrolytes and osmolality during a period of no fluid intake. The duration of the test is generally determined by the patient's age and/or anthropometric measurements; it may be 3–4 hours for an infant, or over 24 hours for an adolescent or adult patient. Weight, clinical status, serum sodium and hemodynamic parameters are closely monitored during the test. Urine osmolality > 750 mOsm/L during a water deprivation test suggests primary polydipsia. Urine osmolality < 750 mOsm/L at the end of the study should be further evaluated with the administration of vasopressin. The production of urine with osmolality below 300 mOsm/L by a patient with a serum osmolality greater than 300 mOsm/L is diagnostic of diabetes insipidus (DI); the response to vasopressin administration distinguishes central DI from nephrogenic DI. A water deprivation test should never be performed on a patient with renal insufficiency, uncontrolled diabetes mellitus, hypovolemia, uncorrected adrenal insufficiency, or uncorrected hypothyroidism. Appropriate supervision in the hospital setting is necessary due to the risk for inducing marked dehydration.

Suggested Reading

Alon US, Srivastava T. (2006) Urolithiasis. In: Kher KK, Schnaper HW, Makker SP. (eds.) *Clinical Pediatric Nephrology*, 2nd ed. Informa HealthCare, Abingdon.

Bagga A, Bajpai A, Menon S. (2005) Approach to renal tubular disorders. *Indian J Pediatr* 72: 771–776.

Filler G, Lepage N. (2003) Should the Schwartz formula for estimation of GFR be replaced by cystatin C formula? *Pediatr Nephrol* **18**: 981–985.

Guignard J-P, Santos F. (2004) Laboratory Investigations. In: Avner ED, Harmon WE, Niaudet P (eds.) *Pediatr Nephrol*, 5th ed. Lippincott Williams and Wilkins, Philadephia.

Hogg RJ, Furth S, Lemley KV, *et al.* (2003) National Kidney Foundation's kidney disease outcomes quality initiative clinical practice guidelines for chronic kidney disease in children and adolescents: evaluation, classification, and stratification. *Pediatr* **111**: 1416–1421.

Levey AS, Eckardt KU, Tsukamoto Y, *et al.* (2005) Definition and classification of chronic kidney disease: a position statement from Kidney Disease: Improving Global Outcomes (KDIGO). *Kidney Int* **67**: 2089–2100.

Milliner DS. (2004) Urolithiasis. In: Avner ED, Harmon WE, Niaudet P. (eds.) *Pediatr Nephrol.* 5th ed. Lippincott Williams and Wilkins, Philadephia.

Schwartz GJ, Brion LP, Spitzer A. (1987) The use of plasma creatinine concentration for estimating glomerular filtration rate in infants, children, and adolescents. *Pediatr Clin North Am* **34**: 571–579.

Schwartz GJ, Furth SL. (2007) Glomerular filtration rate measurement and estimation in chronic kidney disease. *Pediatr Nephrol* **22**: 1839–1848.

Schwartz GJ, Munoz A, Schneider MF, *et al.* (2009) New equations to estimate GFR in children with CKD. *J Am Soc Nephrol* **20**: 629–637.

4

Imaging Techniques

Azam Eghbal and Michael Rubin

Introduction

This chapter will review the various techniques of radiographic imaging involving the urinary tract. Indications for each modality along with benefits and disadvantages will be detailed.

Plain Film

Technique: Usually one upright and one supine image are done with each view extending from the diaphragm to pubic symphysis.

Many reasons exist for taking a preliminary abdominal radiograph as it may alter the next imaging modality.

Indications for plain abdominal radiographs (KUB)

- Abdominal pain
- Mass effect on adjacent structures
- Congenital anomalies
- Urinary tract stone
- Presence of previously administered contrast
- History of surgery

Ultrasound (US)

Technique: Supine and prone images are done with no sedation.

Typically, the exam takes 15–20 minutes with additional 15–20 minutes if duplex vascular study is needed. Ultrasound has become the primary diagnostic method for many renal and urologic processes.

The advantages are that it is noninvasive, painless, safe, relatively inexpensive, and flexible. The disadvantages are that it is operator dependant, and that bones and bowel gas do not transmit sound, obscuring adjacent organs.

Indications for US

- UTI
- Flank pain
- Hematuria
- Obstructive uropathy
- Congenital anomalies
- Differentiating cystic vs. solid masses
- Pyelonephritis
- Nephrocalcinosis
- Renal vascular disease: renal artery stenosis, AV fistula, aneurysm
- Renal transplant
- Neonatal hydronephrosis

Fluoroscopy/VCUG (Voiding Cystourethrogram)

Technique: Foley catheter is placed in the bladder in a sterile fashion while the patient is lying on the fluoroscopy table.

Depending on the age, a 5–8 Fr catheter is used for urethral catheterization. Scout images of the kidneys and bladder are obtained. Then, contrast is instilled by gravity through the catheter, and low-dose fluoroscopic images of the kidneys and bladder are acquired. Voiding images are essential. Finally, images of the kidneys are done postvoid. This exam is done without sedation.

It is predominantly used for the presence or absence of vesicoureteral reflux (VUR). Structural bladder abnormalities such as trabeculation, suggestive of a neurogenic bladder, can also be identified.

The advantage is that no advance preparation is needed. However, the disadvantage is that the need for urethral catheterization and the use of ionizing radiation may create great anxiety for the parent and the child. For this reason, most centers contact the family prior the examination, review the procedure, and make a child-life specialist available the day of the procedure.

Indications for VCUG

- UTI
- Hydronephrosis
- Enuresis
- Voiding dysfunction
- Anatomic abnormalities of bladder and urethra, such as posterior urethral valves, urachal anomalies, etc.

Computed Tomography (CT)

Technique: Depending on the type and reason for the study, the patient is supine or prone on the CT table. IV contrast is only needed for specific reasons.

This test usually takes less than five minutes and typically sedation is not needed in a semicooperative patient. The applications of CT in the evaluation of the urinary tract are widely used in pediatric radiology.

Advantages include no need for advance preparation, the visualization/resolution of extremely small structures, and it is not operator dependent. Its disadvantages are radiation exposure, the fact that it is more costly than ultrasound, the potential contrast allergy/complications, the inability to repeat within a short time interval due to radiation exposure–related fertility concerns, the need for sedation in small children.

Indications for CT

- Urolithiasis (CT with small cross-sections)
- Trauma with hematuria with delayed imaging for renal, ureteral, or bladder injury
- Further characterization of abnormalities seen on US
- Tumors
- Infection including abscesses or any other fluid collection or its complications
- Anatomic abnormalities not resolved by other imaging modalities

- Any vascular abnormalities including renal artery stenosis or aneurysm
- Posttransplant complications including infection, fluid collection or vascular injury

Intravenous Urography (IVU)

Technique: Multiple KUB images are taken at different projections after intravenous contrast administration.

The study can take approximately 20 minutes (normal study) to two hours (obstruction). For many medical conditions, IVU has been replaced by US, CT Urography (CTU), and Magnetic Resonance Urography (MRU). The need for IVU must be determined on a case-by-case basis. It is typically used by a pediatric nephrologist or urologist to solve a specific problem/issue.

The major disadvantages are lack of resolution, finding the underlying cause, and radiation.

Indications for IVU

- Urinary tract stone, specifically when causing obstruction in single or duplex kidneys
- Anatomic anomalies especially ectopic ureter in a patient with continuous wetting
- Postoperative evaluation of urinary tract
- Primary megaureter

Contraindications for IVU

- Severe dehydration and shock
- Renal dysfunction
- Allergy to IV contrast
- Pregnancy
- Newborn state (due to reduced GFR)

Retrograde Urethrography (RUG)

Technique: The tip of a Foley catheter is placed in distal urethra. In adults, the balloon is inflated in Fossa navicularis.

Contrast is slowly instilled in the urethra under fluoroscopy. Because of inadequate filling, the urethra proximal to the external sphincter cannot be evaluated. This technique is primarily used in male patients.

Indications for RUG

- Anterior urethral strictures
- Postoperative status of urethral reconstructions
- *Infrasphincteric rectourethral fistulas* in patients with anorectal malformation
- Anterior urethral injuries

Nuclear Medicine

Two agents used in majority cases: Tc99m Mercaptoacetyltriglycine (MAG3) and Dimercaptosuccinic acid (DMSA)

Indications for MAG3

Technique: Following intravenous administration of Tc99m MAG3, sequential one minute images of the abdomen are obtained for six minutes.

IV furosemide is given during excretory phase and time-activity curves are done. This test requires sedation in young children. It is rapidly cleared by tubular secretion, not retained in the parenchyma of normal kidneys, and provides good assessment of drainage.

Indications for DMSA

Technique: Following intravenous administration of Tc99 DMSA, planar images of the abdomen are obtained in anterior, posterior and oblique projections. Magnified views and/or pinhole images of each kidney are also done.

This test requires sedation in young children. Due to its high affinity for the renal cortex, it evaluates renal morphology.

- Pyelonephritis, especially when not visualized by US
- Evaluate for renal scarring
- Presence or absence of functioning renal tissue; such as multicystic dysplastic kidney, ectopic kidney, etc.
- Determine differential uptake of each kidney

Magnetic Resonance Imaging/Magnetic Resonance Urography (MRI/MRU)

Technique: An IV and Foley catheter are placed. Typically, patient is in the supine position. After initial precontrast images are obtained, IV contrast is given and sequential imaging is acquired.

Younger children need sedation. This is the newest modality available for pediatric radiologists.

Its advantages are that it does not use ionizing radiation, different contrast medium (gadolinium), so it can be used in patients with CT contrast allergy, and superb resolution of soft tissues allows for optimal characterization of abnormalities. Its disadvantages are the higher cost compared to CT or US, need for sedation in small children, potential for nephrogenic systemic fibrosis in patients with renal failure/insufficiency when IV contrast gadolinium is used. Gadolinium is contraindicated in the presence of renal dysfunction. Also, it is more time consuming than CT or US, and has limited availability.

Indications for MR

1. Evaluation of renal masses
2. Further characterization of abnormalities seen on other modalities
3. Vascular abnormalities including renal artery stenosis, central AVM and aneurysm
4. Posttransplant complications in patients who can not have CT with contrast; IV contrast doesn't need to be used in MRI as tissue resolution is superb
5. Any anatomic abnormalities whether in the kidneys, ureter or bladder; such as duplex obstructing kidneys, ectopic ureter, crossed fused ectopia, etc.

Interventional Radiology

Renal angiography

Technique: First, an informed consent is obtained, and an IV and Foley catheter are placed. The typical access route is femoral artery. The artery is cannulated and sequential images are obtained by injecting contrast intravenously.

This test can be used diagnostically; but also can be therapeutic if abnormalities (e.g. vessel stenosis) are detected. This test also requires sedation. There has been significant decline in pediatric angiography due to the emergence of noninvasive modalities including CTA and MRA.

Indications for renal angiography

- Renal artery stenosis diagnosis when CTA or MRA not available, and therapeutic intervention such as stent placement and angioplasty
- Characterization of vasculopathy such as polyarteritis nodosa
- Diagnosis and transcatheter embolization of acute bleeding after renal vascular trauma.

Percutaneous procedures

Percutaneous interventional procedures include needle biopsy, abscess drainage, and nephrostomy catheter placement. The procedures are done under fluoroscopy, US or CT guidance depending on the procedure.

Precautions of Contrast Use

The contrast used for CT, IVU, and angiography is iodine based. Three types of reactions can potentially occur:

1. Mild: Hives, rhinorrhea, sneezing, nausea, and vomiting. It is usually treated with an antihistamine if necessary.
2. Moderate: Not immediately life threatening, vasovagal reaction, tachycardia, mild laryngeal edema. It is treated with bronchodilators, Epinephrine for laryngeal edema, and leg elevation for HTN.
3. Severe: Life threatening, anaphylactic shock, pulmonary edema, seizure, and cardiac arrest. Activate emergency response system.

Contraindications for IV contrast:

- Previous severe reaction to IV contrast
- Acute or chronic renal failure
- Patients presenting with sickle cell crises
- Patients on drugs containing metformin should withhold their medicine for 48 hours postcontrast injection and their renal function should be re-evaluated before resuming medication.

Patients with previous "mild" reaction should be premedicated according to the Radiology department policy. Patients with previous "moderate" allergy should be evaluated for other imaging modalities, and need premedication.

The contrast used for MRI is gadolinium based. The above allergic reactions with gadolinium are extremely rare. However, it is contraindicated in patients with renal insufficiency/failure due to nephrogenic systemic fibrosis.

Guidelines for Initial Imaging Modality

1. Trauma: Abdominal and pelvic CT with IV contrast with delayed images thru bladder
2. Hematuria with flank pain: Unenhanced CT of abdomen and pelvis which evaluates for stone and hydronephrosis
3. Painless hematuria: US
4. UTI: US and VCUG
5. Hypertension: Renal US with Doppler, if limited or positive, need to follow up with CTA or MRA
6. Congenital anomalies: Renal US first, if limited or very complex, need MRI
7. Renal Transplant: Renal US with Doppler. If complex, might need CT or MRI
8. In-utero Hydronephrosis: Renal US 7–10 days postnatally if patient clinically stable.

Suggested Reading

Donnelly LF. (2001) *Fundamental of Pediatric Radiology*, W. B. Saunders Company.

Lim R. (2009) Vesicoureteral reflux and urinary tract infection: evolving practices and current controversies in pediatric imaging, *Am J Roentgenol* **192**: 1197–1208.

Lowe LH, Isuani BH, Heller RM, *et al.* (2000) Pediatric renal masses: Wilms tumor and beyond, *Radiographics* **20**: 1585–1603.

Part II

Fluid Balance in the Pediatric Patient

5

Normal Body Fluid Composition and Compartments

Thomas R. Welch

Introduction

An elementary understanding of the composition and compartmentalization of body fluids is useful in order to understand the principles of fluid therapy. Humans are mostly composed of water. As a percentage of body weight, total body water (TBW) varies somewhat based upon factors such as age and the size of other body compartments, especially fat. A commonly cited range for children beyond the newborn period is 60–65%.

TBW is compartmentalized between that contained within cells (intracellular water) and that outside (extracellular water). By definition, these compartments are separated by the semipermeable cell membrane, through which water generally diffuses to maintain osmolic equilibrium.

The distribution of TBW between these two compartments is difficult to determine with precision. Variations exist based upon the methods of measurement used. A reasonable estimate is that one-third of this water is extracellular and two-thirds is intracellular.

Intracellular Water

The complex membrane which separates the intracellular from extracellular space is freely permeable to water. Consequently, water moves between the two spaces to maintain osmotic equilibrium. This results in changes in cell volume as water movement buffers changes in osmolality.

The osmolar content of intracellular fluid is mainly comprised of potassium and accompanying anions, much of which are macromolecular. Intracellular solutes are regulated by the transcellular transport of ions, mostly via the Na^+/K^+-ATPase pump. Additionally, osmotically active substances can be synthesized in some cells as a mechanism for defending cell volume in response to increases in extracellular osmolality.

Rapid changes in extracellular osmolality produce immediate shifts in intracellular water in order to maintain osmotic equilibrium between the two compartments. The resulting changes in cell volume are generally inconsequential outside the central nervous system (CNS). They can, however, have major clinical consequences in the brain. Sudden drops in extracellular osmolality, for example, result in cell swelling as water influx into cells occurs to equalize osmolality. Within the fixed compartment of the skull, this cell swelling results in brain edema and devastating CNS consequences. Such sudden osmolar shifts can occur, for example, in the treatment of diabetic ketoacidosis or severe uremia. In the former case, too rapid reduction in serum glucose produces osmotic shifts, while in the latter rapid reduction in urea produces a similar effect. The latter situation is referred to as "dialysis disequilibrium."

Extracellular Water

The extracellular water occurs in three compartments, each of which has unique features and importance.

"Transcellular" water

This is the most variable component of extracellular water. In most individuals, it is trivial in amount and importance. It represents fluid within epithelial spaces such as the gut. The fluid within these spaces is secreted and absorbed by the epithelial cell linings. It is not directly exchangeable with the rest of extracellular water, and rarely plays a role in body fluid or electrolyte balance.

In some disruptions of normal physiology, however, enough extracellular water moves into the transcellular compartment that functional volume depletion results. An example of this would be severe gastroenteritis in which losses of fluid into the bowel lumen contributes to dehydration. Thus, while this fluid is still within the "extracellular water" compartment, it is effectively lost from the body. These are the losses which are referred to as "third space."

Plasma water

This is the compartment of extracellular fluid whose composition is regularly measured, and in which changes occur most readily. This compartment is subject to active regulation of its volume and composition by coordinated activity of the renal, central nervous, endocrine, and cardiovascular systems.

Plasma water is separated from interstitial water by capillary walls, structures much more permeable than cell membranes. Thus, water and solute move freely between the plasma and interstitial space. Consequently, the electrolyte content of the two compartments is very similar, with subtle differences accounted for by the relative negative charge of serum proteins (the Gibbs–Donnan distribution).

The plasma also contains proteins, such as albumin, which are much less permeable through the capillary wall. This leads to an oncotic pressure that acts to maintain plasma water in the intravascular space. Reduction in serum proteins, as occurs in nephrotic syndrome, results in movement of plasma water to the interstitium driven by hydrostatic forces.

Interstitial water

While water within the plasma and transcellular compartments is readily measurable and visible, that in the interstitial space is less so. This is the fluid which continuously bathes tissues. It is freely exchangeable with plasma water.

The volume of interstitial water is largely driven by factors within the vascular space. As mentioned above, decreased oncotic pressure consequent to hypoproteinemia results in movement of plasma water to the interstitial space, producing edema. Similarly, dehydration resulting from loss of plasma water results in net movement of fluid from the interstitial space into the vascular space. Since interstitial fluid contributes to cutaneous elasticity, this is the explanation for such signs of dehydration as loss of skin turgor and "sunken" eyes.

Suggested Reading

Chesney RW. (2008) The role of the kidney in protecting the brain against cerebral edema and neuronal cell swelling. *J Pediatr* **152**: 4–6.

Friedman JN, Goldman RD, Srivastava R, Parkin PC. (2004) Development of a clinical dehydration scale for use in children between 1 and 36 months of age. *J Pediatr* **145**: 201–207.

Oh MS, Carroll HJ. (1995) Regulation of intracellular and extracellular volume. In: Arieff AI, Defronzo RA. (eds.) *Fluid, Electrolyte and Acid–Base Disorders*, Churchill Livingstone, New York.

Patel N, Dalal P, Panesar M. (2008) Dialysis disequilibrium syndrome: a narrative review. *Semin Dial* **21**(5): 493–498.

Trachtman H. (2004) Sodium and water. In: Avner ED, Harmon WE, Niaudet P (eds.) *Pediatric Nephrology* (5th ed.) Lippincott, Williams and Wilkins, Philadelphia.

6

Prescribing Fluids to the Pediatric Patient

Thomas R. Welch

Introduction

Much of the history of pediatrics in America has led to the development of our understanding of body fluid compartments and parenteral fluid therapy. Most of this work was done with children suffering from diarrheal dehydration. The basic principles undergirding our current approach to parenteral fluids in children have changed very little over the past several decades. Some current "controversies" in fluid therapy actually result from an apparent misunderstanding of these principles.

The Concept of "Maintenance" Fluids

Simply put, the provision of "maintenance" fluids to a patient means that all ongoing, normal losses of water and solute are being replaced such that a net zero balance is *maintained.* Although we frequently hear of a "maintenance rate" of fluid administration, it must be recognized that there really is no fixed number which defines maintenance. Indeed, any rate at which it is possible to achieve a zero net balance is, by definition, a maintenance rate. The prescription of maintenance fluids cannot be too difficult, since virtually all beings do this for themselves continuously.

By definition, patients with preexisting deficits of fluid or solute, or those with ongoing "abnormal" losses, do not receive "maintenance" therapy. These children require additional fluid to repair existing deficits or to replace ongoing abnormal losses.

The concept of fractions ("half maintenance") or multiples ("twice maintenance") of maintenance fluid, although common clinical shorthand, really makes no sense — and as such, use of this terminology should be discouraged.

Indeed, providing someone with only half the fluid required to maintain zero net balance would not be compatible with life for very long!

Situations in which parenteral maintenance fluids are required

In actuality, there are not too many clinical situations today in which parenteral *maintenance* fluids are required. Children who are not permitted to take oral feedings while awaiting a diagnostic or therapeutic procedure are one such group; another would be those in whom a change in neurologic status has rendered oral intake temporarily impossible. Children unable to take oral feeds while recuperating from surgery would constitute a third group. Keep in mind, however, that some in the latter group will have alterations in their ongoing losses (e.g. nasogastric tube drainage) which would require something other than a "normal" maintenance fluid prescription.

Major components of the need for maintenance fluids

Under most circumstances, there are only two sources of daily fluid loss which must be replaced by maintenance fluid therapy: Insensible water loss ("IWL") and urine. Although there are a few additional sources of loss (as well as one additional input), the magnitude of these in the otherwise well child is so small that they may be ignored.

Although there are a few ways in which IWL and urine losses can be estimated, the most rational is that of *caloric expenditure.* This relates fluid loss to its most fundamental driver, metabolic activity. This method also allows for the use of a convenient, clinical shorthand. One of the classic studies in pediatric fluid therapy first introduced this rule for estimating caloric expenditure in hospitalized patients:

0–10 kg: 100 kcal/kg/d
10–20 kg: 1000 kcal/d + 50 kcal/kg/d for weight >10 kg
>20 kg: 1500 kcal/d + 20 kcal/kg/d for weight >20 kg

IWL requirement

The constant, ongoing evaporative loss of water from skin, and the water vapor contained in exhaled air constitute the IWL. This is *electrolyte-free* water. A reasonable allowance for IWL is about 45 ml/100 kcal, of which about one-third is from the lungs and two-thirds from the skin. The skin component of IWL should not be confused with sweat, which is a source of electrolyte-containing water which is rarely important in hospitalized children.

Urinary water loss requirement

Unlike the relatively fixed requirement for IWL, urine water loss requirements fall within a very broad range. The actual amount is a function of *urine concentration* and *solute load.* Using conservative assumptions for both of these, an allowance of 55 ml/100kcal/d should be adequate.

Combining the normal allowances for IWL and urine, one can estimate a normal maintenance fluid administration rate of 100 ml/100 kcal/d. This is the derivative of the "100–50–20" shorthand by which maintenance fluids are often estimated.

Maintenance requirements for solute

Unlike that for water, there is no true fixed daily requirement for sodium. In fact, the fate of virtually all ingested sodium is to be excreted in the urine. Rather than providing a quantity of this electrolyte on the basis of weight, surface area, or caloric expenditure, the most rational approach is to provide enough sodium so that the tonicity of the infused volume is dilute enough to provide sufficient free water for IWL and solute excretion. Generally, 0.22% sodium chloride in 5% dextrose (D5 ¼ isotonic saline) meets this requirement. Although it has been claimed that some children have developed hyponatremia when receiving maintenance fluid therapy with this solution, careful analysis shows that such children either had unrecognized fluid deficits or abnormally concentrated urine — both of which would really disqualify the child from receiving "normal maintenance fluid."

Ongoing potassium losses in normal children are so trivial that inclusion of potassium in normal maintenance fluid is unnecessary. In the rare circumstances of a child at risk for potassium deficiency requiring maintenance fluids, the addition of 20 mEq/l KCl is safe and reasonable.

Finally, while calcium and phosphate are required for skeletal growth and are routinely included in total parenteral nutrition, they need not be added to brief courses of parenteral maintenance fluid therapy.

Adjustments to normal maintenance fluids

The formula for estimating usual maintenance requirements for water is such that physiologic flexibility permits it to be used safely in a very wide range of circumstances. There are, however, some specific circumstances in which these calculations are inappropriate. Failure to recognize these may result in a fluid prescription which could be dangerous.

Abnormal metabolic rate

Fever, sepsis, or inflammatory disease may lead to an increased metabolic rate and therefore an increase in IWL. A febrile infant provided with "maintenance" fluids by the usual calculation could become dehydrated over a few days. A common correction for this involves increasing the estimated caloric expenditure by 12% for each 1°C elevation of temperature over 37°C. Since daily fluid requirements are tied to caloric expenditure, adjusting this will automatically increase the fluid calculation.

Alteration in IWL

Breathing humidified air may result in a reduction or elimination of the usual lung IWL losses. This, in turn, should lead to a reduction in the total usual maintenance fluid requirement of 15 ml/100 kcal, to 85 ml/100 kcal. Situations which disrupt the barrier function of the skin (e.g. significant burns) may *increase* the IWL from skin, adding to the usual maintenance fluid requirement.

Alteration in requirement for urinary fluid loss

The usual allowance for urinary water (55 ml/100 kcal) is based upon conservative assumptions about the *solute load* requiring excretion (primarily a function of sodium intake and protein metabolism) and the *concentration* of these solutes in urine (i.e. urine osmolality). Since urine osmolality in healthy individuals can range from under 100 mosm/kg to over 900 mosm/kg, the requirement for urinary water can be met by a very wide range of intake.

Problems can develop in situations in which the usual wide range of urine concentration is constrained. This is most often seen in children who are unable to concentrate their urine. This situation could occur in children with anatomic abnormalities such as dysplastic kidneys, genetic disorders such as nephrogenic diabetes insipidus, or acquired disorders such as acute tubulointerstitial. *Increases* in the usual allowance for urinary losses in such conditions is critical; otherwise, dehydration and hypernatremia would result. Adjustments can be based upon urine osmolality. Since the usual 55 ml/100 kcal is based upon a urine osmolality of 300 mosm/kg, a child with a fixed urine concentration of 100 mosm/kg would require *three times* the usual allowance (165 ml/100 kcal). Assuming no change in IWL, this hypothetical child would require a total daily fluid intake of 210 ml/100 kcal — more than twice what would have been provided by simply following the "100–50–20" rule.

The converse of the situation of abnormally dilute urine is the child with persistently concentrated urine. Assuming that unrecognized volume concentration is not present, most such children have non-osmotic signal for vasopressin release ("SIADH"). A child with a consistent urine osmolality of 600 mosm/kg, for example, would require only half of the usual 55 ml/100 kcal) urine water allowance. Assuming unchanged IWL, this child's total maintenance fluid requirement would be 73 ml/100 kcal.

Note that both of these examples allow a much more precise calculation of fluid requirements than that provided by the typical (but unfortunate) "half maintenance"/"twice maintenance" shorthand.

Alteration for unusual continuing losses

Most hospitalized children requiring parenteral maintenance fluids have IWL and urine as their only substantive losses requiring replacement. There are special circumstances, however, in which additional losses are ongoing and large enough to require replacement to maintain homeostasis.

Most often, these losses are gastrointestinal, either as diarrhea or gastric (vomiting or, more commonly, continuous nasogastric suctioning).

Failure to replace these may result in serious electrolyte or hemodynamic disturbances. Typically, such losses are carefully measured over a set time interval and replaced over the next such interval. This replacement is provided in addition to that calculated for the usual maintenance requirement. Although most gastrointestinal losses are approximately half isotonic, if losses are substantial it is safest to measure the actual electrolyte content to determine the ideal replacement solution.

Some surgical drainage losses may contain substantial protein content, which may also need to be replaced to avoid hypoproteinemia and resulting interstitial edema.

Parenteral Fluid Therapy in the Face of Deficits

Some children requiring parenteral fluid therapy will have significant deficits of fluid and electrolytes at initiation of therapy. The most common situation in which this occurs is that of diarrheal dehydration. Such children not only need ongoing maintenance fluid therapy, they also must have their deficits repaired.

For reasons deeply rooted in the ancient history of fluid therapy, it was once taught that such replacement should be "gradual." Not only is there no real rationale for such an approach, it is counterintuitive. In what other clinical situations would one choose to treat hypovolemic shock over 8–24 hours?

Children with dehydration resulting in decreased perfusion should be rapidly rehydrated with an isotonic solution. Either 0.9% NaC1 ("isotonic saline") or lactated Ringer's solution are appropriate for this purpose, although my preference is the latter. The volumes of these fluids needed to restore hydration in a seriously dehydrated child can be as much as 80 ml/kg given in successive 20–40 ml/kg rapid infusions. Dehydration is essentially a clinical diagnosis and improvement in these clinical measures should be immediate with such treatment. There are varying systems to quantitate such clinical measures; an excellent recent example is provided in Table 1.

Once volume deficits are repaired, most children can resume oral feedings. In the event this is impossible, continued maintenance fluids, as described above, should be provided parenterally. If there are continued ongoing losses, one must be sure to account for these. It is probably safest

Table 1. Clinical dehydration scale

Feature	0 Points	1 Point	2 Points
General appearance	Normal	Thirsty, restless, or lethargic, but irritable to stimuli	Drowsy, limp, cold, sweaty, H-comatose
Eyes	Normal	Slightly sunken	Very sunken
Tongue	Moist	Sticky	Dry
Tears	Present	Decreased	Absent

Adapted from Table 1 in Friedman JN *et al.* (2004) Development of a clinical dehydration scale for use in children between 1 and 36 months of age. *J Pediatr* **145**: 201–207.

to provide this fluid as D5 ½ isotonic saline (0.45% NaCl), in the event that residual vasopressin activity is promoting free water retention. A child in whom all deficits are repaired and for whom usual maintenance fluid is appropriate should have a urine osmolality <300 mOsm/kg.

Children recovering from diarrheal dehydration may have potassium deficits, although these are not likely to be consequential in a previously well child. Addition of 20 mEq/l of KCl to the usual maintenance fluid is appropriate.

Special Situations

Postoperative fluid therapy

Children in whom parenteral fluids are being provided in the postoperative period should be treated according to the above principles, but attention must be given to some other details. Additional losses of fluid may occur postoperatively from several sites. Surgical drainage and continuous nasogastric suction are common and easily measurable. Ongoing replacement of each such losses with an appropriate electrolyte solution (either half or fully isotonic) must be added to the usual maintenance allowance. Substantial unrecognized losses may occur into bowel lumen or the interstitium surrounding operative sites. These losses are often referred to as "third spacing" and may be significant enough to compromise perfusion. Precise measurement of such losses is impossible to achieve and replacement needs have to be provided based upon clinical evidence of intravascular volume contraction. Such losses are generally isotonic, and replaced as such. Also, it must be remembered that, with healing, such "compartmentalized" fluid may be taken back up into the circulation, occasionally abruptly.

Another important consideration in the management of fluids postoperatively is regularly assessing the child's tolerance of free water. Occasionally, the combination of pain and medication (e.g. opiates) may stimulate vasopressin, leading to inappropriate antidiuresis (water conservation). Provision of maintenance fluids as quarter isotonic under such circumstances could result in water retention and hyponatremia. Conversely, provision of insufficient free water intake could impair solute excretion, especially in children with increased IWL. The single best way to assess this is with regular determination of urine osmolality. A urine osmolality of <300 mOsm/kg suggests adequate ability of the child to handle free water.

Diabetic ketoacidosis (DKA)

DKA represents a complex state of fluid, electrolyte, and metabolic decompensation. Most centers today have fairly rigid protocols for the fluid management of DKA, something which probably is important to ensuring good outcomes in this life-threatening condition. This section is intended to provide the background to such protocols, rather than substituting for them.

Most such protocols begin with addressing the volume depletion of DKA, which results from the combination of hyperglycemia-induced osmotic diuresis, vomiting, and decreased oral intake. This part of therapy involves rapid volume expansion with an isotonic solution (isotonic saline or lactated Ringer's solution). As serum glucose decreases with insulin therapy, the ongoing drive for osomotic diuresis decreases and retention of infused fluid begins. Therapy at this point is generally provided with a half isotonic solution. Replacement fluids are glucose-free until control of hyperglycemia has been achieved, after which dextrose (5 or 10%) is employed.

Significant potassium deficits may occur in DKA. Provision of potassium in the form of potassium phosphate and/or acetate is begun early in treatment. Control of acidosis occurs gradually as perfusion is restored and ketoacids are metabolized and their production decreases with insulin.

The rare but devastating complication of cerebral edema must be considered as any child is undergoing treatment for DKA. The pathophysiology of this complication is complex and probably involves both rapid osmotic shifts and vasogenic factors. Avoidance of rapid reduction in plasma osmolality may help in prevention, and there is some evidence that a gradual increase in serum sodium as serum glucose decreases is salutary. If a sudden deterioration in neurologic status occurs early in the course of therapy, consideration of increasing plasma osmolality with mannitol should be given.

Parenteral alimentation

Some clinical situations preclude enteral feedings for extended periods of time. It is possible to repair and prevent severe malnutrition in such settings by providing nutrition parenterally. While the details of total parenteral nutrition (TPN) are beyond the scope of this chapter, there are a few very important considerations.

It is very important when prescribing TPN to pay attention to the total solute intake, and to be sure that adequate free water is being provided to excrete this solute. The osmolar load of TPN is derived from its mineral and protein content; fat and carbohydrate do not contribute to osmolar load. The metabolism of a gram of protein produces about 5 mOsm of urea. The solute load of minerals derives directly from their osmolality; 50 mEq of sodium and its accompanying anions, for example contribute 100 mOsm of solute.

Knowing the solute requiring excretion and the urine osmolality provides all the data one needs to calculate the necessary free water. A child with urine osmolality of 300 mOsm/kg and a 300 mOsm TPN solute intake will thus require one liter of water for the urinary excretion of this solute.

Problems with solute excretion in TPN may result from the provision of too much sodium. Unlike calories, there is really no fixed daily biologic requirement for sodium. Unfortunately, some TPN ordering procedures imply this by providing a mEq/kg daily sodium allowance. This unfortunate error should be avoided by aiming for appropriate TPN *tonicity* rather than the provision of a fixed daily sodium requirement. In most circumstances, no more than one quarter isotonic saline is appropriate for this.

Sodium disorders

When diarrheal dehydration is accompanied by *hyponatremia*, it is usually a consequence of avid free water retention stimulated by vasopressin released in response to volume contraction. Neurologic findings in this situation are rare, and once the volume deficit has been restored and the stimulus for vasopressin is gone, the kidneys generally excrete the excess free water and the hyponatremia corrects.

Hyponatremia may also occur in a number of clinical situations in which a non-osmotic stimulus for vasopressin is present. Nephrotic syndrome and end-stage liver disease are such scenarios in children. In general, hyponatremia in such settings develops very gradually and is rarely an emergency. In fact, attempts at correcting the hyponatremia with additional salt can upset what may be a tenuous metabolic compensation. Correcting, or at least modifying, the underlying hemodynamic abnormality will reduce the recurring stimulus and permit correction by renal free water excretion.

Hyponatremia may also occur in situations in which inappropriate secretion of vasopressin occurs ("SIADH"). SIADH is recognized by the presence of plasma hypo-osmolality, concentrated urine (>100 mOsm/kg), euvolemia, and normal renal/adrenal function. When this phenomenon occurs chronically (for example, as a complication of a medication), it is rarely associated with neurologic symptoms and usually responds to elimination of the offending agent and restriction of water intake. The latter can be calculated precisely according to the principles outlined above if the urine osmolality is known.

When hyponatremia from SIADH occurs more suddenly, osmotic shifts in the CNS may produce severe neurologic complications including seizures. A setting in which this could occur would be postoperatively, related to a combination of pain, opiates, or vomiting. In this setting, more rapid correction of hyponatremia with 3% NaCl is appropriate. Although good evidence of the most effective way to accomplish this is lacking, 1–2 ml/kg of 3% NaCl over an hour is likely to be safe, and can be repeated based upon the clinical and biochemical response. Ideally, such rare scenarios can be avoided by careful attention to urine concentrations and avoiding hypotonic fluid in the presence of concentrated urine.

Hypernatremia is a less frequent electrolyte disorder in children. Decades ago, hypernatremia often accompanied diarrheal dehydration. This usually resulted from feedings with high solute remedies (e.g. scalded skim milk), something rarely done today.

The management of hypernatremic dehydration should be guided by the longstanding concern that rapid reduction in serum sodium can result in cerebral injury. This concern, however, should not cause delay in repairing volume deficits with an isotonic solution, as one would do for any dehydrated child. Following this repair phase, if the child is unable to take feedings orally (probably the safest route), maintenance fluid may be provided with a ¾ or ½ isotonic solution, giving careful attention to the rapidity of fall in serum sodium.

Today, a more common setting for hypernatremia is the infant with breast feeding failure. These children may present significantly below birth weight with elevations in BUN and sodium. They are at great risk of decompensation with overly aggressive treatment. Although there are no evidence-based guidelines, a rational approach involves the use of colloid infusions to insure hemodynamic stability, followed by oral formula or breast milk if tolerated. If enteral feeds are not possible, fluids such as recommended for hyponatremic dehydration may be employed.

In both of the above situations, urine should be concentrated. The presence of hypernatremia and *dilute* urine is diagnostic of diabetes insipidus (DI). DI results either from deficits in vasopressin release from the pituitary or from an abnormal renal response to vasopressin. While awaiting definitive diagnosis, it is necessary to supply adequate free water. Again, this can be calculated based upon the system discussed earlier, knowing the urine osmolality.

Suggested Reading

Chesney RW. (2008) The role of the kidney in protecting the brain against cerebral edema and neuronal cell swelling. *J Pediatr* **152**: 4–6.

Ellison DH, Berl T. (2007) The syndrome of inappropriate antidiuresis, *N Engl J Med* **356**: 2064–2072.

Friedman JN, Goldman RD, Srivastava R, Parkin PC. (2004) Development of a clinical dehydration scale for use in children between 1 and 36 months of age. *J Pediatr* **145**: 201–207.

Holliday MA, Segar WE. (1957) The maintenance need for water in parenteral fluid therapy. *Pediatr* **19**: 823–832.

Holliday MA, Friedman AL, Wassner SJ. (1999) Extracellular fluid restoration in dehydration: a critique of rapid versus slow. *Pediatr Nephrol* **13**: 292–297.

Hoorn EJ, Carlotti AP, Costa LA, *et al.* (2007) Preventing a drop in effective plasma osmolality to minimize the likelihood of cerebral edema during treatment of children with diabetic ketoacidosis. *J Pediatr* **150**: 467–473.

Winters RW. (1973) Maintenance fluid therapy. In: Winters RW (ed.) *The Body Fluids in Pediatrics,* Little, Brown and Company, Boston.

Part III

Electrolyte Disorders in the Pediatric Patient

7

Disorders of Sodium and Water Balance

Aaron Friedman

Introduction

Salt and water homeostasis has been a focus for clinicians and scientists for generations. The elegant experiments by Verney describing the role of the central nervous system in diuresis and antidiuresis (antidiuretic hormone); the marvelous description of extracellular fluid and its relationship to the intracellular space by Gamble; and the single author text by Homer Smith are all testaments to the remarkable work done in the middle of the 20th century that set the stage for our understanding of salt and water balance. As our understanding of fluid, electrolytes, and renal physiology expanded, our ability to assist patients with derangements of salt and water balance improved. This chapter will address common sodium and water disorders seen in children.

Hyponatremia and Hypernatremia: Physiology and Pathophysiology

A common laboratory finding is a lower-than-normal plasma sodium concentration (hyponatremia). Less common is a higher-than-normal plasma sodium concentration (hypernatremia). When either occurs, the vast majority of the time, the underlying cause is a disorder of water balance. Thus, when a patient demonstrates hyponatremia, the first question to address is: why is there relatively more water than sodium in this patient compared to the normal steady state? When the patient demonstrates hypernatremia, the opposite question should be asked: why is there relatively less water than sodium in this patient compared to the normal steady state?

To address the questions above it helps to have an understanding of how water balance (homeostasis) is maintained. The key physiologic mechanisms that control the total body water under normal circumstances are thirst (intake); urine output under the influence of hormones such as arginine vasopressin (AVP) also termed antidiuretic hormone (ADH), aldosterone, etc.; and other sources of salt and water loss, such as sweating or water loss in expired air. AVP release is mediated by osmoreceptors in the hypothalamus that "sense" the serum osmolality and increase production or release of AVP when serum osmolality is high or reduce production and release of AVP when serum osmolality is low. A second signal for AVP release is "effective plasma volume" sensed by stretch or baroreceptors in great vessels and transmitted via the nervous system to the hypothalamus. Decreased "effective plasma volume" results in an increase in AVP production and release. A full "effective plasma volume" results in a decrease in AVP production and release. AVP results in the incorporation water channels in the membrane of renal distal tubule and collecting duct cells, which results in increased movement of water from the renal tubular lumen into the interstitium of the kidney and then into vasculature, thus increasing water reabsorption.

Aldosterone influences sodium reabsorption by the kidney. In situations of reduced "effective plasma volume" or reduced blood flow to the kidney, renin release results in increased aldosterone release by the adrenal gland (mediated by angiotensin II). Aldosterone results in the increased reabsorption of sodium by the distal tubule. This along with increased water reabsorption results in an increase in extracellular volume — the desired effect in situations of volume contraction.

A useful tool for consideration of fluid and electrolyte physiology is the distinction between intracellular and extracellular fluid compartments. Total body water (TBW) comprises about 60% of total body weight. Total body water ranges from nearly 50% in some adult females to at least 70% in newborns. After the newborn period, the extracellular fluid compartment is approximately a third of TBW — with interstitial fluid, the fluid between cells in skin, muscle and organs, comprising 75% of total extracellular fluid. Fluid in the vasculature makes up the rest of the total extracellular fluid. Intracellular fluid accounts for approximately

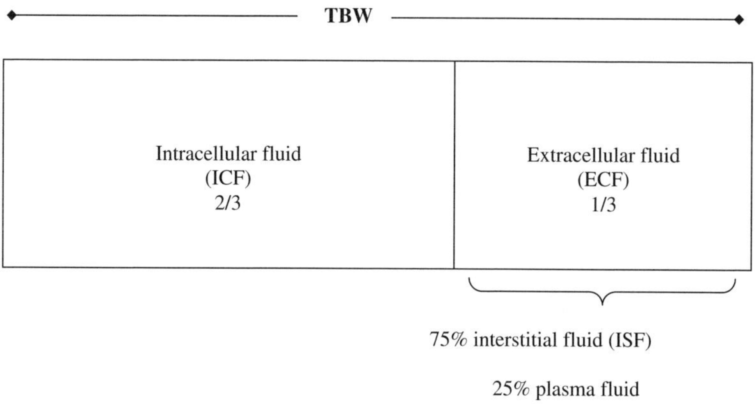

Figure 1. Total Body Water (TBW) 50–60% of total weight in kg.

Table 1. Approximate comparison of most common ions in plasma, interstitial, and intracellular fluid (mmol/l)

		Plasma	Interstitium	Intracellular
	Sodium	140	145	10
Cations	Potassium	4	4	140
	Other	8	5	10
	Chloride	105	115	0
Anions	Bicarbonate	27	30	10
	Phosphate + organic anions	8	<2	110

two thirds of TBW (see Fig. 1). An important element to understanding this model of fluid and electrolyte balance is recognition that water moves essentially freely across cells and across three fluid compartments mostly regulated by osmotic differences (the gradient created by ionic concentrations).

Beside the difference in relative sizes of these compartments, the other important difference is the electrolyte content of the two spaces (see Table 1). Sodium, chloride and bicarbonate are the major electrolytes of extracellular fluid. Potassium, phosphate are the major ions in intracellular fluid. Interstitial fluid contains very little protein; intravascular fluid and intracellular fluid contain proteins.

Hyponatremia – Hypoosmolality

Hyponatremia (a serum sodium below 130 mmol/l) or hypoosmolality (a serum osmolality <280 mOsm/kg H_2O) are most often seen together and nearly always associated with avid renal water retention. Hyponatremic dehydration (extracellular volume depletion) is the most common example. Hyponatremia with extracellular volume expansion occurs with heart failure, renal failure, liver failure, and with AVP excess, known as SIADH (syndrome of inappropriate antidiuretic hormone) release. AVP results in increased water reabsorption but this must be accompanied by the intake of water, or other hypotonic solutions to result in hyponatremia or hypoosmolality. Hyponatremia can be seen disassociated from hypoosmolality. The best example occurs in the setting of hyperglycemia as seen with diabetes mellitus, where for every 100 mg/dl increase in the serum glucose, there is a 1.6 mmol/l decrease in the serum sodium.

A stepwise approach to hyponatremia starts with:

Step 1: Does hyponatremia mean hypoosmolality?

A. Hyponatremia with normal osmolality. This is termed pseudohyponatremia. While commonly seen in textbooks, this finding rarely exists today as present-day laboratory techniques to measure sodium are not altered by hyperlipidemia or hyperproteinemia.
B. Hyponatremia with hypertonicity (osmolality >295 mOsm/kg H_2O). As noted above this is most commonly seen with hyperglycemia. The treatment is first and foremost to reduce the serum glucose. Second, in this situation, extracellular volume contraction is usually seen and volume expansion (isotonic saline) is part of the treatment.

Step 2: Hyponatremia with hypoosmolality

A. With a decrease in osmolality, signs and symptoms vary depending on the severity of the hypotonicity; the presence of extracellular volume depletion and the rapidity with which alteration from normal occurred. Symptoms may range from none to anorexia, malaise, anxiety, agitation, and more significant neurologic changes, such as disorientation, ataxia, decreased mentation, diminished deep tendon reflexes, seizures, coma, and without intervention, death.

B. Determine extracellular volume status. Table 2 describes the signs and symptoms used clinically to determine the degree of volume depletion.

1. Hyponatremia with hypovolemia
This results from the loss of extracellular fluid and replacement of losses with water or hypotonic fluids. This is seen with gastrointestinal losses such as vomiting, diarrhea, burns, ascites, and cystic fibrosis (excessive skin loss of high sodium/chloride sweat). Unless acute renal failure occurs, these patients will demonstrate decreasing urine volume and low urine sodiums with a fractional excretion of sodium (FE_{Na^+}) <1%.

Renal disease results in salt loss and adrenal disease, especially mineralocorticoid deficiency, results in sodium and chloride loss. Like gastrointestinal fluid losses, renal and adrenal diseases can present with hyponatremia and hypovolemia; however, these disorders are associated with a urine sodium that is high and a FE_{Na^+} that may be above 3%.

Table 2. Severity of dehydration

	Mild	Moderate	Severe
Infant (<12 mos)	1–5%	6–9%	>10%
Children	1–3%	4–6%	7–10%
Pulse	Full, normal	Rapid	Rapid, weak
Systolic B.P.	Normal	Normal, low	Very low
Urine output	↓	↓↓	Oliguria (<1 ml/kg/hr)
Skin	Normal	Cool	Cool, pale
Cap refill	≤2 sec	2–3 sec	>3 sec
Buccal mucosa	Sl. Dry	Tacky	Parched
Eyes	Normal	Sunken	Markedly sunken
Ant. fontanelle	Normal	Sunken	Markedly sunken

The approach to treatment should be to first restore extracellular volume (restoration therapy) using 0.9% saline (isotonic) or lactated Ringer's solution. Example: a 20 kg child with 5% dehydration will require 1 liter of restoration fluid (5% of 20 kg = 1 liter). Providing 1 liter of isotonic saline over 6–12 hours will restore previous losses, improve well-being and improve the likelihood that the patient will tolerate oral fluids as a method of ongoing fluid therapy. Oral rehydration solutions are used frequently throughout the world for rehydration in patients with dehydration, including patients with hyponatremic dehydration. The solutions usually prescribed are hypotonic — containing from 45 mmol/l to 90 mmol/l of sodium and chloride, based on World Health Organization recommendations — with the highest sodium concentration utilized in the most seriously ill patients. Over-the-counter preparations for oral use contain ≤40 mmol/l of sodium.

2. Hyponatremia with euvolemia (normal extracellular fluid volume)
   This results from excessive water intake relative to the clinical state. The most common situation is SIADH (syndrome of inappropriate antidiuretic hormone) release. Central nervous system injury or infection is the usual causes, but other conditions can result in excess AVP release (see Table 3). Other less common causes include: glucocorticoid or thyroid deficiency, or psychogenic water intake. SIADH was first described in situations of nonphysiologic AVP release caused by malignancy leading to uncontrolled AVP release by the hypothalamus or actual AVP production by cancer cells. As seen in Table 3, many more clinical situations will result in nonosmotic release of AVP. When SIADH release occurs, the kidney is under constant AVP stimulation resulting in a concentrated urine despite a falling plasma osmolality, which is the usual negative feedback for AVP production and release. The features of SIADH release are: hyponatremia, plasma hypoosmolality, low urine volume, hyperosmolar urine with normal or even high urinary sodium concentration despite euvolemia, or even

Table 3. Causes of SIADH release

Drugs	CNS Disease/Injury	Pulmonary/Chest	Malignancy
Barbituate	Infection	Infection	Adenocarcinoma
Cancer chemotherapy	Hemorrhage	Positive pressure ventilation	Lung
Cystosine arabinoside	Hypoxia		Breast
Vinblastine	Malignancy	Pneumothorax	Pancreas
Vincristine	Thrombosis	Asthma	Duodenum, colon
CNS agents	Trauma	Cystic fibrosis	Leukemia
Amitriptyline	Misc.	Mitral valve repair	Lymphoma
Carbomazepine	Guillain–Barre		Thymoma
Tricyclics	Hydrocephalus		
Narcotics	Idiopathic		
Morphine			
Misc.			
Chloropropamide			
Clofibrate			
Colchicine			
Isoproterenol			
Nicotine			
Others			

hypervolemia. This means that the FE_{Na^+} is often >3% and never <1%. If the FE_{Na^+} is <1% then one must consider unappreciated volume contraction. The clinical signs and symptoms are those of central nervous system changes as noted above. Treatment includes: treatment of the underlying cause and concomitant water restriction (50% of maintenance). In situations of significant central nervous system symptoms, a more rapid increase in the osmolality of extracellular fluid is warranted. Usually central nervous system findings will not occur until the serum sodium concentration is below 125 mmol/l. If significant symptoms are present the use of hypertonic saline (3%) is the recommended approach. 3% saline is 513 mmol/l of sodium and has an osmolality of nearly 1000 mOsm/kg H_2O. Thus, 1 ml of 3% saline contains 0.5 mmol of sodium, the amount of hypertonic saline provided should achieve desired change in serum sodium or serum osmolality, enough to reduce symptoms, but should not exceed a 10 mmol change in serum sodium in 24 hours.

Therefore, an infusion of 1–4 ml/kg of 3% saline over 60–90 minutes, followed by a remeasurement of the serum sodium and a second infusion if needed, (based on symptoms) will help correct the serum sodium and osmolality, but remain safely under the maximum safe correction per 24 hours. An additional therapeutic agent is furosemide, at a dose of 0.5–2 mg/kg IV, which will increase water excretion by the kidney and decrease the risk of hypertension that could occur with the hypertonic saline infusion. Patients with SIADH release do not demonstrate edema even though they may have excessive TBW. A newer approach to SIADH is the use of vaptans, non-peptide arginine vasopressin antagonists. The vasopressin 2 receptor (AVPR2) antagonists-vaptans have been used in adults to induce a hypotonic diuresis without significant electrolyte excretion. Their use in acute treatment as well as chronic treatment of SIADH has been examined in adult patients with some success. Studies in children are lacking.

Hyponatremia (and hypoosmolality) associated with central nervous system injury can indicate cerebral salt wasting as opposed to SIADH release. Both occur following central nervous system injury, infection or surgery. However, cerebral salt wasting usually is associated with high urine volumes and if measurable, a decrease in extracellular volume (this may be difficulty to determine in a patient in the intensive care unit unless symptoms are severe — high pulse, low blood pressure). Table 4 can help with differentiating features. The differentiation is important because water restriction is the therapy for SIADH release and isotonic saline infusion is the treatment for cerebral salt wasting.

C. Hyponatremia with hypervolemia. This occurs because nonosmotic, in particular volume receptor mediated, AVP release continues to occur despite a drop in serum osmolality. These patients present with edema, weight gain and ascites. The clinical conditions most likely to be associated with this picture are heart failure, end-stage liver disease (cirrhosis), and nephrotic syndrome. In all of these, urine volumes are low and the FE_{Na^+} is low

Table 4. Differentiation SIADH release and Cerebral Salt Wasting (CSW)

	SIADH release	CSW[a]
Weight	↑	↓
Extracellular volume	nl or ↑	↓
Hct	nl or sl ↓	↑
Serum sodium	↓	↓
Plasma osmolality	↓	↓
BUN and serum creatinine	nl or ↓	Normal or ↑
Serum albumin	nl or ↓	nl or ↑
Serum uric acid	nl or ↓	nl
Plasma AVP	↑	nl or ↓ [b]
Urine osmolality	↑	↑
Urine sodium	↑	↑↑
Treatment	Fluid restrict	Isotonic saline

[a] In CSW natriuretic peptides (brain and cardiac) are elevated and renin and aldosterone levels are *not* elevated despite volume contraction.
[b] Lack of elevation of AVP levels is not understood.

(urine sodium is low). Patients with ascites, or nephrotic syndrome have low serum albumin and loss of oncotic pressure leading to interstitial edema and often plasma volume contraction. The kidney in these patients is under both AVP stimulation leading to avid water reabsorption and aldosterone stimulation leading to avid sodium reabsorption. The combination results in edema, volume expansion, and hyponatremia especially if typical water intake continues. Patients with severe or end-stage kidney disease may have the same picture although the explanation is slightly different. In these patients, their intake of salt and water exceeds the filtration ability of the kidney to excrete salt and water. In all of the above, the therapeutic approach is salt and water restriction.

Maintenance Fluid Therapy and the Prevention of Hyponatremia

Maintenance fluid therapy is a concept known to pediatricians for more than 50 years. The term maintenance fluid therapy, as described by Holliday and Segar, refers to the anticipated water requirements and estimated sodium, potassium and chloride requirements for the upcoming 24-hour period in euvolemic patients. The authors developed a bedside

Table 5. Maintenance therapy[a] water, electrolyte requirement based on weight (24 hrs or per hr)

Body Weight (kg)	Water (ml)	Sodium (mmol/100ml H_20)	Chloride (mmol/100ml H_20)	Potassium (mmol/100ml H_20)
3–10[b]	100 kg/24 hr or 4 kg/hr	3	2	2
11–20	1000 + 50 kg from 11–20 kg	3	2	2
>20	1500 + 20 kg >20 kg Or 60/hr + 1 kg/hr >20 kg	3	2	2

[a] Another approach — not Holliday and Segar — for water needs is 1500 ml/m^2/24 hr.
[b] For preterm infants, the water needs are ≥150 ml/kg/24 hr.

technique for determining water and electrolyte needs for the upcoming day. This approach is used ubiquitously and is based on tying water needs to caloric expenditure and sensible/insensible losses (see Table 5). Sensible losses are more easily measured (urine), while insensible losses are harder to measure (sweat, water in expired air, etc.).

Using this approach a 15 kg child's needs for maintenance IV fluids for the upcoming 24 hours is:

$$15 \text{ kg} = 1000\text{ml} + 250 \text{ ml or } 1250 \text{ ml } H_2O$$
$$36 \text{ mmol } Na^+, 25 \text{ mmol } K^+$$

In practice this becomes 1250 ml/24 hr of water as D_5W + 0.22 NS (1/4 normal saline or 34 mmol/l NaCl) + 20 mmol/l KCl.

While this calculation is used often, it is important to know this prescription is only for determining the recurring needs of a euvolemic patient. Maintenance therapy is *not* a solution for restoring extracellular fluid loss, such as vomiting, and diarrheal losses. Maintenance fluid is rarely the appropriate fluid for replenishing ongoing losses such as those from nasogastric drainage, fistulas, etc. Maintenance fluid therapy is not the appropriate fluid to induce a diuresis — often needed for chemotherapy, for example. Isotonic saline is more effective. Therefore, considerations of fluid therapy that use multiples (1.5 or 2 or 3 times maintenance) is not appropriate for the above clinical situations.

These inappropriate uses serve as an important reason for the proposed substitution of isotonic saline for the hypotonic solutions of the Holliday–Segar approach. The case for this modification of the solution (not the volume to be delivered) is based on the observation that children have been seriously injured or have died due to the use of maintenance fluid solutions inappropriately, especially in situations of nonosmotic release of AVP or unappreciated volume contraction. The use of isotonic saline versus maintenance fluid to prevent hyponatremia still requires more testing to know if unintended consequences occur. However, we know there are situations where this approach makes sense. In the perioperative (immediately before, during and in the first 12–24 hours after surgery), isotonic saline is more prudent. It is difficult to assess volume status and volume depletion, if it occurs, should it be treated with isotonic saline. Further bolus isotonic saline may be useful to treat hypotension. Anesthetics and pain medication often result in AVP release, so we must anticipate the nonosmotic release of AVP and again, isotonic saline is safer in these situations.

Hypernatremia and Hypertonicity

Hypernatremia (serum sodium >150 mmol/l) or hypertonicity (serum osmolality >295 mOsm/Kg H_2O) usually reflects a water deficit through water loss without adequate water replacement. Hypernatremia always means hyperosmolality. In extremely rare conditions, hypernatremia means increased sodium intake without concomitant water intake or insufficient water intake. Premature babies, neonates and young infants are at particular risk for hypernatremia given relatively large water losses due to large surface area to weight ratio and their dependence on others to provide adequate water. In older children and adults, hyperosmolality (hypernatremia) provides a strong stimulus through the thirst mechanisms in the brain to drink water. A patient with hypernatremia is at least 10% dehydrated meaning the patient has lost at least 10% of body weight. The consequence of this degree of fluid loss is significant cell size shrinkage — as water has left not only the interstitial space, but each individual cell. In infants this cell and interstitial fluid shrinkage can result in brain injury and intracranial bleeding.

The severe degree of dehydration seen with hyperosmolality/hypernatremia is not as clinically apparent as it would be in patients with hypoosmolality or isoosmotic hypovolemia. This is because the loss of water is spread throughout all the fluid spaces — two thirds of which is intracellular, thus, appearing to "protect" plasma volume until the losses exceed 10% and approach 15% of body weight. These patients are critically ill. The signs and symptoms of hypernatremia are irritability, intense thirst, high pitched cry, seizures, and obtundation/coma. As noted above intracranial hemorrhage is a concern as is cranial thrombosis. Patients who present with the signs and symptoms above and low blood pressure require emergent fluid resuscitation.

Approach to hypernatremia/hyperosmolality

In patients with the signs and symptoms noted above, especially those with evidence of extracellular volume depletion, serum sodium will quickly allow one to make a diagnosis of hypernatremia. Hyperglycemia and hypercalcemia may also be seen. The causes of this combination of volume depletion and elevated serum sodium fall into two categories: 1) water loss without adequate replacement — the overwhelmingly most common cause, and 2) increased sodium gain.

Water loss

These losses result from extrarenal and renal causes. The extrarenal causes are usually gastrointestinal — vomiting, diarrhea, GI drainage — all with inadequate replacement which is, in this case, water. Unless the patient is so severely volume depleted that acute kidney injury has ensued, urine assessment will show a high urine osmolality and low urinary sodium with a low FE_{Na}. The treatment for such a patient is isotonic saline with restoration of extracellular volume depletion. Hypernatremia will persist (and should). Then consider a hypotonic solution of (IV) of 0.45 NaCl with 5% dextrose (D_5½NS) infused at a rate that would lower the serum sodium no faster than 0.5 mmol/l/hr or 10–12 mmol/l/24 hours. This calculation to determine the amount of electrolyte-free water needed to lower serum sodium can be done as follows:

$$\text{Free water needed (ml)} = \#\text{ of mmol/l change in serum sodium} \times 4\text{ ml/kg } H_2O \times \text{body wt (kg)}.$$

Example: 15 kg child with serum sodium of 165mmol/l. Reducing serum sodium from 165 → 145 (upper limit of normal) mmol/l = 20 mmol. This amount exceeds the safe level of change/24 hours (10–12 mmol/L/24hrs — see above). Therefore, the free water (electrolyte free) needed is 10 (maximum sodium change/24 hours) × 4 × 15 = 600ml.

Other conditions can result in water loss often with little or no associated electrolyte loss. Examples include: (a) renal water loss due to central or nephrogenic diabetes insipidus, reset osmostats where the release of AVP does not occur until the serum sodium is much higher than normal (b) extrarenal water loss — sweat or other skin loss, respiratory (high respiratory rate especially of unhumidified air). In the example of extrarenal water loss, one would expect urine osmolality to be high; whereas, renal water loss is associated with a low urine osmolality.

Increased sodium gain

In situations of too much sodium intake, the approach to therapy should be removal of the source of too much sodium, the use of diuretics such as furosemide along with careful addition either orally or intravenously of water. With renal impairment, dialysis may be necessary.

Diabetes insipidus

The name diabetes insipidus reflects the high urine volume with a lack of electrolyte or glucose found in the urine. This condition results from too little or no AVP release (central diabetes insipidus) or from an inability to respond to AVP in the kidney (nephrogenic diabetes insipidus). With either form, the signs and symptoms include: polyuria, polydipsia, and large urine volumes despite osmotic, or volume stimuli for AVP release, and the elaboration of a concentrated urine. Polyuria is urine volume of >2000 ml/m^2 or >4 ml/kg/hr.

Central diabetes insipidus can be idiopathic, hereditary or caused by intracranial injury or disease (see Table 6). A decrease in urine volume and an increase in urine osmolality occur with the administration of exogenous AVP. AVP administration today uses the intranasal or oral

Table 6. Central and nephrogenic diabetes insipidus

Central Diabetes Insipidus	Nephrogenic Diabetes Insipidus
Idiopathic	Congenital- hereditary
Hereditary — autosomal dominant, autosomal recessive	AVP receptor — X linked
	Aquaporin defect
Intracranial injury	Renal disease
• Trauma, hemorrhage, thrombosis	• Obstruction
• Infection	• Hypoplasia, dysplasia
• Malignancy, lymphoma, leukemia	• Polycystic kidney disease
• Granulomatous disease	• Medullary cystic disease or nephronophthisis
• Anorexia nervosa	• Urate nephropathy
	Systemic disease
	SLE
	Amyloid
	Sarcoid
	Myeloma
	Metabolic disorder
	Hypokalemia
	Hypercalcemia
	Medications
	Lithium
	Iphosphamide
	Amphotericin
	Aminoglycosides
	Diuretics
	Others

routes with more predictability and potency via the intranasal route. The dose is:

oral dosing:

≤12 years of age: The initial dose should be 0.05mg one to two times a day then titrate to 0.1–0.6 mg/day at one to two times/day.

>12 years of age: 0.05 mg two times/day then titrate to 0.1–1.2mg/day in two to three divided doses.

intranasal dosing:

3 mo ≤12 yrs: 5 microgms/day divided one to two times/day titrate to up to 40 microgms/day.

>12 years: 5–40 microgms/day divided one to two times/day.

Nephrogenic diabetes insipidus is the inability to concentrate urine despite the presence of AVP in the circulation. The hereditary forms of the disease present in infancy or early childhood with polyuria, excessive thirst with a desire for water that exceeds calorie interest, poor weight gain, unexplained fever, and recurrent episodes of hypernatremia. The hereditary forms represent AVP receptor defects with the most common being a defect in AVPR2 or vasopressin 2 receptors. The loss of function or dysfunction mutation of AVPR2 is usually an X-linked recessive as the AVPR2 receptor is on the X chromosome. Autosomal recessive or autosomal dominant presentations usually represent a defect in aquaporin-2 — the water channel normally created when AVP binds to its receptor on the renal tubule epithelium. Nephrogenic diabetes insipidus will *not* respond to exogenous AVP. Acquired forms of nephrogenic diabetes insipidus are more common than hereditary forms. Acquired nephrogenic diabetes insipidus is due to different forms of kidney disease or metabolic derangements, such as hypokalemia (see Table 6).

For idiopathic or hereditary forms of nephrogenic diabetes insipidus, the approach to treatment is multifocal. The reduction in the intake of osmols by salt restriction to 50–100 mmol/day of NaCl and the reduction in protein intake to 1–1.5 gm/kg/day of high-quality protein has been recommended. In the infant and young child, protein restriction must be considered judiciously and under careful dietary guidance. Adequate water intake and access to water is a must. In infants, G-tube or NG tube fluids have proposed. Diuretic use, specifically hydrochlorothiazide 1–2 mg/kg/24 hr divided two times/day or chlorothiazide 25–50 mg/kg/24 hr divided two times/day along with amiloride 0.2–0.4 mg/kg/day (reduces potassium wasting associated with thiazide diuretics) also reduces polyuria. Indomethacin 0.7–1.5mg/kg/day reduces GFR and thereby decreases total water loss.

Suggested Reading

Bartter FC, Schwartz WB. (1967) The syndrome of inappropriate secretion if antidiuretic hormone. *Am J Med* **42**: 790–806.

Decaux G, Soupart A, Vassart G. (2008) Non-peptide arginine-vasopressin antagonists: The vaptans. *Lancet* **371**: 1624–1632.

Deen PMT, Knoers N. (1998) Vasopressin type-2 receptor and aquaporin-2 water channel mutants in nephrogenic diabetes insipidus. *Am J Med Sci* **316**: 300–309.

Finberg L. (1959) Pathogenesis of the lesion in the central nervous system in hypernatremic states: I. Clinical observations of infants. *Pediatr* **23**: 40–45.

Friedman AL, Ray PE. (2008) Maintenance fluid therapy: what it is and what it is not. *Pediatric Nephrol* **23**: 677–680.

Gamble JL. (1950) *Chemical Anatomy Physiology and Pathology of Extracellular Fluid.* Harvard University Press.

Gauer OH, Henry JP. (1963) Circulatory basis of fluid volume control. *Physiol Rev* **43**: 423–481.

Holliday MA, Segar WE. (1957) The maintenance need for water in parenteral fluid therapy. *Pediatr* **19**: 823–832.

Kappy MS, Ganong CA. (1996) Cerebral salt wasting in children: the role of atrial natriuretic hormone. *Adv Pediatr* **43**: 271–307.

Kirchlechner V, Koller DY, Seidl R, *et al.* (1999) Treatment of nephrogenic diabetes insipidus with hydrochlorothiazide and amiloride. *Arch Dis Child* **80**: 548–552.

Moritz ML, Ayus JC. (2003) Prevention of hospital acquired hyponatremia, a case for using isotonic saline. *Pediatr* **111**: 227–230.

Smith HW. (1951) *The Kidney: Structure and Function in Health and Disease.* Oxford University Press, New York.

Vander A. (1985) Control of sodium and water excretion: regulation of extracellular volume and osmolality. In: *Renal Physiology*, 3rd ed. McGraw-Hill, Inc, New York, pp. 136–4016.

Verney EB. (1947) The antidiuretic hormone and factors which determine its release. *Proc R Soc London* (Series B) **135**: 25–106.

Winters RW. (1973) *The Body Fluids in Pediatrics*, Little, Brown and Co, Boston, pp. 95–112.

8
Disorders of Potassium Balance

Laurence Shoemaker

Hypokalemia

Introduction

Hypokalemia, defined as serum potassium (K^+) concentration below 3.5 mEq/L, is commonly encountered in the nephrology clinic and in hospitalized pediatric patients. While mild hypokalemia is well-tolerated in most children, severe hypokalemia may lead to significant morbidity, particularly in those with cardiac disease or neuromuscular dysfunction. Chronic hypokalemia has been associated with metabolic perturbations and nephropathy.

Interpretation of a low K^+ result should include consideration of possible pseudohypokalemia, which is associated with *ex vivo* uptake of K^+ by leukocytes in the specimen tube prior to measurement. Individuals in whom this is identified have normal extracellular K^+ concentration, leukocytosis, and procedural delay in either refrigerating or separating the plasma prior to measurement.

Pathogenesis

Hypokalemia is defined as subnormal K^+ concentration in the extracellular space, wherein only 2% of the total body stores reside. The balance of total body K^+ is intracellular, and numerous homeostatic mechanisms actively maintain this transcellular gradient.

Hypokalemia ultimately results from either 1) total body K^+ deficit, 2) transcellular shift of K^+ from the extracellular to cytosolic space, or 3) a combination of both. Causes can be categorized into 1) insufficient intake, 2) increased cellular uptake, and 3) excessive loss of K^+. Dietary K^+ deficiency is rare in children, although relative deficiency may be encountered in

Table 1. Causes of increased cellular uptake of K^+

Acute alkalosis (metabolic or respiratory)
Insulin therapy
Increased β-adrenergic activity
Hypokalemic periodic paralysis
Increased bone marrow cell production
Barium poisoning

hospitalized diet-restricted children who have not received K^+ for prolonged periods. The causes of increased cellular K^+ uptake are itemized in Table 1. Causes of excessive kaliuresis are numerous and are categorized into those associated with low or normal blood pressure (BP) (see Table 2A), or those associated with elevated BP (and usually mild alkalosis) (see Table 2B). Further sub-categorization of the causes of hypokalemia is based upon urinary Na^+, K^+ and Cl^- concentrations, acid–base status, renin (concentration or activity), and adrenal hormone profile.

Presentation

The clinical features of hypokalemia result from hyperpolarization of cell membranes. Symptom severity varies with the rapidity of development of hypokalemia and the concentration of K^+, calcium, sodium, magnesium, and acid–base status. Affected organ systems include *cardiovascular*, *neuromuscular*, *endocrine organs*, and *kidneys*. Hypokalemia may also be discovered following an evaluation of symptoms unrelated to the K^+ concentration (see Table 3). These may manifest variably, such as polyhydramnios and premature birth, neonatal or infantile failure to thrive, nephrocalcinosis or nephrolithiasis, symptoms related to hypertension, or even failure of normal pubertal development.

Cardiovascular effects include abnormalities in electrical conduction and blood pressure regulation. As plasma K^+ decreases below 3.0 mEq/L, there is diminution in T wave amplitude and U waves develop. At concentrations near 2.5 mEq/L, the ST segment sags, T waves flatten further, and U waves become prominent. At even lower K^+ concentrations, the PR interval lengthens and the QRS complex widens. Patients who have congestive heart failure, take digitalis, or who recently experienced cardiac ischemia are prone to develop supraventricular or ventricular dysrhythmias

Table 2A. Causes of excessive K^+ loss and low-normal blood pressure

Renal loss	Extrarenal loss
Metabolic acidosis:	Sweat loss
Renal tubular acidosis (I and II)	Ostomies and fistulas
Use of carbonic anhydrase inhibitors	VIPoma
Ureterosigmoid diversion	Dialysis
Diabetic ketoacidosis	GI loss
Variable acid–base status	Diarrhea
Polyuric states (concentrating defect, hypercalcemia)	Laxatives
Prolonged (K^+-free) saline resuscitation/diuresis	Pica/geophagia
Magnesium depletion	K^+ binders
Congenital K^+ wasting	
Acquired K^+ wasting	
Leukemia	
Thyrotoxicosis	
Edematous states	
Drugs (carbenicillin, gentamicin, amphotericin B, cis-platinum)	
Metabolic alkalosis with low urine Cl^- concentration ($\leq$15 mEq/L)	
Cl^- Deficient diet	
Gastric Cl^- loss (vomiting, NG tube to suction)	
Sweat Cl^- loss	
Congenital chloridorrhea	
Cl^- secreting villous adenomas (colon and rectum)	
Posthypercapnea	
Postdiuretic effect	
Metabolic alkalosis with normal-high urine Cl^- concentration (>15 mEq/L)	
Recent diuretic effect	
Bartter syndrome	
Gitelman syndrome	
Congenital K^+ wasting	
Severe hypercalcemia	
Familial hypocalcemia (activating CaSR mutation)	
Hypovolemia (and secondary aldosteronism)	

in the setting of severe hypokalemia. *Torsades de pointes* is more likely to develop in hypokalemic children with prolonged QT syndrome, and may manifest as syncope or sudden cardiac arrest.

In predisposed individuals, hypertension may develop or be exacerbated by diets high in sodium and low in K^+. Chronic hypertension is also associated with hypokalemia in several genetic disorders with stimulated mineralocorticoid activity (see Table 3) and with Liddle syndrome.

Table 2B. Causes of excessive (renal) K^+ loss and high blood pressure (and alkalosis)

Low renin	Normal or high renin
High aldosterone; low/normal DOC	Renal parenchymal disease
Adrenal tumors	Renal compression
Adrenal hyperplasia	Renal tumors
Dexamethasone suppressible hyperaldosteronism (FH-I)	Pheochromocytoma
Familial hyperaldosteronism II (FH-II)	Excess exposure to ACTH/ glucocorticoids
Low aldosterone; low/normal DOC	
Excessive exposure to licorice, carbenoxolone, grapefruit juice	
Excessive exposure to ACTH / glucocorticoids	
Exogenous mineralocorticoid exposure	
Apparent mineralocorticoid excess	
Liddle syndrome (pseudoaldosteronism type1, PA-I)	
Mineralocorticoid receptor (MR) activating mutation (PA-II)	
L810 mutation of MR (pregnancy-associated PA-II)	
High deoxycorticosterone (DOC); variable aldosterone	
11-β hydroxylase deficiency	
17-α hydroxylase deficiency	
Glucocorticoid receptor (GR) resistance	
DOC-secreting tumors	

Neuromuscular symptoms include muscle weakness (usually lower extremity), cramps, tetany, and rhabdomyolysis, which can be exacerbated with aminoglycoside use. At progressively lower K^+ concentrations, weakness of quadriceps, truncal muscles, upper extremity muscles, and respiratory muscles occurs. Smooth muscle involvement leads to nausea, vomiting, constipation, postural hypotension, and urinary retention.

Endocrine and metabolic dysfunction is often subclinical, but may manifest as increased symptom severity in children with chronic diseases. For example, hypokalemia may worsen glucose intolerance in prediabetes and diabetic children, and can restrict growth in children with chronic illnesses. Protein catabolism is stimulated by hypokalemia, and may result in hepatic encephalopathy in children with liver disease.

Reversible changes in *renal* function and anatomy may result from chronic hypokalemia. Vasopressin-resistant urinary concentrating defect is characteristic. In chronically hypokalemic individuals who have otherwise normal renal function, urinary concentrating defect is paradoxically associated with a fluid expanded state (sometimes with generalized

Table 3. Inherited disorders associated with kaliuresis

Fanconi syndromes
Cystinosis
Tyrosinemia type 1
Dent disease
Wilson disease
Fructosemia
Mitochondrial disorders
Glycogen storage disease (types I and XI)
Oculocerebral (Lowe) syndrome
Fanconi-Bickel syndrome
Proximal RTA (type II)
Bartter syndrome
Familial hypocalcemia (CaSR activating mutation)
Gitelman syndrome
Distal RTA (type I)
Liddle syndrome (epithelial sodium channel activation, PA-I)
Stimulated mineralocorticoid activity disorders
Adrenal enzymopathies
11-β hydroxylase
17-α hydroxylase
11-β hydroxysteroid dehydrogenase deficiency (AME)
Familial hyperaldosteronism I (GRA)
Familial hyperaldosteronism II
Mineralocorticoid receptor activation (PA-II)
Glucocorticoid receptor inactivation

edema) and mild metabolic alkalosis associated with acidic urine. Renal potassium reabsorptive capacity is conserved. Such patients have polydipsia and polyuria. The complex physiology is associated with stimulated renin release and angiotensin II production, suppressed aldosterone levels, increased proximal tubular salt reabsorption, renal tubular intracellular acidosis, and stimulated ammonium secretion. Cytosolic vacuoles in proximal tubular cells have been described. A persistent nephropathy, characterized by interstitial fibrosis, medullary cyst formation, and atrophic tubular changes may develop in chronic severe hypokalemia.

Diagnosis

Despite numerous causes of hypokalemia, a detailed history will often limit the differential diagnosis. Inquiry should include the duration of hypokalemia, recent medicines, dietary history, surgical history, growth pattern, polyuria, nighttime thirst, recent blood pressures, headaches, muscle cramps, weakness, ease of fatigue, paresthesias, tachycardia, orthostatic symptoms, excessive sweating or heat intolerance, and persistent constipation or diarrhea. A family history of hypokalemia, inherited disease, growth disturbance, or any of the symptoms listed above is helpful.

The examination should focus on blood pressure, heart rate, height percentile, evidence of gastrointestinal or urologic surgery, skin lesions associated with inherited syndromes (such as neurofibromatosis), abdominal mass, adenopathy, edema, weakness, tetany, or abnormal neuromuscular findings, genitourinary abnormalities, and assessment of pubertal development.

After hypokalemia has been discovered, laboratory evaluation should follow and needs to be interpreted in conjunction with the history and examination. A renal function panel, CBC, arterial blood gas, plasma renin activity/concentration, and concurrent spot urinary K^+, sodium, and chloride suffices to evaluate potential pseudohypokalemia, transcellular K^+ shifts, and subcategorize children in whom kaliuresis is the primarily mechanism. An electrocardiogram (ECG) confirms severity and identifies patients requiring urgent therapy.

An algorithm to evaluate hypokalemia is depicted in Fig. 1. This evaluation is best delayed until children have been off IV fluids, since this may mitigate the mechanisms involved in causing hypokalemia leading to misinterpretation of results. However, if hypokalemia persists in children receiving IV fluids containing sodium and K^+, and ongoing gastrointestinal losses are excluded, then a primary renal K^+ wasting condition is implicated.

If recent diuretic use is excluded, causes of extrarenal K^+ loss should be pursued if the urinary K^+ ≤15 mEq/L and adequate distal nephron sodium delivery is assured (urinary Na >25 mEq/L). Transtubular potassium gradient is often helpful. A TTKG >4 in a child with hypokalemia is abnormal and suggests renal potassium wasting. It is calculated as:

$$\mathrm{TTKG} = (K_u/K_p) \times (O_p/O_u)$$

where potassium concentration in urine (K_u) and plasma (K_p) are in mEq/L, and osmolality in urine (O_u) and plasma (O_p) are measured as

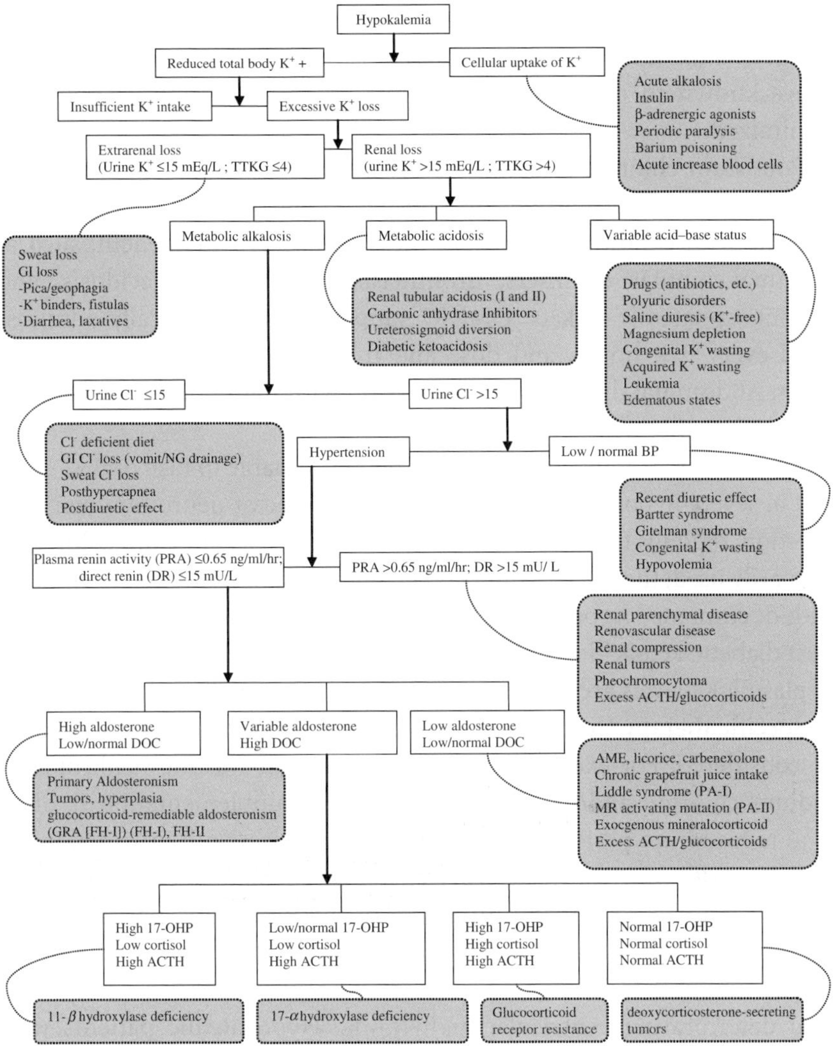

Figure 1

milliosmoles/kg. This parameter is only valid when $O_u > O_p$ and adequate distal nephron sodium delivery is present.

Treatment

The treatment goal is to raise the K^+ above 3.0 mEq/L, using oral potassium salts. Magnesium levels should be checked and supplemented if low. Potassium sparing diuretics are often helpful; amiloride is especially useful because it reduces urinary loss of K^+ and magnesium. Exposure to drugs known to promote hypokalemia (such as diuretics) should be minimized.

Potassium chloride is used most often for supplementation, but gluconate, bicarbonate, citrate, or phosphate salts are generally used in patients with conditions in whom these anions provide benefit, such as proximal tubular disorders, urolithiasis, renal tubular acidosis, and hypophosphatemic rickets. Oral K^+ supplements are typically administered every 3–4 hours, and dose and frequency are titrated to desired levels. Abdominal discomfort may develop with high dosages and should be anticipated.

Intravenous therapy is indicated in patients unable to take oral K^+ salts, and in severe hypokalemia associated with cardiac or neuromuscular dysfunction, digitalis toxicity, and diabetic ketoacidosis. Potassium chloride is primarily used; the use of IV phosphate salt infusions is limited to children with documented hypophosphatemia and hypokalemia, or empirically to treat diabetic ketoacidosis. Cardiac monitoring and frequent measurement of plasma K^+ levels are important.

Specific therapy (in addition to potassium salt administration) should be considered. For example, in children with salt-wasting nephropathy, sodium chloride and/or sodium bicarbonate supplementation is often required; sodium phosphate may be needed in cases with proximal tubular salt wasting. In contrast, hypertensive or edematous patients usually benefit from K^+-sparing diuretics. In hypokalemic patients with hypomagnesemia, magnesium supplementation is indicated, and IV magnesium sulfate is critical to correct *torsades des pointes*, a frequently fatal deteriorating ventricular arrhythmia. Hypokalemic patients with hypertension and normal or high renin values may require renovascular angioplasty or surgery, angiotensin converting enzyme inhibitors, α- and β-adrenergic receptor blockers, potassium sparing diuretics, and other antihypertensive agents. Those children with hypertension and low-renin hypertension may require surgical tumor removal, glucocorticoid therapy, or potassium sparing diuretics. They may also require antihypertensive therapy. Patients with hypokalemic periodic paralysis may require acetazolamide and non-selective β-blockers in addition to K^+ supplementation.

Hyperkalemia

Introduction

Life-threatening cardiac conduction dysfunction is often the only clinical finding in children with hyperkalemia. Elevated potassium (K^+) level should be interpreted cautiously, with consideration of the risk of pseudohyperkalemia, and recognition that normal levels vary with age, and specimen type.

Hyperkalemia is defined as a serum K^+ >6.0 mEq/L in neonates or 5.5 mEq/L in older children and adults. Values from serum may be as much as 0.5 mEq/L higher than from plasma, due to intracellular potassium released during clotting.

Pseudohyperkalemia, an artifactual elevation of measured K^+ concentration, results from release of cytosolic K^+ to the extracellular fluid either *in vivo* at the phebotomy site or *ex vivo* in the blood specimen tube prior to separation from blood cells, from hemolysis due to traumatic capillary blood collection, or after prolonged tourniquet use. It may also be consequent to elevated number of circulating cells (thrombocytosis, leukocytosis, polycythemia), or disorders of red cell membrane permeability. Although measured K^+ levels may be dramatically elevated, the child with pseudohyperkalemia will lack expected electrocardiographic features.

Pathogenesis

Healthy children tolerate acute K^+ loads without developing hyperkalemia due to rapid, hormonally regulated, intracellular uptake into muscle within minutes, and renal excretion over several hours. Chronic intake of a high potassium diet rarely causes hyperkalemia due to intestinal adaptation, increasing stool K^+ loss (up to three-fold), and renal cortical collecting duct secretory adaptation resulting in excretory rates exceeding glomerular K^+ filtration.

Pathologic conditions interfering with physiologic mechanisms of K^+ homeostasis may result in hyperkalemia (see Table 4). Risk factors include acute kidney injury (AKI) and chronic kidney disease (CKD), multi-organ dysfunction [systemic inflammatory response syndrome (SIRS), trauma], comorbid conditions (diabetes mellitus, adrenal suppression), exposure to multiple medications, hypovolemia, and illnesses with known risk of cell lysis (rhabdomyolysis, tumor lysis, hemolysis). Children who develop

Table 4. Causes of hyperkalemia

Exogenous load	
	K^+-containing IVF/TPN
	K^+ supplementation
	Blood or platelet transfusion
	Penicillin potassium salts
	Dietary/herbal sources
Endogenous release	
	Rhabdomyolysis
	Burns
	Tumor lysis syndrome
	Hemolysis
	Exercise
	Prolonged seizure
	Infection
	Trauma
	Intravascular coagulopathy
	Starvation
	Reabsorption of hematoma
	Gastrointestinal bleeding
Extracellular shift	
	Metabolic acidosis
	Hyperosmolarity (mannitol, hypertonic saline)
	Insulinopenia
	Familial hyperkalemic periodic paralysis
	Drugs (see Table 5)
Impaired renal excretion	
	Severe hypovolemia
	Extremely premature neonates
	Acute kidney injury and chronic kidney disease
	Drugs (see Table 5)
	Mineralocorticoid deficiency (see Table 6)
	Mineralocorticoid resistance (see Table 6)
	Primary renal secretory defect (see Table 6)

hyperkalemia have at least one of the following three contributing mechanisms: 1) *excessive load*, 2) *transcellular shift*, and 3) *impaired renal clearance*. Drugs that interfere with potassium disposal or with intracellular uptake are listed in Table 5.

Presentation

Organ systems affected by hyperkalemia include *cardiac*, *skeletal muscle*, and *peripheral nervous system*. Increased tissue excitability initially results

Table 5. Drugs (K^+-free) associated with hyperkalemia

Extracellular Release of K^+	Impaired renal excretion
Non-specific β-blockers (Propranolol, etc.)	NSAIDs (Ibuprofen, etc.)
α-agonists (Phenylephrine, etc.)	Drospirenone
Spironolactone	Spironolactone
ACE-inhibitors	Amiloride
Angiotensin II receptor blockers	Triamterene
Digitalis	Trimethoprim
Succinylcholine	Pentamidine
Sodium fluoride	Azole antifungals
Epsilon-amino caproic acid	ACE-inhibitors
Arginine HCl, Lysine HCl	Arginine
Herbal preparations	Angiotensin II receptor blockers
Lily of the Valley	Cyclosporine
Milkweed	Tacrolimus
Siberian Ginseng	Heparin

from hyperkalemia-induced decreased resting membrane potential that approaches depolarization threshold. Later, there is reduced excitability, as membrane repolarization is impeded.

Cardiac dysrhythmia is the most dangerous consequence of hyperkalemia. Severity is influenced by the K^+ concentration, as well as the concurrent electrolyte and acid–base status. Dysrhythmias are more likely to occur, and more refractory to treatment, following a rapid rise in K^+ level, and with acidosis, hyponatremia, and hypocalcemia. With this variability in mind, ECG changes often correlate to plasma potassium concentration:

Plasma K^+ (mEq/L)	ECG changes
6.5–7	narrow peaked T waves, shortened QT, prolonged PR
7–8	widened QRS, loss of P wave amplitude
>8	sine wave pattern, ventricular fibrillation, asystole

Neuromuscular findings due to hyperkalemia include paresthesias and muscle weakness that may progress to ascending flaccid paralysis. This rare presentation occurs at extremely high potassium concentrations, usually >8 mEq/L. Head, trunk, and respiratory muscles are typically spared.

Diagnosis

A thorough medical history and examination should be performed with particular attention focused on assessment of intravascular volume, drug exposure including over-the-counter supplements, and recent dietary intake of K^+-rich foods. A comprehensive plasma chemistry panel, CBC, and urinalysis are important to assess plasma electrolytes, calcium and bicarbonate buffer status, renal function, and endogenous sources of potassium. An ECG is necessary to determine cardiac toxicity. Other studies may be indicated including concentrations or activities of: creatinine phosphokinase, lactate dehydrogenase, uric acid, plasma osmolality, 8 AM cortisol, renin activity/direct renin assay, aldosterone, 17-hydroxyprogesterone, and urine electrolytes, osmolality, and creatinine. Urinary tract imaging, urinary heavy metal screens, and genetic mutation analysis may be warranted.

The history, exam, and initial laboratory evaluation should identify the cause of hyperkalemia for a majority of patients (see Tables 4–6). Failure to identify the mechanism is usually due to the necessity for prompt therapy with hydration and emergency medications, resulting in delayed laboratory evaluation. If the cause of hyperkalemia is not readily apparent, then calculation of the TTKG (see "Hypokalemia"), at a time when the patient is stable, off diuretics, and off K^+ containing intravenous fluids, is helpful to assess distal renal K^+ handling. Normal renal K^+ excretion is indicated by a TTKG ≥ 5. A value <5 is consistent with mineralocorticoid deficiency or resistance (see Table 6).

Treatment

For all patients, ongoing K^+ intake (enteric or parenteral) and drugs associated with hyperkalemia should be stopped. Isotonic saline should be given as soon as possible in cases of severe hypovolemia.

If adrenal insufficiency is suspected, glucocorticoids should be administered. Urgent therapy is necessary when ECG changes manifest or if plasma K^+ exceeds 7 mEq/L (see Table 7). Euvolemic patients should receive isotonic saline and intravenous furosemide. Patients with generalized edema, without anuria, should receive furosemide (with or without 25% albumin). Higher doses of furosemide are necessary in patients with

Table 6. Hyperkalemic disorders with impaired K^+ excretion without azotemia

Inherited	Acquired
Mineralocorticoid deficient	
21-hydroxylase deficiency	Primary adrenal insufficiency
3β-hydroxysteroid-dehydrogenase deficiency	Secondary adrenal insufficiency
Congenital lipoid hyperplasia (StAR)	Aldosterone synthase deficiency
	Hyporeninemic hypoaldosteronism
Mineralocorticoid sufficent	
Pseudohypoaldosteronism I	Obstructive uropathy
Pseudohypoaldosteronism II	Reflux nephropathy
Antenatal Bartter syndrome (ROMK)	Lead nephropathy
Familial hyperkalemia with hypertension	Sickle cell disease
	Papillary Necrosis
	Systemic lupus erythematosis
	Type 4 distal RTA
	Renal transplant tubulopathy

Table 7. Treatment of hyperkalemia

Therapy	Dose	Onset	Duration
Sodium chloride [isotonic] (IV)	10 mL/kg	Immediate	
Furosemide (IV)	1 mg/kg higher if AKI/CKD	15–60 min	4–6 h
Calcium chloride (IV)	20–25 mg/kg	Immediate	30 min
Calcium gluconate (IV)	100 mg/kg	Immediate	30 min
Kayexalate (PO, NG, PR)	0.5–2.0 g/kg	1–2 h	4-6 h
Sodium bicarbonate (IV)	1–2 mEq/kg	30–60 min	2 h
Insulin [Regular] (IV) + Glucose	0.1–0.3 Units/kg 0.5–2 gm/kg	15–30 min	2–6 h
Albuterol (nebulized)	2.5–5.0 mg	15–30 min	2–4 h
Dialysis	Nephrology consult		

renal dysfunction. Fludrocortisone is helpful in patients with primary mineralocorticoid resistance or with renal disease resulting in this secondarily, as well as mineralocorticoid deficient patients. These interventions maximize delivery of sodium to the distal nephron and promote kaliuresis.

Cell membranes should be stabilized quickly, by correcting acidosis and abnormal plasma concentrations of sodium, calcium, and magnesium.

Calcium salts should be infused to individuals with ECG changes, even if plasma levels are normal. In patients with known cardiac disease, especially those receiving digitalis, cardiology consultation is imperative due to the associated risk of dysrhythmia, which may require antiarrhythmic medication. Although often life-saving, treatment with calcium salts does not lower plasma K^+ levels, hence concurrent treatment to promote K^+ excretion and intracellular redistribution is necessary. Redistributing K^+ to the intracellular space is an effective strategy to temporarily reduce the K^+ level and improve ECG findings. Insulin with glucose, and nebulized albuterol, are both effective. Blood glucose testing is required after giving insulin, and tachycardia often results with albuterol, even though it is a β_2-specific agonist. Sodium bicarbonate is effective primarily in the setting of metabolic acidosis.

K^+ loss may also be achieved from the gastrointestinal tract using sodium polystyrene sulfonate given orally, or as enema. This resin binds K^+ in exchange for sodium in equimolar ratio, and 1 g/kg reduces plasma K^+ concentration approximately 1 mEq/L. Oral doses are more palatable with sorbitol (70%) or dextrose (10%) and require minimal dilution (3–4 ml per 1 g). When used rectally, sorbitol should be avoided and the resin should be diluted 1:5 (v/v) with isotonic saline to avoid colonic injury. Enemas must be retained 15–30 minutes to work.

Dialysis may be necessary in patients with oligoanuria. The establishment of dialysis access may take a significant amount of time; and therefore, an alternate initial potassium lowering regimen may be implemented prior to initiating dialysis. Hemodialysis is preferred due to more rapid K^+ clearance, but peritoneal dialysis is effective in extremely small children, those with limited venous access, and when asymptomatic hyperkalemia is not worsening, nor severe enough to warrant immediate intervention.

Rare genetic causes of hyperkalemia (see Table 6) require treatment tailored for the mechanism involved. Cases associated with defective adrenal steroid synthesis require glucocorticoid or mineralocorticoid replacement. Children with mineralocorticoid resistance require supplementation with both sodium chloride and sodium bicarbonate; fludrocortisone may benefit those with partial resistance. The rare patient with familial hyperkalemia and hypertension should respond to thiazide diuretics.

Suggested Reading

Alfonzo AV, Isles C, Geddes C, Deighan C. (2006) Potassium disorders — clinical spectrum and emergency management. *Resuscitation* **70**(1): 10–25.

Allon M. (1995) Hyperkalemia in end-stage renal disease: Mechanisms and management. *J Am Soc Nephrol* **6**(4): 1134–1142.

Giebisch G, Malnic G, Berliner RW. (1996) Control of renal potassium excretion. In: Brenner BM, Rector FCJ (eds.) *The Kidney*, 5th ed., pp. 371–407, WB Saunders, Philadelphia.

Mack EH, Shoemaker LR. Dyskalemias. (2009) In: Kiessling SG, Goebel J, Somers MJG (eds.), *Pediatric Nephrology in the ICU*, 1st ed., pp. 35–54, Springer-Verlag, Berlin.

Osorio FV, Linas SL. (1999) Woodard disorders of potassium metabolism. In: Schrier RW, Berl T, Bonventre JV (eds.) *Atlas of Diseases of the Kidney, Volume 1: Disorders of Water, Electrolytes, and Acid–Base*, 1st ed., pp. 3.5, 3.5–3.12, Current Medicine, Inc., Philadelphia.

Perazella MA. (2000) Drug-induced hyperkalemia: Old culprits and new offenders. *Am J Med* **109**(4): 307–314.

Rose BD, Post TW. (2001) Hyperkalemia. In: Wonsciewicz M, McCullough K, Davis K (eds.) *Clinical Physiology of Acid–Base and Electrolyte Disorders*, 5th ed., pp. 888–930, McGraw-Hill, New York.

Satlin LM, Schwartz GJ. Metabolism of potassium. (1990) In: Ichikawa I (ed.) *Pediatric Textbook of Fluids and Electrolytes*, 1st ed., pp. 89–98, Williams and Wilkins, Baltimore.

Schwartz GJ. (2004)Potassium. In: Avner ED, Harmon WE, Niaudet P (eds.) *Pediatr Nephrol*, 5th ed., pp. 147–188, Lippincott Williams and Williams, Philadelphia.

West ML, Marsden PA, Richardson RM, *et al.* (1986) New clinical approach to evaluate disorders of potassium excretion. *Miner Electrolyte Metab* **12**(4): 234–238.

9

Acid–Base in Health and Disease

John W. Foreman and Rasheed A. Gbadegesin

Introduction

Hydrogen ion (H^+) is one of the most tightly regulated ions in the body. The normal H^+ concentration in extracellular fluid (ECF) is only 40 nanomolar or 0.00004 meq/L and ranges at most from 0.000035 to 0.000045 meq/L in healthy individuals. Normal extracellular pH is 7.4, and one pH unit change represents a ten-fold change in H^+ concentration. The H^+ concentration changes in diseases compatible with life range from 0.0001 (pH 7.0) to 0.00002 meq/L (pH 7.7).

Maintenance of Acid–Base Balance

Buffers

The first line of defense in maintaining normal pH is body buffers. A buffer is a weak acid or weak base that is partially dissociated: $HA \leftrightarrow H^+ + A^-$, where HA is the undissociated weak acid. If a stronger acid is added to a buffer containing solution, the final H^+ concentration is not as high (or the final pH is not as low) as a pure concentration of the stronger acid alone. Similarly, if a strong base is added to this solution, the OH^- ions from the base will combine with the H^+ ions of the weak acid to form H_2O, causing an equilibrium shift to the right and dissociating HA to form new H^+ ions, minimizing pH change. This relationship is described as

$$\mathrm{pH} = \mathrm{pK} + \log\frac{[\mathrm{A}^-]}{\mathrm{HA}}$$

This equation illustrates that a buffer functions best at a pH equal to the pK, when HA is 50% dissociated.

Body buffers

The body has a number of buffer systems, including plasma proteins, carbonic acid–bicarbonate system, and hemoglobin in the ECF. Principal intracellular buffers include proteins, and phosphate. Plasma proteins are effective buffers because their free carboxyl and amino groups can dissociate. Hemoglobin serves as a buffer by dissociation of the imidizole groups of histidine, which makes it a six-fold greater buffer than plasma proteins. Deoxyhemoglobin is a better buffer than oxyhemoglobin.

The easiest buffer system to measure is the carbonic acid–bicarbonate system, the pK of which is 6.1, which is low to maintain the pH at 7.4. However, the ability to modulate the carbonic acid concentration through changes in pCO_2 makes this buffer system effective. The relationship of these buffer pairs is: $H^+ + HCO_3^- \leftrightarrow H_2CO_3 \leftrightarrow H_2O + CO_2$.

Conversion of carbonic acid to water and CO_2 is quite slow, but the enzyme carbonic anhydrase (CA), found inside many cells and RBCs, rapidly facilitates this interconversion. This interconversion is illustrated in the Henderson–Hasselbalch equation:

$$pH = 6.1 + \frac{\log[HCO_3^-]}{0.03pCO_2}$$

The advantage of the carbonic acid–bicarbonate system is that it is an open system as opposed to a closed system of carbonic acid and bicarbonate. In an open system, the concentration of pCO_2 can be adjusted by the lungs and bicarbonate by the kidneys, minimizing the change in pH for any given acid or alkali load.

Normal respiratory acid removal

Metabolism of carbon containing fuels generates 16,000 to 20,000 mmoles of CO_2 gas per day. In this process, 2000–3000 mmoles of strong acids, such as lactic, tricarboxylic, and keto acids, are formed and further metabolized to CO_2, which poses no threat as normal respiration can easily excrete this CO_2 load, maintaining blood pCO2 at 40 mm Hg. In normal respiration, CO_2 production and excretion are closely matched. Chemoreceptors in the carotid and aortic bodies and in the brainstem sense pCO_2, pO_2, and pH and accordingly adjust minute ventilation.

Changes in pCO_2 lead to changes in CSF pH since pCO_2 freely moves from blood to CSF. Under normal circumstances, minute ventilation is more closely linked to pCO_2 than pO_2.

Normal renal acid excretion

Oxidation of sulfur containing amino acids and organophosphate compounds, such as phosphoserine, generates strong inorganic acids, H_2SO_4 and H_3PO_4. The catabolism of other compounds, such as nucleic acids, generate organic acids, such as uric, oxalic, glucoronic, and hippuric acids, (termed nonvolatile or fixed acids) cannot be combusted to CO_2 and must undergo renal elimination. The typical American diet generates approximately 1 mmol/kg/day of these acids in an adult, and more in children and infants (2–3 mmol/kg/day) due to buffer (OH^- and phosphate) consumption by bone formation. Greater dietary intake of base equivalents through milk, especially human milk offsets acid production in infants and young children.

H^+ generated by this metabolism is initially buffered by body buffers, such as HCO_3^- and is ultimately converted to CO_2 and eliminated from the body by the lungs. However, to maintain acid–base balance, the kidney regenerates an equivalent amount of HCO_3^-. Organic acids not completely metabolized to CO_2 are renally excreted, resulting in HCO_3^- loss that is regenerated by the kidney through renal tubular H^+ secretion and excreted as titratable acids (TA), mostly monobasic phosphate ($H_2PO_4^-$) and ammonium ion (NH_4^+). The distal nephron regenerates HCO_3^- by combining CO_2 and H_2O forming H^+ and HCO_3^-, catalyzed by carbonic anhydrase (CA), which is transported into blood, replacing lost HCO_3^-. The urinary concentration of phosphate, varies minimally; however, NH_4^+ generation and excretion can increase exponentially, especially in conditions of excess acid production. Thus, the major renal response to an acid load is increased NH_4^+ production and elimination.

However, any HCO_3^- loss in the urine diminishes net acid excreted (NAE) by the kidney. This relationship is shown below:

$$NAE = TA + NH_4^+ - HCO_3^- - \text{metabolizable anions}$$

When the urine pH is less than 6.5, there is minimal HCO_3^-. Although many organic anions are directly unmeasurable, their presence is suspected by a significant difference (>100 mosm/L) between the measured urine osmolality and the calculated osmolality:

$$\text{Calculated } U_{osm} = 2 \times U_{Na} + 2 \times U_K + U_{Urea}/2.8 + U_{Glucose}/18.$$

Renal handling of bicarbonate

In normal adults, approximately 4500 mmol/day of bicarbonate must be reclaimed from the glomerular filtrate (180 L/day glomerular filtrate × 25 mmol/L plasma bicarbonate = 4500 mmol). Proximal tubule bicarbonate reabsorption occurs by tubular secretion of H^+ in exchange for Na^+, via the luminal membrane sodium/hydrogen exchanger (NHE3) (see Fig. 1).

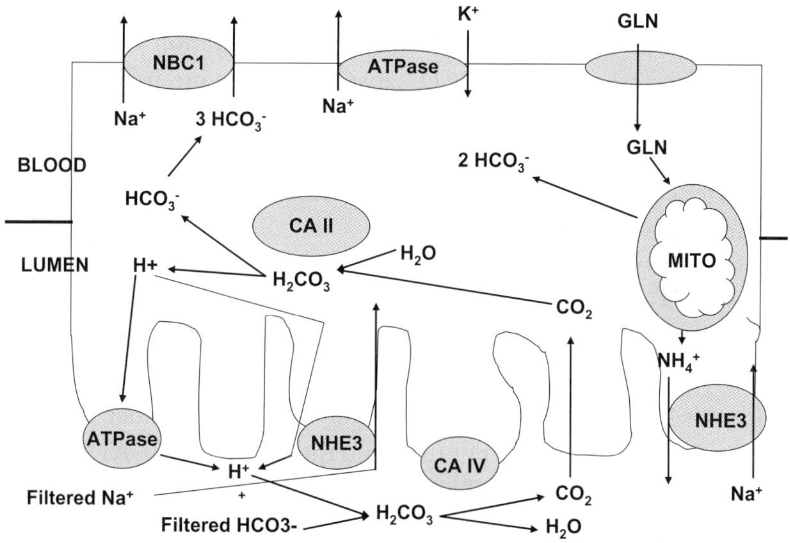

Figure 1. Proximal tubule showing recovery of bicarbonate and sodium from the glomerular ultrafiltrate. Acid–base secretion by the proximal tubule. H^+ generated by CAII exits the cell and enters into the lumen via the Na^+/H^+ exchanger 3 (NH3) and the H^+-ATPase. There it combines with filtered HCO_3 to form CO_2 (facilitated by CAIV) that diffuses back into the cell. HCO_3^- exits the cell and moves into the blood via the Na^+-HCO_3^- cotransporter (NBC1). Glutamine (GLN) enters the cell via a specific transporter where it is metabolized to 2 HCO_3^- and 2 NH_4^+ molecules. NH_4^+ exits the cell via Na^+/H^+ exchanger 3 in place of H^+.

The driving force for this exchange is the basolateral Na^+/K^+-ATPase, where 3 Na^+ are transported extracellularly in exchange for 2 K^+, leading to an electrochemical (low intracellular Na^+ concentration and negative potential charge relative to lumen) gradient favoring Na^+ entry into the cell. The H^+-ATPase pump transports small amounts of H^+ from the tubular cell into the lumen. The hydrogen for this process is generated in the cytosol by reaction of CO_2 and H_2O, catalyzed by CAII. The HCO_3^- generated in this process exits the cell via the Na^+, HCO_3^- exchanger (NBC1) which is coded for by the gene SLC 4A4. The H^+ transported into the proximal tubule lumen combines with filtered HCO_3^- to form carbonic acid and, subsequently, CO_2, a reaction rapidly catalyzed by CAIV, which resides on apical and basolateral membranes of the proximal tubule and thick ascending limb of the loop of Henle (TAL). Approximately 80–90% of the filtered load of HCO_3^- is reabsorbed in the proximal tubule. Factors increasing HCO_3^- reabsorption include increased filtered load, low peritubular pH and high pCO_2, angiotensin II, extracellular volume contraction, and potassium depletion. Acute administration of parathyroid hormone decreases proximal HCO_3^- absorption. The mechanism of bicarbonate reabsorption by the neonatal proximal tubule is similar to that of the adult, but has 1/3 the capacity due to lower activity and abundance of transporter compared to adults. Glucocorticoids stimulate the maturation of bicarbonate absorption.

The TAL reabsorbs a majority of HCO_3^- exiting the proximal tubule (see Fig. 2). Apical Na^+/H^+ exchange mediates most luminal H^+ secretion. The HCO_3^- exits the cell via several transporters including Na^+/HCO_3^- and K^+/HCO_3^- co-transporters and the Cl^-/HCO_3^- exchanger. The distal nephron is responsible for reabsorption of the remainder of filtered HCO_3^-, where H^+ is actively pumped into the lumen via H^+-ATPase pump and H^+, K^+-ATPase pump. Bicarbonate exits the cell distally via the Cl^-/HCO_3^- exchanger (AE1).

Distal tubular acidification

The distal nephron consists functionally of three segments: cortical collecting tubule (CCT), outer medullary collecting tubule (OMCT), and inner medullary collecting tubule (IMCT). The CCT, a low-capacity segment in which acidification is regulated by Na^+ transport, generates

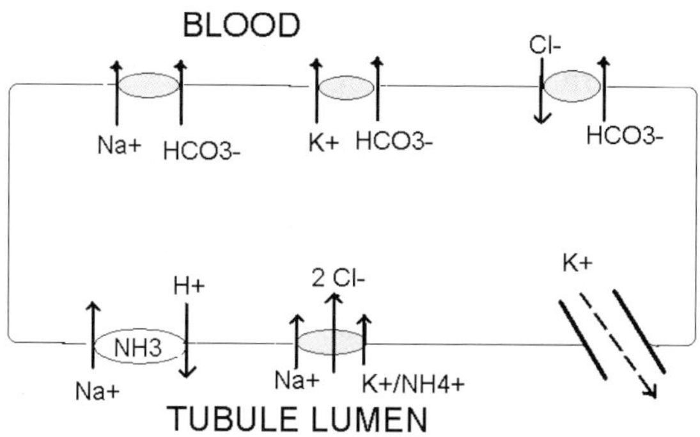

Figure 2. TAL cell showing sodium, chloride, potassium and bicarbonate reabsorption pathways. Acid–base secretion by TAL. The remaining filtered HCO_3^- is reabsorbed by combining with H^+ secreted by the Na^+/H^+ exchanger 3 (NH3). HCO_3^- exits the cell via several transporters, including Na^+, HCO_3^- cotransporter, K^+, HCO_3^- cotransporter, and the Cl^-/HCO_3^- exchanger. NH_4^+ enters the cell in place of K^+ on the $2Cl^-$, Na^+, K^+ transporter for recycling in the medullary interstitium.

a lumen negative membrane potential. The OMCT has high-capacity for H^+ secretion but does not transport Na^+. The IMCT has low capacity for H^+ secretion and is regulated by systemic acid–base and K^+ balances both in terms of net H^+ secretion and NH_4^+ transport. The collecting tubule α-intercalated cell is responsible for H^+ secretion primarily via the H^+-ATPase pump with some by the H^+/K^+-ATPase pump (see Fig. 3). Bicarbonate exits the cell via the basolateral anion exchanger.

Mineralocorticoids play an important role in H^+ secretion, both by Na^+-dependent and -independent mechanisms. Mineralocorticoids in the CCT increase Na^+ absorption, increasing lumen negativity, favoring H^+ secretion. Mineralocorticoids also directly stimulate H^+ secretion in the OMCT and the IMCT. Low systemic pH and high pCO_2 augment distal H^+ secretion. The neonatal CCT has fewer intercalcated cells and lower H^+ secretion compared to the adult, while the MCT has a similar rate. Overall, the neonate has a lower H^+ secretion rate.

Ammonia production and excretion

Excreted H^+ is buffered by ammonia to prevent extreme luminal acidity (see Fig. 4). Ammonia (NH_3) is highly permeable to cell membranes.

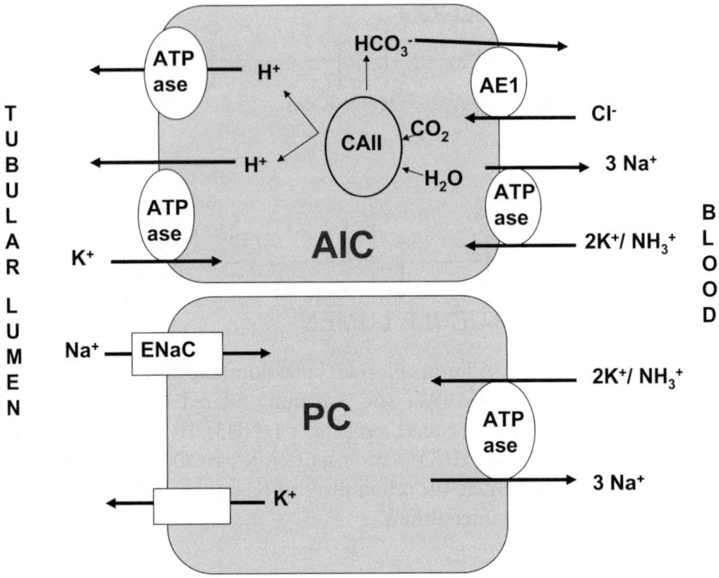

Figure 3. Acid–base secretion in the distal nephron. H^+ is generated from CO_2 by CAII in the α-intercalated cell (AIC) and exits via the H^+-ATPase or the H^+/K^+ exchanger. HCO_3^- exits the cell via the AE1 Cl^-/HCO_3^- exchanger. NH_4^+ can enter the cell from the interstitium by competing with K^+ on the Na^+/K^+ ATPase. Na^+ enters the cell via the sodium channel (ENaC) generating a lumen to cell negative gradient in the principal cell (PC).

Secreted H^+ converts luminal NH_3 to NH_4^+, thus lowering the concentration of NH_3, allowing more NH_3 to diffuse into the lumen. NH_4^+ is relatively impermeable to cell membranes and thus, is "trapped" in the lumen. The higher H^+ concentration in the lumen of the distal nephron compared to medullary interstitium further favors the transfer of NH_3 into the distal lumen.

Most ammonia is generated in the proximal tubule cell by amino acid metabolism, principally glutamine, yielding two NH_4^+ ions and α-ketoglutarate (α-KG). Further metabolism of α-KG yields two "new" HCO_3^- ions that are transported out of the cell across the basolateral membrane into the blood to replace the [HCO_3^-] lost in buffering acid. The rate limiting steps in glutamine metabolism are glutaminase and phosphoenolpyruvate carboxykinase (PEPCK). However, NH_4^+ must be eliminated from the body to remove H^+. If NH_4^+ enters the blood stream, it is transported to the liver, where it combines with 2 HCO_3^- to form urea with

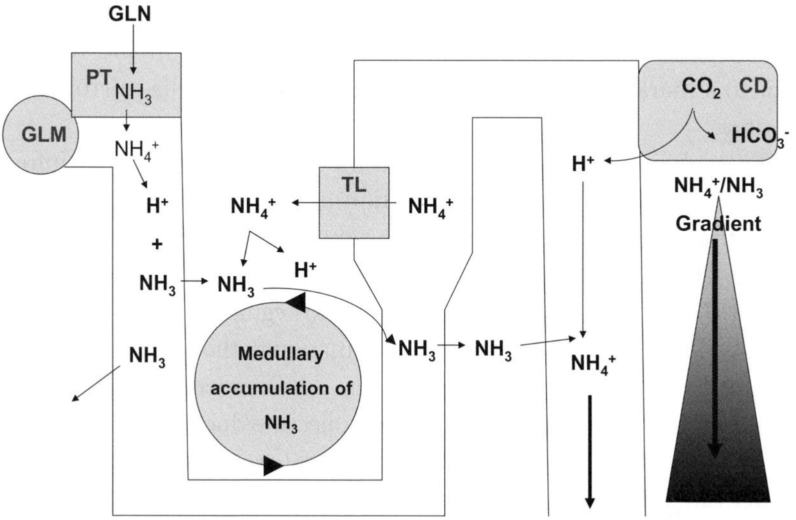

Figure 4. Renal ammonia metabolism. NH_4^+ is generated from glutamine in the proximal tubule cell. As the tubular fluid travels down the thin limb of the loop, water abstraction concentrates the luminal HCO_3^-, increasing the luminal pH favoring NH_3. NH_3 diffuses out of the lumen and into the medullary interstitium. The $2Cl^-$, Na^+, K^+ transporter can also actively transport NH_4^+ out of the lumen. Both of these processes lead to NH_4^+/NH_3 accumulation in the medulla and an increasing concentration favoring ammonia entry into the MCT.

no net addition of HCO_3^- to the body. To accomplish this, NH_4^+ is preferentially secreted across the apical membrane by the Na^+/H^+ antiporter. In the proximal straight tubule, the low luminal pH compared to that of the cell traps diffused NH_3 as NH_4^+. Acidosis stimulates glutamine release from muscles, uptake by the proximal tubule cells, and metabolism to NH_4^+. Acidosis also increases glucocorticoid levels, which in turn also stimulates ammoniagenesis. Hypokalemia stimulates ammoniagenesis and hyperkalemia inhibits it. Angiotensin II increases ammoniagenesis and proximal tubule secretion of NH_4^+.

As fluid leaves the proximal tubule, a number of processes lead to high medullary ammonia-ammonium concentrations. Water abstraction from the thin descending limb of the loop of Henle alkalinizes tubular fluid by concentrating luminal HCO_3^- favoring NH_3 efflux into the interstitium. In the TAL, NH_4^+ is actively transported into the cell by the $Na^+/2Cl^-/K^+$ cotransporter by substituting for K^+. Approximately a third of NH_4^+ transport in the TAL is paracellular. This arrangement of transporters in the loop of Henle and slow flow in the *vasa recta* leads to a marked concentration gradient in the medulla mirroring that for urea.

The high interstitial NH_3 concentration facilitates diffusion into the ICMT, where it is "trapped" by secretion of H^+ to form NH_4^+. NH_4^+ also enters the collecting tubule lumen by substituting for K^+ on the Na^+/K^+-ATPase. This interaction of K^+ and NH_4^+ on the $Na^+/2Cl^-/K^+$ cotransporter and Na^+/K^+-ATPase is another mechanism to regulate NH_4^+ excretion. The net excretion of NH_4^+ is dependent on formation in the proximal tubule cell, transport into the proximal tubule lumen, development of high interstitial medullary gradient, and trapping in the collecting duct by H^+ secretion.

The neonate has all the enzymes necessary for ammoniagenesis but has a lower rate under normal conditions, with reduced compensation ability. Reduced ammoniagenesis, H^+ secretion, and bicarbonate reabsorption place neonates and young infants at greater risk for acidosis during times of stress.

Systemic Response to Changes in Acid–Base Changes

Respiratory acidosis and alkalosis

Respiratory system disturbances alter CO_2 production and excretion, leading to abnormal pCO_2 levels. Hyperventilation leads to an abnormally low pCO_2, a raised pH, and respiratory alkalosis (see Tables 1 and 2). Hypoventilation causes the opposite changes in pCO_2 and pH, resulting in respiratory acidosis (see Table 3).

Plasma HCO_3^- decreases slightly with decreases in pCO_2 and rises slightly with increases in pCO_2 due to buffering by non-carbonate buffers.

Table 1. Definitions

	pH	$[HCO_3^-]$	pCO_2
Respiratory acidosis	↓	↓	↑
Respiratory alkalosis	↑	↓	↓
Metabolic acidosis	↓	↓	↓
Metabolic alkalosis	↑	↑	↑

Table 2. Acid–Base disturbances and expected compensation

Disturbance	Cause	pH	Compensatory response	Expected compensation	Limits of compensation
Acute respiratory acidosis	↑pCO_2	↓	↑ renal $[HCO_3^-]$ reabsorption	$[HCO_3^-]$↑ 0.1 meq/L for each 1 mmHg pCO_2 ↑	$[HCO_3^-]$ 38 meq/L
Chronic respiratory acidosis	↑pCO_2	↓	↑ renal $[HCO_3^-]$ reabsorption	$[HCO_3^-]$ 0.25–0.5 meq/L for each 1 mmHg pCO_2 ↑	$[HCO_3^-]$ 45 meq/L
Acute respiratory alkalosis	↓pCO_2	↑	↓ renal $[HCO_3^-]$ reabsorption	$[HCO_3^-]$ ↓ 0.25 meq/L for each 1 mmHg pCO_2 ↓	$[HCO_3^-]$ 18 meq/L
Chronic respiratory alkalosis	↓pCO_2	↑	↓ renal $[HCO_3^-]$ reabsorption	$[HCO_3^-]$ ↓ 0.0.4–0.5 meq/L for each 1 mmHg pCO_2 ↓	$[HCO_3^-]$ 15 meq/L
Metabolic acidosis	↓$[HCO_3^-]$	↓	↑pCO_2	$pCO_2 = 1.5\ [HCO_3^-] +$ 8 mmHg pCO_2 = last 2 digits of pH $pCO_2 = 15 + [HCO_3^-]$	pCO_2 15 mmHg
Metabolic alkalosis	↑ $[HCO_3^-]$	↑	↓pCO_2	$pCO_2 = 40 + 0.7$ $([HCO^-_{3\ measured}] -$ 24) mmHg $pCO_2 = 15 + [HCO_3^-]$	pCO_2 55 mmHg

Plasma $[HCO_3^-]$ increases approximately 0.1 meq/L for each 1 mmHg increase in pCO_2 and decrease 0.25 meq/L for each 1 mmHg decrease in pCO_2 to a maximum of 4–5 meq/L. Acute hypocapnia also increases organic acid production, especially lactic and citric acids, decreasing blood $[HCO_3^-]$.

With chronic changes in pCO_2 the kidney is recruited to alter blood $[HCO_3^-]$ and return pH towards normal, "compensation." Persistent hypocapnia causes decreased proximal tubule HCO_3^- reabsorption and decreased distal tubule acidification lowering blood bicarbonate by 0.4–0.5 meq/L for each mmHg decrease in pCO_2. This compensation takes hours to days to achieve and lowers the pH towards, but not to 7.4. Simultaneously,

Table 3. Common acid–base disturbances — respiratory disturbances

Acidosis	Alkalosis
CNS depression	CNS stimulation
Airway obstruction	Anxiety
Pulmonary disease	Fever
Pleural disease	Hypoxia/high altitude
Neuromuscular disease	Pregnancy
Obesity	Salicylates
Chest wall injury	CHF
Mechanical hypoventilation	Asthma
	Pulmonary embolism
	Sepsis
	Hepatic failure
	Urea cycle disorders

Increased AG	Normal AG
Metabolic acidosis	
Diabetic ketoacidosis	Diarrhea
Alcoholic ketoacidosis	Renal tubular acidosis
Starvation ketoacidosis	Early renal failure
Lactic acidosis	Early diabetic ketoacidosis
Organic acidemias	Glue sniffing (Toluene)
Methymalonic	
Proprionic	
Isovaleric	
Uremia	D-lactic acidosis
Salicylism	TPN (HCl amino acid salts)
	NH_4Cl
	$CaCl_2$
Ethylene glycol	Ureterosigmoidostomies
	Small intestinal ostomies
Methanol	Chlolestyramine
	Sevelamer
	CA inhibitors
	Acetazolamide
	Topiramate
	Dilutional

(*Continued*)

Table 3. (*Continued*)

Low Urine Cl^- Saline responsive	High Urine Cl^- Saline unresponsive	High Urine Cl^- Saline responsive
Metabolic alkalosis		
Pyloric stenosis	Cushing disease	Bartter syndrome
Nasogastic suction	Steroid therapy	Gitelman syndrome
Loop diuretics	Primary hyperaldosteronism	Loop diuretics
Thiazide diuretics	Renovascular stenosis	
Hypokalemia	Malignant hypertension	
Congenital chlorrhea	Cirrhosis	
Villous adenoma	CHF	
Non-reabsorbable anions	Alkali excess in CKD	
Penicillin	Glucocorticoid remedial hyperaldosteronism	
Carbenicillin	Apparent mineralocorticoid excess	
Magnesium deficiency	Glycyrrhizin	
	(Licorice, chewing tobacco)	

plasma Cl^- rises due to a shift of Cl^- from red blood cells, ECF volume contraction, and increased renal reabsorption.

Chronic hypercapnia causes the opposite renal changes that take several days for completion. With full compensation, the plasma [HCO_3^-] rises by 0.25 to 0.5 meq/L for each mmHg rise in pCO_2. Elevated pCO_2 causes increased [H^+] secretion by both proximal and distal renal tubules. The elevated blood pCO_2 raises cortical pCO_2 and enhances proximal tubule $HCO3^-$ reabsorption and distal tubule NH_4^+ excretion. Hypercapnia causes systemic vasodilation and decreases effective circulating volume, enhancing HCO_3^- reabsorption. Hypercapnia decreases NaCl reabsorption further compromising effective circulating volume and stimulating [HCO_3^-] reabsorption. In the distal nephron, hypercapnia increases insertion of H^+ pumps, H^+-ATPase and H^+/K^+-ATPase in the apical membrane, increasing H^+ secretion.

Metabolic acidosis and alkalosis

Metabolic acidosis, the gain of H^+/loss of HCO_3^-, causes changes in respiratory CO_2 excretion. Decreased arterial pH is sensed by chemoreceptors controlling respiration causing increased ventilation, lowering pCO_2 and blunting the pH fall from an acid load or bicarbonate loss. This response occurs relatively quickly with maximal effect by 10–14 hours. The pCO_2 falls by 1.25 mm Hg for every 1 meq/l fall in $[HCO_3^-]$ (see Table 2). Predicted pCO_2 for a given $[HCO_3^-]$ can be estimated as $pCO_2 = 1.5 [HCO_3^-] + 8$ ($\pm$ 2 mm Hg). In mild to moderate metabolic acidosis, the last two digits of the pH approximate pCO_2. Ultimately, correction requires renal excretion of acid load or restoration of lost bicarbonate by increased proximal tubule resorption of HCO_3^- and distal excretion of TA and NH_4^+. Soon after an acid load, urine pH decreases to 4.5, but ammonia production and excretion increases in response. In older infants, children, and adults ammonium excretion rises from 30–40 meq/day to > 300 meq/day to increase pH to nearly 6.

Changes in pCO_2 also compensate for metabolic alkalosis (see Table 2). A rise in arterial pH is sensed by the chemoreceptors controlling respiration, thereby decreasing respiration, raising pCO_2, and blunting the increase in pH. This compensatory response is limited by the concomitant fall in pO_2 which stimulates respiration. The pCO_2 rises 0.7 mmHg for every 1 meq/L rise in $[HCO_3^-]$ to a maximum of 55 mmHg. A quick calculation of this compensation is made by adding 15 to serum $[HCO_3^-]$.

Dissection of Acid–Base Disorders

The first step in diagnosing an acid base disorder is to carefully review the patient's history, medications, and physical examination which often give important clues to type of acid–base disturbance, especially in those with a mixed acid–base disturbance. Blood pH, serum HCO_3^-, and pCO_2 should be measured simultaneously (see Fig. 5). All three components are necessary to accurately assess presence and type of acid–base disturbance. Serum HCO_3^- should be measured soon after obtaining the blood sample to prevent falsely low HCO_3^- concentration from prolonged contact with red cells. Capillary blood draws, prolonged tourniquet time, and excessive "dead space" in the specimen tube may also falsely lower HCO_3^-.

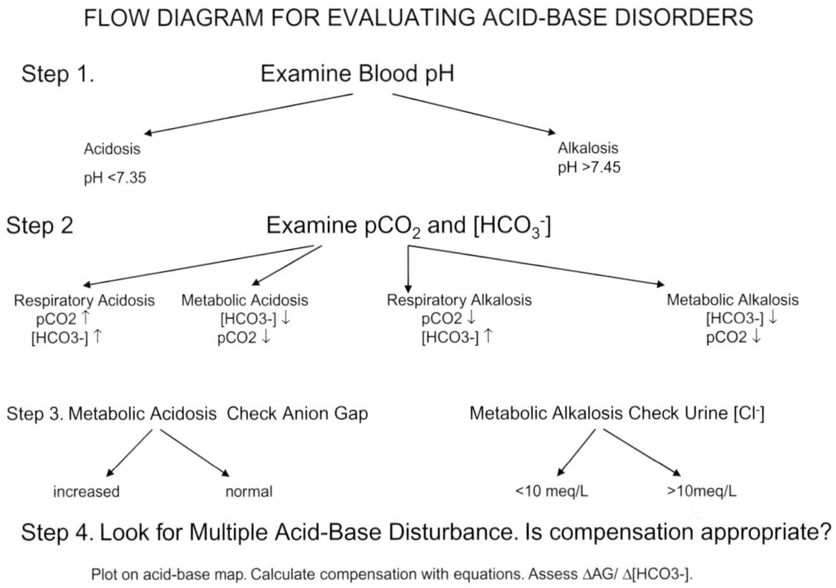

Figure 5. Flow diagram for evaluating acid–base disorders.

The presence of acidosis or alkalosis should be assessed by blood pH, with subsequent analysis of serum HCO_3^-, and pCO_2 to differentiate metabolic and respiratory disturbances. Respiratory acidosis is associated with an elevated pCO_2 and plasma HCO_3^- while respiratory alkalosis has opposite values. Metabolic acidosis is associated with low plasma HCO_3^- and a low pCO_2. Metabolic alkalosis has the opposite HCO_3^- and pCO_2 values. Common causes of these disturbances are shown in Tables 2 and 3.

Respiratory acidosis and alkalosis

Respiratory acidosis is caused by hypoventilation, which can originate in the brainstem respiratory centers, nerves innervating respiratory muscles, the respiratory muscles, the pleura, airway, or lung parenchyma and circulation. Respiratory alkalosis arises from hyperventilation, due to many conditions, including anxiety, fever, pregnancy, hepatic failure, sepsis, hypoxia, acute cardiopulmonary disease, central nervous system disease, and drugs.

Metabolic acidosis

Metabolic acidosis occurs due to either the loss of bicarbonate, through the GI tract or kidney; or gain of acid from an exogenous source, such as parenteral nutrition solutions. Other etiologies include abnormal metabolism causing organic acid generation, such as β-hydroxybutyrate in diabetic ketoacidosis (DKA) or methylmalonate in methylmalonic aciduria. Failure to excrete the usual acid load due to nephron loss [chronic kidney disease, or renal tubular acidosis (RTA)] can cause metabolic acidosis.

Anion gap

In metabolic acidosis, anion gap (AG) should be determined: AG = Na^+ – (HCO_3^- + Cl^-). A normal AG (AG = 8–16 mEq/L) acidosis is most commonly seen with diarrhea or RTA. An elevated AG usually indicates an increased concentration of unmeasured anion with a concomitant increase in plasma [Na^+]. The normal anion gap assumes normal amounts of unmeasured anions (PO_3^{3-}, SO_4^{2-}) in plasma and negative charges on plasma proteins (albumin). Albumin contributes significantly to the anion gap: for every 1 g/dL albumin decrease from 4.5 g/dL, the anion AG should be decreased by 2.5 meq/L. Corrected AG = (measured AG + 2.5 (4.5 – measured albumin)). For example, if the plasma albumin is 1.5 g/dL the normal AG should be 5 meq/L. If the AG is 10 meq/L, which is in the normal range, then the corrected AG is 17 meq/L, suggesting a metabolic acidosis. Severe alkalosis increases the negative charge of albumin leading to increased AG.

Other considerations in assessing AG include changes in plasma cations and elevations in plasma IgG (plasma cell dyscrasias). Marked increases in plasma calcium and magnesium can lower AG and marked decreases have the opposite effect. IgG carries a cationic charge and very high levels lower the AG. Abnormal cations, such as lithium (Li^-) also decrease AG. Hyperviscosity or hyperlipidemia may cause under-measurement of the plasma [Na^+] and bromide (Br^-) intoxication causes an overestimation of the plasma [Cl^-], falsely lowering AG. Newer methods of measuring serum [Cl^-] have led to higher values, tending to lower the normal range for AG in some laboratories.

With a normal plasma albumin, a raised AG is usually due to the addition of a nonchloride containing acid, such as in lactic acidosis due to decrease in the GFR, limiting urinary excretion of lactate. Alternatively, β-hydroxybutyrate and acetoacetate in DKA are typically lost in the urine (unless there is underlying renal dysfunction). Calculation of the Δ/Δ is useful in looking for multiple acid–base disturbances in a patient: $\Delta/\Delta = (AG - 12)/(24 - [HCO_3^-])$. A $\Delta/\Delta < 1$ suggests a greater fall in $[HCO_3^-]$ than the AG, potentially caused by combination acidosis, such as diarrhea in a patient with renal failure. A $\Delta/\Delta > 2$ suggests a smaller deviation of $[HCO_3^-]$ from normal compared to the increase in AG, indicating a mixed disturbance, such as lactic acidosis from sepsis in a patient on nasogastric suction.

Urine anion gap

Urinary ammonium excretion is the prime renal defense against an acid load. Determination of urine NH_4^+ excretion is useful in assessing renal ability to excrete acid, especially in normal AG acidosis. Indirectly, urine ammonium can be estimated by urine net charge = $Na^+ + K^+ - Cl^-$ (anion gap). Urinary cations, Na^+, K^+, NH_4^+, Ca^{2+}, and Mg^{2+}, must balance urine anions Cl^-, HCO_3^-, PO_4^-, SO_4^-, and organic anions. Urine Ca^{2+}, Mg^{2+}, PO_4^-, and SO_4^- are usually in low and fixed concentrations and can be ignored. If urine pH is < 6.5, urinary HCO_3^- concentration is very low, signifying low urine organic anion concentrations. Major urine ions are Na^+, K^+, NH_4^+, and Cl^-; of which Na^+, K^+, and Cl^- can be easily measured.

Metabolic acidosis, usually associated with a negative urine net charge ($[Cl^-] > [Na^+] + [K^+]$), indicates normal renal response to metabolic acidosis by increasing NH^{4+} excretion as NH_4Cl. A positive urine anion gap suggests RTA or chronic kidney disease causing reduced NH_4^+ excretion. Occasionally, the urine net charge is positive with an appropriate renal response of increased NH_4^+ excretion, because NH_4^+ is excreted with an organic anion other than Cl^-. Examples include glue-sniffing where the NH_4^+ is excreted with hippurate and DKA where NH_4^+ is excreted with β-hydroxybutyrate and acetoacetate. If this is suspected, the difference between calculated urine osmolality and measured osmolality detects the presence of unmeasured anions and estimates NH_4^+ excretion. A difference of more than 100 mosm/kg (normal < 100 mosm.kg) represents a significant concentration of an organic anion, such as β-hydroxybutyrate or hippurate. One half of this difference can be used as an estimate of the ammonia concentration.

Metabolic alkalosis

Increased acid loss causes metabolic alkalosis. With normal renal function, an exogenous alkali load is rapidly excreted with only short term acid–base effects. Exogenous alkali load can cause systemic alkalosis in patients with renal impairment when the load exceeds renal excretion capacity. Exogenous administration of sodium citrate (i.e. anticoagulation in continuous renal replacement therapy) is one example.

The respiratory response, hypoventilation, is less predictable than in metabolic acidosis. An estimate of compensatory rise in pCO_2 is made by adding 15 to the serum [HCO_3^-] within the range of 25–40 meq/L. The respiratory compensation is limited by decrease in pO_2.

The clinical approach should focus on etiology of alkali generation and renal excretion ability. Metabolic alkalosis can be divided into "saline responsive" (chloride loss syndromes) and "saline resistant" due to increased sodium reabsorption and ECF expansion. Chloride deficiency often results from gastric fluid loss, where HCO_3^- added to the blood by stomach parietal cells is not balanced by intestinal absorption of the secreted H^+, generating alkalosis, which is then maintained by volume contraction from NaCl loss. This volume contraction reduces GFR, stimulates aldosterone secretion, and enhances proximal bicarbonate reabsorption. Aldosterone stimulates the H^+/K^+ -ATPase in α-intercalated cell and the Na^+, K^+-ATPase and luminal sodium channel, ENaC, in the principal cell of the collecting duct. This increases H^+ and K^+ excretion, maintaining alkalosis. During active vomiting when new bicarbonate is added to the ECF, not all is reabsorbed, in spite of the enhanced proximal and distal tubule HCO_3^- reabsorption, leading to alkaline urine. With vomiting cessation without volume repletion, the enhanced proximal and distal tubule reabsorption is maintained and the increased filtered load of bicarbonate from the high serum bicarbonate is completely reabsorbed resulting in acidic urine. Both situations are associated with urine [Cl^-] < 10 meq/L. During active vomiting or nasogastric suction, with urinary bicarbonate loss, urine [Na^+] is relatively high and decreases with a decrease in urine bicarbonate.

Hypokalemia also maintains alkalosis by increasing ammoniagenesis and transport in the proximal tubule, TALH, and medullary collecting duct, all increasing H+ excretion. Chronic hypokalemia reduces GFR independent of volume contraction through increased production of the vasoconstrictors, angiotensin II, and thromboxane. Hypomagnesemia induces metabolic alkalosis by stimulating renin and ultimately aldosterone secretion, causing distal nephron urine acidification. Large doses of nonreabsorbable anions, such as penicillins, also enhance distal acidification and metabolic alkalosis by increasing distal tubule luminal negative charge, facilitating H^+ and K^+ excretion.

Other pediatric causes of metabolic alkalosis include cystic fibrosis (CF), congenital chloridorrhea, villous adenomas, Bartter syndrome, Gitelman syndrome, and primary hyperaldosteronism. Hyperreninemic hypertension, with or without renovascular disease, causes mild metabolic alkalosis via aldosterone secretion.

Exogenous corticosteroids commonly cause metabolic alkalosis and mimic hyperaldosteronism. Cortisol interacts with the mineralocorticoid receptor, and is in abundance compared to aldosterone. Intracellular 11 β-hydroxysteroid dehydrogenase (11 β-HD) converts cortisol to cortisone which does not interact with the receptor. High levels of cortisol overwhelm 11 β-HD and interact with the mineralocorticoid receptor, causing a hyperaldosterone-like state. In apparent mineralocorticoid excess, 11 β-HD is defective causing a similar effect. This enzyme is inhibited by glycyrrhizin, which is found in licorice. Another cause of saline-resistant metabolic alkalosis is Liddle syndrome, an autosomal dominant defect in either the gene coding for the β or the γ subunit of the CCT luminal sodium channel (ENaC). These defects maintain the channel in an open position and interfere with channel recycling, leading to increased sodium reabsorption, potassium and hydrogen secretion, hypertension, and metabolic alkalosis.

Mixed disturbances

Multiple acid–base disorders can occur simultaneously. For example, a patient with CF and chronic respiratory acidosis treated with loop diuretics causes metabolic alkalosis with respiratory acidosis. As in simple acid–base disorders the first step is obtaining a good history, with special attention to recent medications, and the physical examination. A quick

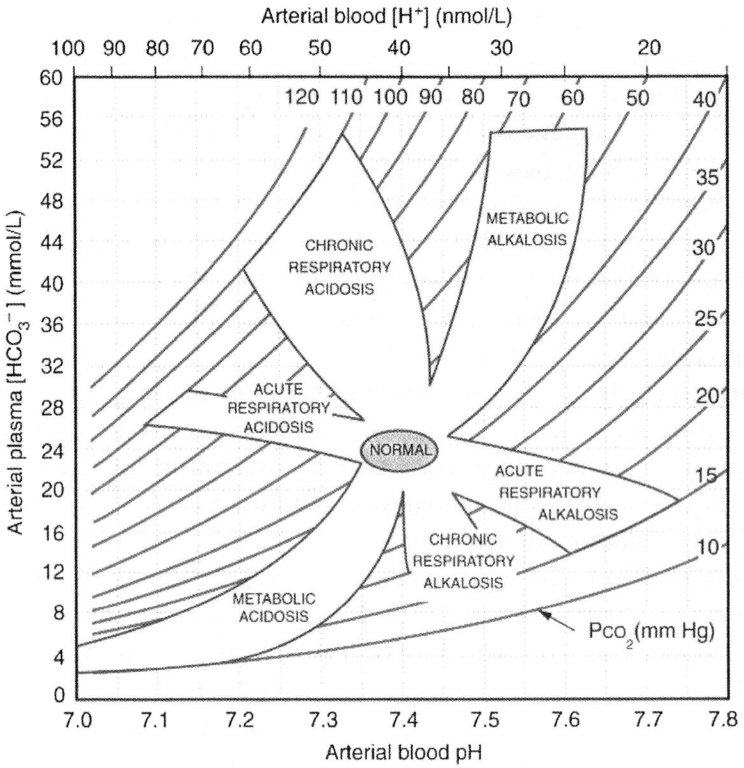

Figure 6. Acid–base map. Shaded areas represent 95% confidence limits of the normal respiratory and metabolic compensations for primary acid–base disturbance. Data falling outside of the shaded area denote a mixed disorder if a laboratory error is not present. Reprinted with permission from Brenner BM, ed. (2008) *Brenner and Rector's The Kidney.* (2008) 8th ed. Saunders, Philadelphia.

approach is to place the patient's acid–base values on a "map" (see Fig. 6). Another approach is to calculate the expected compensation (see Table 2) and compare this to the patient. However, acute and chronic compensation may differ and duration of respiratory disturbance is not clear.

Normal plasma [HCO_3^-] does not exclude metabolic abnormality. A patient with chronic respiratory acidosis who develops lactic acidosis may have normal plasma [HCO_3^-] but still has acidosis that is detected by increased anion gap and lower than expected [HCO_3^-] for the pCO_2. In looking for a mixed disturbance one should keep in mind that a mildly raised anion gap normally occurs in alkalosis from an increase in the negative charges on albumin and alkalosis-induced increase in lactate.

Calculating the $\Delta AG/\Delta[HCO_3^-]$ can detect a mixed disturbance. A $\Delta/\Delta < 1$ indicates normal AG acidosis as well as a raised AG acidosis and a $\Delta/\Delta > 2$ suggests a metabolic alkalosis in addition to the raised AG acidosis.

Other Methods of Dissecting an Acid–Base Disturbance

Whole-blood buffer base and base excess method

Base excess (BE) is often reported, and is based on the whole blood buffer base concept. Normal whole blood buffer base in adults is 48 meq/L and is mainly composed of serum HCO_3^-, plasma proteins, and based on hemoglobin concentration of 15 g/dL. The standard HCO_3^- (24 mEq/L) which is the bicarbonate concentration in a blood sample at 38°C, fully saturated with O_2 and equilibrated with $pCO_2 = 40$ mmHg, eliminates the respiratory component. BE is the amount of acid or base that must be added to a liter of blood that is fully oxygenated and equilibrated to a pCO_2 of 40 mmHg at 38°C to achieve a pH of 7.40. Adults with hemoglobin of 15 g/dL and a serum $[HCO_3^-]$ of 24 meq/L will have a BE = 0. Normal infants with a lower serum $[HCO_3^-]$ and hemoglobin have BE = −3. A positive BE indicates metabolic alkalosis and negative component indicates metabolic acidosis. BE does not add information not already apparent from the pH, pCO_2, and $[HCO_3^-]$. Using BE without considering compensatory changes in chronic conditions leads to erroneous interpretations. For example, a patient with chronic respiratory disease and a pCO_2 of 80 mmHg with normal renal function, will have a serum $[HCO_3^-]$ of 40 meq/L, a standard $[HCO_3^-]$ of 32 meq/L, and a BE of +11 meq/L. Interpretation by the BE method would imply a significant metabolic alkalosis as opposed to expected compensation. If this patient develops DKA such that the $[HCO_3^-]$ decreases to 29 meq/L and the pH to 7.18, the standard bicarbonate would be 23 meq/L and the BE would be 0 meq/L. The base excess method would miss a significant metabolic acidosis in addition to respiratory acidosis.

Treatment

Respiratory acidosis and alkalosis

Principal treatment is aimed at correcting the underlying disorder. Medications suppressing respiratory drive, such as opiates, should be avoided and electrolyte abnormalities impairing respiratory muscle function, such as hypokalemia, hypomagnesemia, and hypocalcemia, should be corrected. Alkali does not treat respiratory acidosis, but patients with severe disease may require respiratory support. If diuretics are used, adequate KCl should be provided to avoid metabolic alkalosis.

In patients with hyperventilation, a rebreathing bag often corrects the problem. In other disorders, such as liver failure or subarachnoid hemorrhage, the metabolic alkalosis is minor part of a much larger problem.

Metabolic acidosis

Treatment of the underlying cause is imperative, especially in reversible cases such as lactic acidosis or DKA. In severe acidosis, defined as a serum pH of <7.10, impaired myocardial contractility and catecholamine responsiveness, increased cardiac arrhythmias, and hypotension can occur. Many clinicians administer bicarbonate (0.5 to 1 meq/kg of $NaHCO_3$) to acutely raise the pH to 7.2 as part of the overall management.

Bicarbonate therapy is not without risk. Exogenous bicarbonate may increase pCO_2 and induce hypernatremia and hypervolemia. Hypokalemia can be unmasked or worsened by rapid correction of acidosis. Acidosis correction may increase tissue hypoxia because increasing pH increases hemoglobin oxygen affinity and decreases oxygen tissue unloading. Raising blood pH may precipitate tetany in hypocalcemic patients by increasing albumin binding. Bicarbonate therapy is a risk factor for cerebral edema development in patients with DKA, so bicarbonate administration should be considered only if pH is <6.90 or in life-threatening hyperkalemia.

Less severe acidosis may require treatment if the underlying process is irreversible and acidosis is persistent, leading to poor growth, bone mineralization and increased muscle-wasting, especially when associated with chronic kidney disease or RTA. In these disorders, patients usually require buffer equal to daily acid production (2–3 mEq/kg/day).

Metabolic alkalosis

In patients with metabolic alkalosis and low urine chloride, volume expansion enhances renal alkali excretion. Correction of potassium losses may be necessary to fully correct acidosis. Volume status should be optimized if alkalosis cannot be corrected rapidly. Depending on etiology, other agents utilized to correct metabolic alkalosis include supplemental KCl, potassium sparing diuretics (amiloride, triamterene, spironolactone), and nonsteroidal anti-inflammatory agents. Hyperreninemic states should be corrected. Acetazolamide is useful in volume expansion states such as congestive heart failure. In extremely rare situations, dilute (0.1N) HCl or NH_4Cl can reduce blood pH to 7.5. Hemodialysis with a high chloride, low bicarbonate bath is effective in patients with renal failure and metabolic alkalosis. Patients on continuous renal replacement therapy with citrate anticoagulation often develop metabolic alkalosis responsive to bicarbonate removal from replacement fluid. Rarely, these patients require infusion of 0.1N HCl postfilter.

Suggested Reading

Androgue HJ, Madias NE. (1998) Medical progress: management of life-threatening acid–base disorders: first of two parts. *N Engl J Med* **338**: 26–34.

Androgue HJ, Madias NE. (1998) Medical progress: management of life-threatening acid–base disorders: second of two parts. *N Engl J Med* **338**: 107–111.

Badrick T, Hickman E. (1998) The anion gap: a reappraisal. *Am J Clin Pediatr* **98**: 249–252.

Carlisle EJF, Donnelly SM, Halperin ML. (1991) Renal tubular acidosis (RTA): recognize the ammonium defect and pHorget the urine pH. *Pediatr Nephrol* **5**: 242.

Core HE. (2005) Bench-to-bedside review: fundamental principles of acid–base physiology. *Crit Care* **9**: 184–192.

Edelmann CM, Jr, Biochis H, Rodriguez Soriano J, *et al.* (1967) The renal response of children to acute ammonium chloride acidosis. *Pediatr Res* **1**: 452.

Edelmann CM, Jr, Rodriguez Soriano J, Biochis H, *et al.* (1967) Renal bicabonate and hydrogen ion excretin in normal infants. *J Clin Invest* **46**: 1309.

Narins RG, Emmitt M. (1980) Simple and mixed acid–base disorders: a practical approach. *Medicine* **59**: 161–187.

Quigley R, Baum M. (2004) Neonatal acid base balance and disturbances. *Seminars in Perinatology* **28**: 97–102.

Schlictig R, Grogono AW, Severinghaus JW. (1998) Human $PaCO_2$ and standard base excess compensation for acid–base imbalance. *Crit Care Med* **26**: 1173–1179.

10

Disorders of Calcium Balance

Farah N. Ali and Craig B. Langman

Hypocalcemia

Introduction

The importance of calcium to cellular function is highlighted by the fact that it is the most abundant mineral in the body. It is essential for most metabolic functions of the cell, as well as for normal skeletal development. Its regulation is complex, involving numerous hormones and interplay between the gastrointestinal tract, kidneys, and the skeletal system (see Fig. 1). Dietary calcium is absorbed from the gut under the influence of $1{,}25(OH)_2D$, or calcitriol. This hormone is formed in the proximal tubule of the kidney under the influence of 1-alpha-hydroxylase.

Ninety-eight percent of total body calcium resides in the bony skeleton, less than 1% in the circulation, and the remainder located in intracellular and extracellular fluid spaces. In the serum, 50% of calcium exists in the ionized and active state; 40% is protein bound, mainly by albumin, and 10% is chelated to anions such as phosphate or carbonate. Calcium that is not protein bound is freely filtered across the glomerulus and thus the renal tubules must reabsorb most of this calcium in order to maintain homeostasis (see Fig. 2).

Pathogenesis

Hormonal regulation of calcium is affected by the interplay between the extracellular calcium-sensing receptor (eCaSR), parathyroid hormone (PTH), and $1{,}25(OH)_2D$. The highest cell surface expression levels of the eCaSRs are found in parathyroid tissue. This receptor is a member of the G-protein coupled receptor (GPCR) family, and is located on

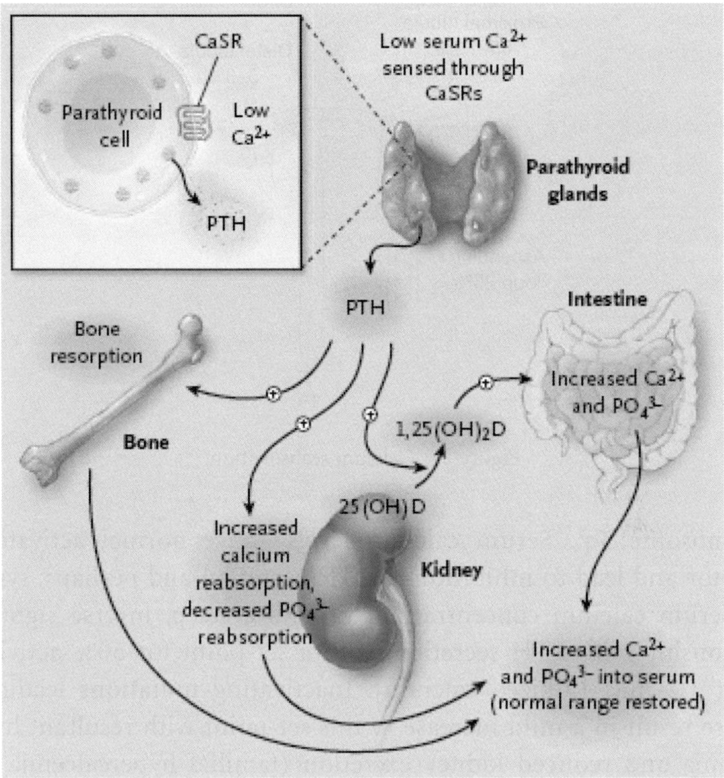

Figure 1. Control of mineral metabolism by parathyroid hormone.

Levels of serum ionized calcium (Ca^{2+}) are tightly controlled through the action of parathyroid hormone (PTH) and 1,25-dihydroxyvitamin D (1,25[OH]$_2$D). Both the rate and magnitude of changes in the serum ionized Ca^{2+} concentration are detected by extracellular calcium-sensing receptors (CaSRs) expressed on parathyroid cells. When ionized Ca^{2+} levels decrease, the release of PTH secretion is triggered. Conversely, when ionized Ca^{2+} levels increase, PTH secretion is suppressed. PTH stimulates bone resorption, which delivers calcium and phosphorus (PO_4^{3-}) into the circulation. In the kidney, PTH stimulates renal reabsorption of calcium and promotes phosphate excretion. PTH also enhances the conversion of 25-hydroxyvitamin D (25[OH]D) to the active vitamin D metabolite 1,25(OH)$_2$D, which increases the transepithelial transport of calcium and PO_4^{3-} through actions in intestinal cells. In concert, these steps restore ionized Ca^{2+} levels to the normal range, and, through the actions of PTH and other factors (e.g., fibrolast-derived growth factor 23) in the kidney, reset the level of serum PO_4^{3-} within the normal range. When the actions of PTH are reduced or lost, all subsequent steps in the maintenance of homeostasis are impaired, resulting in hypocalcemia, hyperphosphatemia, and hypercalciuria.

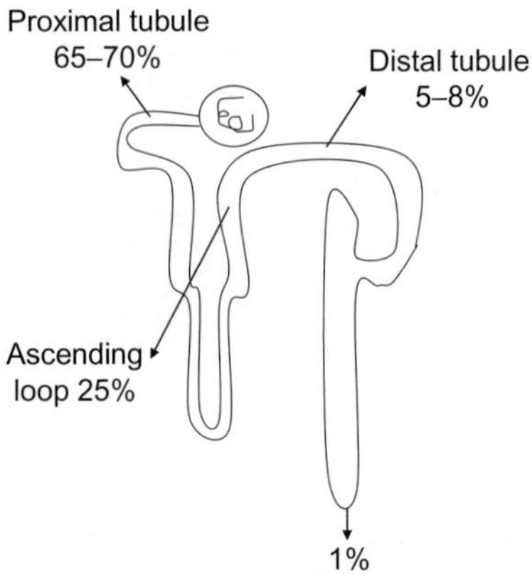

Figure 2. Calcium reabsorption.

chromosome 3q[1]. Serum calcium levels above normal activate the receptor and lead to inhibition of PTH secretion and perhaps, synthesis. Serum calcium concentration displays a steep, inverse sigmoidal relationship with PTH secretion, with a set-point for 50% activity at about 1.2 mM [ionized calcium]. Inactivating mutations leading to disease result in a mild increase in this set-point with resultant hypercalcemia and reduced kidney excretion (familial hypercalcemia with hypocalciuria).

PTH is released in response to serum ionized calcium levels below normal. This hormone promotes bone resorption of calcium (and phosphorus), decreases urinary calcium excretion, enhances conversion of 25(OH)D to $1,25(OH)_2D$, and increases phosphate excretion. In the setting of hypocalcemia, $1,25(OH)_2D$, enhances calcium absorption from the intestine, increases bone resorption, and reduces calcium excretion in the kidney allowing preservation of serum calcium. Figure 1 depicts the interplay of hormonal control of calcium homeostasis, and Fig. 2 shows sites of reabsorption of calcium along the nephron.

Clinical presentation

Hypocalcemia is defined as having low serum levels of ionized calcium or albumin-corrected total calcium. Measured serum calcium must be adjusted for serum albumin levels. The corrected total calcium (mg/dL) = measured total calcium + 0.8 [4.0 – serum albumin (g/dL)]. Therefore, hypocalcemia is defined when the corrected total calcium level is less than 7 mg/dL for preterm infants, less than 8 mg/dL for term infants, and less than 8.8 mg/dL children. Extracellular fluid pH also affects binding of calcium to albumin; for each 0.1 decrease of pH, ionized calcium increases about 0.2 mg/dL.

Symptoms of hypocalcemia are determined by the duration of abnormality, the rate of development of the problem, and the severity of the hypocalcemia. The most prominent symptoms are usually related to neuromuscular dysfunction. This may include altered mental status or seizures; paresthesias, carpopedal spasm, tetany, cramps and/or twitching; a prolonged QT, decreased myocardial contractility, or heart failure; and stridor, or laryngospasm/bronchospasm.

Chvostek's sign may be elicited by tapping the cheek over the path of the facial nerve, resulting in twitching of the ipsilateral upper lip. Trousseau's sign elicits a painful carpal spasm upon inflation of a sphygmomanometer, placed on the upper arm for three minutes, to a value midway between the systolic and diastolic pressures.

Diagnosis

Diagnostic possibilities include rarely, deficiency of calcium intake or more commonly, nutritional vitamin D deficiency. Inherited or other acquired disorders of vitamin D metabolism are a more unlikely possibility. In vitamin-D dependent rickets type 1, mutations in the 25-hydroxyvitaminD-1-alpha-hydroxylase prevents conversion of 25(OH)D to $1{,}25(OH)_2D$, thereby resulting in hypocalcemia. This condition is inherited in an autosomal recessive manner, and is also known as pseudo-vitamin D-deficient rickets. Vitamin D-dependent rickets type 2 is similarly inherited in an autosomal recessive fashion, but occurs as a result of end organ resistance to the actions of $1{,}25(OH)_2D$, due to one of several mutations in the vitamin D receptor. These children have rickets and alopecia.

Kidney failure is also a cause of hypocalcemia. As kidney disease advances, hypocalcemia results from loss of the ability to convert 25(OH)D to the activated form, $1{,}25(OH)_2D$. This is associated with rising PTH levels and serum phosphorus as well. The entity has been termed chronic kidney disease bone mineral disorder (CKD-MBD), and evidence-based medicine guidelines have recently been issued for its diagnosis, prevention, and treatment.

Magnesium abnormalities must be considered in the differential diagnosis of hypocalcemia. Adequate magnesium stores are vital to proper PTH functioning; hypomagnesemia leads to impaired PTH secretion, in addition to end-organ PTH resistance. Rarely, magnesium excess may also lead to hypocalcemia by inducing functional hypoparathyroidism.

Hypoparathyroidism also results in hypocalcemia. The DiGeorge anomaly is one diagnostic possibility, associated with chromosome 22q11 deletions. This disorder affects approximately 1 in 4000–5000 live births, and affected children may have facial dysmorphism, cardiac anomalies, and aplasia/hypoplasia of both the parathyroid and thyroid glands. Autoimmune polyglandular syndrome 1 (autoimmune-polyendocrinopathy-candidiasis-ectodermal dystrophy) is another disorder associated with hypoparathyroidism, as well as adrenal insufficiency, chronic mucocutaneous candidiasis, hypothyroidism, hypogonadism, pernicious anemia, type 1 DM, vitiligo, and alopecia. Acquired causes of hypoparathyroidism include postthyroidectomy, parathyroidectomy, or radical neck dissection, which usually result in hypoparathyroidism due to damage to glands or their blood supply. Finally, infiltration of the gland from iron (hemochromatosis), copper (Wilson's disease), or metastatic infiltration by tumor may lead to hypoparathyroidism.

Pseudohypoparathyroidism includes another group of disorders leading to hypocalcemia. These disorders are characterized by hypocalcemia but in the setting of elevated PTH. In type 1 disease, genetic mutations occur in the alpha subunit of the G stimulatory protein. Type 1a is termed Albright's hereditary osteodystrophy. Patients with this disorder have obesity, short stature, round faces, short metacarpals/metatarsals, mental retardation, and subcutaneous calcifications. When the calcium level is normal, this is termed pseudopseudohypoparathyroidism. Patients with type 1b disease have a normal phenotype, with isolated PTH resistance in the kidney. Type 2 pseudohypoparathyroidism involves defects beyond the PTH-receptor complex; urinary cAMP levels are normal in response to the infusion of PTH (as opposed to low cAMP levels in type 1).

Autosomal dominant hypocalcemia may present with a wide clinical spectrum from symptomatic hypocalcemia in the neonate to asymptomatic presentation in adulthood. Hypocalcemia in this disorder is associated with hypoparathyroidism, hyperphosphatemia, and hypercalciuria. This is a result of gain of function of the eCaSR due to activating mutations. Treatment should be limited to symptomatic patients since attempts to normalize the serum calcium may exacerbate hypercalciuria and increase stone formation. Hydrochlorothiazide has been used successfully in this setting.

Treatment

The treatment of hypocalcemia must be guided by the symptoms and the severity of hypocalcemia, factored by its pathogenesis. Oral calcium is a mainstay of therapy, but in severe cases intravenous calcium (as calcium gluconate or calcium chloride) may be necessary. Intravenous calcium formulations must be used with caution through peripheral lines as extravasation of the drug can lead to tissue damage. Correction of hypomagnesemia is also necessary if present; magnesium sulfate can be given intravenously. Hypocalcemia in CKD-MBD should be approached differently, with consideration of limitation of dietary calcium supplements due to the possibility of increasing vascular calcification.

In many cases, the use of vitamin D is also necessary. Nutritional, or 25(OH)D, deficiency should be addressed with ergocalciferol therapy.

Table 1. Delineatation of the biochemical features of differing causes of hypocalcemia

Causes of hypocalcemia	Phos	PTH	25(OH)D	$1,25(OH)_2D$	Mg	Urine Ca
Magnesium deficiency	N	L or N	N	L	L	H
Vitamin D deficiency	L or N	H	L	L,N, or H	N	L
Vitamin D dependent rickets type 1	L or N	H	N	L	N	L
Vitamin D dependent rickets type 2	L or N	H	N	H	N	L
Hypoparathyroidism	H	L	N	N or L	N	L
Pseudo-hypoparathyroidism	H	H	N	N or L	N	L
Kidney failure	H	H	N	L	N,H	L
CASR defect	H or N	L or N	N	N or L	N	H

Treatment should continue until a normal level is achieved, and then maintenance therapy ensured with a minimum daily dose of 400 units.

Calcitriol is also necessary for acute hypocalcemia to prevent adverse symptoms, such as seizures or laryngospasm, as well as in conditions such as hypoparathyroidism, pseudohypoparathyroidism, kidney failure, etc., in which activated vitamin D is deficient as part of the pathophysiologic process. Long-term monitoring for hypercalciuria, nephrocalcinosis, and nephrolithiasis is very important in patients requiring prolonged calcitriol therapy.

Hypercalcemia

Pathogenesis

Hypercalcemia develops if the amount of calcium entering the circulation from sites of calcium transport, such as the bone, kidneys, and intestine, exceeds the kidney's capacity for excretion. It is defined as serum calcium value above 10.6 mg/dL or ionized calcium value above 1.4 mmol/L.

Clinical presentation

The symptoms of hypercalcemia tend to be nonspecific and also depend upon on the severity of disturbance and rate of increase. Neurologic symptoms may be mild, from fatigue, headache, and muscle weakness, to more profound effects such as confusion, stupor, or coma. Gastrointestinal effects include anorexia, nausea, vomiting, abdominal pain, and constipation. Kidney manifestations include decreased urinary concentrating ability, kidney stones, nephrocalcinosis, or kidney failure, and cardiovascular symptoms such as arrhythmias, bradycardia, and hypertension may also occur. Bone pain and arthralgias are possible symptoms as well.

Diagnosis

Diagnostic possibilities include hyperparathyroidism. This entity is rather uncommon in children below adolescent age. However, if present, consideration for a diagnosis of multiple endocrine neoplasia (MEN) I or II should be made.

Malignancy is in the differential diagnosis of hypercalcemia, which in this circumstance may result from increased bone resorption due to release of factors from tumor cells that activate osteoclasts. Alternatively, PTH related peptide (PTHrP) production can induce hypercalcemia by increasing osteoclastic bone resorption and the renal tubular reabsorption of calcium. Biochemical findings resemble those of primary hyperparathyroidism (PHP), but serum PTH is markedly suppressed. In addition, ectopic 1,25$(OH)_2$D production may occur, leading to hypercalcemia. This mechanism of hypercalcemia can also be found in sarcoidosis and other granulomatous diseases, wherein 1,25$(OH)_2$D is produced by macrophages, and has systemic effects discussed above.

Other causes of hypercalcemia likely account for fewer than 10% of all causes of hypercalcemia. Table 2 contains a detailed list of other causes of hypercalcemia.

There are a few heritable disorders associated with mutations in the eCaSR that bear specific mention. Loss of eCaSR function due to inactivating mutations can result in Familial Hypocalciuric Hypercalcemia (FHH). In this disorder moderate hypercalcemia and hypocalciuria are associated with an inappropriately normal PTH. It is inherited in an autosomal dominant manner with heterozygous CaSR mutations occurring in affected individuals. Such affected individuals are usually asymptomatic despite their hypercalcemia, or may note nonspecific symptoms, such as fatigue, weakness, joint pain, or headache. Treatment of FHH appears unnecessary.

In Neonatal Severe Primary Hyperparathyroidism (NSHPT) mutations in the eCaSR are homozygous most typically. Here, marked hypercalcemia occurs associated with elevated PTH levels. Infants with this condition present in the neonatal period with poor feeding, failure to thrive, hypotonia, and respiratory distress associated with rib cage deformities. Total parathyroidectomy may be needed for survival.

Treatment

Hypercalcemia leads to volume depletion due to the "diuretic effects" of the metabolic derangement. The kidney increases sodium reabsorption to counter this effect, but thereby also increases calcium reabsorption,

Table 2. Causes of hypercalcaemia

Malignancy-associated hypercalcaemia
Local osteolytic hypercalcaemia
Humoral hypercalcaemia of malignancy
Ectopic production of $1{,}25(OH)_2$ vitamin D
Other humoral factors
Parathyroid Hormone (PTH) mediated hypercalcaemia
Autonomous hyperparathyroidism
Primary (isolated or within the context of syndromes)
Tertiary hyperparathyroidism
Parathyroid carcinoma
Familial benign hypocalciuric hypercalcaemia
Granulomatous disorders
Sarcoidosis
Tuberculosis
Leprosy
Candidiasis
Histoplasmosis
Wegener's granulomatosis
Crohn's disease
Drugs
Thiazides
Lithium
Vitamin D
Vitamin A
Aluminium intoxication in renal failure
Miscellaneous
Thyrotoxicosis
Adrenal insufficiency
Pheochromocytoma
VIP-producing tumour
Milk-alkali syndrome
Parenteral nutrition
Renal failure (acute, chronic)
Immobilization
William's syndrome

worsening the problem. Thus initial steps should include volume expansion with normal saline; indeed administration of physiological saline is the cornerstone in the treatment of hypercalcemia of any cause.

Traditionally, loop diuretics have been recommended in hypercalcemia management because they result in increased urinary calcium excretion.

However, scientific evidence to support their use is lacking, and in addition, if loop diuretics are given in the setting of volume depletion, they may even worsen the hypercalcemia.

The treatment of choice for malignancy associated hypercalcemia is bisphosphonate therapy. This class of medications has direct inhibitory action on bone resorption, thereby acting at the source of the hypercalcemia, increased osteoclastic bone resorption. The use of corticosteroids may be helpful in some situations, such as hypercalcemia related to ectopic production of 1,25$(OH)_2$D. In addition, calcimimetics (e.g. cinacalcet) may be useful in the setting of hypercalcemia associated with secondary hyperparathyroidism in kidney failure or after kidney transplantation.

Suggested Reading

D'Souza-Li L. (2006) The calcium-sensing receptor and related diseases. *Arq Bras Endocrinol Metabol* **50**: 628–639.

Jacobs TP, Bilezikian JP. (2005) Clinical review: rare causes of hypercalcemia. *J Clin Endocrinol Metab* **90**: 6316–6322.

Kher KK, Schnaper HW, Makker SP. (2006) *Clinical Pediatric Nephrology*, 2nd ed., Informa Healthcare, London.

Kidney Disease: Improving Global Outcomes (KDIGO) CKD-MBD Work Group. (2009) KDIGO clinical practice guideline for the diagnosis, evaluation, prevention, and treatment of Chronic Kidney Disease-Mineral and Bone Disorder (CKD-MBD). *Kidney Int Suppl* **113**: S1–S130.

Makras P, Papapoulos SE. (2009) Medical treatment of hypercalcaemia. *Hormones (Athens)* **8**: 83–95.

Shoback D. (2008) Clinical practice. Hypoparathyroidism. *N Engl J Med* **359**: 391–403.

Umpaichitra V, Bastian W, Castells S. (2001) Hypocalcemia in children: pathogenesis and management. *Clin Pediatr (Phila)* **40**: 305–312.

11

Disorders of Phosphorus Balance

Farah N. Ali and Craig B. Langman

Introduction

Inorganic phosphate is the most abundant anion in the body, and is the major component of bone in the mineral phase as hydroxyapatite. In addition, phosphorus is an essential part of nucleic acids, integral as a cell membrane component, and vital to numerous cellular processes, including intracellular signaling and maintaining cellular energy, in the form of ATP.

Approximately 85% of the total body phosphorus is in the skeleton and teeth, with about 15% present in the soft tissue components. A small remainder is found in the extracellular fluid. While the healthy adult maintains a zero phosphorus balance, a positive phosphorus balance is necessary in children in order to meet the needs of skeletal growth.

Within the plasma, phosphorus is found as organic compounds, including phospholipids and phosphate esters, inorganic phosphates, and complexed with cations, such as calcium and magnesium. Of the total plasma inorganic phosphorus, 10–15% is bound to protein, and thus only the remaining component is filtered by the glomerulus.

In order to minimize the effect of dietary factors on serum phosphorus levels, it is best to obtain specimens for blood phosphorus levels in the AM-fasted state. In addition, clinicians must be aware of the normal circadian rhythm governing serum phosphorus levels, as phosphorus decreases early in the morning, has a nadir before noon, and peaks after midnight. Normal values of the mineral in the blood vary with age; adult levels are significantly lower than those found in infants and older children.

Phosphorus homeostasis results from the balance of intestinal absorption, kidney excretion, and equilibration between extracellular and intracellular and bone stores (see Fig. 1). Net intestinal absorption, primarily by passive diffusion along paracellular pathways is extremely high in infants, exceeding 90% at times, and this decreases to 60–65% by adulthood. Active gastrointestinal absorption through sodium-dependent transcellular processes occurs when luminal phosphorus concentrations are low.

The majority of filtered phosphorus is resorbed by the proximal tubule and the kidney component of excretion or reclamation is the main determinant of chronic phosphorus equilibrium. Figure 2 depicts the sites of

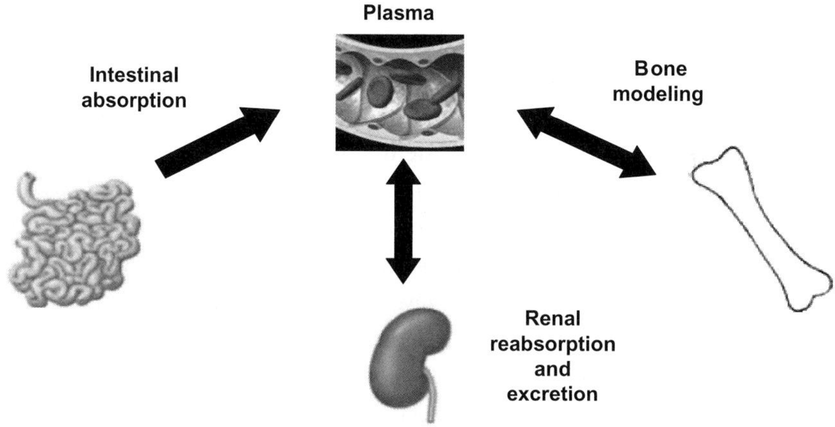

Figure 1. Phosphorus balance.

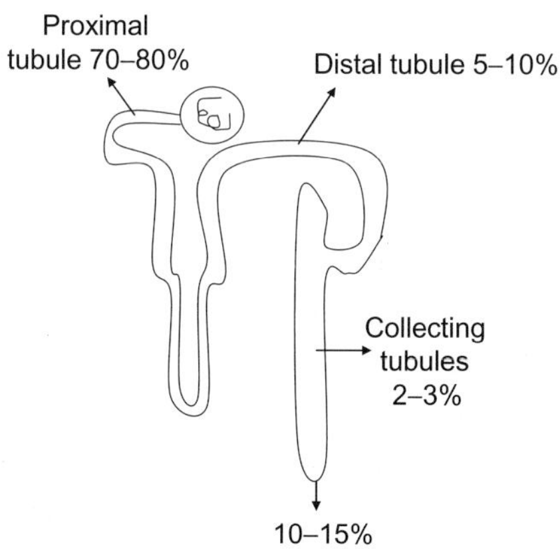

Figure 2. Phosphorus reabsorption.

phosphorus reabsorption along the nephron: 70–80% within the proximal tubule, 5–10% in the distal tubule, and 2–3% in the collecting tubule. In the proximal tubule, sodium-phosphate cotransporters types IIa and IIc are primarily responsible for phosphorus reabsorption. They allow delivery of one phosphate ion along with three sodium ions from the lumen into the tubular cells. This transport utilizes the existing sodium gradient, which is maintained by the basolateral Na^+/K^+-ATPase.

Hormonal regulation of phosphorus involves interplay between vitamin D, PTH, and the phosphatonins (see below). Hypophosphatemia, by increasing intrinsic production of $1,25(OH)_2D$ thereby leading to a rise in blood levels of the hormone, leads to increased intestinal absorption of phosphorus (and calcium) as well as increased phosphorus (and calcium) mobilization from bone. The combined effect of these processes is an increase in phosphorus (and transiently, calcium). Elevated serum calcium, acting through the extracellular calcium-sensing receptor, reduces PTH secretion, which then limits bone resorption of calcium and phosphorus, increases phosphorus reabsorption in the kidney, and reduces calcium reclamation by the kidney. Hypophosphatemia also directly increases calcium excretion in the kidney. The net result of all of these hormonal changes in the setting of hypophosphatemia is an increase of serum phosphorus towards normal, with relatively little change in serum calcium long-term. Opposite effects occur in hyperphosphatemia, which reduces levels of $1,25(OH)_2D$, increases PTH levels, thereby decreasing the serum phosphorus by limiting gastrointestinal absorption and increasing losses through the kidney.

New to the homeostatic picture of phosphorus balance are the hormones called "phosphatonins." Phosphatonins encompass a group of proteins, including at least three that have been identified as acting to decrease serum phosphorus: secreted frizzled protein 4 (sFRP4), matrix extracellular phosphoglycoprotein (MEPE), and fibroblast growth factor 23 (FGF23). At present, the best understood actions are those related to FGF23.

FGF23 is a 251 amino acid-containing protein which is produced by bone. This hormone (see Fig. 3) acts on the proximal tubule to promote phosphaturia by decreasing expression of sodium-phosphate transporters at the brush border membrane, and by decreasing proximal tubular production of $1,25(OH)_2D$, and increasing its degradative enzyme, with an overall net effect of decreasing intestinal phosphorus absorption.

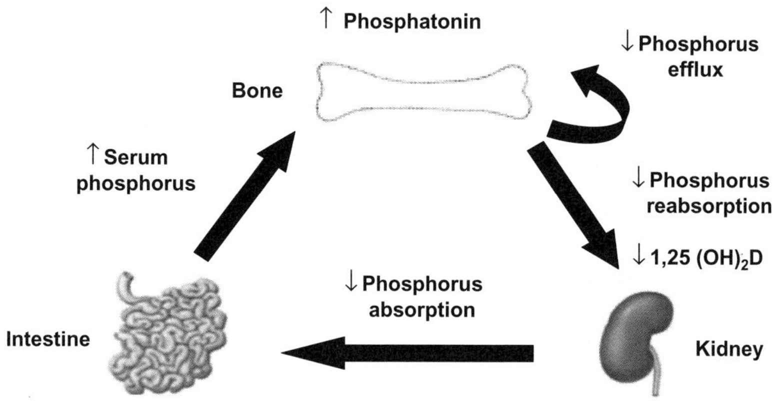

Figure 3. Phosphatonin actions.

Other factors that may increase phosphorus excretion are volume expansion, acidosis, glucose infusions, calcitonin, mannitol, loop diuretics, thiazides, and glucocorticoid therapy. Increased phosphate preservation by the tubules may occur in the setting of dietary phosphorus restriction, alkalosis, insulin therapy, thyroid hormone therapy, and with growth hormone therapy, through stimulation of the sodium-phosphorus cotransporter and/or independent actions of IGF-1.

Hypophosphatemia

Pathogenesis

Hypophosphatemia may result from dietary deficiency or impaired intestinal absorption, and include malnutrition, eating disorders, use of antacids that bind phosphorus in the intestinal tract, malabsorptive processes, defective vitamin D metabolism that reduces circulating levels or actions of 1,25$(OH)_2$D, or intravenous hyperalimentation with an insufficient phosphorus additive.

Intracellular shift of phosphate may explain hypophosphatemia in certain settings. These settings may include infusion of large quantities of carbohydrate, respiratory alkalosis, cellular incorporation of phosphorus due to hungry bone syndrome, leukemic blast crises, sepsis, or refeeding in malnutrition, and hormonal factors such as insulin, catecholamines, glucagon, or calcitonin.

There are many situations where hypophosphatemia may be explained by renal phosphate wasting. Such disorders include proximal renal tubular acidosis, primary hyperparathyroidism or secondary hyperparathyroidism in early chronic kidney disease, metabolic acidosis, diabetic ketoacidosis, and postrenal transplantation, as well as with therapeutic agents that include diuretics, glucocorticoids, mineralocorticoids, sodium bicarbonate, or during volume expansion. Inherited disorders of kidney phosphate wasting will be discussed below.

Clinical Presentation

Clinical manifestations of hypophosphatemia usually are a result of decreased intracellular ATP levels and do not typically occur with mild hypophosphatemia. Severe hypophosphatemia may be associated with hematologic manifestations, including hemolysis and impaired phagocytosis; muscle function abnormalities, including weakness, respiratory failure or heart failure, and rhabdomyolysis. Skeletal manifestations of long-standing hypophosphatemia include rickets or osteomalacia.

Diagnosis

The most straightforward approach in diagnosis of disorders of hypophosphatemia is to start with assessment of the urinary phosphorus excretion. The fractional excretion of phosphorus ($FE_{PO_4^{3-}}$) can be calculated using the following formula:

$$FE_{PO_4^{3-}} = \frac{U_{PO4} \times P_{Cr}}{P_{PO4} \times U_{Cr}} \times 100$$

The normal value in children for the fractional excretion of phosphorus is 15–20%, but the value should be much less than 20% in the setting of hypophosphatemia. The fractional excretion of phosphorus can be used to calculate the tubular reabsorption of phosphate or TRP. The TRP represents the amount of filtered phosphorus that is reabsorbed by the renal tubules:

$$TRP = 1 - FE_{PO_4^{3-}}$$

The normal range for the TRP in children is greater than 0.80, with higher expected values in infants and growing children. These tests may be done on random urine samples, but are more reliable specimen would be a short timed collection under fasting conditions. Figure 4 suggests an algorithm for the evaluation of hypophosphatemia.

There are several clinical conditions and syndromes that must be considered in the category of selective renal phosphate wasting disorders.

Hereditary hypophosphatemic rickets with hypercalciuria (HHRH) is a genetic disorder associated with rickets, short stature, phosphaturia, hypercalciuria despite normal serum calcium, and high 1,25(OH)2D levels (as opposed to low or normal 1,25(OH)2D seen in the other conditions below).

X-linked hypophosphatemic rickets (XLH) is an inherited condition associated with a mutation in the phosphate-regulating gene with homologies to endopeptidases on the X-chromosome (PHEX), leading to overproduction and excess circulating levels of FGF23 and prevention of proteolysis of MEPE. It typically manifests during late infancy when a child begins walking, and can lead to bowing of long bones, widening of the metaphyseal regions, prominence at the costochondral junction (rachitic rosary), decreased growth velocity, short

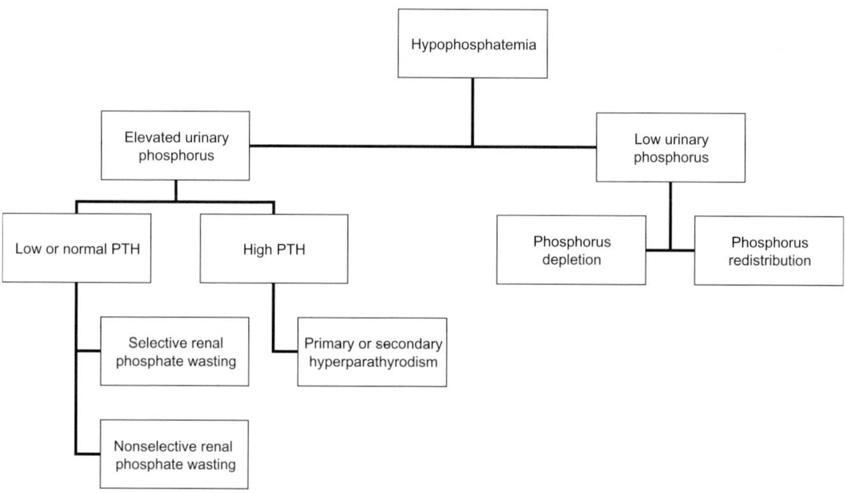

Figure 4. Evaluation of hypophosphatemia.

stature, and later in life, osteomalacia, degenerative joint disease, and dental disease.

Autosomal dominant hypophosphatemic rickets (ADHR) was first described in 1971 and presents with skeletal defects (bowing of the long bones and widening of metaphyseal regions). This condition has a variable onset, with incomplete penetrance and occurs as a result of a mutated FGF23, leading to hypophosphatemia from isolated renal phosphate wasting.

Autosomal recessive hypophosphatemic rickets (ARHP) has similar clinical features to the above disorder, with rickets and skeletal deformities, but in addition dental defects are present. It is due to a mutated dentin matrix protein 1 (DMP1) leading to over-expression of FGF23 in bone. Table 1 goes over the biochemical and genetic features of these inherited hypophosphatemic disorders.

Tumor induced osteomalacia is a paraneoplastic syndrome due to production of phosphatonins/FGF23. Most cases are associated with small benign mesenchymal tumors. Although surgical removal leads to complete cure, locating tumor may be difficult.

Hypophosphatemic rickets associated with McCune–Albright syndrome/fibrous dysplasia of bone results from over-expression of FGF23 in bone. These children have additional findings of abnormal skin pigmentation and premature sexual development.

Table 1. Biochemical and genetic features of inherited hypophosphatemic disorders

	FGF23	TRP	$1,25(OH)_2D$	PTH	Serum calcium	Urinary calcium	Mutation
XLH	High inappropriately normal	Low	Low-normal	High-normal	Normal	Normal	PHEX
ADHR	High inappropriately normal	Low	Low-normal	High-normal	Normal	Normal	FGF23
ARHP	High inappropriately normal	Low	Low-normal	High-normal	Normal	Normal	DMP1
HHRH	High inappropriately normal	Low	High	Low	Normal/elevated	High	NPT2c

Treatment

It is important to differentiate acute hypophosphatemia found generally in inpatient hospital settings from chronic hypophosphatemia, found generally in outpatients with inherited abnormalities of kidney phosphate handling or gastrointestinal disorders. The former needs prompt attention, while the latter needs chronic therapy, but rarely if ever, parenteral phosphorus administration.

In adults severe acute hypophosphatemia is consistently associated with poor clinical outcomes in hospitalized patients as well as in-hospital mortality.[6] In children untreated hypophosphatemia is associated with skeletal defects and growth failure;[5] thus treatment is essential, but on a chronic outpatient basis.

For the treatment of mild or chronic hypophosphatemia of any cause, use of oral sodium and potassium phosphate preparations is indicated. Examples of such preparations include: Neutra-Phos®, Neutra-Phos K®, or an oral solution of sodium or potassium phosphate. The addition of calcitriol therapy in patients with disorders associated with low or inappropriately normal $1,25(OH)_2D$ levels is necessary. In severe or symptomatic hypophosphatemia, intravenous phosphorus may be necessary, but caution should be used in this setting to avoid potential complications of over-treatment, including renal failure, tetany from hypocalcemia, hypotension, hyperphosphatemia, and EKG abnormalities.

Hyperphosphatemia

Pathogenesis

A thorough approach to hyperphosphatemia involves examining the interplay between intake and absorption, extracellular shift of phosphorus, and kidney excretion of phosphorus. Artifactual hyperphosphatemia should also be excluded, and can occur with hemolysis of the sample, or in the setting of paraproteinemias or hypertriglyceridemia. Increased intake of exogenous phosphorus may occur with some therapeutic interventions, such as use of phosphate-containing enemas, bisphosphonate therapy, vitamin D toxicity, or parenteral nutrition containing excess phosphate. Excess endogenous phosphorus may lead to hyperphosphatemia in the setting of hemolysis, rhabdomyolysis, tumor lysis syndrome, or malignant hyperthermia. Hyperphosphatemia may also result from extracellular shift of phosphorus as a result of acidosis, or intravenous calcium infusion.

Most commonly, however, increased serum phosphorus occurs in the setting of impaired kidney excretion, as there is large capacity to increase the fractional excretion of phosphorus in the setting of normal kidney function. This is easily apparent in the settings of acute kidney injury and chronic kidney disease, but impaired renal phosphate excretion can also occur with hypomagnesemia, tumoral calcinosis, endosteal hyperostosis, and several endocrinopathies, such as hypoparathyroidism, pseudohypoparathyroidism, acromegaly, and hypothyroidism.

Clinical Presentation

Hyperphosphatemia may often be clinically silent and symptoms usually result from hypocalcemia associated with the elevated serum phosphorus. These symptoms may include paresthesias, seizures, tetany, or arrhythmias. When the calcium-phosphorus product is above normal, precipitation of calcium-phosphorus in the soft tissue and vasculature is of concern, with resultant arteriosclerosis, metastatic tissue calcification or painful necrosis due to calciphylaxis.

Diagnosis

Measurement of serum creatinine and determination of the tubular reabsorption of phosphorus are essential in the evaluation of hyperphosphatemia. Redistribution and increased absorption of phosphorus are associated with increased urinary phosphorus, whereas reduced urinary phosphate levels limit the differential diagnosis as detailed above. If kidney function is normal, then serum calcium and PTH levels also aid in the diagnostic process. Disorders associated with hypocalcemia are discussed in another section.

The diagnosis of tumoral calcinosis bears special mention. This condition, associated with inactivating mutations in FGF23 or GALNT3, leads to a destabilized, dysfunctional FGF23. The resultant hyperphosphatemia, is associated with increased tubular reabsorption and inappropriately elevated $1{,}25(OH)_2D$ levels in the setting of normal serum calcium. Klotho, a distal nephron derived protein, is a necessary coprotein for FGF23 kidney actions on phosphorus excretion. KLOTHO mutations are now reported, leading to resistance of the actions of FGF23, and tumoral calcinosis. From any mutation leading to tumoral calcinosis, the patient suffers from periarticular calcifications along the extensor surfaces; nephrolithiasis and dental abnormalities may occur.

Treatment

All attempts should first focus on treating the underlying etiology of hyperphosphatemia if possible. Dietary phosphorus should be restricted and the use of enteral dietary-phosphorus binders may be necessary to prevent absorption of dietary phosphate in the setting of chronic kidney disease, or in deficient FGF23 action. In severe symptomatic cases, especially in the setting of impaired of kidney function, dialysis may be necessary.

Suggested Reading

Bastepe M, Juppner H. (2008) Inherited hypophosphatemic disorders in children and the evolving mechanisms of phosphate regulation. *Rev Endocr Metab Disord* **9**: 171–180.

Brenner BM, Rector FC. (2008) *Brenner and Rector's The Kidney*, 8th ed., Saunders Elsevier, Philadelphia.

Brunelli SM, Goldfarb S. (2007) Hypophosphatemia: clinical consequences and management. *J Am Soc Nephrol* **18**: 1999–2003.

Fukumoto S. (2008) Physiological regulation and disorders of phosphate metabolism — pivotal role of fibroblast growth factor 23. *Intern Med* **47**: 337–343.

Garabedian M. (2007) Regulation of phosphate homeostasis in infants, children, and adolescents, and the role of phosphatonins in this process. *Curr Opin Pediatr* **19**: 488–491.

Kher KK, Schnaper HW, Makker SP. (2006) *Clinical Pediatric Nephrology*. 2nd ed., London: Informa Healthcare.

12

Disorders of Magnesium Balance

Farah N. Ali and Craig B. Langman

Introduction

Magnesium is the second most prevalent intracellular cation and the fourth most abundant cation in the body. As a cofactor for many enzymes, magnesium is fundamental to intracellular processes that subserve signal transduction and diverse metabolic processes. The skeletal system houses the majority, about 60%, of body stores of magnesium as part of the hydroxyapatite crystalline structure. This provides a buffer for extracellular levels, which make up less than 1% of the total magnesium stores. The remainder of magnesium stores resides in the intracellular compartments of muscle and soft tissue.

Magnesium balance involves a complex interplay between intestinal absorption, exchange with bone, and final balance determined at multiple sites in the kidney for either excretion or reclamation. Both passive paracellular and active transcellular absorption/resorption occur in intestinal and kidney tubular systems, respectively. Intestinal absorption may be enhanced by vitamin D, parathyroid hormone (PTH), and increased sodium absorption. Factors that decrease intestinal magnesium absorption include increased dietary or luminal calcium or phosphate, and increased intestinal motility. As an isolated example, the extent of intestinal absorption varies inversely with body stores of magnesium, but directly with its dietary content.

The majority, 70–80%, of the circulating fraction of magnesium is ultrafilterable, while the remaining 20–30% is protein bound, and thus non-ultrafilterable. 90% of the ultrafilterable fraction is in an ionized/dissociated form and is biologically active, while the remainder is complexed to anions, phosphate, or citrate, and likely inert.

On a normal diet, the fractional excretion of magnesium is 3–5%, and the healthy kidney has the ability to decrease this to <1% in the setting of extrarenal causes of hypomagnesemia (see below).

While there is some resorption of magnesium in the proximal tubule (approximately 15–20%), the majority is resorbed in the loop of Henle (65–75%) (see Fig. 1). A small fraction of magnesium is resorbed by diffusion in the thin descending limb of the loop, with the majority reabsorbed by a paracellular pathway in the thick ascending limb. Tight junction proteins claudin 16 (paracellin-1) and claudin 19 appear to control this paracellular permeability. The remaining filtrate of magnesium undergoes resorption by a transcellular pathway in the distal tubule; the "transient receptor potential melastatin 6" (TRPM6) channel, which is expressed apically, is important in this process. Figure 1 depicts the sites of magnesium reabsorption along the human nephron.

There are additional factors that affect magnesium handling in the kidney. The basolateral calcium-sensing receptor can detect elevated plasma magnesium levels as well, and resulting in decreased resorption in the tubules. Hormones, such as PTH, calcitonin, glucagon, and vasopressin, stimulate magnesium transport. Acidosis is associated with renal wasting of magnesium and alkalosis has the opposite effect. Medications such as tacrolimus and cyclosporine cause magnesium wasting. In addition, loop

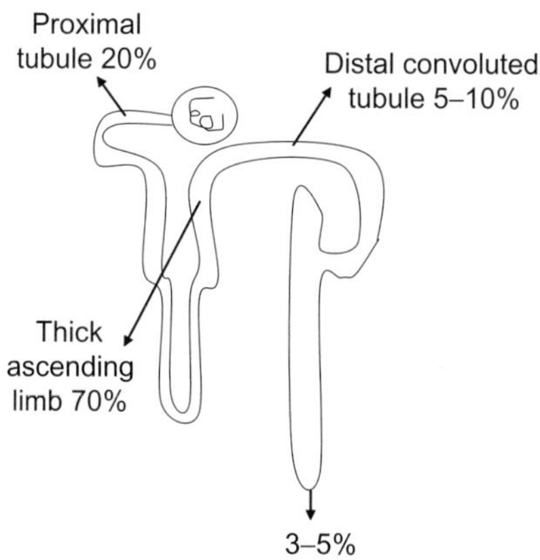

Figure 1. Magnesium reabsorption.

diuretics inhibit the Na–K–2Cl transporter and reduce transepithelial voltage, thereby diminishing paracellular resorption of magnesium in the loop.

Hypomagnesemia

Pathogenesis

Hypomagnesemia results from a net negative magnesium balance which involves interplay between intake, output (through gastrointestinal and kidney systems), and shifting between cellular compartments. Factors that may lead to insufficient intake include dietary deficiency or prolonged intravenous fluid therapy with insufficient magnesium supplementation. Increased losses may be due to gastrointestinal malabsorptive states, such as those seen with chronic diarrhea or celiac disease. In addition, increased losses may be of kidney origin, such as in the setting of diuretic therapy, primary aldosteronism, hyperparathyroidism, states of diuresis (e.g. postobstructive, following renal transplant, or with acute tubular necrosis), and use of nephrotoxic agents such as aminoglycosides, amphotericin B, cyclosporine, tacrolimus, or cisplatin. Finally a shift from the extracellular to the intracellular compartment (as occurs during respiratory alkalosis, or treatment of diabetic ketoacidosis with insulin) may also result in hypomagnesemia.

Acquired disorders are the most common explanation for hypomagnesemia seen clinically, but hereditary disorders in renal magnesium handling, though rare, do exist (see Table 1).

Clinical Presentation

Hypomagnesemia is defined as a serum level of magnesium <1.8 mg/dL. Symptoms increase with the depth of hypomagnesemia, and include progressive neuromuscular irritability, which may manifest as lethargy, weakness, tremor, carpopedal spasm, muscle cramps, tetany, or seizures. In addition, cardiac arrhythmias including atrial and ventricular tachycardia, prolonged QT interval, and torsades de pointes may occur. Hypomagnesemia is frequently associated with other abnormalities including hypocalcemia and hypokalemia. While there is a general trend

Table 1. Hereditary causes of hypomagnesemia, and the affected genes and proteins

Hereditary cause of hypomagnesemia	OMIM® reference	Gene	Chromosome	Protein
Familial hypomagnesemia with hypercalciuria and nephrocalcinosis	603959	*CLDN16*	3q27–29	Paracellin-1 (claudin-16), found at tight junctions in thick ascending limb of the loop of Henle and distal convoluted tubule
Familial hypomagnesemia with hypercalciuria and nephrocalcinosis with ocular manifestation	610036	*CLDN19*	1p34.2	Claudin-19, found at tight junctions in the thick ascending limb of the loop of Henle and to a much lesser extent in the distal convoluted tubule
Autosomal dominant hypomagnesemia with hypocalciuria	154020	*FXYD2*	11q23	γ subunit of basolateral Na^+/K^+-ATPase in distal convoluted tubule
Isolated recessive hypomagnesemia with normocalciuria	NA	*EGF*	4q25	The pro-EGF-Pro1070Ala mutation leads to impaired basolateral sorting of pro-EGF, resulting in decreased stimulation of the EGF receptor, which is localized at the basolateral membrane of distal convoluted tubule
Hypomagnesemia with secondary hypocalcemia	602014	*TRPM6*	9q22	TRPM6 is expressed in distal convoluted tubule and in intestine
Activating mutations of the extracellular Ca^{2+}/Mg^{2+}-sensing receptor	601199	*CASR*	3q13.3–q21	Ca^{2+}/Mg^{2+}-sensing receptor in chief cells of parathyroid gland and basolateral membrane in thick ascending limb of the loop of Henle and distal convoluted tubule
Gitelman syndrome	263800	*SLC12A3*	16q13	NCCT in distal convoluted tubule
Antenatal Bartter syndrome type 1	601678	*SLC12A1*	I5q15–q21.1	NKCC2 in thick ascending limb of the loop of Henle
Antenatal Bartter syndrome type II	241200	*KCNJ1*	11q24	ROMK in thick ascending limb of the loop of Henle
Classic Bartter syndrome type III	607364	*CLCNKB*	1p36	CLCKB in thick ascending limb of the loop of Henle
Bartter syndrome with sensorineural deafness type IV	602522	*BSND*, or *CLCNKA* plus *CLCNKB*	1p31, 1p36	Barttin acts as an essential β subunit for CLCKA and CLCKB, which are located in the basolateral membrane of thick ascending limb of the loop of Henle

Abbreviations: CLCKA and CLCKB, renal chloride channels; EGF, epidermal growth factor; NA, not available; NCCT, sodium–chloride cotransporter; NKCC2, Na^+–K^+–$2Cl^-$ cotransporter; OMIM, Online Mendelian Inhentance in Man® (Johns Hopkins University. Baltimore, MD, www.ncbi.nlm.nih.gov/sites/entrez?db=OMIM); pro-EGF, epidermal growth factor precursor protein; ROMK, renal outer medulla potassium channel; TRPM6, transient receptor potential cation channel, subfamily M, member 6.

for increasing symptomatology with worsening hypomagnesemia, it is important to note that the degree of symptoms may not always correlate with the serum level. This is perhaps explained by the fact that magnesium is largely an intracellular cation, and thus measured serum levels may not accurately reflect reductions in total body stores.

Diagnosis

Evaluation of hypomagnesemia should start with a careful history and physical examination, with particular attention to dietary intake, use of offending medications, and findings of neuromuscular irritability, including Trousseau and Chvostek signs.

Laboratory testing should include serum magnesium, phosphorus, calcium, and measures of kidney glomerular and tubular functions. Urinary magnesium quantification is extremely helpful to determine kidney versus extrakidney magnesium losses. The fractional excretion (FE) of magnesium can be calculated with the following formula:

$$100 \times \frac{\text{Urine [Mg]} \times \text{P [Creat]}}{\text{P [Mg} \times 0.7] \times \text{Ur [Creat]}}$$

In the formula above, since only 70% of measured plasma (P) magnesium is ultrafilterable, the plasma magnesium is multiplied by 0.7 to account for this.

If an extrakidney disease is the source of a patient's hypomagnesemia, the FE of magnesium will be <2%; conversely the FE of magnesium is usually >4% if urinary losses account for the hypomagnesemia.

The differential diagnosis of hypomagnesemia includes both hereditary forms (see Table 1) and acquired causes. Table 2 lists many of the acquired causes of hypomagnesemia. A brief discussion of the hereditary causes of hypomagnesemia follows.

Familial hypomagnesemia with hypercalciuria and nephrocalcinosis is an autosomal recessive disorder with urinary wasting of magnesium and calcium. The disorder is caused by mutations in the CLDN16 gene encoding the tight junction protein paracellin-1. The cardinal feature of nephrocalcinosis occurs with normal serum calcium, but hypercalciuria. It often presents in early childhood with urinary tract infection, stones,

Table 2. Common acquired causes of hypomagnesemia

Intracellular shift

- Respiratory alkalosis
- Hungry bone syndrome postparathyroidectomy or vitamin D therapy of rickets
- Refeeding syndrome in malnutrition
- Insulin therapy

Insufficient intake or poor absorption

- Malnutrition (alcoholism, parenteral nutrition)
- Malabsorption (celiac disease, inflammatory bowel disease, intestinal resection)
- Chronic diarrhea
- Selective intestinal magnesium absorption defect

Urinary magnesium wasting

- Drug use (aminoglycosides, amphotericin B, cyclosporine, cisplatin, dopamine, loop and thiazide diuretics, pentamidine)
- Diuresis (postobstructive, acute tubular necrosis, volume expansion, postrenal transplant, osmotic)
- Miscellaneous conditions (hypoparathyroidism, phosphate deprivation, hypercalcemia, hyperthyroidism)

polyuria, polydipsia, and failure to thrive. Patients progress to chronic kidney disease by adolescence. Mutations in the CLDN19 gene, encoding claudin-19, a tight junction protein in the thick ascending limb of the loop of Henle, are responsible for familial hypomagnesemia with hypercalciuria and nephrocalcinosis with ocular manifestations as well.

Hypomagnesemia with secondary hypocalcemia is an autosomal recessive disorder that involves impairment of both intestinal and renal magnesium transport related to mutations in TRPM6. This condition presents in the newborn period with seizure, tetany, and muscle spasms. Hypocalcemia is related to parathyroid hormone secretory failure from sustained magnesium deficiency.

Activating mutations of the calcium/magnesium-sensing receptor present in infancy with hypomagnesemia and hypocalcemia with concomitant urinary wasting. Defects in the gene encoding the extracellular calcium/magnesium-sensing receptor in the parathyroid gland are implicated. This activating mutation shifts the set-point of the receptor and enhances the affinity of the receptor for calcium and magnesium, thereby diminishing PTH secretion and reducing renal tubular reabsorption of calcium and magnesium.

Hereditary salt-wasting nephropathies may also be associated with hypomagnesemia. Gitelman syndrome is an autosomal recessive condition caused by a mutation in the gene encoding the Na–Cl co-transporter, or thiazide-sensitive cotransporter, in the distal convoluted tubule. The disorder is characterized by metabolic alkalosis, hypokalemia, hypomagnesemia with increased urinary losses of magnesium, and hypocalciuria. Patients may present during childhood or adolescence, display normal growth, and often are asymptomatic but can have episodes of weakness or tetany due to the hypomagnesemia. Bartter syndrome is an autosomal recessive disorder, but with poor growth in addition to metabolic alkalosis, hypokalemia, hyperreninemia, and normal BP. Classically Bartter syndrome is not associated with hypomagnesemia, but may be found in some genetic variants.

Autosomal dominant hypomagnesemia with hypocalciuria is another hereditary disorder that may be distinguished from Gitelman by a normal potassium level and the absence of alkalosis. It can present in the neonatal period or early childhood. Isolated recessive hypomagnesemia with normocalciuria also exists as a hereditary entity.

Treatment

Increased dietary intake may be sufficient for treatment of mild hypomagnesemia related to dietary deficiency, but oral or intravenous supplementation is necessary for symptomatic patients. Magnesium salts available for supplementation include magnesium oxide, magnesium chloride, magnesium lactate, and magnesium sulfate. Diarrhea is a common side effect of oral magnesium supplementation. In patients who are symptomatic or in these with severe hypomagnesemia (levels <0.5 mg/dL), intravenous therapy with magnesium sulfate may be necessary. Careful cardiac monitoring in these patients is advised.

Hypermagnesemia

Hypermagnesemia is defined by a serum level >2.5 mEq/L. The kidney has a large capacity for magnesium excretion; due to this, hypermagnesemia rarely occurs in patients with normal kidney function, except from toxic ingestion. Even in the setting of chronic kidney disease, normal serum levels are usually maintained until creatinine clearance falls below 20 mL/min/1.73 m^2.

Initial manifestations of hypermagnesemia may include hypotension, facial flushing, nausea, vomiting, ileus, and urinary retention. Untreated hypermagnesemia may lead to progressive neurologic symptoms, including hyporeflexia, flaccidity, lethargy, confusion, and coma, as well as cardiac abnormalities, such as prolongation of the PR interval, widened QRS, heart block, and cardiac arrest.

Just as in hypomagnesemia, evaluation should include a careful history and physical exam as well as testing the serum and urine calcium and magnesium levels. Differential diagnoses include identifying sources of excess magnesium load, such as laxatives (milk of magnesia), magnesium sulfate enemas, antacids, and magnesium therapy. Patients with gastrointestinal disease, including inflammation, obstruction, or perforation, may be at higher risk of hypermagnesemia with administration of enteral magnesium salts. The treatment of preeclampsia in the pregnant mother with magnesium sulfate can give rise to hypermagnesemia in the neonate. In addition, Addison disease, hypothyroidism, milk-alkali syndrome, and lithium therapy may be associated with mild elevations in serum magnesium.

Treatment of hypermagnesemia varies with the clinical condition of the patient. In the setting of normal kidney function with mild hypermagnesemia related to excess supplementation, cessation of the magnesium supplements may resolve the situation. Intravenous calcium salts may provide temporary aid in the setting of hypermagnesemia-related cardiac toxicity. Magnesium excretion may be enhanced with the use of saline diuresis or loop diuretics, such as furosemide. Dialysis may be necessary for patients with severe hypermagnesemia and renal failure.

Suggested Reading

Alexander RT, Hoenderop JG, Bindels RJ. (2008) Molecular determinants of magnesium homeostasis: insights from human disease. *J Am Soc Nephrol* **19:** 1451–1458.

Brenner BM, Rector FC. (2008) *Brenner and Rector's The Kidney*, 8th ed., Saunders Elsevier, Philadelphia.

Kher KK, Schnaper HW, Makker SP. (2006) *Clinical Pediatric Nephrology*, 2nd ed, Informa Healthcare, London.

Naderi AS, Reilly RF, Jr. (2008) Hereditary etiologies of hypomagnesemia. *Nat Clin Pract Nephrol* **4**: 80–89.

Schlingmann KP, Konrad M, Seyberth HW. (2004) Genetics of hereditary disorders of magnesium homeostasis. *Pediatr Nephrol* **19**: 13–25.

Unwin RJ, Capasso G, Shirley DG. (2004) An overview of divalent cation and citrate handling by the kidney. *Nephron Physiol* **98**: 15–20.

Part IV

Abnormal Urinary Findings

13

Hematuria

Alyssa A. Riley and Deepa H. Chand

Classification

Hematuria, defined as >5 red blood cells (RBCs) per high-powered field on microscopy from a freshly centrifuged urine sample, is present in 3–6% of all children on evaluation of a single urine specimen; on repeat urine specimen, prevalence decreases to 0.5–1%.

Macroscopic hematuria, also called gross hematuria, is visible discoloration of the urine. Pink/red urine is usually extraglomerular in etiology and tea- or cola-colored urine is usually glomerular in origin. The presence of hematuria by dipstick should be confirmed by the presence of RBCs on microscopy to exclude other etiologies such as hemoglobinuria and myoglobinuria, which may result in a dipstick positive for blood. Drugs, toxins, and foods may result in discoloration of the urine; however urine dipstick will be negative for blood.

Microscopic hematuria is the presence of red blood cells on urine microscopy; however, the urine is clear without visible discoloration. Hematuria can be classified as either glomerular or extraglomerular. Glomerular hematuria is often evidenced on microscopy by deformed, misshapen RBCs and RBC casts. Additionally, proteinuria, hypertension, and renal dysfunction are suggestive of glomerular cause. Extraglomerular hematuria is suggested by the presence of normal RBCs on microscopy, blood clots in the urine, and/or initial or terminal blood in the urinary stream. Tables 1–3 outline the various classifications of hematuria.

Evaluation

The initial evaluation of hematuria should include history and physical examination with particular attention to blood pressure and temperature.

Table 1. Nonheme causes of red/brown urine

Red food coloring
Beets
Rhubarb
Blackberries
Rifampin
Levodopa
Doxorubicin
Nitrofurantoin
Ibuprofen
Phenolphthalein
Porphyrins
Urate crystals

Table 2. Differentiating glomerular vs. extraglomerular hematuria

Glomerular hematuria	Extraglomerular hematuria
Dysmorphic RBCs	Blood clots
RBC casts	Normal erythrocyte morphology
Proteinuria	Blood in initial or terminal part of urinary stream
Hypertension	
Renal insufficiency	

Table 3. Causes of microscopic hematuria

Glomerular etiologies	Extraglomerular etiologies
IgA nephropathy	Urinary tract infection
Postinfectious glomerulonephritis	Urolithiasis
Thin basement membrane disease	Hypercalciuria
Benign familial hematuria	Sickle cell nephropathy
Membranoproliferative glomerulonephritis	Coagulopathy
Lupus nephritis	Malignancy
Henoch–Schönlein purpura	Cystic kidney disease
Alport syndrome	Loin pain hematuria syndrome
Anti-GBM disease	Nutcracker syndrome

If history and/or exam is suggestive of trauma, then urology should be consulted for evaluation and treatment. Symptoms warranting prompt diagnostic imaging, such as renal ultrasound and/or abdominal CT, include flank pain or dysuria suggesting urolithiasis, abdominal mass suggestive of malignancy, or unremitting gross hematuria suggestive of life threatening bleeding. Urology consult should be obtained if evaluation reveals the presence of stones greater than 5 mm in size, there is concern for renal vascular, or congenital malformation, or if life threatening bleeding exists. Physical exam findings meriting prompt evaluation for intrinsic renal disease include hypertension and edema.

Hematuria, micro- or macroscopic, should always be confirmed by the presence of RBCs on microscopy. Examination of urinalysis and microscopy should include particular attention to the presence of white blood cells (WBC), nitrites, and leukocyte esterase since a urinary tract infection (UTI) is the most common cause of hematuria. A urine culture should also be performed for confirmation. In the presence of a UTI, urinalysis should be repeated after treatment to evaluate for ongoing hematuria.

Concurrent proteinuria on urinalysis should raise suspicion for glomerular disease, and a first morning void should be evaluated to rule out orthostatic proteinuria as well as to quantify proteinuria. Persistent proteinuria is pathologic, and warrants further evaluation for glomerular disease. Renal function should be evaluated with serum creatinine and BUN, as well as electrolytes. Serum albumin level is helpful in the setting of proteinuria to better assess degree of protein loss. Additional laboratory evaluation includes complement levels (C3, C4) and antinuclear antibody (ANA) to assess for hypocomplemententemic glomerular disease, such as membranoproliferative glomerulonephritis (MPGN) or lupus nephritis; hemoglobin electropheresis to evaluate for sickle cell nephropathy (if newborn screen results are unavailable); and antistreptolysin O titer if postinfectious glomerulonephritis is suspected. A renal ultrasound is useful to assess anatomic and architectural appearance. Proteinuria should be quantified via urine protein-to-creatinine ratio on first morning void, and if greater than 0.2 mg/mg, further investigation a renal biopsy should be considered.

In the setting of isolated hematuria, careful attention to history and physical exam will often reveal urgent issues. In the absence of significant signs or symptoms, the urinalysis can be repeated weekly over 2–3 weeks to confirm persistent hematuria. Once persistent hematuria is confirmed, the investigation should include renal ultrasound, laboratory assessment (serum creatinine, BUN, and electrolytes). A urine calcium-to-creatinine ratio can be obtained on a random sample. If urine calcium-to-creatinine ratio is greater than 0.2 mg/mg, or history is suggestive of possible urinary mineral abnormality/nephrolithiasis, a 24-hour urine collection for calcium, citrate, urate, oxalate, magnesium, sodium, cystine, and creatinine should be obtained. The patient should be reassessed if the hematuria becomes macroscopic. The evaluation of macroscopic hematuria, microscopic hematuria without proteinuria, and microscopic hematuria with proteinuria, are depicted in Figs 1–3.

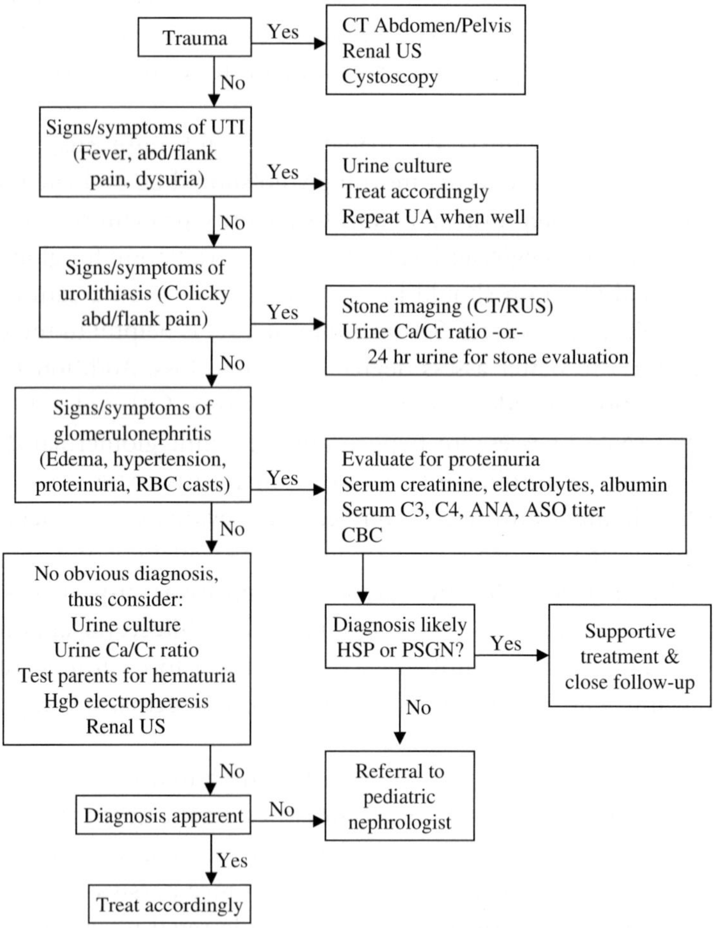

Figure 1. Macroscopic Hematuria.

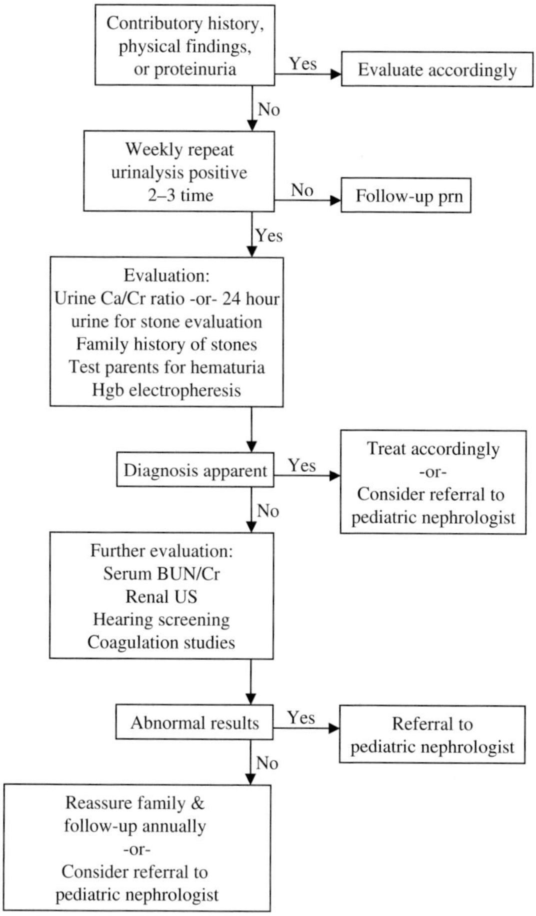

Figure 2. Isolated Microscopic Hematuria without Proteinuria.

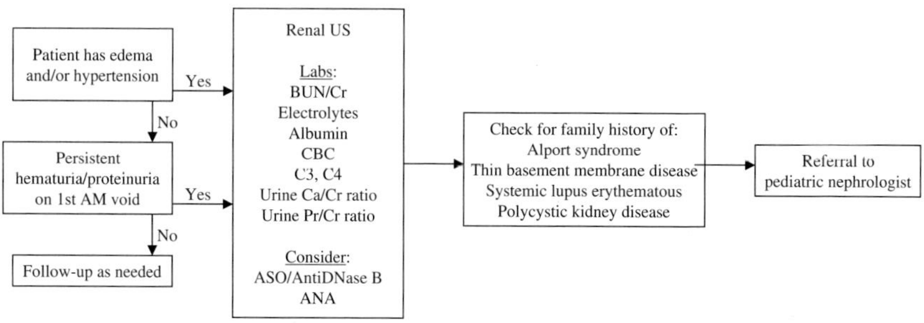

Figure 3. Isolated Microscopic Hematuria with Proteinuria.

Urinary Tract Infection

UTIs are the most common cause of hematuria, macro- or microscopic. Twenty to twenty-five percent of patients with UTI will have macroscopic hematuria at presentation. Patients presenting with hematuria should always be evaluated for fever, dysuria, urgency, frequency, and flank or suprapubic pain. Attention should be made to the presence of leukocyte esterase, nitrites, and white blood cells on urinalysis with microscopy. A urine culture should be considered in all patients presenting with hematuria to evaluate for infection. Studies for viral infections, such as adenovirus, should also be considered as hemorrhagic cystitis is a common symptom. Patients with hematuria and UTI should have follow-up urinalysis performed after completion of infection therapy to evaluate for persistent hematuria.

Urolithiasis

Urolithiasis is detailed elsewhere in this manual, but a brief synopsis is presented here. Urolithiasis most typically presents with colicky flank pain; however, younger children tend to report nonspecific abdominal pain. Macroscopic hematuria is often a presenting feature. Risk factors for stone formation include excess calcium intake, medication usage such as loop diuretics, urinary tract infections, ketogenic diets, and metabolic defects, such as hyperoxaluria and cystinuria. Stones may be composed of calcium phosphate, calcium oxalate, struvite (magnesium, ammonium, and phosphate), cystine, uric acid, or purines. Stone composition should be evaluated whenever possible. Urine pH should be determined, and urine inspected by microscopy to evaluate for crystal presence. If the stone is available, it should be sent for analysis. Additionally, 24-hour urine collection should be analyzed for calcium, oxalate, citrate, uric acid, magnesium, cystine, and creatinine. A patient who presents with renal colic should be evaluated with renal ultrasound and/or spiral abdominal CT for the presence of urolithiasis to rule out acute obstruction. In the acute setting, care includes hydration and pain control. If a stone is obstructive or greater than 5 mm in diameter, the patient requires urological evaluation. Therapy will be directed at the etiology of urolithiasis, however all patients should maintain adequate hydration to minimize recurrence.

Hypercalciuria

Hypercalciuria without overt nephrolithiasis may result in painless gross hematuria or asymptomatic hematuria identified during routine screening. Evaluation for hypercalciuria includes a spot urine calcium-to-creatinine ratio, with subsequent confirmation by 24-hour urine collection if suggestive of hypercalciuria. Individuals with hypercalciuria are at increased risk for stone formation. Therapy includes maintaining adequate hydration, thiazide diuretics to increase calcium reuptake in the distal tubule, and citrate therapy to alkalinize urine and prevent precipitation.

Postinfectious Glomerulonephritis (PIGN)

PIGN typically presents as new onset of tea- or cola-colored urine and/or edema and hypertension following a recent infection. The most commonly implicated infection is group A β-hemolytic streptococcus, with presentation 1–2 weeks after throat infection or 3–6 weeks after skin infection. Impairment of renal function at presentation is common. Due to salt and water retention with resultant edema and hypertension, in severe cases, a patient may also present with pleural effusions, ascites, and congestive heart failure. When PIGN is suspected, urinalysis will typically show proteinuria and urine microscopy will show dysmorphic RBCs and RBC casts. Mild to moderate proteinuria is common, and may persist for a few months after initial presentation.

A suspected diagnosis of PIGN is confirmed by positive throat or skin culture for group A β-hemolytic streptococcus or bloodwork demonstrating elevated antistreptolysin O or anti-DNase B levels. Complement levels showing low C3 with normal C4 is consistent with PIGN and low C3 levels typically return to normal within eight weeks of diagnosis. Lupus nephritis and membranoproliferative glomerulonephritis should be considered if the complement level does not normalize in this timeframe. Indications for confirmatory diagnosis via renal biopsy include atypical range or prolonged proteinuria, increasing serum creatinine, or depressed complement levels for greater than three months.

The mainstay of treatment for PIGN is supportive care, including salt and water restrictions along with diuretic therapy until hypertension and edema resolve. In the presence of positive skin or throat cultures, antibiotic treatment should be directed accordingly; however, the use of antibiotics will not affect the renal course.

IgA Nephropathy

Presentation of IgA nephropathy is variable and may include macroscopic hematuria, asymptomatic microscopic hematuria, microscopic hematuria with acute nephritis, nephritic syndrome, or a mixed nephritic-nephrotic syndrome. Recurrent macroscopic hematuria is often coincident with illness, usually an upper respiratory infection. This is in contrast to PIGN, in which the hematuria occurs 1–2 weeks after the acute illness. IgA nephropathy is the most common glomerular disease in adolescents. Disease occurs 2–6-fold more frequently in males than females. At presentation, patients should be evaluated for proteinuria, acute kidney injury, and hypertension. Laboratory evaluation should include blood chemistry panel with BUN and creatinine, complement levels to rule out PIGN and MPGN, and urine protein-to-creatinine ratio. Approximately 25% of patients will reach ESRD within 20 years of diagnosis following a slow, progressive decline in renal function. Poor prognostic indicators include older age at onset, absence of macroscopic hematuria, hypertension, persistent proteinuria, and renal dysfunction at presentation. Therapeutic interventions include corticosteroids, immunosuppressants, such as azathioprine or cyclophosphamide, plasmapheresis, and fish oil. Clinical response and resultant outcomes to these vary and risks/benefits need to be reviewed on an individual basis. Renal transplant remains an option; however, recurrence has been reported.

Henoch–Schönlein Purpura

Henoch–Schönlein purpura (HSP) is a systemic vasculitis presenting with palpable purpuric lesions, most prominent on the buttocks and lower extremities. Greater than half of affected patients will present with gastrointestinal symptoms, including abdominal pain, vomiting, hematemesis, hematochezia, and melena. An equal number may also have transient arthralgias.

Nearly one quarter to half of affected patients will also exhibit renal involvement. Both micro- and macroscopic hematuria at presentation is typically transient. Patients should be evaluated for the presence of proteinuria, hypertension, and renal dysfunction, as presentation with nephritis or nephrotic syndrome does occur. Patient with such presentation or with persistent hematuria and proteinuria following resolution of primary illness should have a renal biopsy performed for treatment and prognosis. The histological appearance of renal biopsy is consistent with that of IgA nephropathy, with mesangial IgA deposition.

Most patients require only supportive therapy during the acute phase of illness. Patients should be reassessed weekly at presentation with particular focus to blood pressure, and urinalysis assessment. The patient may require antihypertensive treatment, or support of acute nephrosis. In the presence of rapidly progressive glomerulonephritis, plasmapheresis or immunosuppression may be warranted. Corticosteroid therapy is often indicated for relief of abdominal pain or arthralgias; however, it has insignificant impact on the renal course. In the presence of persistent or more severe renal involvement, patients are treated for chronic IgA nephropathy.

Membranoproliferative Glomerulonephritis (MPGN)

A comprehensive review of MPGN is presented elsewhere in this manual. Hence, only a brief description is presented in this section. MPGN may present with acute gross hematuria in up to 25% of cases, however microscopic hematuria is more common. Patients will also have proteinuria and RBC casts in their urine. Approximately half of patients with MPGN will present with nephritic syndrome, and a quarter will have edema and/or hypertension. Affected patients usually have normal renal function; however, mild hypoalbuminemia is common. Low complement C3 level is suggestive of the diagnosis, particularly in the absence of antecedent infection or elevated ASO titer. The diagnosis is confirmed by renal biopsy, and subdivided into type I, II, or III. MPGN can be idiopathic or associated with systemic lupus erythematous, rheumatoid arthritis, hepatitis B, hepatitis C, and subacute bacterial endocarditis, thus these etiologies should be considered during the diagnostic evaluation.

Corticosteroids are often the mainstay of treatment, dependent on the subtype of MPGN, which is determined by renal biopsy. The prognosis also depends on the subtype.

Alport Syndrome

Alport syndrome, also known as hereditary nephritis, is X-linked in 85% of cases. Hence, boys are more likely to be significantly affected clinically. Persistent microscopic hematuria is the initial presenting symptom, and is usually identified when an affected individual undergoes screening urinalysis because other family members are affected. Female carriers may also exhibit microscopic hematuria. The condition is also associated with sensorineural hearing loss and anterior lenticonus. When family history reveals individuals with hematuria, renal dysfunction, and hearing loss, Alport syndrome must be considered. The disease is gradually progressive, with eventual onset of proteinuria, hypertension, and chronic kidney disease. Typically, an affected male develops ESRD by the second to third decade of life. Affected females, with autosomal inheritance, may only have microscopic hematuria, and over a lifetime only 10–15% will develop chronic kidney disease. Although a variety of immunosuppressants have been utilized in an attempt to delay progression, none have been found to show consistently reproducible results. Once the patient has reached ESRD, renal transplantation is an effective therapy. Of note, approximately 3% of transplanted males will develop de novo anti glomerular basement antibody disease post transplant.

Nutcracker Syndrome

Nutcracker syndrome is characterized by flank pain and hematuria without definable etiology. Typically, a patient undergoes complete evaluation to rule out infection, urolithiasis, hypercalciuria, etc., and has normal renal function. The syndrome is due to compression on the left renal vein at the point of passage between the aorta and the superior mesenteric artery. The diagnosis is made by Doppler ultrasound, with emphasis on the peak velocities in the left renal vein.

Familial Benign Essential Hematuria/Thin Basement Membrane Disease

Familial benign essential hematuria and thin basement membrane disease is manifested by the presence of persistent microscopic hematuria without proteinuria. In familial benign essential hematuria, inheritance is autosomal dominant and affected family members have no other sequelae of renal disease. Patients have normal renal function without proteinuria. Renal ultrasound is normal as well. Obtaining a urinalysis on the mother and father often shows presence of isolated microscopic hematuria in one parent. Previously renal biopsies were performed in these children with light microscopy from renal biopsy showing normal renal tissue. Immunofluorescence may show small granular C3 deposits, and electron microscopy shows regular and diffuse thinning of the basement membrane of at least 50% of the capillary walls. Renal biopsy is not currently indicated in this clinical scenario. This condition is benign by definition without progression to chronic kidney disease. This diagnosis, however, should be made cautiously, and only after thorough evaluation so as not to misdiagnose the patient.

Sickle Cell Nephropathy

The renal abnormalities associated with sickle cell disease and traits vary considerably. The manifestations can include microscopic hematuria, gross hematuria, renal infarction, papillary necrosis, and renal medullary carcinoma. The hematuria occurs more often from the left kidney, due to the longer length of the renal vein, and its compression between the aorta and superior mesenteric artery causing increased pressures (nutcracker syndrome).

When sickling occurs, the kidneys are more prone to renal infarction and papillary necrosis due to ischemia. Papillary necrosis may present as painless gross hematuria. Infarcts may present clinically with hematuria, flank pain, and hypertension (renin-mediated).

Many children have an inability to concentrate the urine, which results in polyuria. The mechanism involved is triggered by sickling in the *vasa rectae*, which then inhibits the countercurrent multiplier in the inner medulla, causing a decrease in free water reabsorption. In younger children, this can be reversed by blood transfusions, but this effect is not seen in older patients. Similarly, children may develop renal tubular acidosis, often associated with aldosterone independent hyperkalemia. This is usually mild, and may be exacerbated by intravascular volume depletion, rhabdomyolysis, or potassium/acid loading. Some children may also have proximal tubular dysfunction.

Children with sickle cell nephropathy are at increased risk for acute kidney injury as well as chronic kidney disease. Specific causes of AKI include rhabdomyolysis, sepsis, drug induced nephrotoxicity, renal vein thrombosis, hepatorenal syndrome (hemosiderosis-induced hepatic failure), urinary tract obstruction secondary to blood clots, and papillary necrosis.

Children often exhibit hyperfiltration, and hence, have higher than normal glomerular filtration rate (GFR), and renal blood flow. Over time, this decreases and as adults, many patients may develop CKD.

Suggested Reading

Diven, SC, Travis LB. (2000) A practical primary care approach to hematuria in children. *Pediatr Nephrol* **14**(1): 65–72.

Feld LG, Meyers KE, Kaplan BS, Stapleton FB. (1998) Limited evaluation of microscopic hematuria in pediatrics. *Pediatr* **102**(4): E42.

Massengill SF, Hematuria. (2008) *Pediatr Rev* **29**(10): 342–348.

Stapleton FB. (1994) Hematuria associated with hypercalciuria and hyperuricosuria: a practical approach. *Pediatr Nephrol* **8**(6): 756–761.

14

Proteinuria

C. Frederic Strife

Introduction

Isolated proteinuria (proteinuria in the absence of hematuria) in children and adolescents is common and most often transient or orthostatic. However, persistent proteinuria, defined as ≥1 + protein by dipstick on multiple measures, or the combination of persistent proteinuria and hematuria can be a marker of chronic kidney disease. Screening of urine from healthy school children detected 10% with proteinuria in at least one of four samples. However, in Korea where a first morning urinalysis is performed on all school children, the incidence of proteinuria is approximately 0.2%. Children of any age with both proteinuria and hematuria are much more likely to have significant renal pathology than those with isolated proteinuria. Thus, the primary care physician must determine if proteinuria is benign or represents chronic kidney disease (CKD).

Pathogenesis

Protein excretion in normal children

In normal individuals the glomerular capillary wall prevents all but a very small amount of protein from entering the proximal renal tubule (see Table 1). Most filtered proteins are then reabsorbed resulting in a final excretion of <150 mg per 24 hours, which is usually not detectable by the standard urine dipstick. About half of the proteins in normal urine are secreted by the tubular epithelium (Tamm–Horsfall protein — also called uromodulin). The other half are proteins filtered from plasma. Most of these are low molecular weight proteins such as albumin and amino acids.

Table 1. Methods to measure urine protein and normal values

Method (comment)	Normal Value
Dipstick (primarily detects albumin) (false positive with high urine pH)	Negative to trace
Sulfosalicylic acid (precipitation of all proteins) (false positive with several drugs)	Negative
24-hour urine total protein	<150 mg/24 hrs <100 mg/m^2 BSA <300 mg/m^2 BSA (in neonates)
Short-timed urine total protein	<4 mg/m^2 BSA/hr
Random urine protein to creatinine ratio	<0.2 mg/mg (6–24 months <0.5 mg/mg)

BSA body surface area

Mechanisms for proteinuria

Persistent proteinuria in children is most commonly the result of an abnormality of the glomerular capillary wall (glomerular proteinuria) (see Table 2). Other mechanisms include proteinuria due to inability of the proximal tubules to reabsorb filtered low molecular weight proteins (tubular proteinuria) and proteinuria due to excessive production of low molecular weight proteins (overflow proteinuria), such as seen with multiple myeloma in adults.

Glomerular proteinuria

Loss of the negative charge on the glomerular basement membrane (GBM)

Loss of the normal negative charge of the GBM is thought responsible for the massive albuminuria (also negatively charged) that occurs with idiopathic nephrotic syndrome of childhood.

Disruption of the glomerular basement membrane by inflammation, breaks in the GBM or immune complexes

Immune complex deposition within the glomerular capillary wall or disruption of the GBM from necrosis as seen in pauci immune glomerulonephritis

Table 2. Mechanisms responsible for proteinuria

Glomerular:

1. Loss of the negative charge on the glomerular basement membrane
   — Primarily albuminuria
   — Associated with idiopathic nephrotic syndrome
2. Disruption (damage) to the glomerular capillary wall
   — Immune complex glomerulonephritis
   — Pauci immune glomerulonephritis
   — Hereditary glomerulonephritis
3. Increased venous pressure
   — Congestive heart failure
   — Venous thrombosis
4. Altered podocyte proteins
   — Mutations
   - Nephrin (NPHS 1) — autosomal recessive FSGS
   - Podocin (NPHS2) — autosomal recessive FSGS
   - Alpha-actin-4 — dominant FSGS
   - CD2-associated protein (CD2AP) — dominant FSGS

   — Acquired

Tubular

1. Genetic tubular dysfunction: Fanconi syndrome with proximal renal tubular acidosis, Dent disease
2. Acquired tubular dysfunction: drug toxicity, tubulointerstitial nephritis

leads to loss of the integrity of the natural glomerular barrier, resulting in proteinuria and most often hematuria. Epimembranous deposits, such as seen in idiopathic membranous nephropathy, can be associated with isolated proteinuria.

Increased venous pressure

Patients with congestive heart failure or venous thrombosis may develop proteinuria which, in some, can be severe enough to cause heavy (nephrotic range) proteinuria. This mechanism may be responsible for "orthostatic" or "postural" proteinuria as well. The hypothesis for causality of orthostatic proteinuria is that increased abdominal pressure in the upright position leads to increased venous pressure and proteinuria, which is not seen in the supine position.

Altered podocyte proteins

Podocyte proteins in the area of the slit pores are critical for maintaining permselectivity and preventing proteinuria. These may be genetically abnormal or altered by acquired disorders leading to podocyte structural changes in the cytoskeleton and resulting proteinuria. The number of podocyte proteins associated with genetic and possibly acquired proteinuria is growing rapidly, and leading to an understanding of evolution of focal segmental glomerulosclerosis (FSGS).

Tubular proteinuria

Renal tubular disorders as a cause of proteinuria are rare and are associated with low molecular weight proteins, usually amino acids, which may not be detected by dipstick urinalysis. Inherited tubular abnormalities are commonly associated with Fanconi syndrome (renal tubular acidosis, phosphaturia, glycosuria, and aminoaciduria). Dent disease (sex-linked recessive nephrolithiasis) is associated with nephrocalcinosis, or recurrent kidney stones. Acquired tubular damage from drug or heavy metal toxicity or interstitial inflammation can also lead to proteinuria.

Clinical Presentation

Transient

Proteinuria in children is most often found on routine urinalysis. Most of these patients are asymptomatic or have an acute febrile illness and the proteinuria will be transient (see Table 3). In the absence of hematuria, a repeat urinalysis, preferably on first morning voided urine, after the acute illness has subsided should be done. If proteinuria is persistent or is associated with microscopic hematuria a careful history, physical assessment, and a logical plan for evaluation should be developed.

Orthostatic or postural proteinuria

Protein excretion increases in normal people when in an up-right position, but not enough to give an abnormal urinalysis. However, a common observation in adolescents and occasionally younger children (>7 years

Table 3. Causes of proteinuria in children and adolescents

	Appropriate test
Transient	Repeat dipstick urinalysis
— Fever	
— Exercise (postseizure)	
— Extreme cold exposure	
Orthostatic or postural	First morning urine dipstick
Persistent	≥1 + multiple measures
Structural renal abnormalities	Renal ultrasound
Glomerular abnormalities	Renal function
— Focal segmental	Serum albumin
Glomerulosclerosis	24-hour urine total protein
— Membranous nephropathy	(or random urine protein to creatine ratio)
— Genetic	C3, C4, ANA
— Glomerulonephritis	

old) is the presence of protein in urine samples collected during the daytime (upright position) but no significant protein in first morning urine collected immediately upon waking. If the absence of protein in first morning urine samples is clearly confirmed no additional tests are necessary. These are generally healthy adolescents who are often thin and tall. Some have exaggerated lordotic posturing. History and physical exam are usually normal. The cause of postural proteinuria is not known but is suspected to be an alteration in glomerular permeability due possibly to increased venous pressure that occurs in the upright position. In most patients postural proteinuria will eventually stop such that it is rare to continue after age 30 years. Although long-term follow-up has confirmed no association with chronic kidney disease, a normal yearly urinalysis on a first morning sample will reassure the absence of CKD.

Persistent proteinuria

Children and adolescents with persistent proteinuria (nonorthostatic) may be entirely asymptomatic with no clinical signs of nephrotic syndrome or glomerulonephritis (hematuria, hypertension). Alternatively, children may present with heavy proteinuria (≥1000 mg/m^2 BSA/24 hours, ≥40 mg/m^2BSA/hour) and a history of acute onset of swelling suggestive of nephrotic syndrome. It is important to note that any form of glomerulonephritis can be associated with nephrotic syndrome. Thus, the evaluation must try to distinguish the child with idiopathic nephrotic syndrome from the patient with glomerulonephritis.

Diagnosis

Persistent proteinuria in children and adolescents suggests the presence of kidney disease. In the presence of hematuria (microscopic or gross), persistent proteinuria is likely of glomerular origin (glomerulonephritis). However, in the absence of hematuria, the diagnostic possibilities with isolated proteinuria are limited and listed in Table 3.

Structural renal abnormalities

Patients with renal dysplasia, a scarred kidney from previous pylonephritis, cystic kidney disease, or obstructive uropathy can have proteinuria. A renal ultrasound or alternative renal imaging study will help to identify these structural abnormalities.

Glomerular abnormalities

If the renal ultrasound reveals no structural abnormality, it is likely that persistent proteinuria is of glomerular origin.

Asymptomatic patient

In patients with no symptoms, a decision will need to be made whether to proceed with a renal biopsy. It is important to recognize that a renal biopsy will only evaluate a small percentage of glomeruli. Glomerular lesions, such as FSGS, may not be present in the glomeruli evaluated, especially early in the disease process. Thus, prior to recommending a renal biopsy, measures of renal function, serum albumin, C3 and C4, and quantitative test for proteinuria (first morning urine for protein and creatinine) should be performed in addition to a careful history and physical examination. Unless indicated by abnormal tests, a renal biopsy is reserved for those patients with persistent quantified proteinuria >1.0 mg/mg based on protein to creatinine ratio, or those with a history suggestive of kidney disease (diabetes mellitus, sickle cell disease, massive obesity). The purpose of doing a renal biopsy is to determine the source of persistent proteinuria to determine the best treatment option. In children and adolescents with persistent proteinuria, the biopsy may reveal membranous nephropathy, FSGS, or show only fusion or flattening of the podocytes, a nonspecific finding. Many times a biopsy will be completely nonrevealing. In asymptomatic patients with mild proteinuria and normal renal function, close observation is the usual follow-up plan.

Symptomatic patient

In patients with hematuria in addition to proteinuria, hypertension, renal impairment, hypoalbuminemia, and/or nephrotic syndrome the evaluation must proceed more rapidly. In patients with proteinuria associated with acute glomerulonephritis, a definitive diagnosis is preferred either by evaluation of laboratory tests, or renal biopsy. In instances when a patient is rapidly improving, a definitive diagnosis can be deferred.

Children who fit the clinical criteria for nephrotic syndrome (anasarca, hypoalbuminemia, heavy proteinuria, hypercholesterolemia) are usually given a trial of four to six weeks of high dose corticosteroids (usual dosing is 2 mg/kg/day divided BID). If there is complete response, as would be expected for more than 85%, the patient is assumed to have idiopathic (steroid responsive) nephrotic syndrome. However, if the patient continues with proteinuria after the trial with corticosteroids, further evaluation including a renal biopsy is usually done to guide recommendations for additional treatment.

Treatment

The treatment for patients with persistent proteinuria of glomerular origin usually involves a specific treatment directed at the disease process (such as prednisone for nephrotic syndrome), and, in those whose proteinuria persists, nonspecific treatment directed at reducing proteinuria. Although not proven in children, studies in adults suggest that proteinuria alone may hasten glomerular damage and reduction of proteinuria may slow this process. Angiotensin converting enzyme inhibitors (ACEi) and angiotensin receptor blockers (ARB) can be used alone or in combination to reduce proteinuria. Other nonspecific treatments to slow the progression of CKD associated with proteinuria include aggressive management of hypertension, and hyperlipidemia.

Prognosis

The prognosis for most children with isolated proteinuria is very good. The vast majority will be found to have transient or orthostatic proteinuria with no evidence for CKD. In those with nephrotic syndrome, most (>85%) will respond to steroids which then predicts a very good long-term prognosis.

However, in the child or adolescent with nephrotic syndrome unresponsive to steroids or with significant persistent proteinuria (urine protein to creatinine ratio > 1.0), the finding of FSGS on renal biopsy indicates a poor prognosis for most. Only a small percentage of such patients will respond fully to further treatments and most will progress to CKD. Unfortunately, up to 40% of these patients will have recurrence of the disease in a kidney transplant. The pathologic finding of FSGS appears to be the final glomerular response to a number of possible insults (genetic, reflux nephropathy, hyperfiltration). As the mechanisms leading to the focal sclerotic lesions are better understood, more specific treatments are likely to be found and the prognosis will improve.

Suggested Reading

Cho BS, Kim SD. (2007)School urinalysis screening in Korea. *Nephrol (Carlton)* 12 Suppl 3: S3–S7.

Eknoyan G, Hostetter T, Bakris GL, *et al.* (2003) Proteinuria and other markers of chronic kidney disease: a position statement of the National Kidney foundation (NKF) and the National Institute of Diabetes and Digestive and Kidney Diseases (NIDDK). *Am J Kidney Dis* **42**: 617–622.

Gagnadoux MF. (2009) Evaluation of proteiunuria in children. In: UpToDate

Hogg RJ, Portman RJ, Millner D, *et al.* (2000) Evaluation and management of proteinuria and nephrotic syndrome in children: recommendations from a pediatric nephrology panel established at the National Kidney Foundation conference on proteinuria, albuminuria, risk, assessment, detection, and elimination (PARADE). *Pediatr* **105**(6): 1242–1249.

Kunz R, Friedrich C, Wolbers M, Mann JF. (2008) Meta-analysis: effect of monotherapy and combination therapy with inhibitors of the renin angiotensin system on proteinuria in renal disease. *Ann Intern Med* **148**(1): 30–48.

Rytand DA, Spreiter S. (1981) Prognosis in postural (orthostatic) proteinuria: Forty to fifty year follow-up orsix patients after diagnosis by Thomas Addis. *N Engl J Med* **305**: 618.

Springberg PD, Garrett LE Jr., Thompson AL Jr., *et al.* (1982) Fixed and reproducible orthostatic proteinuria: results of a 20-year follow-up study. *Ann Intern Med* **97**(4): 516–519.

Trachtman H, Berwerk A, Gauthier B. (1994) Isolated proteinuria in children. Natural history and indications for renal biopsy. *Clin Pediatr (Phila)* **33**(8): 468–472.

Vehaskari VM, Rapola J. (1982) Isolated proteinuria: analysis of a school-age population. *J Pediatr* **101**(5): 661–888.

Part V

Glomerulopathies: Renal Limited

15

Steroid Sensitive and Steroid Resistant Nephrotic Syndrome

Robert P. Woroniecki, Brian Becknell and William E. Smoyer

Introduction

Definition

Nephrotic syndrome (NS), or nephrosis, encompasses a group of kidney diseases characterized by histologic picture of glomerular exudation and proliferation in contrast to inflammation (nephritis). The clinical and biochemical description of NS includes a constellation of findings:

1) *Massive Proteinuria*, defined as urinary loss of >40 mg/m^2/hr of protein in children, and >3.5 g/d in adults. Measurement of protein to creatinine ratios in first-morning spot urine sample in both adults and children has strongly correlated with 24-hour urine protein measurements. As such, urinary protein:creatinine ratio >3.5 mg/mg is consistent with nephrotic range proteinuria in adults. However, in children a urinary protein:creatinine ratio >2.0 mg/mg is considered nephrotic range proteinuria.
2) *Hypoalbuminemia*, defined as serum albumin concentration <2.5 g/dL, occurs due to inability of hepatic albumin synthesis to compensate for the massive urinary losses of albumin.
3) *Edema*, defined as swelling in areas of low tissue resistance (i.e., periorbital, scrotal, and labial regions) which can become generalized (anasarca) and is gravity dependent, involving sacral area in supine position, and lower extremities in upright position. Edema generally becomes apparent when fluid retention exceeds 3–5% of body weight.

4) *Hyperlipidemia*, defined by elevated serum concentrations of cholesterol, triglycerides, and lipoproteins.

Since NS may have a remitting and relapsing clinical course, edema, proteinuria, hypoalbuminemia, and hyperlipidemia may not all be present during some stages of disease.

Classification

Nephrotic syndrome in children can be classified based on etiology (see Table 1) or clinical responsiveness to steroids.

1) Etiology:
   a. Primary/idiopathic (~90% of cases)
      i. Minimal change nephrotic syndrome (MCNS)
      ii. Focal segmental glomerulosclerosis (FSGS)
      iii. Membranous nephropathy (MN)
      iv. Membranoproliferative glomerulonephritis (MPGN)
      v. Mesangial proliferative glomerulonephritis (Mes PGN)
   b. Secondary (~10% of cases)
2) Steroid response:
   a. Sensitive
   b. Resistant

The International Study of Kidney Diseases in Childhood (ISKDC) reported that 84.5% of children with primary NS had minimal-change nephrotic syndrome (MCNS), 9.5% had focal segmental glomerulosclerosis (FSGS), 2.5% had mesangial proliferation, and 3.5% had membranous nephropathy or another cause of disease.

Steroid Response

The clinical response to a 4–6 week trial of high-dose (60 mg/m^2 of body surface area, up to 80 mg/day) prednisone therapy is generally used to characterize NS as either steroid responsive or steroid sensitive (SSNS; disappearance of proteinuria), or steroid resistant (SRNS; persistence of

Table 1. Etiologies of nephrotic syndrome

Primary (~90% of cases)	Secondary (~10% of cases)	
MCNS	Infections	HIV Hepatitis B, C Malaria Toxoplasmosis Syphilis Streptococcus Other bacteria/viruses/sepsis
FSGS (Idiopathic)	Obesity	FSGS
Genetic causes of nephrotic syndrome NPHS1 (Nephrin) NPHS2 (Podocin) PLCE1 TRPC6 ACTN4 CD2AP	Toxins/drugs	Gold NSAIDs Interferon Lithium Heroin Mercury Pamidronate
	Malignancies	Lymphoma Leukemia
Membranous nephropathy	Vasculitis	Wegener granulomatosis Churg–Strauss syndrome Polyarteritis nodosa Microscopic polyangiitis Henoch–Schönlein purpura
	Other renal diseases	IgA nephropathy MPGN Alport syndrome Postinfectious glomerulonephritis Crescentic glomerulonephritis Reflux nephropathy
	Other systemic diseases	SLE nephritis Diabetic nephropathy Sarcoidosis Thyroiditis Sickle Cell disease Hypertensive nephrosclerosis

proteinuria). Remission is defined as complete disappearance of proteinuria with resolution of edema. Steroid response is considered the best predictor of renal outcome, even better than renal histology. Steroid sensitivity is associated with a good prognosis, whereas steroid resistance is associated with progression to end-stage renal disease (ESRD).

Steroid sensitive nephrotic syndrome (SSNS)

The vast majority of SSNS is due to minimal change nephrotic syndrome (MCNS). Often called "nil disease" (i.e., no changes seen on light microscopy, but diffuse podocyte foot process effacement on electron microscopy), MCNS accounts for 85% of NS cases in children, but only 22% in adults. In children, about 95% with MCNS are steroid sensitive, whereas only 25% with FSGS are steroid responsive. Children with SSNS relapse in 60–70% of cases; they rarely develop ESRD.

The etiology of MCNS remains unknown. One hypothesis is clonal expansion of lymphocytes resulting in production of cytokines which increase the permeability of the glomerular filtration barrier to proteins. Evidence supporting this hypothesis includes: absence of immune complexes in glomeruli, rapid response to steroids, association of NS with Hodgkin's disease, and observation that MCNS often enters remission following measles infection — a condition known to suppress cell-mediated immunity. The potential role of T cells in MCNS is further supported by the fact that cyclosporine A induces remission in many children with this disease. Inhibition of T cell activation by cyclosporine A results in decreased cytokine expression thereby decreasing T cell dysfunction thought to be important in the pathogenesis of proteinuria. However, mechanisms by which T cells might increase glomerular permeability are unclear. Alterations in various circulating cytokines in the serum and urine which may alter glomerular permeability to albumin have been reported. Recently, a humanized animal model of idiopathic NS was developed by injecting CD34+ stem cells or CD34+ peripheral blood mononuclear cells from patients with MCNS or FSGS into immunocompromised mice. The injection of CD34+ stem cells induced albuminuria and podocyte foot process effacement, suggesting that immature cells which undergo differentiation into T cells may be responsible for pathogenesis of MCNS and FSGS.

Steroid resistant nephrotic syndrome (SRNS)

Children with SRNS are most often found to have focal segmental glomerulosclerosis (FSGS), although about 5% of children with MCNS are also steroid resistant. Controversy exists whether MCNS and FSGS represent a spectrum of the same heterogeneous disease process. It should be noted that FSGS is a histologic, rather than clinical entity, and can be present in many primary and secondary renal diseases. FSGS is characterized histologically by focal (not all glomeruli), and segmental (involving only part of the glomerulus) glomerular sclerosis. The juxtamedullary glomeruli are affected first. The histologic classification of FSGS includes five major variants: perihilar, cellular, tip, collapsing, and not otherwise specified (NOS). Of these, FSGS-NOS is the most common lesion. The tip lesion has been associated with steroid responsiveness and a favorable prognosis, whereas the collapsing variant has been associated with podocyte proliferation, human immunodeficiency virus (HIV) infection, disease progression, and poor prognosis. In contrast to MCNS, FSGS usually affects older children and young adults. The etiology in the majority of idiopathic FSGS cases remains unknown. In up to 25% of patients with idiopathic FSGS, mutations in genes encoding proteins that play structural or functional roles in podocytes are responsible for the phenotype (see Table 2). Patients carrying these mutations do not respond to steroids and thus, have a poor prognosis.

Membranous nephropathy (MN) is a less common cause of NS in children that is associated with SRNS. In MN, the glomerular blood vessel walls become thickened due to deposition and accumulation of protein and immune complexes in the subepithelial space. In this disease, antigen-antibody complexes can develop *in situ* by binding of circulating antibodies to endogenous renal antigens, or by deposition of circulating antigen-antibody complexes. In secondary forms of MN due to SLE and hepatitis, concomitant mesangial and/or subendothelial deposits may also be present. Hepatitis B surface antigen and hepatitis E antigens have been identified in immune deposits, and in patients with thyroiditis, thyroid antigens have been identified. The majority of cases of idiopathic MN have recently been identified as being due to antiPLA_2 receptor autoantibodies of the IgG4 subclass. Studies of idiopathic MN have shown significant increases in IgG4 production, increased B cell surface antigen CD20 mRNA expression and increased urinary excretion of complement

Table 2. Changes in proteins and genes causally associated with nephrotic syndrome

Protein	Gene	Disease
Nephrin	*NPHS1*	Finnish-type congenital NS
Podocin	*NPHS2*	Autosomal recessive FSGS
Alpha-actinin-4	*ACTN-4*	Autosomal dominant FSGS
Transient receptor potential cation 6	*TRPC6*	Autosomal dominant FSGS [24]
Phospolipase epsilon C	*PLCE1*	Case reports of familial FSGS and diffuse mesangial sclerosis [25]
CD2-associated protein	*CD2AP*	Single case reports of sporadic familiar FSGS
Wilm's tumor protein 1	*WT1*	Frasier syndrome: FSGS with pseudohermaphroditism; normal female external genitalia, and XY karyotype, and frequently develop gonadoblastoma, but not Wilm's tumor Denys–Drash syndrome: Diffuse mesangial sclerosis with pseudohermaphroditism, Wilm's tumor, and hypertension
*β*2 laminin	*LAMB2*	Pierson syndrome: Congenital nephrotic syndrome with extreme nonreactive narrowing of the pupils (microcoria) due to aplasia or atrophy of the dilatator pupillae muscle
LIM homeobox transcription factor 1 beta	*LMX1B*	Nail-patella syndrome: Congenital nephrotic syndrome with dysplasia of the nails and absence or hypoplasia of patellae
Undetermined	?	Galloway–Mowat syndrome; Congenital microcephaly with hiatus hernia and nephrotic syndrome

membrane attack complexes (C5b-9, or MAC), supporting the hypothesis that altered functions of both T cells and B cells play a role in the immune response and pathogenesis of idiopathic MN. While MN is not a common pediatric glomerular disease, it is the most common lesion identified in adult patients with idiopathic NS.

Epidemiology

Primary (idiopathic) NS has a reported incidence of 2.7 new cases per 100,000 children per year, and a cumulative prevalence rate of 16 per

100,000 children in the United States. In childhood MCNS, the male to female ratio is approximately 2:1, but this difference disappears by adolescence. There is also an increased familial incidence of disease. A medical history of asthma, and/or environmental allergies is reported by as many as 50% of children who present with MCNS. The mean age at onset of MCNS is 3.4 years in Asians and 4.2 years in Europeans.

Membranous nephropathy also has a predilection for males over females, with a male to female ratio of 2:1. The incidence of secondary forms of MN varies by region, and is often influenced by the varying regional prevalence of hepatitis. In contrast to FSGS, there is no increased incidence of MN reported in African Americans.

Pathogenesis

Pathogenesis of proteinuria

Understanding the pathogenesis of NS begins with appreciation of the molecular composition of the glomerular filtration barrier, comprised of podocytes, an extracellular glomerular basement membrane (GBM), and fenestrated capillary endothelium. Each of these components exerts an important and synchronous role in glomerular filtration and permeability.

The glomerular filtration barrier separates blood from the urinary space and under physiologic conditions permits selective ultrafiltration of solutes, while preventing excessive leakage of large molecules, such as albumin and clotting factors, with molecular weight >40,000 Daltons. The glomerular filtration barrier is believed to become incompetent and "leaky," leading to massive proteinuria during NS. Normally, low-molecular–weight proteins (<40,000 Daltons) such as beta 2 microglobulin and retinol binding protein are freely filtered through the glomerulus and reabsorbed by the proximal tubule. With massive leakage of protein across the glomerular filtration barrier, tubular injury develops and leads to inability to reabsorb these proteins with resultant urinary losses.

Proteinuria seen in MCNS is usually selective (>85% of urine protein fraction comprised of albumin). However, nonselective proteinuria (glomerular leakage of all plasma proteins) may also be observed.

Podocytes

Podocytes are terminally differentiated epithelial cells with a cell body and numerous foot processes extending outward contacting adjacent podocytes through interpodocyte connections called slit diaphragms. All genetic defects identified to date in patients with hereditary forms of NS affect gene transcription or assembly of critical podocyte structural proteins. These, in turn, regulate the slit diaphragm, the actin-based cytoskeleton and adhesion complexes (see Table 2). These genes include nephrin (*NPHS1*), podocin (*NPHS2*), alpha-actinin-4 (*ACTN-4*), CD2-associated protein (*CD2AP*), Wilm's tumor gene (*WT1*), and transient receptor potential cation 6 (*TRPC6*).

Recently, mutations in the gene encoding phospolipase epsilon C have been identified as a cause of early-onset NS which progresses to ESRD, with the histologic findings of diffuse mesangial sclerosis and FSGS. Notably, all but one patient was reported to be steroid resistant.

Glomerular basement membrane

The presence of highly negatively charged heparan sulfate proteoglycans in the GBM is thought to prevent passage of negatively charged macromolecules, such as albumin. Experimental reduction of these negative charges in animals by *in situ* perfusion of heparitinase results in proteinuria. Further evidence of GBM involvement in proteinuria includes mutations of β2 laminin in the GBM which were associated with congenital NS in Pearson syndrome (see Table 2). Additionally, mutations in the alpha-5 chain of type IV collagen in the GBM are responsible for proteinuria in X-linked Alport's syndrome.

Endothelial cells

Glomerular endothelial cells are fenestrated with numerous openings of 70–100 nm in diameter. They constitute a physical barrier to the passage of macromolecules from the plasma into Bowman's space of glomeruli. Injury of the glomerular endothelium (endotheliosis), mediated by vascular endothelial growth factor (VEGF), has been reported in preeclampsia, HIV-associated nephropathy, and collapsing FSGS.

Pathogenesis of edema

While several mechanisms contribute to edema formation during NS, the primary cause for fluid retention is increased renal sodium reabsorption. It has recently been demonstrated that glomerular leakage of plasminogen into the urinary space leads to its intratubular conversion to plasmin, which in turn cleaves and activates the γ subunit of the epithelial sodium channel (ENaC) located in the distal tubule, leading to stimulation of sodium retention. Sodium retention can sometimes be observed before the serum albumin level starts falling. With massive proteinuria, protein loss from the blood leads to low intravascular oncotic pressure that, by Starling's forces, results in fluid shifts from the intravascular space into the interstitial space. The resulting intravascular volume depletion leads to renal hypoperfusion and stimulation of the renin-angiotensin-aldosterone (RAA) system. However, there is no consistent experimental evidence of intravascular volume depletion. In fact, intravascular volume has been reported to be normal or even increased in some patients with NS. Other studies have failed to demonstrate consistent elevation of RAA hormones in NS patients. Another important contributing factor in edema formation is increased capillary permeability. This condition is especially apparent in children and during acute respiratory tract infections which are frequently associated with NS relapses.

Pathogenesis of hyperlipidemia

Several mechanisms contribute to hyperlipidemia during NS. Low serum albumin concentrations stimulate hepatic synthesis of albumin and lipids, resulting in high concentrations of cholesterol, triglycerides, and lipoproteins. Another factor is impaired hepatic catabolism of apolipoprotein B and VLDL chylomicrons. Of note, the hyperlipidemia has a strong temporal association with hypoalbuminemia. In relapsing forms of NS which lack prolonged states hypoalbuminemia, there is no conclusive evidence of increased atherosclerosis and ischemic complications. In contrast, in patients with persistent SRNS, where hypertension and chronic kidney disease are present, accelerated atherosclerosis becomes a clinically significant problem.

Immune system in nephrotic syndrome

MCNS has been widely associated with immune system abnormalities. These include suppressed cell-mediated immunity, defective opsonization, decreased serum levels of complement factors D and B, and abnormal humoral immunity (thought primarily due to loss of IgG). Other abnormalities in MCNS include: decreased delayed-type hypersensitivity reactions, markedly reduced responses to mitogenic stimulation, abnormal antibody-dependant cellular cytotoxicity, abnormal reticuloendothelial function, and abnormal lymphocyte surface marker expression. Clinically, these above immunologic abnormalities are likely responsible for the well-documented increased risk of infections during active NS (i.e., during relapse). Indeed, infection remains a leading cause of death in children with NS.

Coagulation system in nephrotic syndrome

Nephrotic syndrome is also associated with increased risk for thromboembolism. During active NS, patients are hypercoagulable due to significant urinary losses of anticoagulants (protein S, and antithrombin III) and increased hepatic synthesis of procoagulants (factors V and VIII, and fibrinogen) as a consequence of hypoalbuminemia.

Clinical Presentation

The diagnosis of NS is based on a combination of the history, physical examination and laboratory investigations.

History

History is the most important component in correctly diagnosing and classifying NS. A variety of key historical findings can suggest specific etiologies for NS (see Table 3). In addition, new-onset NS often presents with a history of insidious development of periorbital edema, most commonly shortly following an upper respiratory infection, thus it is often confused with allergic disease.

Table 3. History-based approach to nephrotic syndrome

History	Association with NS
Vertically acquired HIV	HIV-associated nephropathy
Hepatitis B, C	MPGN
Facial rash with joint symptoms	SLE nephritis
Fetal hydrops, or edema in first three months of life	Congenital nephrotic Syndrome of the Finnish type (CNF)
Recent (within weeks) throat, impetigo, and brown-colored urine	Postinfectious glomerulonephritis
URI or throat infection concurrent with macroscopic hematuria	IgA nephropathy
IV drug use and/or risky sexual behaviors	HIV-associated nephropathy
Morbid obesity	FSGS
Family history of nephritis	Alport's syndrome
Preschool age and edema	MCNS
African American teenager with normal growth and hypertension	FSGS
Association with asthma, eczema, atopy	MCNS

Physical examination

In addition to the presence of edema, children with NS may present with signs of intravascular volume depletion, such as tachycardia, hypotension or hypertension, poor peripheral perfusion, decreased urine output, metabolic acidosis, or even acute kidney injury. These signs usually resolve with intravascular volume repletion with colloid infusion, most often with 25% albumin.

Since the presence of edema confirms that these children are total body fluid overloaded, administration of IV saline may be harmful and predispose to increased sodium retention, worsening edema and/or hypertension. The presence of persistent hypertension suggests a disease other than MCNS.

Additional evaluation

Serum sodium levels may be mildly low, due to a combination of decreased intravascular volume resulting in increased secretion of antidiuretic hormone, and fluid shifts into the interstitial compartment. Serum calcium concentration is usually low due to hypoalbuminemia (calcium is ~55% bound to albumin), but ionized calcium is usually normal.

The role of renal biopsy

Following initial steroid treatment, if patients are either steroid resistant from the onset of disease, or develop it during the course of the disease, a renal biopsy in usually performed. As a general rule a renal biopsy is indicated in the following circumstances:

a) Steroid resistance
b) Acute kidney injury (if intrinsic cause is suspected)
c) Atypical presentation (hypertension; persistent or gross hematuria)
d) Decreased serum C3/C4 levels
e) Positive serum ANA

Complications

While mortality in NS is generally low, morbidity related either to primary disease, or more commonly to treatment toxicity, is common. Complications of NS include infection, thromboembolism, and acute kidney injury (AKI) (see Table 4). Serious infections continue to be the most common complication associated with mortality in NS. Thromboembolism has been reported in 1.8–9.2% of children with idiopathic NS, in contrast to the much higher incidence in adults (20–30%). Its incidence may approach 10% during the first six months following presentation with NS. Recently several independent risk factors for thromboembolism in children with NS have been identified, including age >12 years at disease onset, severity of proteinuria, and history of thromboembolism preceding diagnosis of NS. Lastly, AKI has become more common in recent years. This may be due to increased use of calcineurin inhibitors to treat difficult cases of NS. These medications, cyclosporine A and tacrolimus, are known to induce vasoconstriction thereby reducing renal blood flow. Other long-term complications in children with frequently relapsing (>4 relapses/year) MCNS include growth delay and reproductive system impairment.

Treatment

The initial treatment of children >1 year of age presentating with NS is corticosteroids. Failure to achieve complete remission (resolution of proteinuria) following this treatment course identifies a patient subset at

Table 4. Complications of nephrotic syndrome

	Complication	Description
Infection	Pneumonia (most common) Peritonitis Sepsis	Infection usually caused by encapsulated bacteria: Pneumococcus due to alterations in immune response, opsonization, and urinary immunoglobulin losses
Thromboembolism	Venous (more common) and/or arterial (less common) thrombosis	Multifactorial in origin: Urinary loss of antithrombin III and plasminogen Increased concentrations of clotting factors, especially factors I, VII, VIII, and X is associated with deep vein and renal vein thrombosis
Drug-induced toxicity	Steroids	Cushingoid features Gastritis Stomach ulcer Neurobehavioral disturbances Osteoporosis and pathological fractures Infection
	Cyclophosphamide (Cytoxan)	Gonadal toxicity Infection
	MMF/purine inhibitors	Diarrhea Vomiting Infection
	Calcineurin inhibitors (Cyclosporine A and Tacrolimus)	Nephrotoxicity Seizures Acute renal failure Hypertension
	Rituximab	Infection
Renal failure	Prerenal	In SSNS, usually prerenal and related to decreased intravascular volume
	Intrarenal	In SRNS, may be related to fibrosis, glomerular sclerosis, or tubulointerstitial damage
Bone disease	Pathologic fractures	Development of bone disease due to malabsorption of calcium from GI tract due to low serum vitamin D levels and urinary loss of vitamin D-binding proteins
Hyperlipidemia	Atherosclerosis in SRNS	Increased hepatic synthesis of lipids and lipoproteins, and diminution of lipid catabolism caused by reduced plasma levels of lipoprotein lipase

higher risk for progressive renal disease, and prompts consideration for a renal biopsy. Subsequent treatment strategies are best divided into categories based on the child's initial response to oral corticosteroid treatment.

Steroid sensitive nephrotic syndrome

Current steroid treatment regimens are based largely on studies from the German collaborative group Arbeitsgemeinschaft für Padiatrische Nephrologie and recently endorsed by a U.S. consensus panel. Treatment begins with prednisone at a dose of 2 mg/kg/day (maximum 60 mg/day) for six weeks, followed by alternate-day dosing of 1.5 mg/kg/day (maximum 40 mg/day), given as a single morning dose for another six weeks. No taper is required at the conclusion of this 12 week regimen. Prospective, randomized trials have documented the value of initial prolonged steroid treatment, associating such regimens with complete remission and prolonged duration of remissions, compared to short-term steroid treatment. Most children (~75%) enter remission within approximately two weeks of initiation of prednisone treatment, and 90–95% of children with steroid responsive disease enter remission within the initial four weeks of treatment. Only a small percentage of children not responding within the initial weeks enter remission if steroids are continued for up to 12 weeks.

Steroid dependent and frequently relapsing nephrotic syndrome

The majority of children with NS (50–70%) develop one or more relapses. In some, these relapses may be transient, with spontaneous remission occurring within 4 to 14 days. However, despite prolonged initial steroid use, about 40–50% of children with complete remission subsequently develop either frequent relapsing NS (FRNS) or steroid dependent NS (SDNS). Frequent relapsing NS is defined as four or more episodes of NS in any 12 month period, while SDNS is defined by patients who enter complete remission, but relapse either during their steroid taper or within two weeks of discontinuation. Several factors appear to be associated with an increased risk for relapse, including age <5 years old at presentation and male gender. The relapse risk is high during intercurrent infections, as approximately 70% of relapses have been reported to be preceded by an upper respiratory tract infection. In addition, a multicenter study in children identified a direct correlation between the number of relapses in the first six months of diagnosis and risk of subsequent relapse.

Management of relapses generally includes reinstitution of oral daily steroids at a dose of 2 mg/kg/day divided bid (maximum 60 mg/day) until the urine protein is trace or negative for three consecutive days, followed by tapering of the steroids to 1.5 mg/kg as a single dose on alternate mornings, and gradual taper over approximately the following six weeks (~0.25 mg/kg/dose/week until off). Among children with FRNS, the initial taper to 1.5 mg/kg on alternate mornings is often continued for two weeks, and then very gradually tapered off over 5–6 months to try to reduce the relapse frequency. Nonetheless, children with SDNS relapse either prior to, or within two weeks of, discontinuation of the steroids. Relapses are usually treated with prednisone in a manner similar to other relapses except that the patients are not usually tapered off steroids, but rather tapered to the lowest alternate-day dose which historically has kept that child in remission (usually 10–20 mg/dose, or 15–20 mg/m2/dose). This "prophylactic" dosage can be continued for 6–18 months, and then tapered by 0.25 mg/kg/dose every two weeks until discontinuation of therapy. The use of low-to-moderate doses of alternate-day steroids is generally not associated with significant side effects, although a decreased growth velocity is sometimes seen in adolescents. Overall, these treatment strategies are directed at a balance between minimizing the overall steroid exposure for children with SSNS, and minimizing the frequency of relapses.

Steroid-sparing agents

Many frequently relapsing and steroid-dependent children either fail to have an adequate response to the above approaches or develop significant steroid side effects. In this situation, alternative treatments are frequently used, including alkylating agents, cyclosporine A, and mycophenolate mofetil. Due to absence of placebo-controlled randomized clinical trials, there is no clear second-line therapy for these children.

Alkylating agents

Cyclophosphamide (2 mg/kg/day for 8–12 weeks) and chlorambucil (0.2 mg/kg/day for 8–12 weeks) have both been reported to induce long-term remissions in approximately 75% of children with FRNS. However, these agents induced long-term remission in only 30–35% of children with SDNS. Both cytotoxic agents have well-known dose-related toxicities, including leukopenia, hair loss, thrombocytopenia, seizures (chlorambucil), hemorrhagic cystitis (cyclophosphamide), severe bacterial infections, malignancies, and fatalities. Given the comparable efficacy of both agents and the unique risk for seizures and increased incidence of severe bacterial infections with chlorambucil, the lower toxicity profile associated with cyclophosphamide has led to its more widespread use. Of note, cumulative cyclophosphamide doses >200–250 mg/kg are associated with gonadal toxicity, particularly in males. These considerations generally result in the use of alternative agents if a single 12-week course of 2 mg/kg/day cyclophosphamide (cumulative dose 168 mg/kg) does not induce long-term remission. More recent reports suggest that cyclophosphamide can be equally effective, with less toxicity, in both FRNS and SDNS patients, if given as six-monthly intravenous infusions of 500 mg/m2/dose compared with daily oral dosing for 12 weeks. The mechanism of action of alkylating agents in NS is unknown, although they are presumed to act via inhibition of immune cells and their secreted cytokines.

Cyclosporine A

Cyclosporine A (CsA) is a known inhibitor of calcineurin, a critical enzyme for T lymphocyte activation. While its mechanism in NS is largely unknown, it has been reported to enhance stability of the actin cytoskeleton in podocytes. The introduction of CsA to the treatment of NS has resulted in a reduction in the frequency of relapses in SDNS, with ~85% of children responding to therapy. However, many children relapse when CsA is tapered or stopped. CsA has proven a very useful alternative agent in children suffering from steroid toxicity. CsA therapy is associated with side effects, such as hypertension, mild azotemia, hyperkalemia, gingival overgrowth, and hypertrichosis. However, its major drawback is risk of nephrotoxicity, which manifests as interstitial fibrosis. In one study, tubulointerstitial lesions attributed to CsA were found in 11% of children with MCNS treated with CsA for <24 months, but in 58% of those continued on this medication >2 years. Since interstitial fibrosis is irreversible and can develop without an apparent decline in renal function, a renal biopsy is often performed prior to initiation of treatment, as well as every two years thereafter as long as treatment is continued. As a general rule, identification of significant interstitial fibrosis on follow-up renal biopsy should prompt consideration of an alternative therapy from CsA.

Mycophenolate Mofetil

Mycophenolate mofetil (MMF) is an alternative agent in children with FRNS and SDNS. While its mechanism of action remains unknown, MMF inhibits lymphocyte DNA synthesis and proliferation via inhibition of a key enzyme in purine biosynthesis, inosine monophosphate dehydrogenase (IMPDH). These effects are selective for T and B lymphocytes. Several reports have demonstrated the usefulness of MMF in reducing the frequency of relapses in children with FRNS and SDNS, permitting a significant reduction in total steroid exposure. The typical treatment dose used for MMF has been 600 mg/m2/dose given twice daily (maximum dose 1000 mg bid). Side effects of MMF include nausea, vomiting, diarrhea, constipation, headache, edema, bone marrow suppression, anemia, and gastrointestinal bleeding.

Two recent studies highlight the potential usefulness and limitations of MMF in children with FRNS. A randomized controlled trial of MMF versus CsA in 31 children with FRNS and biopsy-proven MCNS demonstrated a higher relapse rate for children treated with MMF (0.83 relapses/year) compared to CsA (0.08 relapses/yr). In a separate prospective, open-label, multicenter study of 33 children with FRNS, a 6-month course of MMF (with a tapering doses of alternate-date prednisone) maintained remission in 75% of children, and reduced relapses from once every two months to once every 14.7 months. However, only 33% had a sustained remission after discontinuing MMF. Thus, while MMF can be effective in reducing relapses in children with FRNS and has preferable side effect profile, it is not as effective as CsA in reducing relapses.

Steroid resistant nephrotic syndrome

Despite optimal management, approximately 10% of children will prove to be steroid-resistant and require alternative therapies. Before concluding that the patient is steroid-resistant, it is important to verify adherence to the treatment regimen, consider whether the patient is able to absorb the medication, rule out underlying infection, and consider the possibility of occult malignancy. Resistance to steroid therapy identifies children at dramatically increased risk for ESRD and extrarenal complications of NS. The risk for development of CKD or ESRD in this population is >40% within five years from the time of diagnosis, and SRNS is the underlying cause for >10% of all children who develop ESRD. Given these ominous statistics, a variety of alternative therapies have been utilized to try to induce remission. However, the majority of data are derived from uncontrolled clinical trials, leading to a lack of consensus among pediatric nephrologists about the optimal treatment for SRNS.

In general, the management of SRNS can be divided into three major categories: 1) Supportive therapy, 2) Immunosuppressive therapy, and 3) Nonimmunosuppressive therapy.

Supportive and adjunctive therapies

Supportive therapy includes meticulous general medical care, dietary adjustments, alteration of immunizations, management of edema, and management of hyperlipidemia.

General medical care

Careful general medical care plays an important role in the management of children with refractory NS. Cutaneous infection and cellulitis can rapidly evolve in an edematous patient and skin breakdown should be identified and treated early. Development of pain or asymmetric swelling of an extremity, respiratory distress, acute oliguria or gross hematuria, or neurologic symptoms may indicate venous thrombosis, and require urgent treatment. Abdominal pain may be due to peritonitis and needs prompt attention. Hypovolemia and hypotension are usually responsive to intravascular volume expansion by a colloidal solution, such as 5% albumin given as a bolus intravenously or a 25% albumin solution given IV more slowly. Intravenous albumin infusions can be complicated by the acute development of hypertension or respiratory distress if infused too rapidly.

Immunizations

Prior to steroid initiation, each patient should undergo tuberculin testing with a PPD to exclude tuberculosis, and immunity to varicella should be verified. Treatment of such infections should occur prior to initiation of steroid therapy. In general, routine immunizations, in children with NS should be delayed until the child has entered stable remission and tapered to low-dose alternate-day steroids — due to suboptimal vaccine responsiveness in immunosuppressed patients. Live virus vaccines are not recommended by the American Academy of Pediatrics for patients who have received corticosteroids, at a dose of 2 mg/kg/day of prednisone or its equivalent for >14 days, until the patients have been off of steroids for >4 weeks. In contrast, children who are on lower doses of steroids (less than 20 mg/day) or alternate-day steroids can generally receive live virus immunizations. For nonimmune children exposed to varicella while on immunosuppressive therapy, prophylactic VariZIG™ (if available) is recommended to prevent or minimize the severity of infection. To be effective, however, it must be given within 96 hours after exposure, and earlier treatment is more efficacious. If unavailable intravenous immunoglobulin (IVIG) can be considered. Although a rare risk for induction of relapses by immunizations exists, children with NS being treated with either no or alternate-day steroids can be effectively immunized with minimal risk. Thus, there does not appear to be a contraindication to immunization in most children with NS (i.e., those on no or alternate day steroids), since most can be expected to respond to routine immunizations, and the benefits of immunization generally far outweigh the risks of relapse.

Management of edema

General strategies for the management of edema in NS include salt restriction, and judicious use of diuretics and/or fluid restriction. In hospitalized patients, severe anasarca or disabling edema can be relieved by intravenous infusion of 25% albumin at a dose of 1 g/kg/dose, given over 3–4 hours, followed immediately by intravenous furosemide (1 mg/kg/dose) usually given slowly to avoid ototoxicity. This therapy may be cautiously repeated in severely edematous patients. The risk of aggressive albumin infusion therapy is sudden mobilization of interstitial fluid into the intravascular compartment with resultant congestive cardiac failure and pulmonary edema. In general, gradually increasing the serum albumin level to approximately 2.8 g/dl is sufficient to restore intravascular oncotic pressure and volume; little additional clinical benefit results from further increasing the albumin level to normal values.

The most commonly used diuretic is furosemide, which acts by inhibiting the Na-K-2Cl transporter in the thick ascending limb of the loop of Henle. Several factors may impair the efficacy of furosemide during NS, including hypoalbuminemia (leading to reduced delivery of furosemide to proximal tubular cells responsible for its secretion into the urinary space), and proteinuria (leading to increased association of furosemide with urinary albumin and decreased availability at the site of action). A variety of approaches have been developed to overcome the furosemide resistance, including increased diuretic dosage, coadministration with albumin, and coadministration with distal tubular diuretics (thiazides). While these strategies can improve the efficacy of furosemide, they also increase the risk for inducing complications, as evidenced by the recent identification of furosemide as the major iatrogenic risk factor for the development of thrombosis in children with NS. Moreover, loop diuretics have other side effects, including hypokalemia and metabolic alkalosis, hypercalciuria, nephrocalcinosis, and ototoxicity. Thus, chronic outpatient use of diuretics in children with NS should generally be avoided. Lastly, nonpharmacologic management of edema can also be clinically useful. Elevation of the extremities to the level of the heart or higher increases the tissue hydrostatic pressure, returning fluid to the intravascular space and thus reducing the edema.

Management of hyperlipidemia

Treatment of hyperlipidemia in children with refractory NS reduces the risk for cardiovascular complications later in life. A few uncontrolled trials have demonstrated the safety and potential utility of hydroxymethylglutaryl CoA (HMG CoA) reductase inhibitors (statins) in children with SRNS, with reductions in total cholesterol, LDL and triglyceride. However, placebo controlled studies are needed to clarify the efficacy and safety of statin therapy in pediatric NS. Additional dietary recommendations include maintenance of protein intake of 130–140% of the recommended daily allowance (RDA) for age, and avoidance of saturated fats, to avoid worsening hyperlipidemia.

Immunomodulatory therapies

Early identification and treatment of complications, management of edema and hyperlipidemia, alterations of immunizations, and dietary considerations described above are all essential to optimize the supportive management of children with refractory NS. However, the primary management goal in children with SRNS should be directed at induction of remission.

Pulse Intravenous Methylprednisolone

Methylprednisolone pulses have been used for many years in the management of SRNS. The most widely known protocol for IV pulse methylprednisolone was first proposed by Mendoza and Tune in 1990 and included IV methylprednisolone (30 mg/kg) in the following schedule: alternate days for two weeks, then weekly for eight weeks, then every other week for eight weeks, then monthly for nine months, then every other month for six months. This treatment was accompanied by oral prednisone, and if needed, cyclophosphamide or chlorambucil. In long-term follow-up (mean = 6.3 years) of 32 children with steroid-resistant FSGS treated with this protocol, 21 children (65.6%) were in complete remission, three (9.4%) had mild proteinuria, two (6.2%) had moderate proteinuria, and six (19%) remained nephrotic. The reported side effects included cataracts (22%), impaired growth (17%), hypertension (17%), leukopenia (19%), and gastrointestinal distress, which was common. Despite impressive clinical response with modest side effects, IV pulse methylprednisolone remains highly controversial, due primarily to concerns about long-term side effects of corticosteroids in children.

Alkylating agents

Alkylating agents, such as cyclophosphamide and chlorambucil, have been widely used in the treatment of SRNS. Investigators have gravitated toward the use of six months of pulse IV rather than oral cyclophosphamide, due to reports of lower cumulative doses and higher rates of complete remission with IV cyclophosphamide. Several reports have also highlighted the potential clinical importance of primary versus secondary steroid resistance in the likelihood of response to IV pulse cyclophosphamide therapy, with increased risk for unresponsiveness to IV cyclophosphamide among children with primary steroid resistance.

Cyclosporine A

A recent meta-analysis of all randomized controlled trials for the treatment of childhood SRNS found that, compared to placebo or no treatment, treatment with CsA resulted in a relative risk for persistent NS of 0.69 [95% confidence intervals (CI) 0.47–0.88)]. Thus the available literature overall suggests that CsA is similarly effective to IV pulse methylprednisolone therapy in the management of SRNS, and is among the most effective therapies currently available. Because children with SRNS often require long-term CsA use, it is important to note that the risk for interstitial fibrosis appears to increase with increasing duration of therapy. Other factors found to correlate with increased risk for CsA nephrotoxicity include previous impairment of renal function, histologic diagnosis (FSGS >MCNS), dosage >5.5 mg/kg/d, and duration of heavy proteinuria >30 days. In summary, while CsA appears to be clinically very helpful for many children with SRNS, the long-term risk for CsA nephrotoxicity underscores the importance of efforts to taper and/or transition children to alternate forms of therapy within two years of starting CsA whenever possible.

Mycophenolate mofetil

Few reports to date have evaluated the efficacy of MMF in children with SRNS. While MMF may have a moderately beneficial role in the management of SRNS, it is not very effective in inducing complete remission in these children, and may thus be most useful as an adjunct to the other alternative therapies for the maintenance of remission.

Tacrolimus

Tacrolimus is among the newer immunosuppressive medications to be used for SRNS. Similar to CsA, tacrolimus acts via inhibition of calcineurin, but its mechanism of action in NS is unknown. Tacrolimus monotherapy (i.e., without steroids or other immunosuppressive medications) has resulted in partial or complete remission in patients with SRNS. Like CsA, withdrawal of therapy resulted in early relapses, which have responded well to reintroduction of tacrolimus. Far fewer children have been reported for tacrolimus compared to IV methylprednisolone or CsA, so limited data are available regarding long-term outcomes and dose-related toxicity. A recent single-center retrospective study of children with SRNS reported that tacrolimus induced complete remission in 15 of 16 patients (94%) after a median of 120 days of therapy. Two of 24 (8%) patients were found to have increased tubulointerstitial fibrosis on follow-up biopsies after a median of 24 months. Of note, children with higher trough tacrolimus levels were found to have more extensive tubular atrophy and interstitial fibrosis, suggesting that risk of prolonged tacrolimus usage is similar to that of CsA.

Monoclonal antibodies

Very recent studies have reported that monoclonal antibody therapy is also capable of inducing remission in a subset of children with NS. A recent multicenter experience with rituximab, a humanized monoclonal antibody targeting the CD20 B lymphocyte surface antigen with SDNS or SRNS. After receiving 2–4 rituximab infusions, 3 of 7 patients (43%) with proteinuria at the time of administration entered complete remission, and at least one immunosuppressive medication was able to be withdrawn in 19 patients (85%) without triggering a relapse or need for increased dosing of other immunosuppressive drugs. Adverse effects were reported in 45% of patients but most were mild and transient. Another multicenter prospective trial of single-dose rituximab in 12 children with refractory SDNS found that those who were in remission at the time of treatment, were able to discontinue steroids after a median of 74 days. Over the six months following rituximab infusion, these patients enjoyed a longer steroid-free interval and reduced relapse frequency, compared to the six months prior to treatment. Seventy-five percent of patients relapsed after a median of 129 days, and 7 of 9 received another rituximab infusion due to steroid dependency. Of note, similar to the above study, relapse was associated with recovery of the B cell count. Only 25% of patients experienced a sustained remission of >1 year. While no severe adverse effects were observed in this study, the recent report documented severe and even fatal pulmonary toxicity in two NS patients following rituximab therapy. To date, prognostic factors for favorable response to rituximab and risk factors associated with severe toxicity are both unclear. Moreover, lack of controlled randomized studies raises a concern of publication bias, i.e., that more positive outcomes are reported at the expense of negative results that are often considered less noteworthy.

Nonimmunomodulatory therapy: ACE inhibitors and angiotensin receptor blockers (ARBs)

Angiotensin-converting enzyme inhibitors (ACEIs) and angiotensin receptor blockers (ARBs) are being increasingly used in the management of SRNS. Several uncontrolled studies involving both children and adults with SRNS have reported significant reductions in proteinuria in response to ACEI. Among the side effects noted with ACEI therapy are transient acute renal failure, hyperkalemia, cough, hypotension, and rarely angioedema. These agents should be used cautiously in adolescent females due to teratogenicity.

Prognosis

The initial response to corticosteroids is the single best indicator of the long-term prognosis for a child presenting with NS, since children who fail to respond to an 8-week course of oral corticosteroids have a relatively poor prognosis. In a major international study, 80% of children with SSNS were in remission at eight years. In addition, 75% of those children who remained relapse-free for the initial six months after presentation either continued in remission during their entire course or had only rare relapses. These findings suggest that while the majority of children (60%) with NS experience one or more relapses, most patients experience a gradual decrease in the frequency of relapses over time. In addition, children with SSNS have no apparent increase in malignancies, atopic diseases, clinical defects in cell-mediated immunity, or cardiovascular diseases over more than two decades of follow up. Furthermore, relapsing NS during childhood does not appear to place children at increased risk for cardiovascular morbidity or mortality as adults compared with the general population.

In contrast, there is significant heterogeneity in the clinical course of FSGS. Some children experience progressive disease within the first few years from presentation, whereas others progress more slowly. Importantly, however, the prognosis in children with steroid resistant FSGS is always guarded, as the risk for progressive disease is high and these children are also at increased risk for recurrence of FSGS in a future renal transplant. Indeed, recurrence rates as high as 50% for pediatric first renal allograft recipients has been reported. Of note, while a pathogenetic plasma-circulating factor has not yet been definitively identified, the use of plasmapheresis has been shown to be helpful both in prolonging renal function in the native kidneys and in preventing recurrence of FSGS in transplanted kidneys.

Summary

Nephrotic syndrome is one of the most common types of kidney disease seen in children. Because neither its pathogenesis nor the mechanism of action of the drugs which effective treat it have been well-defined, it remains a very challenging and intriguing problem for pediatric nephrologists. Despite this, the long-term prognosis is generally excellent for children with NS unless they develop resistance to steroid therapy. Unfortunately, children with SRNS are often unresponsive to even the newest therapies that have been attempted, which leaves them at increased risk for both ESRD and death. Further research on both the pathogenesis of NS and the mechanisms of action of the identified therapies for it is needed to permit the development of more effective and less toxic therapies.

Suggested Reading

Gipson DS, Massengill SF, Yao L, *et al.* (2009) Management of childhood onset nephrotic syndrome. *Pediatrics* **124**(2): 747–757.

Guigonis V, Dallocchio A, Baudouin V, *et al.* (2008) Rituximab treatment for severe steroid- or cyclosporine-dependent nephrotic syndrome: a multicentric series of 22 cases. *Pediatr Nephrol* **23**(8): 1269–1279.

Iijima K, Hamahira K, Tanaka R, *et al.* (2002) Risk factors for cyclosporine-induced tubulointerstitial lesions in children with minimal change nephrotic syndrome. *Kidney Int* **61**: 1801.

International Study of Kidney Disease in Children. (1981) Primary nephrotic syndrome in children: clinical significance of histopathologic variants of minimal change and of diffuse mesangial hypercellularity. A Report of the International Study of Kidney Disease in Children. *Kidney Int* **20**(6): 765–771.

Kamei K, Ito S, Nozu K, *et al.* (2009) Single dose of rituximab for refractory steroid-dependent nephrotic syndrome in children. *Pediatr Nephrol* **24**(7): 1321–1328.

Kerlin BA, Blatt NB, Fuh B, *et al.* (2009) Epidemiology and risk factors for thromboembolic complications of childhood nephrotic syndrome: a Midwest Pediatric Nephrology Consortium (MWPNC) study. *J Pediatr* **155**(1): 105–110.

Passero CJ, Mueller GM, Rondon-Berrios H, *et al.* (2008) Activates Epithelial Na+ Channels by Cleaving the γ Subunit. *J Biol Chem* **26**; **283**(52): 36586–36591.

Valentini RP, Smoyer WE. (2007) In: Kher K, Schnaper HW, Makker SP (eds.) *Clinical Pediatric Nephrology*. Informa UK Ltd.

Woroniecki RP, Kopp JB. (2007) Genetics of focal segmental glomerulosclerosis. *Pediatr Nephrol* **22**(5): 638–644.

16

Postinfectious Glomerulonephritis

Michael C. Braun

Introduction

Postinfectious glomerulonephritis (PIGN) is the most common cause of acute nephritis in the pediatric population. It occurs more frequently in males than females, and incidence peaks in children between 5 and 12 years of age. It rarely occurs in children under age 2 and in adults over age 60. A wide range of infectious agents have been associated with PIGN (Table 1), including bacterial, viral, parasitic and fungal pathogens. The vast majority of these infectious agents are endemic in the developing world, and are rarely seen in the United States or Europe. Overall, the rate of PIGN has declined over the past several decades in the developed world. While reasons for this are unclear, it is likely related to improvements in hygiene, the wide-spread use of vaccination, and increase in antibiotic use. This discussion will focus on renal injury associated with group A beta-hemolytic streptococcal infections as it is the predominate cause of PIGN in the United States.

Clinical Presentation

Typically, there is a latent period following the acute infectious process which varies depending on the agent and site of infection. For PIGN following streptococcal infections, this ranges from 7–14 days after pharyngitis, to 2–3 weeks after cutaneous infection. PIGN occurs sporadically, in epidemics related to seasonal outbreaks of pharyngitis, and in an endemic form. The classical presentation is marked by the abrupt onset of dark or tea colored urine, edema, hypertension and varying degrees of renal dysfunction. The wide spectrum of clinical presentation can range from isolated hematuria and proteinuria without renal impairment to

Table 1. Postinfectious renal diseases in children

Pathogen	Infectious presentation	Renal presentation	Renal pathology
Alpha-hemolytic *Streptococcus*	Pharyngitis/ pyoderma	GN	Proliferative GN
Staphylococcus aureus	Endocarditis	GN proteinuria	Proliferative GN
Staphylococcus epidermidis	VA/VP shunt infections	GN/nephrotic syndrome/ hematuria/proteinuria	MPGN
Treponema pallidum	Secondary Syphilis	Nephrotic syndrome/GN	Proliferative GN
Leptospirosis	Weil's syndrome	Proteinuria/pyuria	Tubulointerstitial disease/ATN
Mycobacterium tuberculosis	Pulmonary TB	Sterile pyuria	Caseating granulomas
Hepatitis B	Chronic hepatitis	Proteinuria/nephrotic syndrome	Membranous
	Polyarteritis Nodosa	Hypertension/proteinuria	Renal arteritis/GN
Hepatitis C	Chronic hepatitis/ cirrhosis	Proteinuria/nephrotic syndrome	MPGN/Membranous
Schistosoma mansoni	Diarrhea/fever	Nephrotic syndrome	MPGN/Membranous/ proliferative GN
Plasmodium falciparum	Malaria	GN/nephrotic syndrome/gross hematuria	Proliferative GN/ ATN

Table 2. PIGN clinical features at presentation

Common	Less Common	Rare
Gross Hematuria	Encephalopathy	Nephrotic syndrome
RBC casts	Seizures	RPGN
Hematuria/proteinuria	anuria	
Oliguria	Congestive heart failure	
Hypertension		
edema		

acute kidney injury (AKI) requiring renal replacement therapy (RRT) (see Table 2). Typically the proteinuria, while heavy, is not in the nephrotic range. A fresh urine sample will often reveal the presence of RBC casts and large numbers of white blood cells early in the disease course. The severity of salt and fluid retention drives many of the clinical features at presentation, ranging from mild edema, to frank volume overload with congestive heart failure. Hypertension is very common and may progress to encephalopathy and seizures. While some degree of renal impairment is frequently seen, only a small minority of patients will present with overt renal failure.

Rates of PIGN following pharyngitis are estimated at 8–14% to less than 5% following an episode of pyoderma. One study of asymptomatic siblings of individuals with PIGN indicated that up to 15% had clinical or laboratory findings consistent with PIGN. In addition, a study of patients with pyoderma reported that up to 50% of patients had evidence of sub-clinical glomerular injury. Overall it has been estimated that there are 3–4 times more individuals with asymptomatic disease compared to those that seek medical attention.

Differential Diagnosis

Any disease which can cause acute nephritis needs to be considered when evaluating a patient for PIGN. A complete detailed history and physical examination is essential. Commonly considered diagnoses include: IgA nephropathy, Henoch–Schönlein Purpura (HSP), Lupus Nephritis (SLE), Hemolytic Uremic Syndrome (HUS), systemic vasculitis (e.g. ANCA diseases), Goodpasture disease, Alport syndrome, membranoproliferative glomerulonephritis (MGPN), and the acute presentation of a chronic glomerular disease. As discussed elsewhere, the clinical and laboratory features of many of these diseases can often be readily distinguished from PIGN.

Table 3. Differential diagnosis of acute GN

Postinfectious glomerulonephritis	IgA nephropathy
Goodpasture disease	Henoch–Schönlein purpura
Alport syndrome	Systemic lupus erythematosus
Systemic vasculitis (ANCA diseases)	Hemolytic uremic syndrome
Acute presentation of chronic disease	Membranoproliferative glomerulonephritis

Laboratory investigation

There is no single specific diagnostic test for PIGN. The presence of an infectious prodrome may be difficult to identify and given the long latent

Table 4. Laboratory features of streptococcal associated PIGN

Prodrome	ASO	Anti-DNase B	C3	C4
Pharyngitis	Elevated	Elevated	Low	Normal
Pyoderma	Often normal	Elevated	Low	Normal

period, signs of cutaneous infection may have resolved. Throat and skin cultures are negative in a majority of patients as the acute infectious process has resolved at the time of presentation. Screening studies for recent streptococcal infections typically include measurements of anti-streptolysin O (ASO) antibody titers alone or a Streptozyme® assay which measures anti-streptolysin O, anti-streptokinase, anti-DNAse B, and anti-hyaluronidase antibodies (Table 4). While ASO titers peak 2–4 weeks after an acute episode of pharyngitis, antibody titers can remain elevated for up to 6 months after infection. The height of the antibody response can also be attenuated with antibiotic treatment, and streptococcal skin infections frequently fail to elicit a strong ASO antibody response. It is thought that anti-DNAse B antibodies are a more sensitive screening test for cutaneous streptococcal infections. Overall the specificity of most antibody tests for acute or post-streptococcal infections is approximately 90%. Thus, screening for host antibody responses to streptococcal infections should be viewed as supportive but not conclusive evidence of PIGN. Serum complement (C3 and C4) levels should be obtained. C3 levels are depressed in PIGN and C4 levels are almost always normal (see Table 5). A CH50, which is a measure of overall complement activity, may be low due to complement consumption. Up to 10% of patients with PIGN may have normal complement studies depending when in the disease course these studies are obtained. Neither the height of the antibody response nor the degree of C3 depression correlates with disease severity. As thrombocytosis, mild anemia, and an elevated white blood cell count are frequently seen in PIGN; a CBC should also be obtained. Baseline measures of electrolytes, albumin, BUN, serum creatinine, as well as urinary protein excretion should also be performed. Additional laboratory studies should be considered depending on the history and physical examination. If there is any evidence of multisystem organ involvement, an atypical presentation or clinical course, an alternative diagnoses should be rigorously pursued.

Table 5. Differential diagnosis of hypocomplementemic nephritis

Low C3 and Normal C4	Low C3 and Low C4
PIGN	SLE
MPGN II	Cryoglobulinemia
MPGN III	MPGN I
	Nephritis of chronic bacteremia

Pathology

The vast majority of patients with a clinical diagnosis of PIGN are never biopsied. Those that are biopsied have distinctive pathologic findings. Light microscopy generally shows uniformly enlarged glomeruli, commonly filling Bowman's capsule. The glomeruli are very proliferative with a marked increased in mesangial and endothelial cell number. Infiltration of the glomerular space by leukocytes is also very common. The glomerular capillary loops may be narrowed by infiltrating cells or as a result cellular proliferation. Typically there is little evidence of tubulointerstitial disease beyond mild focal cellular infiltrates. In severe cases, glomerular crescents are often seen and can be both cellular and fibro-cellular. Immunofluorescence staining for C3 and IgG is usually in a fine granular pattern involving both the glomerular capillary loops and the mesangium. Staining for C4, IgA, or IgM is commonly negative. Ultrastructural analysis of the glomerular basement membrane (GBM) using electron microscopy demonstrates the hallmarks of PIGN: the presence of rounded deposits that extend from the outer layer of the GBM under the epithelial foot process, so called "subepithelial humps", which are unique to PIGN. The GBM is intact, and there may be effacement of the podocytes with sub-endothelial or mesangial deposits of varying degrees.

Pathogenesis

The development of PIGN from group A streptococcal infections is primarily limited to the M-type, although rare cases have been reported with groups C and G. Strains of *Streptococcus* that are linked to PIGN are termed "nephritogenic". Nephritogenic types differ with sites of primary infection; type 12 is a common isolate in PIGN following an episode of pharyngitis, while type 49 is more common in PIGN following cutaneous infections. Several potential mechanisms have been proposed to explain why some strains are nephritogenic and not others. A number of putative streptococcal antigens have been indentified in nephritogenic strains that have been shown to induce disease in animal models, and it has been argued that neuraminidase produced by some strains alters the native protein structure of human IgG making it immunogenic. Two other possible pathogenic mechanisms have been also proposed: firstly that these epitopes on nephritogenic strains of *Streptococcus* that cross-react with antigens present in normal human glomeruli leading to local immune complex formation; and secondly that *Streptococcus* can act as a "superantigen" and that the hyper-activation of the immune system mediates the renal injury nonspecifically. None of these potential mechanisms have been conclusively proven.

Circulating immune complexes (CIC) can be detected in most individuals with PIGN. It is presumed that these immune complexes are deposited in the kidney by one of two mechanisms. One hypothesis is that preformed CIC are thought to be nonspecifically trapped by glomerular endothelial or mesangial cells forming localized deposits. Alternatively, low molecular weight antigens diffuse across the GBM where they are trapped and immune complexes reform on the inner portion of the GBM generating subepithelial "humps". The presence of IgG staining and deposit formation in the glomerulus favors the hypothesis that PIGN is an immune complex disease, however the pattern of complement activation argues against this. Serum C4 levels are usually normal in patients with PIGN and there is a lack of C4 deposition in the kidney. The low levels of C3 and lack of C4 or C1q deposition in the glomerulus suggests that the alternative pathway of the complement system is preferentially activated in PIGN, and not the classical pathway as one would expect in prototypical immune complex diseases.

Regardless of the precise pathogenic mechanisms that mediate PIGN, local deposition of immune complexes and activation of the complement system are thought to be the primary mediators that drive the host inflammatory response, mesangial and glomerular endothelial cell proliferation, and leukocyte recruitment, which in turn results in an acute change in glomerular perfusion and reduction in GFR. It is also evident that host specific immune responses also play a critical role in the development of

PIGN as some individuals infected with nephritogenic strains of *Streptococcus* develop PIGN while others do not.

Treatment

There is no specific therapy for PIGN, and antibiotic therapy is not indicated. The use of corticosteroid therapy for the vast majority of pediatric patients with PIGN has been shown to be of little benefit. Medical care therefore should be directly toward detailed and comprehensive management of the acute kidney injury (AKI). Volume overload and resulting hypertension should be treated aggressively as much of the morbidity from PIGN arises from malignant hypertension. Fluid and sodium restriction combined with diuretics and antihypertensive medication are the mainstays of therapy. Angiotensin converting enzyme (ACE) inhibition or angiotensin receptor blockade should be used only with extreme caution in the acute setting as these agents may precipitate a sudden reduction in GFR and ensuing hyperkalemia. AKI requiring dialysis is atypical in PIGN but can occur in up to 5% of patients, particularly in those with rapidly progressive glomerulonephritis (RPGN). RPGN, characterized by rapid deterioration in renal function and the development of oligoanuria, is widely viewed as an indication for renal biopsy and the use of imunomodulatory therapy. At present there is no consensus regarding the optimal therapy for RPGN. High dose pulse IV methylprednisolone is the most commonly used agent in pediatric RPGN. Additional therapeutic agents such as cyclophosphamide and plasmapheresis have also been employed, although their efficacy in PIGN remains controversial. A recent case series of 27 patients with severe PIGN with RPGN from New Zealand failed to demonstrate a clear benefit from immunosuppressive therapy. Most of the reports regarding the treatment of crescentic GN associated RPGN are observational, nonrandomized, trials of heterogeneous patient populations. It should be remembered that RPGN is a clinical diagnosis that can be seen in many different pathologic processes including SLE, HSP, and MPGN among others.

Prognosis

For the vast majority of patients, PIGN is self-limited. Mortality rates from PIGN have been reported as high at 1–3%, however these estimates are based largely on case series from the 1960' and 1970's. There is little recent data to support these estimates and the current risk of mortality is undoubtedly much lower. Typically renal function returns to normal within 4–6 weeks. In 50% of patients serum C3 levels return to normal within 3 weeks, and in nearly all patients by eight weeks. The failure of C3 levels to normalize within this time frame suggests that the episode of nephritis may not be due to PIGN, but rather MPGN, and renal biopsy may be indicated. Gross hematuria may persist for several weeks following presentation, and microscopic hematuria can continue for up to 2 years. The severity of proteinuria should decline in proportion to the improvement in renal function, although non-nephrotic range proteinuria can persist for as long as 2 years after presentation. In a minority of patients, intermittent proteinuria can continue for much longer periods.

A number of pediatric studies dating back to the 1960's indicate that most patients have an excellent prognosis. For those individuals without underlying renal disease, persistent nephrotic syndrome or severe AKI, there were little long-term complications. The largest series of patients from Trinidad with long term follow-up of both epidemic and sporadic forms of PIGN showed a roughly 8% incidence of persistent hematuria and proteinuria and a 2% incidence of chronic hypertension.

For those patients with severe disease requiring dialysis or those with RPGN, the long-term consequences are less clear. In a recent report from Australia of 37 patients with PIGN, of the 3 patients who required dialytic therapy, 1 had persistent hypertension, and reduced GFR six years following presentation. Furthermore data from India on 11 patients with crescentic PIGN indicated that 7 patients progressed to end-stage renal disease and another 2 patients developed chronic kidney disease. As part of a larger study of pediatric patients with RPGN, the Southwest Pediatric Nephrology Study Group reported that approximately 50% of children with crescents in 50% or more glomeruli progress to ESRD. While it has not been possible to clearly identify predictors of long-term renal injury, based on the this report and others it appears that poor prognosis is associated with a high percentage of fibro-cellular crescents, evidence of chronic renal injury on biopsy, and the persistence of nephrotic range proteinuria.

Suggested Reading

Berrios X, Lagomarsino E, Solar E, *et al.* (2004) Post-streptococcal acute glomerulonephritis in Chile — 20 years of experience. *Pediatr Nephrol* (Berlin) **19**: 306–312.

Blyth CC, Robertson PW, Rosenberg AR. (2007) Post-streptococcal glomerulonephritis in Sydney: a 16-year retrospective review. *J Paed and Child Health* **43**: 446–450.

Clark G, White RH, Glasgow EF, *et al.* (1988) Poststreptococcal glomerulonephritis in children: clinicopathological correlations and long-term prognosis. *Pediatr Nephrol* (Berlin) **2**: 381–388.

Dodge WF, Spargo BH, Bass JA, Travis LB. (1968) The relationship between the clinical and pathologic features of poststreptococcal glomerulonephritis. A study of the early natural history. *Med* **47**: 227–267.

Dodge WF, Spargo BH, Travis LB, *et al.* (1972) Poststreptococcal glomerulonephritis. A prospective study in children. *New Eng J Med* **286**: 273–278.

Nissenson AR, Mayon-White R, Potter EV, *et al.* (1979) Continued absence of clinical renal disease seven to 12 years after poststreptococcal acute glomerulonephritis in Trinidad. *Am J Med* **67**: 255–262.

Rose GM, Cole BR, Robson AM. (1981) The treatment of severe glomerulopathies in children using high dose intravenous methylprednisolone pulses. *Am J Kidney Dis* **1**: 148–156.

Roy S, 3rd, Stapleton FB. (1990) Changing perspectives in children hospitalized with poststreptococcal acute glomerulonephritis. *Pediatr Nephrol* (Berlin) **4**: 585–588.

Southwest Pediatric Nephrology Study Group. (1985) A clinico-pathologic study of crescentic glomerulonephritis in 50 children. A report of the. *Kidney Int* **24**: 450-458

Srivastava RN, Moudgil A, Bagga A, *et al.* (1992) Crescentic glomerulonephritis in children: a review of 43 cases. *Am J Nephr* **12**: 155–161.

Tasic V, Polenakovic M. (2003) Occurrence of subclinical post-streptococcal glomerulonephritis in family contacts. *J Paed and Child Health* **39**: 177–179.

Wong W, Morris MC, Zwi J. (2009) Outcome of severe acute post-streptococcal glomerulonephritis in New Zealand children. *Pediatr Nephrol* (Berlin) **24**: 1021–1026.

Yoshizawa N, Suzuki Y, Oshima S, *et al.* (1996) Asymptomatic acute poststreptococcal glomerulonephritis following upper respiratory tract infections caused by Group A streptococci. *Clin Nephrol* **46**: 296–301.

17

Membranoproliferative Glomerulonephritis

Michael C. Braun

Introduction

Membranoproliferative glomerulonephritis (MPGN) is a rare disease. The annual incidence of MPGN based on registry data in the United States, Europe and Australia is roughly 1–2 per million pediatric patients per year. MGPN accounts for about 3% of all pediatric end-stage renal disease (ESRD) patients in the NAPRTCS database, and about 0.5% of all ESRD patients in the United States. However, due to its heterogeneous and often subtle clinic presentation, MPGN must be considered in the differential diagnosis of nearly all acquired kidney diseases. The classification of MPGN has undergone many evolutions over time. In the 1970s and early 1980s, it was often referred to mesangiocapillary glomerulonephritis (MCGN). By the mid 1980s, MCGN had been supplanted in the literature by the use of MPGN, which in turn was classified as type I (MGPN I), type II (MPGN II), and type III (MPGN III). Recently, it has been proposed to designate MGPN II as Dense Deposit Disease (DDD) in an attempt to emphasize the unique nature of the glomerular basement membrane abnormalities and the pathogenic mechanisms that distinguish it from MPGN I, or MPGN III.

Clinical Presentation

MPGN cannot be distinguished from other forms of glomerulonephritis based on clinical presentation. MPGN varies greatly in its presentations, including asymptomatic hematuria with or without proteinuria, isolated proteinuria, gross hematuria, acute glomerulonephritis, nephrotic syndrome, rapidly progressive glomerulonephritis (RPGN), chronic glomerulonephritis, or even ESRD. There is considerable overlap between all three types of MPGN at clinical presentation although larger case series have suggested that some presentations predominate for each type of MPGN. Asymptomatic presentation is most common in MGPN I and MPGN III, with more than 50% of patients having asymptomatic hematuria, proteinuria, or both. This is much less frequent in MPGN II, usually comprising less than 25% of patients. Nephrotic syndrome is seen in about 30% of patients with MPGN I, and in as many as 50% of MPGN II patients. Acute nephritis is seen in roughly 50% of type II patients and about 25–30% of patients with MPGN I. Nephrotic syndrome or acute nephritis is less frequent in MPGN III accounting for less than a third of patients in most series.

It is therefore essential to consider MPGN in the differential diagnosis for any patient who presents with signs of glomerular injury. The initial step in the laboratory evaluation of MPGN is measurement of serum complement levels, specifically C3 and C4 levels. More than 80% of patients will have low serum C3 levels at presentation. A normal C3 level, however, does not exclude the diagnosis of MPGN. The degree of C3 depression is variable, although patients with MPGN III typically have the most severely depressed C3 levels. Serum C4 levels are depressed in the majority of patients with MPGN I, are occasionally low in MPGN III, and universally normal in patients with MPGN II (see Table 1). Interpretation of serum C4 levels is often confounded by the relatively high frequency of partial C4 deficiency in the US population.

The differential diagnosis of hypocomplementemic (low serum C3 levels) nephritis is limited (see Table 2). The measurement of C3 and C4 levels combined with a careful history and physical examination, and a limited number of laboratory studies, should be sufficient to narrow the diagnostic possibilities to a specific type of MPGN.

Table 1. Clinical and laboratory features of MPGN

MPGN	Relative frequencies	Most common presentation	C3 levels	C4 levels
Type I	36%–78%	Hematuria/proteinuria	Low	Low
Type II	5%–34%	Nephrotic syndrome Acute nephritis	Low	Normal
Type III	14%–41%	Hematuria/proteinuria	Low	Low occasionally

Table 2. Differential diagnosis of hypocomplementemic nephritis

Low C3 and Normal C4	Low C3 and Low C4
Post infectious glomerulonephritis (PIGN)	Systemic lupus erythematosus (SLE)
MPGN II	Cryoglobulinemia
MPGN III	MPGN I
	Nephritis of chronic bacteremia

Secondary MPGN

Worldwide, MPGN is a much more common disease than in the developed world. This can largely be ascribed to the endemic presence of infectious diseases in the developing world that are associated with MPGN type I, including hepatitis B, hepatitis C, malaria, and schistosomiasis. While hepatitis C associated MPGN is reported in the adult US population, the single study looking at serologic evidence of hepatitis in a cohort of children with idiopathic MPGN was unable to identify a single positive individual. Other common causes of secondary MPGN I include B cell lymphoma, chronic lymphocytic leukemia, essential cryoglobulinemia, and chronic bacteremia. The nephritis of chronic bacteremia is typically seen in two settings, individuals with endocarditis and patients with vertriculo-atrial shunt infections, so called shunt nephritis. Identification and treatment of the source of the bacteremia is essential. Another rare, but easily recognized cause of secondary MPGN II is partial lipodystrophy. There are some 150 reports of other diseases associated with the development of MPGN ranging from gastric adenocarcinoma to Turner syndrome; the vast majority of these are single case reports and may be nothing more than fortuitous associations.

Laboratory Investigation of MPGN

In patients with MPGN type I, clinical and laboratory investigation should focus on excluding secondary causes of MPGN (see Fig. 1). Individuals with persistent fevers should have a complete evaluation for chronic bacterial infections including serial blood cultures, and an echocardiogram to rule out endocarditis. Hepatitis B and C should be excluded by both antibody testing, and more sensitive PCR screening. The measurement of circulating immune complexes, or cryoglobulins can be pursued, although

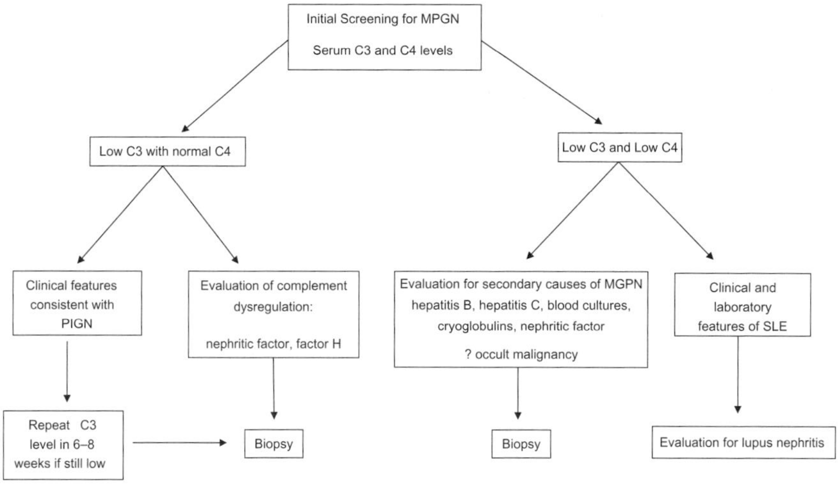

Figure 1. Laboratory evaluation of MPGN.

most clinical tests are insensitive and technically difficult. A detailed travel history should be obtained to identify exposure to pathogens endemic in the developing world. In individuals with signs of systemic illness investigation for occult malignancy, although rare in pediatrics, should be undertaken.

Patients diagnosed with MPGN II, require a detailed genetic and functional analysis of components of the alternative pathway of the complement system. Factor H levels and genetic analysis of factor H should be measured as normal protein levels do not indicate that the factor H is functional. Additional investigation for mutations in other components of the C3 convertase, Factor B and C3 among others, may be indicated, although these studies are not yet available commercially.

While the presence of nephritic factors should be sought in all individuals with MPGN, these tests are typically available in research labs only.

Pathologic Classification of MPGN

The defining histologic features of all forms of MPGN are expansion of the mesangial matrix, mesangial cell proliferation, and disturbance of the normal structure of the glomerular capillary loops. There are differences in the degree of mesangial proliferation seen in the MPGN. Typically

MPGN I has the most severe and diffuse proliferation, while mesangial proliferation in MPGN III tends to be much more focal in nature. MPGN II commonly has an intermediate phenotype, although depending on the severity and acuity of onset this can vary substantially. However, these differences are not absolute, and there is clear overlap between types in regard to the degree of proliferation. The subdivision of MPGN into the individual types is dependent on a combination of patterns of immunofluorescence (IF) staining, and analysis of the glomerular basement membrane (GBM) using electron microscopy (EM).

Immunofluorescence microscopy with staining for C3, C4, and IgG is very useful for provisional classification of the MPGN subtypes (Table 3). While C3 staining is universal in all forms of MPGN, there can be subtle differences in the pattern of C3 staining between the types. In MPGN I, C3 staining is typically along the glomerular capillary loops in a so-called "fringe" pattern. In MGPN II, the C3 staining is strongly positive along the capillary loops and often distinct ring-like structures can be seen along the GBM; in addition C3 staining of the mesangium and Bowman's capsule are common findings. In MPGN III, C3 staining also localizes to the capillary loops, and the mesangium, although it is typically more granular and less intense than that seen in MPGN II. The pattern of C4 staining readily distinguishes MPGN I from MPGN II or MPGN III. In MPGN I, C4 staining is strongly positive and colocalizes along the glomerular capillary loops with C3. C4 staining is not seen in MPGN II, and while weak C4 staining can be seen in MPGN III, it does not colocalize with C3 staining. Similar to C4, IgG staining is strongly positive and colocalizes with C3, and C4 in MPGN I. IgG staining is typically not found in MPGN II, and if present in MPGN III does not colocalize with C3 deposition. Staining for other immunoglobulins IgA, IgM, or IgE, is typically negative in all forms of MPGN.

Table 3. Histologic and immunofluorescence findings in MPGN

MPGN	Mesangial proliferation	C3 staining	C4 staining	IgG staining
Type I	Marked	Positive	Positive	Positive
Type II	Varying	Positive	Negative	Negative
Type III	Focal	Positive	Positive	Weakly Positive/Negative

Table 4. Ultrastructural features of MPGN

MPGN	Sub-endothelial deposits	Sub-epithelial deposits	GBM
Type I	Yes	Variable	Intact
Type II	No	No	Dense deposits
Type II	Yes	Yes	Thickened/disrupted

While IF staining is often suggestive of a specific type of MPGN, the defining pathologic features for each type of MPGN resides in the analysis of the ultrastructure of the GBM (see Table 4). Each form of MPGN has unique patterns of findings on EM. For MPGN I, these typically include an intact GBM with abundant subendothelial deposits. Subepithelial deposits can also be seen in variable amounts. In MPGN II, the GBM is abnormal with large electron dense deposits scattered within the GBM; this is the ultrastructural feature that defines MPGN II. The EM findings in MPGN III are the most complex. While dense deposits are never seen, abundant subendothelial and subepithelial deposits are common, and the GBM appears to be thickened or disrupted with laminations.

Pathogenesis

The pathogenic mechanisms that mediate MPGN I remain to be discovered. However, the preponderance of clinical and experimental data suggests that MPGN I is an immune complex disease. Circulating immune complexes can be detected in some patients with type I, and there is an increased frequency of MPGN type I in individuals with chronic hepatitis C, or chronic bacteremia, or individuals with abnormal levels of antibody production such as patients with B cell lymphomas. The depression in serum C4 levels is a hallmark of antibody dependent activation of the classical pathway of complement activation. Furthermore, the colocalization of C3, C4, and IgG at the site of glomerular injury also supports this hypothesis. Specific genetic risk factors, or deficiency states that increase the risk for developing MPGN I have not been identified.

Over the past decade, there has been an explosion in our understanding of the pathogenesis of MPGN II. It is now clear that MPGN II is the result of dysregulation of the alternative pathway of complement activation. The critical step in the regulation of the alternative pathway occurs at the level of C3 convertase. C3 convertase is a multicomponent enzyme, composed of C3b, and factor B that functions to cleave C3. The activity of this convertase is regulated by multiple components of the complement system including factor I, factor H, and factor B. Mutations affecting the functional activity of factor H to inactivate this convertase as well as mutations in C3 which alter the stability of the convertase have been associated with MPGN II. In addition, it has been known for decades that some individuals with MPGN type II have a circulating auto-antibody, referred to as nephritic factor, which acts to stabilize the C3 convertase. Recently, another set of auto-antibodies has been discovered that block factor H activity. These findings are consistent with the clinical features of MPGN II, namely the normal serum C4 levels, and the lack of C4 or IgG deposition in the kidney, and indicate that unregulated activation of the alternative pathway of the complement system is the primary pathogenic determinate in MPGN II. It is unclear, however, why systemic complement activation results in such disproportionate renal injury compared to other tissues exposed to complement activation products.

Little is known regarding the pathogenesis of MPGN type III. The lack of IgG deposition in the kidney and the lack of C4 colocalization argue against an immune complex-like mechanism. Similar to MPGN type II, reports of a nephritic factor have been found in some patients with type III. This nephritic factor does not appear to stabilize the C3 convertase, but rather C5 convertase, the enzymatic complex that cleaves C5. There have been no specific genetic defects or risk factors that have been linked to MPGN III.

Treatment

There is no clear consensus regarding the optimal therapy for patients with MPGN. Over the years, a host of therapeutic agents have been employed, including cyclophosphamide, aspirin, dipyramidole, nonsteroidal anti-inflammatory drugs (NSAIDS), cyclosporine, azathioprine, corticosteroids; and more recently tacrolimus, and mycophenolic acid. Almost without exception, reports of these treatment trials have been severely hampered by small sample sizes, heterogeneous patient populations, inclusion of patients who had received prior therapy, lack of adequate control populations, and very limited long-term follow-up. To date there has been only one randomized placebo controlled treatment trial in MPGN — the ISKDC study of alternate day high dose prednisone published in 1992. This study included 80 patients with biopsy proven MPGN treated for five years with 40 mg/m^2 on alternate days of prednisone or placebo control. At the end of the study, 33% of the prednisone treated group had failed therapy; defined as a 30% increase in serum creatinine above baseline or an absolute increase of 0.4 mg/dl. In comparison 55% of the placebo group had met criteria for treatment failure. While the response to prednisone of the MPGN cohort as a whole did not meet statistical significance ($p = 0.07$), subset analysis of the type I and type II patients suggested that they did have a significant response to prednisone therapy ($p = 0.035$). Studies by McEnery *et al.* have also supported the use of high dose alternative day prednisone (2 mg/kg on alternate days with a maximum of 80 mg for period of up to two years) in patients with MPGN. Over a period of decades, these uncontrolled treatment trials of all types of MPGN have reported an overall renal survival of 84% at 10 years and 54% at 20 years. More recent reports from the same group have raised questions as to the responsiveness of patients with MPGN II or III to this treatment regimen. The prolonged use of high-dose prednisone has been a matter of much controversy. A number of papers argue that the side effects of this therapy, growth failure, hypertension, and cataracts outweigh the benefits, and propose a more restricted and limited use of corticosteroids. Despite these reservations, corticosteroids remain the primary treatment modality in MPGN. Recently therapies directed toward the complement system have been proposed. These include the use of plasmapheresis, B cell immunomodulatory therapy to reduce nephritic factor production, and plasma infusion to replenish factor H deficiency. Currently, no treatment trials demonstrate the efficacy of these approaches. The use of conservative therapy common to all forms of progressive chronic kidney disease (CKD), such as angiotensin converting enzyme (ACE) inhibition or angiotensin II receptor blockade to reduce proteinuria and control blood pressure, has also been widely employed.

MPGN and Renal Transplantation

MPGN presents a difficult problem in renal transplantation. It became evident in the early 1970s that MPGN recurs with a very high frequency in renal transplants. For patients with MPGN I, rates of recurrence have ranged up to 50%, with graft failure rates from to recurrence as high as

27%. MPGN II has the highest reported recurrence rates with histologic disease recurrence approaching 100%. Allograft failure rates from MPGN II recurrence have varied from 0% to 38%. There is little data on recurrence or failure rates in MPGN III.

Suggested Reading

Andresdottir MB, Assmann KJ, Hoitsma AJ, *et al.* (1997) Recurrence of type I membranoproliferative glomerulonephritis after renal transplantation: analysis of the incidence, risk factors, and impact on graft survival. *Transplantation* **63**: 1628–1633.

Appel GB, Cook HT, Hageman G, *et al.* (2005) Membranoproliferative glomerulonephritis type II (dense deposit disease): an update. *J Am Soc Nephrol* **16**: 1392–1403.

Braun MC, Stablein DM, Hamiwka LA, *et al.* (2005) Recurrence of membranoproliferative glomerulonephritis type II in renal allografts: The North American Pediatric Renal Transplant Cooperative Study experience. *J Am Soc Nephrol* **16**: 2225–2233.

Braun MC, West CD, Strife CF. (1999) Differences between membranoproliferative glomerulonephritis types I and III in long-term response to an alternate-day prednisone regimen. *Am J Kidney Dis* **34**: 1022–1032.

Licht C, Fremeaux-Bacchi V. (2009) Hereditary and acquired complement dysregulation in membranoproliferative glomerulonephritis. *Thrombosis and haemostasis* **101**: 271–278.

McEnery PT, McAdams AJ, West CD. (1980) Membranoproliferative glomerulonephritis: improved survival with alternate day prednisone therapy. *Clin Nephrol* **13**: 117–124.

Smith RJ, Alexander J, Barlow PN, *et al.* (2007) New approaches to the treatment of dense deposit disease. *J Am Soc Nephrol* **18**: 2447–2456.

Tarshish P, Bernstein J, Tobin JN, Edelmann CM, Jr. (1992) Treatment of mesangiocapillary glomerulonephritis with alternate-day prednisone — a report of the International Study of Kidney Disease in Children. *Pediatr Nephrol* (Berlin) **6**: 123–130.

West CD. (1992) Idiopathic membranoproliferative glomerulonephritis in childhood. *Pediatri Nephrol* (Berlin) **6**: 96–103.

West CD. (1994) Nephritic factors predispose to chronic glomerulonephritis. *Am J Kidney Dis* **24**: 956–963.

18

Immunoglobulin A Nephropathy

Gaurav Kapur

Epidemiology

Immunoglobulin A nephropathy (IgAN; aka Berger disease) was first described in 1968 by Berger and Hinglais. It is currently recognized as the most common primary glomerulopathy accounting for nearly 10% of patients reaching end-stage renal disease (ESRD) in many countries. Of the primary glomerulopathies, IgAN is reported in nearly 50% of the cases in Asia (Japan, Singapore), and Australia (including New Zealand), 20–30% of primary glomerulopathies in Europe and 2–10% in North America. This difference could be related to genetic/environmental influence or difference in patient selection based on varying thresholds for renal biopsies. The latter is important as asymptomatic hematuria detected on routine urinalysis is further evaluated by a renal biopsy in Asian countries, which report a high incidence of IgAN. However, this is not the practice in North America. Nearly 3–16% of the patients without clinical symptoms of IgAN have renal biopsy features consistent with IgAN. Detailed characterization of this latent form is important for evaluating the underlying gene polymorphisms associated with IgAN. Also, this points to different processes/triggering factors accounting for IgA deposition in the kidney and glomerular injury.

Pathogenesis

IgAN is an immune complex disease characterized by circulating IgA immune complexes with a propensity for deposition in the renal mesangium. Subsequent course is influenced by various factors including genetics, removal of IgA complexes by the reticuloendothelial system and or mesangium, and the renal response to injury favoring glomerulosclerosis as compared to resolution without sequelae.

IgA deposits

Despite elevated serum levels of IgA (both monomeric, and polymeric), abnormalities of the IgA molecule may be primarily responsible for the disease. Alteration of the galactosylation of the hinge region leads to decreased hepatic clearance of the IgA molecule, increased tendency to self-aggregates, formation of antigen-antibody complexes (with antibodies directed against the hinge epitopes), and increased binding in the renal mesangium have been suggested as possible mechanisms leading to IgA localization within the renal mesangium.

Defective immunity

Hematuria episodes associated with upper respiratory tract infections, polymeric IgA1 deposits in the renal mesangium, presence of antibodies to dietary antigens, viral/bacterial antigens in IgAN patients, and association with gastrointestinal (GI), and respiratory tract syndromes, led to the hypothesis that abnormalities of mucosal immunity underlie IgAN. However, recent studies show that the overproduction of polymeric IgA1 may be secondary to an aberrant systemic, and not a mucosal, immune response to antigen exposure. IgAN patients have been found to have increased levels of IgA autoantibodies such as rheumatoid factor (about 50% of the patients), antinuclear antibodies, antimesangial cell antigens and anticollagen antibodies. Antirheumatoid factor may have a role in impaired solubilization; however, the increase may represent a polyspecific increase rather than true antigen specific autoimmunity.

The role of defective clearance of immune complexes is debatable as some investigators hypothesize that the defective clearance is more likely secondary increased immune complex load.

Glomerular injury

The mechanisms responsible for glomerular injury in IgAN are poorly understood. In the absence of marked cellular infiltration in IgAN, it is

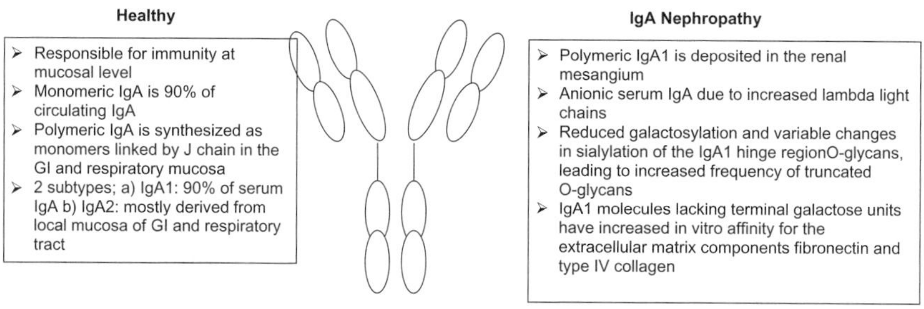

Figure 1. Immunoglobulin A facts: healthy children vs. patients with IgA nephropathy.

hypothesized that resident glomerular cells mediate glomerular injury. Polymeric IgA may elicit mesangial cell phenotypic transformation leading to cellular proliferation, and secretion of extracellular matrix component. In addition, polymeric IgA has a stimulatory effect on pro-inflammatory and pro-fibrotic molecules in the kidney. Immunoglobulin A is unable to activate the complement cascade, however polymeric mesangial IgA is hypothesized to activate the alternative complement system. This is based on demonstration of C3 in renal mesangium by immunohistology, and demonstration of the membrane attack complex.

Genetics

Family studies on IgAN patients have provided supportive evidence for importance of genetic factors in pathogenesis of IgAN. Various gene polymorphisms especially of the renin angiotensin system have been implicated; however the associations have been inconsistent.

Clinical Features

IgAN commonly occurs between the second and third decades of life. It is preponderant in males, with a male to female ratio of 2:1. Studies from Japan have reported a lower male age at diagnosis (9.3 years in boys and 10.3 years in girls) with a male to female ratio of 3:2.

Macroscopic hematuria is the most common initial presentation in nearly 50% of cases. These episodes are closely related to upper respiratory infection (URI), and hence also termed synpharyngitic nephritis. This contrasts with postinfectious glomerulonephritis wherein renal involvement occurs 2–3 weeks after the URI episode. Less commonly, hematuria may follow GI or urinary tract infection. In severe cases, acute nephritis may be associated with acute kidney failure.

Microscopic hematuria is the second most common clinical presentation (30–40%). In countries where routine urine screening is done in school-age children (e.g. Japan), microscopic hematuria, and asymptomatic proteinuria are the most common features. Recurrent gross hematuria is regarded as the hallmark of IgAN accounting for nearly 25% of the patient population; in these patients, microscopic hematuria, and proteinuria persist between episodes of gross hematuria.

Patients with nephritic or nephrotic syndrome at presentation have been reported to have the most severe glomerular damage. IgAN associated glomerular damage has been associated with a number of systemic diseases. These include Henoch–Schönlein purpura (HSP), celiac disease, dermatitis herpetiformis, HIV infection, Crohn disease, Reiter syndrome, and leprosy.

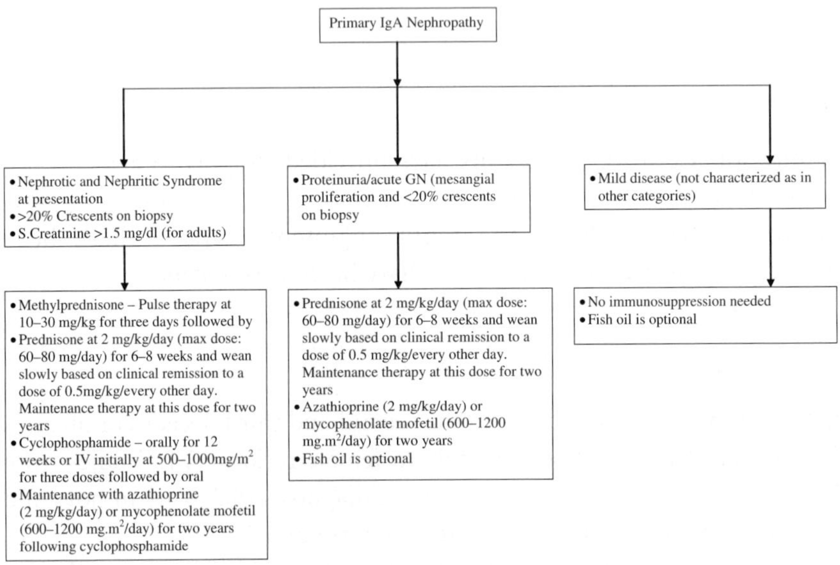

Figure 2. Proposed treatment for IgA nephropathy based on presentation.

HSP and IgAN

The relationship between IgAN and HSP nephritis is supported by reports of both disease entities in family members, including identical twins and occurrence of HSP in patients with biopsy proven IgAN. It has been suggested that HSP may be a systemic form of IgAN, or conversely IgAN is renal limited form of HSP. A better understanding of the factors involved in the deposition of IgA in the kidney will help in elucidating the heterogeneity in the clinical expression of IgA and HSP nephropathy patients.

Laboratory Investigations

No serologic or laboratory tests are diagnostic for IgAN. Raised IgA levels are not specific for IgAN, hence are not performed routinely. IgA-fibronectin complexes, which were initially thought to be significant for IgAN, have not been proven to be a clinically significant test for disease activity.

Serum complement levels, including C3, C4, C1q, and C2-9, are usually normal, but can be elevated. This is true despite the fact that complement activation occurs in this nephropathy as evidenced by elevated C3 fragments (50–70% of the patients) and C4 binding protein concentrations in renal biopsy samples. This suggests that the rate of complement production matches or exceeds its rate of consumption thereby resulting in normal serum levels.

The utility of skin biopsy in patients with IgAN is debatable. Sensitivity of 75% and specificity of 88% has been reported for detection of IgA in dermal capillaries of IgAN patients. It should be noted that dermal IgA along with C3, properdin and fibrin deposits have been reported in IgAN. By contrast, the presence of IgG and IgM in conjunction with IgA in dermal biopsy should raise the suspicion for other causes of glomerulopathy, such as lupus nephritis (LN).

The results of the urinalysis, serum chemistries, and renal function tests in children with IgAN are as expected based on the clinical presentation of the child. Namely, those with clinical nephrosis would be expected to have marked proteinuria likely with hematuria on urinalysis, and hypoalbuminemia, and those with acute nephritis would have hematuria/proteinuria, and possibly azotemia on laboratory assessment.

Pathology

Immunofluorescence microscopy

The definitive diagnosis of IgAN is confirmed by the presence of IgA as the predominant immunoglobulin by immunochemistry on renal biopsy. The glomerular staining pattern is usually in the mesangium with extension into the capillary walls, near the mesangiocapillary junction. Increasing deposits in the peripheral capillary walls have been associated with severe clinical manifestations and poor outcome. The presence of other antibodies (IgG [30%], IgM [8%)] or both [11%]) may be present in conjunction with IgA in a similar staining pattern, but with decreased intensity and frequency to that of IgA. C3 deposits are reported in similar distribution in 64% of the cases, while the earlier components of the complement (C4 or C1q) pathway are absent. Intense staining for earlier complement components should raise the possibility of LN rather than IgAN. A feature that appears to be distinct for IgAN is the more intense staining for lambda light chains than kappa light chains in comparison to other glomerulopathies.

Light microscopy

Mesangial enlargement due to mesangial cell proliferation and increased mesangial cell matrix is characteristic, and the most common finding of IgAN. Mesangial hypercellularity is usually seen in initial biopsies in comparison to increased mesangial matrix; the latter is found in instances associated with a long interval between disease onset and renal biopsy. The histological variability of IgAN has prompted various classification systems (see Table 1), mainly with an aim to predict renal survival. These classification systems have been shown to be clinically relevant, and that chosen by renal pathologists is more due to personal preference rather than superiority of one system over another.

Electron microscopy

The most common characteristic feature of IgAN is electron deposits in the mesangium. These are commonly located at the interface of the glomerular basement membrane with the mesangial matrix (paramesangium).

Table 1. Proposed histological classification systems for IgA nephropathy

WHO Classification	Classification by Lee	Classification by Haas
1. Minimal glomerular lesions • Mostly normal glomeruli with a few showing increased mesangial matrix • Mesangial cells per peripheral mesangial are <3 • Small foci of tubular atrophy and interstitial infiltrate in some patients	Grade I • Mostly normal glomeruli with occasional mesangial thickening with or without hypercellularity • No tubulointerstitial changes	Class 1: Minimal histologic lesion • Glomeruli only show minimal increase in mesangial cellularity without necrosis, crescents, or sclerosis
	Grade II • <50% of glomeruli with localized mesangial proliferation • Rare small crescents • No tubulointerstitial changes	Class II: Focal segmental glomerulosclerosis-like • Glomeruli have focal and segmental sclerosis with minimal increase in mesangial cellularity and no crescents
2. Focal mesangial proliferation • Up to 80% glomeruli with moderate to severe mesangial proliferation (>3 cells per peripheral mesangial area) • Crescents <20% of the glomeruli (segmental capillary collapse is usually associated) • Tubulointerstitial changes in form of atrophy, fibrosis and infiltration are frequent but not extensive • Capsular adhesions are frequent with crescents	Grade III • Diffuse mesangial proliferation with focal and segmental variation • Occasional small crescents and adhesions • Focal interstitial edema and infiltrate rare tubular atrophy	Class III: Focal proliferative glomerulonephritis • Hypercellularity in ≤50% glomeruli (includes mesangial, or endocapillary hypercellularity, crescents, or necrosis) • Usually segmental; however, global hypercellularity may be present as long as ≤ glomeruli involved
3. Diffuse mesangial proliferation • >80% glomeruli with moderate to severe mesangial proliferation • Crescents <50% of the glomeruli • Frequent tubulointerstitial changes and extensive in 10% of the patients • Capsular adhesions may be present without crescents	Grade IV • Marked diffuse mesangial changes • Crescents <45% of glomeruli • Tubular atrophy, interstitial inflammation and occasional foam cells	Class IV: Diffuse proliferative glomerulonephritis • Similar to class III but >50% of the glomeruli are involved
	Grade V • Similar to IV, but crescents in >45% of glomeruli • More severe tubulointerstitial changes	Class V: Advanced chronic glomerulonephritis • Global sclerosis in 40% or more glomeruli and/or >40% estimated tubular atrophy or loss in cortex • If class V criteria are met, then biopsy is graded as such regardless of other histologic features

These deposits have uniform density with no specific substructure. Peripheral glomerular capillary deposits (nearly 30% of the patients) may be noticed in the subendothelial (more common), and subepithelial regions.

Treatment

Currently there is no disease specific treatment option or consensus on treatment of IgAN. Due to this, patient selection for the available treatment options is of paramount importance. This is guided by the reported prognostic factors and potential for cumulative toxicity of the treatment agent given the chronic ongoing nature of IgAN. Patients with poor prognostic factors (see Table 2) on presentation are at risk for chronic kidney disease and worse prognosis and therefore most appropriate candidates for immunosuppressive treatments. Of the prognostic factors listed in Table 2, tubulointerstitial scarring is the strongest predictor, and also the one that has been shown to independently predict progression to end-stage renal disease (ESRD). Hence, the classification systems as proposed by Lee, Haas, and WHO are not good independent predictors of ESRD progression as they focus more on glomerular pathology. Currently efforts are underway to establish a consensus histopathologic classification of IgAN, which is a better predictor of renal outcome than those in current use.

Table 2. Poor prognostic factors in IgA nephropathy

Clinical and Laboratory Features

- Elevated serum creatinine >2.5 mg/dl
- Hypertension usually associated with proteinuria and biopsy changes of arteriosclerosis and tubulointerstitial injury
- Persistent proteinuria >500–1000 mg/day

Histological Features of progression

- Most common; glomerulosclerosis and tubulointerstitial disease
- Immune deposits in capillary loops and mesangium
- Crescent formation
- Vascular disease

Acute kidney injury with gross hematuria, with a renal biopsy showing IgA nephropathy with segmental crescents only (<25% glomeruli involved) with marked acute tubular necrosis (ATN): This is considered benign as the severe renal failure is secondary to ATN due to RBC casts, and patients improve with supportive treatment alone.

Routine immunofluorescence and electron microscopy findings have little value in predicting clinical outcome.

The treatment options available for IgAN can be broadly divided into two categories: 1) Immunosuppressive/cytotoxic agents and 2) Nonimmunosuppressive agents

1) Immunosuppressive agents
    - Corticosteroids: The use of corticosteroids is restricted to patients with evidence of inflammation (hematuria, and persistent proteinuria with a renal biopsy showing proliferative and necrotizing glomerulonephritis). Patients with mild/stable IgAN or renal biopsy showing chronic damage with severe tubulointersitial damage, and glomerulosclerosis are not candidates for chronic steroid therapy owing to potential toxicity.
    - Cyclophophamide: Cyclophophamide in IgAN is used along with steroids for patients with crescentic nephritis or moderate to severe disease activity on kidney biopsy.
    - Azathioprine/Mycophenolate mofetil: These are used for maintenance immunosuppression (up to 1–2 years) for patients receiving combined immunosuppression with steroids and cyclophosphamide once the serum creatinine has stabilized and proteinuria has decreased. They may also be used in patients with persistent proteinuria not responding to nonimmunosuppressive agents (see below).
2) Nonimmunosuppressive treatment options
    - Angiotensin-converting enzyme (ACE) inhibitors/angiotensin receptor blockers (ARB): They are primarily used for reducing proteinuria and management of hypertension (preferred antihypertensive agents), thereby minimizing secondary glomerular injury. These agents may also be used as the only treatment options for patients with stable renal function and mild proteinuria. ARB is usually started after an ACE inhibitor for additional antiproteinuric effect.
    - Fish oil: Currently the benefit of antiinflammatory properties of fish oil for IgAN has not been established.
    - Tonsillectomy: This has been proposed as a possible option for IgAN patients as tonsils are considered the source of abnormal IgA

secondary to tonsillitis. Retrospective reports suggest possibly improved renal survival in patients undergoing tonsillectomy in addition to immunosuppressive therapy. However, in view of lack of randomized trials and reports of no benefit with tonsillectomy, the same is not routinely done in IgAN patients. Currently its use is guided by individual preferences or institutional protocols.

- Low antigen diet: The rationale for a diet low in gluten, dairy, and eggs meats is to decrease the activation of the gastrointestinal IgA. This has been reported by a single study and the benefits have not been confirmed by others.

Prognosis

Overall better outcomes have been reported for children with IgAN compared to adults. The most likely explanation for this is earlier diagnosis during disease course in children, unlike adults. Studies from Japan (n = 169) have reported chronic renal failure in 9% of the pediatric patients over a follow up period of 15 years. Two studies from USA have reported 1) 15% ESRD in IgAN patients followed for at least four years (n = 80) and 2) actuarial renal survival of 87% at ten years and 70% at 20 years.

Retrospective studies have reported recurrence rate of 21–58% of IgAN allograft biopsies secondary to graft dysfunction, and a graft loss rate of 46–71% in patients with graft dysfunction secondary to recurrent IgA. Due to genetic factors implicated in pathogenesis of IgAN, concerns have been raised about donor source for renal transplant in IgAN patients. Current evidence does not suggest poor graft survival in living related donors of patients with ESRD secondary to IgAN and the same is not contraindicated. Recurrence of IgAN in the transplanted kidney does not preclude subsequent renal transplantation.

Suggested Reading

Haas M. (2007) IgAN and Henoch–Schonlein purpura nephritis. In: Jennette JC OJ, Schwartz MM, Silva FG. (eds.) *Heptinstall's Pathology of the Kidney*, Lippincott, Williams and Wilkins, Philadelphia. pp. 423–486.

Julian B. (2001) IgAN and related disorders. In: Greenberg A. (ed.) *Primer on Kidney Diseases*, 3rd ed., Academic Press, San Diego. pp. 165–167.

Yoshikawa N. (2004) Immunoglobulin A nephropathy. In: Avner ED, Harmon WE, Niaudet P. (eds.) *Pediatric Nephrology*, 5th ed., Lippincott, Williams and Wilkins, Philadelphia. pp. 615–628.

19

Alport Syndrome

Gaurav Kapur

Alport Syndrome (AS) is an inherited disorder of basement membrane collagen characterized by involvement of the kidneys (always), ears (often), and eyes (occasionally). This form of inherited nephritis with sensorineural hearing loss was first described by Cecil Alport, in a family in which affected males died in adolescence. AS is a heterogenous disorder phenotypically, secondary to the genetic and molecular heterogeneity of the inherited collagen defect.

Prevalence

The estimated gene frequency for collagen IV mutation associated with AS is 1:5000. AS accounts for nearly 1% of end-stage renal disease (ESRD) in Europe and approximately 2% in the US. However, this may be an underestimation due to the diagnostic difficulties associated with AS.

Pathogenesis

Collagen IV, the major structural component of all basement membranes is composed of hetrotrimers (protomers) of α chains. Six distinct genes encoding for α chains have been identified. These are located in pairs on the chromosomes 13q34 (COL4A1, COL4A2), 2q35 (COL4A3, COL4A4) and Xq22 (COL4A5, COL4A6). Gene defects of α chain lead to impaired/abnormal protomer assembly, which subsequently leads to the phenotypic features characteristic for AS. Mutations in COL4A5 result in X-linked dominant AS; while COL4A3 or COL4A4 mutations lead to autosomal recessive or dominant AS, respectively.

Clinical Features

X-linked dominant AS

This is the inheritance pattern seen in nearly 85% of the AS families and usually presents with family history of hematuric nephritis associated with ESRD and progressive hearing loss.

Hematuria

This universal symptom of AS is usually detected in childhood or even at birth. In one series ($n = 58$), nearly 74% of the patients had manifestation of hematuria by the age of six years. Patients without macroscopic hematuria may be detected with microscopic hematuria in adulthood only. Male patients have worse prognosis with progression to ESRD either by age 20 years (juvenile type) or ESRD by age of 40 years or higher (non-progressive, or adult type). The differentiation between the two groups is not usually possible. The progression to chronic kidney disease (CKD) is characterized by increasing proteinuria with worsening nephritis and development of hypertension in later stages of renal dysfunction. Female patients have variable clinical course secondary to random inactivation of the X-chromosome. Hematuria (usually microscopic) is detected in almost all female carriers with asymptomatic carriers being rare. Proteinuria (75% in one series of AS) may be absent, mild or intermittent and may increase with age. It is difficult to predict renal survival in female members of the families with AS; however, presence of gross hematuria in childhood, increasing proteinuria with development of nephrotic syndrome, presence of hearing loss, and diffusely thickened glomerular basement membrane (GBM) on renal biopsy are associated with worse prognosis. The risk of progression appears to increase after 60 years of age in female patients.

Bilateral hearing loss (sensorineural) in AS is not congenital and develops over the first decade, with boys being more severely affected. Some AS families with progressive nephritis having no hearing loss have been identified as COL4A5 mutation variants.

AS has been associated with ocular changes involving the lens, retina, and cornea. Progressive anterior lenticonus is more common in male patients and exceptionally rare in female patients. Asymptomatic perimacular yellowish flecks in the retina and nonspecific corneal lesion have also been reported. Leiomyomas are benign tumors of the visceral smooth muscle, have been reported in 2–5% of patients and carriers of AS, and are associated with distinct mutation of the COL4A5-COL4A6 genes. Diffuse leiomyomatosis when present is fully penetrant in female patients, unlike AS. The association of AS, mental retardation, midface hypoplasia, and elliptocytosis is now recognized as X-linked contiguous gene syndrome.

Autosomal recessive AS

Autosomal recessive AS accounts for around 15% of the AS cases and is associated with homozygous or heterozygous mutations involving COL4A3 or COL4A4. Clinical features of autosomal recessive AS are similar to X-linked dominant AS. Severe disease in females, history of consanguinity in the family, and hematuria in the father of an affected male patient are indicative of autosomal recessive inheritance. Progression to ESRD and hearing impairment is constant and present in both sexes in these patients. The heterozygote carriers have a broad spectrum ranging from asymptomatic, persistent hematuria to ESRD in some patients.

Autosomal dominant AS

Autosomal dominant AS account for nearly 5% of the AS cases and is characterized by similar disease severity in both male and female patients. The disease phenotype is milder in autosomal dominant patients with ESRD usually occurring after 50 years. Audiologic manifestations are common though late (like ESRD), while ocular involvement is rare.

Renal Biopsy

Light microscopy

Renal biopsies obtained early in the course of AS, show normal glomeruli, or minimal change with podocyte hypertrophy, irregular mesangial stalk enlargement, and focal thickening of the GBM. Thickening of the capillary walls becomes more prominent with disease progression. Progression is associated with increasing thickening of the GBM and the mesangial stalk, associated with hyaline deposits and collapse of the capillary walls. These progress to complete sclerosis and hyalinosis of the glomerular tuft.

Immunoflorescence microscopy

Immunoflorescent staining using antibodies to immunoglobulins and complement proteins is usually negative. Disease progression is associated with focal deposits of IgM, C3 or C1q (nonspecific and no prognostic value).

Electron microscopy

Changes in GBM observed on electron microscopy (EM) are characteristic of AS. The typical lesion seen on EM is the thickening of GBM with splitting and fragmentation. Splitting and fragmentation of the GBM increases with age, and may not be present in young male patients. In these patients, AS can be identified by absence or abnormal distribution of immunostaining with α 3, 4, or 5 type IV collagen.

Diagnosis of AS

Family history of renal failure and deafness raises the suspicion for AS. The diagnosis can be confirmed by genetic testing, or biopsy (renal or skin).

Genetic testing

Molecular genetic testing of the COL4A5 gene is challenging due to the large size of the gene, and the high GC content of genomic DNA. Because identification of the mutation may provide helpful prognostic information, it is often pursued. Some of these challenges can be overcome by analysis of the mRNA, which can be obtained from skin/hair roots allowing for a relatively noninvasive method for diagnosing AS. Information on molecular testing for AS is available at www.genereviews.org. Molecular testing is indicated in prenatal diagnosis of AS, in patients with renal failure wherein family and pedigree history in inconclusive for inheritance patterns, and patients with nonconfirmatory biopsies.

Skin biopsy using commercially available monoclonal antibody against $\alpha 5$ collagen IV subtype is a less invasive method of diagnosing X-linked AS compared to renal biopsy. The skin biopsy should demonstrate complete absence of protein in a male and a mosaic/uneven distribution in a female. In cases of suspected AS in whom $\alpha 5$ collagen IV subtype protein is detected on skin biopsy, further testing in the form of renal biopsy or genetic testing as indicated will be required.

Differential Diagnosis

Thin basement membrane nephropathy

Thin basement membrane nephropathy (TBMN) describes the ultrastructual finding of diffuse attenuation of GBM (normal width 300 nm–400 nm, in TBMN 150 nm–225 nm) on EM in patients with persistent microscopic hematuria. The major clinical presentation is asymptomatic microscopic hematuria, with no/minimal proteinuria and no hypertension. The long-term prognosis is excellent with TBMN; however, slowly progressive renal failure has been reported in a small percentage. Some of these have been identified has having sporadic AS. In other patients, poor prognosis with TBMN has been linked to positive family history of renal failure, and presence of proteinuria. Studies have shown that these patients are more likely to have focal segmental glomerulosclerosis. Therefore, the recent recommendations are to follow up patients with asymptomatic microscopic hematuria, and suspected TBMN, to detect patients with progressive nephritis.

Epstein and Fechtner syndromes

These autosomal dominant disorders are characterized by hereditary nephritis, deafness and macrothrombocytopenia (Epstein). Fechtner syndrome in addition has leukocyte inclusions (blue) and cataracts. Initially considered as variants of AS due to similar EM findings in GBM (focal usually), these are now recognized as distinct entities, with normal immunostaining for type IV collagen and mutations for gene encoding for nonmuscle myosin (mapped to chromosome 22).

Management

There is no definite management of AS. Supportive measures to manage progressive CKD, such as management of hypertension, anemia, hyperphosphatemia, and acidosis are indicated. Patients with severe proteinuria usually benefit from angiotensin blockade (additional blood pressure control). The benefit of cyclosporine in reducing proteinuria, and retarding progression of renal failure has not been conclusively proven, and as such is not routinely indicated. Invariably the patients progress to ESRD, requiring dialysis and renal transplantation. It is important to note that approximately 3% of AS patients develop anti-GBM nephritis following renal transplantation. Overall, renal transplantation has an excellent prognosis in AS.

Suggested Reading

Clinical manifestations, diagnosis and treatment of hereditary nephritis (Alport syndrome). [URL: http://www.uptodate.com/online/content/topic]

Gregory MC. (2001) Alport's Syndrome and related disorders. In: Greenberg A. (ed.) *Primer on Kidney Diseases*, 3rd ed. Academic Press, San Diego. pp. 308–312.

Gubler MC, Heidet L, Antignac C. (2007) Alports syndrome, thin basement membrane nephropathy, Nail-Patella syndrome, and type III collagen nephropathy. In: Jennette JC, Schwartz MM, Silva FG (eds.) *Heptinstall's Pathology of the Kidney*, Lippincott, Williams and Wilkins, Philadelphia. pp. 488–515.

Part VI

Glomerulopathies Associated with Systemic Disease

20

Systemic Lupus Erythematosus

Elahna Paul and Michael J.G. Somers

Introduction

Systemic lupus erythematosus (SLE) is an autoimmune disorder caused by a complex array of environmental and genetic factors dysregulating the immune system leading to both systemic and organ-specific disease. Autoantibodies and antigen-antibody immune complexes are prominent features of the disease and are at least partly responsible for inflammatory changes that produce the diagnostic signs and symptoms of SLE including lupus nephritis (LN) (see Table 1).

The annual worldwide incidence of SLE ranges from 0.5–9 cases per 100,000 individuals, depending on the group at risk. Adult onset SLE is nearly ten times more common in females than in males, and approximately three times more common in African American than Caucasian American females. Higher rates are also found in Asian and Hispanic females. Lupus related mortality from renal failure, infections and extrarenal disease manifestations reaches 10–20% by 5–10 years after diagnosis.

A range of 20–80% of SLE patients manifest overt renal disease that has been associated with increased long-term morbidity and mortality. Moreover, approximately 2–4% of all end-stage renal disease (ESRD) in the U.S. is attributed to SLE. The actual prevalence of LN may be even higher since up to 90–95% of biopsy specimens in multiple studies have shown histologic changes. Such "silent" nephritis underscores how urinary changes are not a prerequisite for renal disease. Additionally, some patients present with lupus-like nephritis years before they meet American College of Rheumatology (ACR) criteria for SLE.

Childhood onset accounts for 20% of all SLE cases, most commonly diagnosed in adolescence, and rarely before five years of age. The marked

Table 1. American College of Rheumatology (ACR) criteria for the diagnosis of SLE. A diagnosis of SLE requires a minimum of 4 of 11 criteria to be present either simultaneously or serially during any period of observation.

1.	Malar rash	fixed malar erythema, flat or raised, usually with sparing of nasolabial folds
2.	Discoid rash	raised erythematous patches with keratotic scaling and follicular plugging
3.	Photosensitivity	skin rash in reaction to sunlight
4.	Mucocutaneous ulcers	oral or nasal; usually painless
5.	Arthritis	nonerosive; involving two or more peripheral joints
6.	Serositis	pleuritis or pericarditis
7.	Renal disorder	cellular casts or persistent proteinuria >3 + by dipstick or >0.5 g/day
8.	Neurologic disorder	seizures or psychosis (in absence of other causes)
9.	Hematologic disorder	hemolytic anemia or leukopenia (WBC <4000 at least twice) or lymphopenia (<1500 at least twice) or thrombocytopenia (<100,000 in absence of offending drugs)
10.	Immunologic disorder	anti-dsDNA antibodies or anti-Sm[a] antibodies or antiphospholipid antibodies(via anticardiolipin titers or positive lupus anticoagulant or false-positive VRDL[b])
11.	Antinuclear antibody	abnormal ANA titer[c] in the absence of drugs associated with a drug induced lupus syndrome

[a] dsDNA and Sm are the autospecificities most strongly associated with lupus nephritis.
[b] False-positive VRDL is associated with lupus anticoagulant (antiphospholipid/anticardiolipin autoantibody) which gives prolonged PTT in the lab but thrombosis and consumptive thrombocytopenia in the patient.
[c] Highly sensitive but not specific; the higher the titer the more specific.

female gender predilection in adults is reduced in adolescents (five females for each male) and in prepubertal children (two females for each male). Pediatric onset SLE is often more aggressive than adult disease, partly due to increased renal involvement. Approximately 20–50% of children with lupus nephritis progress to ESRD.

Pathogenesis

The autoimmunity of SLE manifests as excessive production of abnormal antibodies specific for nuclear and cytoplasmic antigens that become extracellularly exposed to the immune system primarily during apoptotic cell death (see Table 2). When autoantibodies bind to their antigens, they form multimeric immune complexes that precipitate and trigger local inflammatory responses. When immune complexes deposit either within or around glomerular capillaries, they activate intra-renal inflammation in

Table 2. Lupus laboratory evaluations

Chemistries	Routine chemistries will help evaluate for acute and/or chronic renal insufficiency.
Hematology	Check CBC with differential to assess the status of cellular lineages, any of which may be depressed due to autoantibodies. Thrombocytopenia may also point to thrombotic microangiopathy and anemia may be an indicator of chronic renal dysfunction.
Acute phase reactants	ESR and CRP are often elevated with lupus activity.
Complement	C3 and C4 are often both depressed in active disease.
IgM, IgG, IgA	Generalized hypergammaglobulinemia is a common feature of lupus; isolated IgA elevation is not.
ANA	Antinuclear antibody titers are nonspecifically elevated in >95% of patients with SLE and also in patients with other inflammatory conditions. A homogeneous nuclear ANA staining pattern correlates with a specificity for dsDNA which is more suggestive of lupus.
Anti-DNA antibodies	Autoantibodies specific for double stranded DNA (dsDNA, native DNA) are elevated in 40–90% of patients with SLE and are often associated with lupus nephritis. In contrast to ANAs, anti-DNA antibodies are fairly specific for SLE.
Antihistone antibodies	Elevated antihistone titers are seen in drug induced lupus (e.g. hydralazine, procainamide). This specificity is not routinely tested in many centers.
Antiriboprotein antibodies	Elevated anti-Sm titers are rare (<30% of patients) but are fairly specific for lupus nephritis. Autoantibodies against Ro (SSA) La (SSB) are associated with neonatal lupus and antibodies to RNP are associated with lupus-like syndromes, sometimes referred to as mixed connective tissue diseases.
Anticardiolipin antibodies	These antiphospholipid antibodies (once known as lupus anticoagulants) are elevated in 25–50% of SLE patients and are associated with antiphospholipid syndrome and thrombotic microangiopathy.

Note: The presence of specific autoantibodies contributes to a diagnosis of SLE but the rise and fall of autoantibody titers does not reliably correlate with disease activity.

a number of ways. Not only do glomerular immune complexes trigger the complement cascade and recruit inflammatory infiltrates, but they also directly activate glomerular cells to proliferate, elaborate extracellular matrix, and further secrete pro-inflammatory chemokines and cytokines. Acute inflammation can be associated with acute kidney injury (AKI). Progressive or recurrent glomerular inflammation can lead to fibrosis and glomerular sclerosis with evolution of chronic kidney disease (CKD) and eventual ESRD.

The source of the pathogenic autoantibodies remains unclear and the complexity of the immune system makes multiple etiologies plausible. For instance, some individuals prone to SLE have hyperactive B cells or abnormal regulatory T cells so autoimmune responses are easily triggered or poorly silenced. Others may have difficulty processing apoptotic debris safely or problems distinguishing apoptotic self antigens from similar nucleic acid, protein, and lipid antigens also found in pro-inflammatory micro-organisms. Genetic risk factors associated with SLE include mutations or polymorphisms altering extracellular molecules or their receptors (e.g. complement proteins, cytokines, Fc receptors) or cytoplasmic signaling molecules or nuclear transcription factors within professional immune cells (e.g. B cells, T cells, antigen presenting cells) or within resident renal cells. Environmental risk factors include allergic reactions and microbial infections that activate the immune system and trigger inflammatory cascades. Until specific pathogenic mechanisms are better understood so that preventive measures can be implemented, SLE therapy relies on fairly broad immunosuppressive or cytotoxic agents to induce remission, prevent ongoing renal injury and slow progression to ESRD.

Diagnosis

Although SLE is often diagnosed by a rheumatologist, nephrologists may diagnose the condition, especially when the patient presents primarily with renal findings. Exceedingly rare in pre-school–aged children, LN should be considered in any pediatric patient presenting with overt glomerulonephritis, and especially in adolescent girls. LN more commonly presents with microscopic hematuria or low-grade proteinuria and less commonly with macroscopic hematuria, hypertension, nephrosis, or AKI.

There may be a component of noneosinophilic interstitial nephritis, or rarely, an overt tubulopathy. Catastrophic presentation with rapidly progressive glomerulonephritis is rare, and concomitant antiphospholipid antibody mediated microangiopathy should be considered, especially in the setting of thrombocytopenia.

For a new patient, the history and physical should encompass the ACR diagnostic criteria for SLE (see Table 1) and should be used in conjunction with urine microscopy to guide further laboratory testing. Urine protein should be quantified. Laboratory screening for electrolytes, BUN, creatinine, albumin, CBC with differential, ESR, complement C3, C4, total immunoglobulins, and ANA is warranted when lupus is part of the differential diagnosis. While no single laboratory test is diagnostic, a patient with a normal C3 complement level is not likely to have active lupus nephritis. If lupus is strongly suspected at presentation (e.g. 15-year-old girl with hypertension and cellular casts), or following initial evaluation (e.g. hypocomplementemia and hypergammaglobulinemia), or if the renal acuity is high (e.g. active sediment and renal impairment), then additional evaluation would include testing for antidouble stranded DNA (dsDNA), antiSm and other autoantibodies (see Table 2).

Not only are autoantibody and complement measurements important in the general diagnosis of SLE, but anti-dsDNA and antiSm antibodies in particular have been associated with LN. Furthermore, serial serologic testing is often used to monitor disease activity because rising autoantibody titers and falling complement levels may precede renal flares. It is critical to realize, however, that titers rise just as often without a renal flare, and patients can flare without serologic warning. While serologic evaluation contributes to the overall assessment of a patient's lupus activity (along with nonspecific markers of inflammation, such as ESR, or CRP), it should never drive the management of lupus nephritis in the absence of explicit renal findings.

If necessary, screening for other immune mediated nephritides such as antiglomerular basement membrane (GBM) disease, antineutrophil cytoplasmic antibody (ANCA)-positive disease or postinfectious glomerulonephritis, hepatitis B or C, HIV or can help eliminate or indirectly corroborate a diagnosis of LN. Renal imaging contributes little diagnostically, often revealing diffuse, nonspecific increase in parenchymal echogenicity with loss of corticomedullary differentiation. All children with lupus should be comprehensively evaluated by a pediatric rheumatologist for extrarenal manifestations of SLE.

Renal Biopsy

Renal biopsies are indispensable for diagnosing lupus nephritis, assessing renal prognosis, and guiding medical management both at initial presentation and in event of treatment failure, or subsequent renal flare. However, a single tissue core may not always reflect the complete histopathology and biopsy findings are only a histologic snapshot in a continuous disease process that changes readily over time.

Light microscopy

H&E, PAS, trichrome and silver stains are commonly used to evaluate LN. The glomerular and extraglomerular lesions visible by light microscopy are often scored for activity and chronicity in a standardized semiquantitative manner (see Tables 3 and 4). Patients with high activity indices are at risk for progressive CKD but have reasonable chances of responding to

Table 3. Activity and chronicity of renal lesions

	Activity Index	Scoring	Chronicity Index	Scoring
Glomerular lesions	cellular proliferation	0–3	glomerular sclerosis	0–3
	cellular crescents	(0–3) × 2	fibrous crescents	0–3
	necrosis/ karyorrhexis	(0–3) × 2		
	hyaline thrombi/ wire loops	0–3		
	leukocyte infiltration	0–3		
Tubulointerstitial lesions	leukocyte infiltration	0–3	tubular atrophy	0–3
	interstitial	0–3		
			fibrosis	
Possible scores		0–24		0–12

Table 4. Histologic terminology

Active lesions	**Glomerular:** endocapillary hypercellularity (proliferative or inflammatory); crescents (cellular or fibrocellular); subendothelial deposits (identifiable as wire loops by light microscopy);intracapillary hyaline thrombi; karyorrhexis; necrosis; GBM* rupture **Tubulointerstitial:** tubulitis; degeneration/ necrosis; inflammation (mostly T cells and monocytes) **Vascular:** hyaline deposits/ thrombi; necrotizing arteritis; microangiopathy (associated with antiphospholipid antibodies)
Cellular crescents	Proliferation of at least three epithelial cell layers lining Bowman's capsule and occupying at least one fourth of the glomerular capsular circumference
Chronic lesions	**Glomerular:** glomerular sclerosis (segmental or global); fibrous adhesions to Bowman's capsule; fibrous crescents **Tubulointerstitial:** tubular atrophy, fibrosis **Vascular:** sclerosis
Diffuse lesions	Lesions involving ≥50% of all glomeruli
Endocapillary proliferation	Endocapillary hypercellularity due to proliferation of mesangial and Endothelial cells with narrowing the glomerular capillary lumina
Extracapillary proliferation	See cellular crescents
Exudative lesions	Leukocyte infiltration/inflammation
Focal lesions	Lesions involving <50% of all glomeruli
Global lesion	A lesion involving more than half of a glomerular tuft
Hyaline thrombi	Intracapillary homogeneous eosinophilic material (luminal immune deposits)
Karyorrhexis	Apoptotic, pyknotic and fragmented nuclei
Mesangial hypercellularity	≥3 mesangial cells per mesangial region in a 3-micron thick section
Necrosis	Nuclear fragmentation and/or GBM disruption associated with fibrin-rich material
Segmental lesion	A lesion involving less than half of a glomerular tuft
Wire loops	Light microscope appearance of GBM thickened by subendothelial deposits

* GBM glomerular basement membrane

immunosuppressive and cytotoxic therapy. In contrast, high chronicity scores are associated with a worse long-term course because these lesions generally denote irreversible changes that remain unaffected by standard therapies currently in use.

Immunofluorescence microscopy

The composition of immune deposits is determined by staining tissue sections with fluorescently tagged antibodies. Immunostaining is usually performed for IgM, IgG and IgA immunoglobulins and for complement components C3 and C1q. A glomerular staining pattern positive for all five of these reactivities is sometimes referred to as a "full house" and is pathognomonic for LN. Additional immunoreagents can identify kappa and lambda immunoglobulin light chains, as well as albumin and fibrin in glomerular deposits. Tubular deposits are also fairly common but are not part of the histologic classification system.

Electron microscopy

Electron microscopy (EM) is most useful for localizing immune complexes within mesangial, subendothelial and subepithelial regions of the glomerular tuft, which is important for histologic classification. Furthermore, dual presence of subendothelial and subepithelial deposits is diagnostic of LN, as is visualization of tubulo-reticular structures within glomerular endothelial cells which are detected almost exclusively in SLE, and in HIV nephropathy.

Histologic classification

The World Health Organization (WHO) first standardized the histologic classification of LN over three decades ago. Shown to correlate with prognosis, the WHO classification system became an essential tool in diagnosis and management. Most recently updated in 2003 by joint proceedings of the International Society of Nephrology (ISN) and the Renal Pathology Society (RPS), the ISN/RPS 2003 classification system primarily considers glomerular pathology. The location of mesangial, subendothelial, and/or

Table 5. ISN/RPS 2003 histologic classification of lupus nephritis (LN)

Class I:	**Minimal mesangial LN**	
Class II:	**Mesangial proliferative LN**	
Class III:	**Focal LN** (involving <50% of all glomeruli)*	
	Class III(A): Active lesions	
	Class III(C): Chronic lesions	
	Class III(A/C): Active and chronic lesions	
Class IV:	**Diffuse LN** (involving ≥50% of all glomeruli)*	
	Diffuse segmental LN	Diffuse global LN
	Class IV-S(A): Active lesions	IV-G (A): Active lesions
	Class IV-S(C): Chronic lesions	IV-G (C): Chronic lesions
	Class IV-S(A/C): Active and chronic lesions	IV-G (A/C): Active and chronic lesions
Class V:	**Membranous LN** (+/− class III or class IV)	
Class VI:	**Advanced sclerosing LN**	

* The pathology report is meant to indicate the proportion of glomeruli with active lesions, sclerotic lesions, fibrinoid necrosis and cellular crescents.

subepithelial immune complex deposits is particularly important (see Table 5). Tubulointerstitial and vascular lesions are also graded as mild, moderate, or severe in all LN biopsy evaluations.

Mesangial cell injury resulting in mesangial matrix expansion and mesangial cell proliferation predominates in LN classes I and II. Cellular casts are rare and GFR is usually normal. In terms of specific histologic features:

- Class I (minimal mesangial LN) has normal glomeruli by light microscopy, but mesangial immune deposits can be seen by IF and EM.
- Class II (mesangial proliferative LN) is notable for mesangial hypercellularity by light microscopy with neither global nor segmental glomerular scars. The mesangial lesions may be focal or diffuse. There are mesangial immune deposits by IF and EM, and rare subepithelial or subendothelial deposits may be visible exclusively by IF, or EM but not by light microscopy.

In classes III and IV, endothelial cell injury predominates and is associated with inflammatory infiltrates and endocapillary proliferation, with or without extracapillary proliferation or crescents. Focal subendothelial immune deposits seen by IF and EM can appear as wire loops by light microscopy. Mesangial alterations usually accompany these lesions. Specific differences between these classes include:

- Class III (focal proliferative and/or sclerosing LN) involves <50% of glomeruli. Usually segmental, the focal lesions of class III are characterized as active (A) or chronic (C) or both (A/C).
- Class IV (diffuse proliferative and/or sclerosing LN) involves ≥50% of glomeruli and is subclassified as either diffuse segmental (IV-S) or diffuse global (IV-G) when ≥50% of the involved glomeruli have segmental lesions or global lesions, respectively. The diffuse lesions are characterized as active (A), or chronic (C), or both (A/C).

Epithelial cell injury predominates in LN class V where histologic lesions are usually nonproliferative and noninflammatory. Epithelial cell injury is clinically associated with nephrotic range proteinuria. Specific histologic features include:

- Class V (membranous LN) is characterized by subepithelial immune deposits, either segmental or global, that are visible by light, IF, and electron microscopy, with or without mesangial alterations.
- A dual diagnosis of class III + V or IV + V is made if there are either focal, or diffuse subendothelial deposits, or residual scars from prior proliferative, necrotizing, or crescentic lesions in addition to subepithelial deposits that involve ≥50% of the glomerular tuft in ≥50% of all glomeruli.

Class VI (advanced sclerosing LN) is diagnosed only when ≥90% of glomeruli are globally sclerosed without active lesions.

Prognosis

Renal survival in SLE depends largely on the histologic class. Proliferative disease carries the worst renal prognosis in a "dose dependent" manner such that LN class IV is worse than class III, and class V + III or V + IV is worse than class V alone. The combination of high activity and chronicity indices also increases the risk of progressive renal disease, as does reduced GFR, high-grade proteinuria, and anemia. Genetic background affects renal outcome in unknown ways so that Caucasian patients fare better than Hispanic and African American patients in whom ESRD is more likely. Resistance to therapy and recurrent renal flares after response to therapy are also poor prognostic indicators for renal survival. Note that nearly all of these prognostic indicators are in fact manifestations of disease rather than predictors of disease, underscoring the need for useful biomarkers.

Treatment

Ideally, pediatric nephrologists and rheumatologists confer to individualize and optimize treatment plans for each patient affected by both renal and extrarenal disease. This chapter presents only renal-specific treatment guidelines, predicated on the assumption that LN is diagnosed by renal biopsy. The importance of the renal biopsy to tailor therapy cannot be overstressed. For practical purposes, LN can be separated into categories whose risks of progressing to ESRD are low (classes I and II), moderate (classes III and V), and high (classes IV, V + III and V + IV) and patients are treated according to risk (see Table 6).

Table 6. Pragmatic view of ESRD risk and therapeutic options

Risk[a]	Histology	ACE-I/ ARB[b]	HCQ[c]	GC	MMF[d]	ivCY[e]
Lower	• Class I or II	+	+	+/−	+/−	−
↑	• Class III (C)	+	+	+	+/−	−
	• Class III (A) or (A/C)					
	• Class V	+	+	+	+	−
↓	• Class IV	+	+	+	+	+/−
Higher	• Class V+III or V+IV	+	+	+	+	+

[a] For any given biopsy class, manifestations including hypertension, azotemia, nephrosis, nephrotic range proteinuria, resistance to therapy or relapse increase the risk of progression and hence the need for more aggressive therapy.
[b] ACE-I/ARB therapy is not indicated in absence of proteinuria or hypertension.
[c] Usually prescribed for extrarenal SLE with possible renal benefit as well.
[d] Some use MMF as a steroid-sparing agent; some use AZA instead of MMF.
[e] Treatment failure prompts consideration of alternative agents such as rituximab.

Low risk

Children and adolescents with LN class I or II are considered low risk as long as they are free of hypertension, nephrotic range proteinuria, azotemia or impaired GFR. Based on clinical consensus, patients with uncomplicated class I or II lupus nephritis may warrant treatment with angiotensin blocking agents, including ACE-inhibitors (ACE-i), or angiotensin receptor blockers (ARB), as well as hydroxychloroquine (HCQ), and perhaps glucocorticoid (GC) therapy. The intensity of GC therapy can range from prednisone 0.25 mg/kg on alternate days to 2 mg/kg/day, with a daily oral maximum of 60 mg (see Table 7).

Moderate risk

Treatment recommendations for patients with class III or V lupus nephritis are controversial. Clinical studies are limited and the difficulty predicting which class III cases will progress to class IV, which class V patients will acquire proliferative disease, and which children will be best served simply by minimizing medication-induced toxicities, makes treatment standardization problematic. Minimal therapy usually consists of ACE-I/ARB, HCQ, and oral GC, with rapid addition of the antiproliferative immunomodulators- azathioprine (AZA), or mycophenolate mofetil (MMF) either as steroid-sparing agents or in cases of steroid resistance (see Table 7). Monthly intravenous steroid pulses, and/or intensified therapy with cytotoxic agents may be justified in nonresponders, in cases complicated by high grade proteinuria, hypertension, or renal failure and in cases of nonadherence.

One recent prospective study enrolled patients (ages 13–60 years) with proteinuria >2 g/day due to pure class V lupus nephritis to test three treatment regimens: prednisone alone for 12 months (40 mg/m^2 po on alternate days for eight weeks then tapered weekly by 5 mg down to 10 mg/m^2 po on alternate days), prednisone with twice daily cyclosporine (CSA), and prednisone with alternate month intravenous cyclophosphamide (ivCY). The CSA and ivCY arms were both more effective than prednisone alone at inducing remission, but relapses were more rapid and more common following withdrawal of CSA versus ivCY. After one year, reciprocal crossover treatment with CSA and ivCY

Table 7. Common medications in lupus nephritis

Agents	Considerations
ACE-i/ ARB*: Variable	1. Titrate dose to antiproteinuric effect by serial urinary protein/creatinine ratios 2. Monitor for hypotension and hyperkalemia 3. Avoid in AKI
Calcineurin inhibitors: Cyclosporine; tacrolimus	1. Consider as rescue agents for nonresponders 2. Target drug levels are poorly defined
Cyclophosphamide (ivCY): **NIH induction:** 500–1000 mg/m^2 iv monthly × 6 doses **NIH maintenance:** 500–1000 mg/m^2 IV quarterly × 4–6 doses **Euro-Lupus induction:** 500 mg iv or q2wks × 6 doses	1. Dilute ivCY in 150 ml of normal saline and infuse over 60 minutes. 2. Bladder protection: a. Prehydrate to urine specific gravity <1.010. b. Ensure brisk urine output with oral IV fluid at twice maintenance for 4–24 hours. (Consider furosemide in case of fluid retention; consider continuous bladder irrigation if oliguria is present. c. Give MESNA before ivCY and then q3hrs (max of four doses; each IV dose is 20% of total ivCY dose). 3. Premedicate with ondansetron; continue as needed for 2–4 days. 4. See Tables 8 and 9.
Glucocorticoids (GC): **Prednisone:** 2 mg/kg or 60 mg/m^2 poqday, with taper; (max 60 mg daily) **Methylprednisolone:** 750–1000 mg/m^2 IV daily × 3 doses or monthly × 6 doses (max 1000 mg/dose)	1. Risks of long term GC therapy include avascular necrosis of the hip, cataracts, gastritis, growth suppression, hypertension, infection, osteopenia. 2. High dose oral GC is not recommended beyond eight weeks; weekly tapering by 5 mg or 10% is common; maintenance dose is usually determined by extrarenal disease. 3. GC pulses are rarely complicated by acute hypertension and even less commonly by acute psychosis.
Hydroxychloroquine: 3–5 mg/kg po qday (max 200 mg po bid)	1. Usually prescribed for extrarenal SLE with possible renal benefit. 2. Monitor for ocular toxicity

(*Continued*)

Table 7. (*Continued*)

Agents	Considerations
Methotrexate: Variable	1. Usually prescribed for arthritis 2. Weekly oral dosing is used rarely for LN maintenance therapy; monthly parenteral dosing has been reported for rescue therapy 3. Adjust dose for GFR 4. Supplement with folic acid
Purine synthesis inhibitors: **Azathioprine (AZA):** 2–3 mg/kg po q day (max 200 mg daily) **Mycophenolate mofetil (MMF):** 600 mg/m^2 po bid (max 3000 mg/day)	1. Monitor for bone marrow suppression and liver transaminase abnormalities 2. Target drug/ metabolite levels are poorly defined 3. GI toxicity with MMF may be reduced by converting to TID dosing
Rituximab: 375 mg/m^2 IV weekly × 4 doses	1. Premedicate with acetaminophen, diphenhydramine and glucocorticoids 2. Recommended depletion target varies from <5 CD19 cells/microliter to <10% of baseline CD19 counts. 3. Depletion failure may relate to induction of human antichimeric antibodies (HACA) 4. B cells repopulate any time from 3–12 months 5. Known risks include hypogammaglobulinemia, infection and progressive multifocal leukoencephalopathy
Statins: Various	Hyperlipidemia and cardiovascular disease are significant comorbidities in SLE

* ACE-i angiotensin converting enzyme inhibitor; ARB angiotensin receptor blocker.

subsequently induced remission in some of the previous nonresponders, suggesting that rescue therapy should be considered when standard therapy fails. A similar study enrolling patients (ages 12–75 years) with proteinuria >2 g/day and either class III or class V lupus nephritis found equivalent responses to six months of oral prednisone combined with either ivCY or oral MMF. In view of the known drug toxicity profiles, the results of these studies justify the use of MMF plus GC as first line

Table 8. ivCY-associated adverse events are generally dose dependant

Acute toxicity occurs with each dose and may drive adjustment of subsequent doses:	
Nausea/ vomiting	Premedicate with ondansetron; continue as needed
Hemorrhagic cystitis, mediated by direct contact of ivCY metabolites with bladder wall	Minimized with MESNA and with forced diuresis or bladder irrigation
Myelosuppression	WBC nadir generally at 10–14 days
Infection	Consider *Pneumocystis jiroveci* prophylaxis
Alopecia	Occasional
SIADH	Rare
Long term risks increase with cumulative dose:	
Gonadal toxicity:	
Amenorrhea/ovarian failure azospermia/infertility	Consider hormonal prophylaxis therapy after menarche; consider sperm banking
Malignancy	Especially bladder
Interstitial pulmonary fibrosis	

agents for treating moderate risk lupus nephritis, with subsequent escalation to ivCY or CSA as needed for patients who fail to respond (see Table 8).

High risk

Aggressive therapy of children and adolescents with LN class IV, class V + III or class V + IV is warranted to prevent progression to ESRD. Treatment guidelines for high risk patients are largely based on prospective studies initiated by the NIH in the 1980s. Since then, the incorporation of cytotoxic agents into the treatment of proliferative LN has improved survival rates. More specifically, the NIH trials demonstrated that treatment with ivCY significantly improves long term renal survival compared to high dose oral prednisone or intravenous methylprednisolone alone, and with fewer side effects than oral cyclophosphamide.

The NIH regimen recommends a six-month induction period of monthly ivCY followed by a 12–18-month maintenance period of quarterly ivCY. Predating the MMF era, this schedule is truncated only in the event of acute toxicity and is accompanied by oral prednisone at slowly tapering doses. See Tables 7 and 9 for dosing details. Approximately 50%

of patients respond to this prescription within 3–4 months, but fewer than 10% will attain full remission of their nephritis. As many as 25% will fail or will not tolerate this regimen. Response rates vary with ethnicity (reduced in Hispanic- and African-descent patients compared to Caucasian- and Asian-descent patients) and are also lower for patients starting with substantial renal impairment. Patients who relapse at any time during or after therapy are at increased risk for poorer, long-term outcome. Patients who relapse should be rebiopsied and if indicated by histologic findings, retreated with another full course of induction and maintenance ivCY, up to a total of three full courses. Patients who relapse after three courses and nonresponders who fail the initial induction should also be rebiopsied and considered for rescue therapy.

The Euro-Lupus Nephritis Trial (ELNT) compared the NIH induction regimen to a lower dose ivCY induction protocol in patients with proliferative lupus nephritis. All of the predominately Caucasian patients in this study were given three daily doses of iv methylprednisolone followed by oral prednisone, and were treated either with ivCY monthly for six doses and quarterly for two doses or with ivCY every two weeks for six doses. In all cases, ivCY was followed by oral AZA as maintenance therapy and most patients were also treated with ACE-I/ARB agents. There were no significant differences in renal responses or adverse events between the low and high dose ivCY-treated patients within ten years of follow-up. As a result, this regimen could be initiated in otherwise low risk patients (e.g. Caucasians with normal GFR and minimal proteinuria) and then converted to the more intense NIH prescription if needed. See Tables 7 and 9 for dosing details.

Following several case reports, retrospective reviews and small prospective trials all touting the promise of MMF, a recent study by the Aspreva Lupus Management Study Group (ALMS) enrolled over 300 lupus patients with proliferative nephritis and compared the NIH monthly ivCY regimen with 24 weeks of MMF induction. All patients were also treated with oral prednisone (see Table 9). In contrast to the lower risk Caucasian and Asian populations that displayed no significant differences in response to either regimen, higher risk patients of African or Hispanic descent responded significantly better to 24 weeks of MMF induction than monthly ivCY. A recent meta-analysis comparing MMF to ivCY noted similar efficacy with both agents, but distinct adverse event profiles: MMF

Table 9. RCT based treatment protocols for proliferative LN*

Regimen	Medications	Comments
NIH regimen	**ivCY:** 500–1000 mg/m^2 monthly for six months (induction) then quarterly for 12–24 months (maintenance)	1. Give 750 mg/m^2 as first ivCY dose when GFR is normal; 500 mg/m^2 for GFR <50%. Adjust subsequent doses by + 250 mg/m^2 to achieve a 10–14 day WBC nadir of 1500–3000 cells/mm^3.
	prednisone: 0.5 mg/kg po qday for four weeks then taper weekly by 5 mg/ alternate days to maintenance dose of 0.25 mg/kg po alternate days	2. Extrarenal disease may limit the lowest prednisone doseachievable. 3. Renal relapse any time after initial response is re-treated with another full induction for a total of three courses.
Euro-Lupus regimen	**ivCY:** 500 mg q 2 weeks for six doses (induction), followed by **azathioprine:** 2 mg/kg po daily (maintenance)	NB: intravenous medication doses are not adjusted for patient size in this protocol
	methylprednisolone: 750 mg IV daily for three days, followed by **prednisolone:** 0.5 mg/kg po qday for four weeks then taper every two weeks by 2.5 mg to maintenance dose of 5 mg po qday	
ALMS regimen (MMF induction)	**MMF:** 500 mg po bid for one week, then 1000 mg po bid for one week, then 1500 mg po bid for six months	1. The 2009 prospective trial was unable to detect a difference between MMFand ivCY induction therapy for patients with class III, IV or V lupus nephritis.
	prednisone: 60 mg po qday tapered by 5–10% every 1-2 weeks down to 10 mg po qday	2. For adverse events including diarrhea, MMF can be . adjusted to TID dosing and/orreduced by 30%

* **adjunct therapy** including antacids, vitamin D and calcium supplements, ACE-I and/or ARB antiproteinuric agents and other antihypertensives, hydroxychloroquine, etc., should be individualized for each patient. NSAIDs should be avoided.

is most commonly associated with diarrhea whereas ivCY is associated with leukopenia and amenorrhea.

With the caveat that pediatric lupus patients are under-represented even in the larger trials, study results may justify the use of MMF and oral GC as first line agents to induce remission. Frequent physical and laboratory monitoring are imperative, so that disease progression, relapse or adverse events can be detected promptly and therapeutic regimens adjusted on a case-by-case basis. In those children and adolescents at risk of nonadherence the advantage of intermittent infusions for remission induction should be considered, possibly with subsequent transition to oral agents once adherence issues are no longer problematic.

Rescue therapy

Patients who fail standard therapy, are unable or unwilling to tolerate medication toxicity or are unable to comply with dosing instructions may benefit from alternative therapies. Some patients refractory to MMF and ivCY may remit with the calcineurin inhibitors — cyclosporine or tacrolimus. No role for intravenous immunoglobulin, or plasmapheresis has been demonstrated.

The anti-CD20 monoclonal antibody rituximab is a B cell depleting agent that is being used increasingly for LN induction, maintenance and rescue therapy. Uncontrolled observational studies in both adult and pediatric patients variably report reduction in serum creatinine, proteinuria and histologic activity indices along with increases in serum complement levels. While intuitively appealing to clear B cells in the setting of immune complex mediated disease, it is important to note that mature, antibody-producing plasma cells do not express CD20 and are therefore spared by this agent, as are the stem cell precursors of B lymphocytes. Nonetheless, renal responses and relapses seem to generally but not uniformly correlate with the depletion and re-population of circulating B cells that are quantified by flow cytometry as $CD19^+$ cells. LUNAR, the one prospective trial reported patients who were treated with rituximab infusions at weeks 1, 3, 24, and 26, unfortunately failed to demonstrate significant renal response at the 24 or 52 week time points. Additional prospective evaluation of rituximab's efficacy and safety is still needed, especially in trials with larger components of pediatric patients.

Co-morbidities and treatment risks of SLE nephritis

The medications used to treat LN have many side effects, most notably immunosuppression and its concomitant risk of life-threatening infection. Patient and family education combined with a high index of clinical suspicion for infection and a low threshold to provide antimicrobial therapy are important. Prophylactic therapies against specific pathogens, such as *Pneumocystis jiroveci* (previously known as *Pneumocystis carinii*) and varicella zoster, should be considered for patients with impaired cellular immunity. Routine live vaccines should be evaluated on an individual basis and in general, avoided during immunosuppressant administration.

Steroid associated osteopenia is a drug-induced risk of concern. Calcium and vitamin D supplementation should be prescribed routinely for children on chronic GC therapy. Additional medication-related issues are highlighted in Tables 7 and 9.

Extrarenal features of SLE impart additional renal risks to lupus patients. Autoantibody associated antiphospholipid syndrome can cause microangiopathy with renovascular microthrombi, hypertension, and/or loss of GFR, all independent of LN. Thrombotic microangiopathy can increase the risk of thrombosis. Lupus patients also have an increased incidence of hyperlipidemia and ischemic heart disease that develops at a younger age than the general population. Pediatric nephrologists must therefore anticipate and modulate hypertension and dyslipidemia with timely medical intervention and counseling regarding healthy lifestyle choices.

Renal replacement therapy in SLE

Traditionally, preemptive renal transplantation has been delayed in SLE with the hopes of "burning out" the disease during a year of maintenance dialysis. This approach has been rendered obsolete by more than two decades of outcomes data, although most would still avoid transplanting a lupus patient in the midst of an active disease flare. For pediatric patients in particular, the benefits of early transplant likely outweigh the risks of recurrent renal disease, especially if the disease is in remission. Although recurring LN has been detected in as many as 50% of allograft biopsies that are fully evaluated by IF and EM in addition to routine light microscopy, most recurrences are clinically silent and only 2–8% lead to eventual graft failure.

There are conflicting reports as to whether graft survival and indeed patient survival is better, worse or the same in SLE versus non-SLE transplant recipients. Studies analyzing national databases including the USRDS (United States Renal Data System) and the UNOS (United Network of Organ Sharing) renal registry report equivalent outcomes between adult patients with SLE and with other causes of ESRD. Studies limited to pediatric populations also find equivalent allograft outcomes, but a modest and unexplained increase in mortality. It is interesting to note that increasing age among adult recipients correlates with increasing rates of graft survival, whereas the converse is true in pediatrics: the closer to adolescence, the shorter the graft survival.

Suggested Reading

Appel GB, Contreras G, Dooley MA, *et al.* (2009) Mycophenolate mofetil versus cyclophosphamide for induction treatment of lupus nephritis. *J Am Soc Nephrol* **20**: 1103–1112.

Austin HA, 3rd, Boumpas DT, Vaughan EM, Balow JE. (1994) Predicting renal outcomes in severe lupus nephritis: contributions of clinical and histologic data. *Kidney Int* **45**: 544–550.

Austin HA, 3rd, Illei GG, Braun MJ, Balow JE. (2009) Randomized, controlled trial of prednisone, cyclophosphamide, and cyclosporine in lupus membranous nephropathy. *J Am Soc Nephrol* **20**: 901–911.

Austin HA, 3rd, Muenz LR, Joyce KM, *et al.* (1983) Prognostic factors in lupus nephritis. Contribution of renal histologic data. *Am J Med* **75**: 382–391.

Bartosh SM, Fine RN, Sullivan EK. (2001) Outcome after transplantation of young patients with systemic lupus erythematosus: a report of the North American pediatric renal transplant cooperative study. *Transplantation* **72**: 973–978.

Boumpas DT, Austin HA, 3rd, Vaughn EM, *et al.* (1992) Controlled trial of pulse methylprednisolone versus two regimens of pulse cyclophosphamide in severe lupus nephritis. *Lancet* **340**: 741–745.

Bunnapradist S, Chung P, Peng A, *et al.* (2006) Outcomes of renal transplantation for recipients with lupus nephritis: analysis of the Organ Procurement and Transplantation Network database. *Transplantation* **82**: 612–618.

Gipson DS, Ferris ME, Dooley MA, *et al.* (2003) Renal transplantation in children with lupus nephritis. *Am J Kidney Dis* **41**: 455–463.

Hochberg MC. (1997) Updating the American College of Rheumatology revised criteria for the classification of systemic lupus erythematosus. *Arthritis Rheum* **40**: 1725.

Houssiau FA, Vasconcelos C, D'Cruz D, *et al.* (2004) Early response to immunosuppressive therapy predicts good renal outcome in lupus nephritis: lessons from long-term followup of patients in the Euro-Lupus Nephritis Trial. *Arthritis Rheum* **50**: 3934–3940.

Houssiau FA, Vasconcelos C, D'Cruz D, *et al.* (2009) The 10-year follow-up data of the Euro-Lupus Nephritis Trial comparing low-dose versus high-dose intravenous cyclophosphamide. *Ann Rheum Dis.*

Illei GG, Austin HA, Crane M, *et al.* (2001) Combination therapy with pulse cyclophosphamide plus pulse methylprednisolone improves long-term renal outcome without adding toxicity in patients with lupus nephritis. *Ann Intern Med* **135**: 248–257.

LUNAR. [URL:http://www.gene.com/gene/news/press-releases/display.do?method=detail&id=11947] Accessed 2009.

Mak A, Cheak AA, Tan JY, *et al.* (2009) Mycophenolate mofetil is as efficacious as, but safer than, cyclophosphamide in the treatment of proliferative lupus nephritis: a meta-analysis and meta-regression. *Rheumatology (Oxford)* **48**: 944–952.

Nwobi O, Abitbol CL, Chandar J, *et al.* (2008) Rituximab therapy for juvenile-onset systemic lupus erythematosus. *Pediatr Nephrol* **23**: 413–419.

Pepper R, Griffith M, Kirwan C, *et al.* (2009) Rituximab is an effective treatment for lupus nephritis and allows a reduction in maintenance steroids. *Nephrol Dial Transplant.*

Pons-Estel GJ, Alarcon GS, McGwin G, Jr., *et al.* (2009) Protective effect of hydroxychloroquine on renal damage in patients with lupus nephritis: LXV, data from a multiethnic US cohort. *Arthritis Rheum* **61**: 830–839.

Tan EM, Cohen AS, Fries JF, *et al.* (1982) The 1982 revised criteria for the classification of systemic lupus erythematosus. *Arthritis Rheum* **25**: 1271–1277.

Tucker LB, Uribe AG, Fernandez M, *et al.* (2008) Adolescent onset of lupus results in more aggressive disease and worse outcomes: results of a nested matched case-control study within LUMINA, a multiethnic US cohort (LUMINA LVII). *Lupus* **17**: 314–322.

Weening JJ, D'Agati VD, Schwartz MM, *et al.* (2004) The classification of glomerulonephritis in systemic lupus erythematosus revisited. *Kidney Int* **65**: 521–530.

21

ANCA Associated Kidney Diseases

David Kershaw

Introduction

In children, the diseases of the kidney associated with antineutrophil cytoplasmic antibodies (ANCA) are the small vessel vasculitides. These are relatively rare causes of glomerulonephritis (GN) but are important causes of rapidly progressive glomerulonephritis (RPGN). These vasculitides are microscopic polyangiitis (MPA), Wegener's granulomatosis (WG), renal limited, pauci-immune GN, drug-induced ANCA associated disease and Churg–Strauss syndrome (CSS) in roughly descending order of occurrence.

Pathogenesis

The presence of antineutrophil cytoplasmic antibodies usually reflects antibodies to proteinase 3 (PR3-ANCA) or myeloperoxidase (MPO-ANCA). Typically c-ANCA (so named for its cytoplasmic staining pattern on indirect immunofluorescence of alcohol fixed neutrophils) is associated with WG and p-ANCA (perinuclear staining pattern on indirect immunofluorescence) is associated with MPA or renal limited, pauci-immune glomerulonephritis. Several lines of evidence indicate that ANCA antibodies may be pathologic rather than merely markers of disease. Clinically, removal of ANCA with plasma exchange has been associated with improved outcomes, and *in vitro*, ANCA can induce neutrophil activation and MPO-ANCA can activate myleoperoxidase. Finally, injection of MPO-ANCA into mice induces a pauci-immune GN, and mice lacking myeloperoxidase do not develop disease when injected with MPO-ANCA. Several investigators have demonstrated that these models of MPO-ANCA induced disease depend on a functional alternative complement system. Taken together, the evidence supports a pathogenic role for ANCA antibodies.

Clinical Presentation

ANCA associated renal disease in children can present with a RPGN with or without pulmonary hemorrhage. RPGN is the development of acute kidney injury (AKI) with hematuria and proteinuria over a course of weeks to months. This presentation constitutes a medical emergency, and warrants rapid diagnostic evaluation (e.g. renal biopsy), and treatment. RPGN can be caused by a number of glomerular diseases; these are usually classified as immune complex mediated diseases (postinfectious GN, IgA GN, lupus nephritis), pauci-immune [ANCA (+)], and anti-glomerular basement membrane (anti-GBM) (Goodpasture syndrome). Although ANCA associated renal disease is rare in children, it is a common cause of RPGN in children and adults. Overall, the percent of pediatric patients with ANCA associated renal disease that present with RPGN is hard to judge since the nephrology literature is skewed by case series involving severe presentations whereas the rheumatology literature includes those with mild or later presentations which may miss fulminant or renal limited presentations.

The clinical presentation of pediatric ANCA associated vasculitis was well detailed in a recent single center series of 48 pediatric patients by Akikusa *et al.* (2007). This series reviewed demographic information, symptoms at presentation, time to diagnosis, and serologic testing. These results will be separated into the ANCA associated disease states below.

Wegener's Granulomatosis

In this study by Akikusa *et al.* (2007), 25 patients with WG were identified with 79% testing positive for ANCA (three quarters of these testing positive for PR3-ANCA). The patients had a mean duration of symptoms of two months prior to diagnosis. The male to female ratio was 1:4. The presenting symptoms were typically constitutional (fever, arthralgias, or weight loss in 96%). Other common nonrenal symptoms at presentation included ears, nose, or throat involvement in 84%, pulmonary involvement in 80%, and eye involvement in 52%. Only 32% of patients had skin involvement manifesting as purpura. Renal involvement at presentation was present in 88%. Glomerulonephritis was diagnosed in all patients with renal involvement. Dialysis was required at presentation in 20% of patients.

Renal Limited, Crescentic Pauci-Immune ANCA Positive Glomerulonephritis and Microscopic Polyangiitis

Some patients present with an idiopathic renal limited crescentic pauci-immune ANCA positive GN. In the series by Akikusa *et al.* (2007), 5 of 45 patients presented in this fashion; 12 of 45 children presented with MPA. Many authorities place these two diseases as part of a continuum. In a retrospective multicenter report from the Japanese Society for Pediatric Nephrology on ANCA associated GN in children, 34 patients with ANCA positive biopsy proven pauci-immune complex GN were identified. Only 3 three cases were associated with WG with 21 cases associated with MPA. Ten of 34 patients had idiopathic pauci-immune complex GN. Only 3 of 10 of the renal limited patients had constitutional symptoms at presentation while consistent with other series 18 of 21 MPA patients had constitutional symptoms at diagnosis.

Drug-induced ANCA Associated disease and Churg–Strauss Syndrome

Drug-induced ANCA associated disease and CSS are extremely rare causes of ANCA associated renal disease in children. The medication with the strongest association with the development of ANCA associated disease in children and adults is propylthiouracil. Churg–Strauss syndrome usually initially presents with asthma and later develops eosinophilia with eosinophilic pneumonia, or gastroenteritis. Finally, a systemic vasculitis with skin involvement develops in two thirds of patients; involvement of cardiac, lung, kidney, lymphatics, and muscle has also been reported.

Diagnosis

The diagnosis of ANCA associated renal disease is suspected with the presence of hematuria and proteinuria in the setting of a positive ANCA test.

Clinically, it is important to realize not all patients will have a positive ANCA test at the time of diagnosis. Associated constitutional symptoms or evidence of systemic vasculitis syndrome are common but not required for a diagnosis. Confirmation of the diagnosis is made by renal biopsy. In the setting of RPGN, rapid diagnosis and treatment are required.

The renal biopsy typically shows a necrotizing, crescentic GN. The immunofluorescence microscopy shows a lack of staining (pauci-immune). The nature of the crescents may range from early cellular to later fibrous crescents. Granulomas or vasculitis is rarely seen on renal biopsy.

Current consensus criteria for the diagnosis of childhood vasculitides from the European League Against Rheumatism (EULAR) help define childhood WG. The diagnosis of WG requires the presence three of the six criteria shown in Table 1.

MPA is defined as a necrotizing, pauci-immune small vessel vasculitis than may involve the skin, lungs, and kidney. Patients commonly present with pulmonary hemorrhage and GN; however, other organ involvement can occur including gastrointestinal, neurologic, ocular, and musculoskeletal systems (see Table 1).

Table 1.

WG	MPA	CSS
3 of 6 criteria (EULAR)	Eular modified Chapel Hill Concensus Criteria	4 of 6 criteria (ACR)
ANCA		
PR3-or C ANCA	MPO or P ANCA	MPO or p ANCA (not a criteria)
UA hematuria + significant proteinuria	Necrotizing vasculitis, with few/no immune deposits, affecting small vessels	Asthma
Granulomas or necrotizing pauci-immune GN	Necrotizing pauci-immune glomerulonephritis	Positive biopsy
Nasal sinus inflammation	Necrotizing arteritis of small & medium-sized arteries	Pulmonary infiltrates (non-fixed)
Abnormal CXR or CT	Pulmonary capillaritis	Eosinophilia
Subglottic, tracheal, or endobronchial stenosis		Sinusitis Neuropathy

CSS is diagnosed on the basis of the 1990 American College of Rheumatology criteria. The presence of four of six criteria (asthma, eosinophilia (>10%), mono or polyneuropathy, nonfixed pulmonary infiltrates, paranasal sinus abnormalities and extravascular eosinophils on tissue biopsy) yielded a diagnostic sensitivity of 85% and a specificity of 99.7% (adults). Approximately 50% of adults with CSS have a positive p-ANCA (Table 1).

Treatment

The treatment of ANCA associated kidney disease in children is modeled after studies performed in adults. The initial goal of treatment is the induction of disease remission followed by therapy to maintain remission while minimizing side effects.

Induction

The best studied agents for inducing remission are cyclophosphamide and corticosteroids. Typically cyclophosphamide is given orally at 2 mg/kg per day for 3–6 months in the induction phase. This is combined with prednisone 1 mg/kg/day initially tapering to 0.25 mg/kg by 8 weeks. The use of intravenous versus oral cyclophosphamide has recently been studied in adults with WG and MPA and showed equivalent rates of remission induction at 3 and 6 months; however, there has been reported a slightly higher relapse rate with intravenous cyclophosphamide in some analyses.

For patients with mild disease, alternative induction with methotrexate (MTX) has been studied in adults. In comparison to cyclophosphamide induction therapy, the rate of remission with methotrexate induction was equivalent at 6 months (~90%) but the time to remission was longer (median 2 vs. 3 months) and time to relapse was shorter (13 vs. 15 months). The authors concluded that MTX was less effective in patients with extensive disease or pulmonary involvement.

In the setting of oliguric renal failure it is difficult to give oral cyclophosphamide safely due to the risk of hemorrhagic cystitis and the use of intravenous cyclophosphamide with bladder irrigation is preferable.

Adjunctive therapy in severe disease with renal impairment has been studied and has included pulse methylprednisolone (1 g/day for three days in adult), and plasmapheresis (seven exchanges). In a comparison of pulse methylprednisolone and plasmapheresis, the survival at 12 months was similar at ~75 % but the plasmapheresis group had a lower rate of end-stage renal disease (19 versus 43%). Both therapies entail serious adverse effects in close to 50% of patients. In patients with RPGN or significant pulmonary involvement, adjunctive therapy with plasmapheresis should be considered.

Adjunctive therapy with a soluble TNF-α inhibitor (etanercept) in a cyclophosphamide-based regimen has been studied in a rigorous fashion and shown to provide no benefit compared to placebo. In addition, the etanercept group had an elevated rate of malignancies. In short, etanercept has no role in the treatment of ANCA associated kidney disease.

Maintenance therapy

Remission can usually be achieved by 3–6 months of cyclophosphamide therapy; however, prolonged use of cyclophosphamide beyond induction of remission adds considerably to the toxicity of treatment. To maintain remission with lower toxicity, azathioprine (2 mg/kg) has been used and has been shown to have a comparable relapse rate to oral cyclophosphamide. Patients with a reduced activity of the enzyme that metabolizes azathioprine, thiopurine methyltransferase (TPMT) can have severe leucopenia, and hepatoxicity. Before initiating azathioprine therapy TPMT activity testing should be considered. In the maintenance phase, the dose of prednisolone is typically gradually diminished and after a year may be below 0.1 mg/kg. The duration of maintenance is controversial and needs to be adjusted to the clinical situation but a minimum of two years is recommended. Patients with WG have a higher relapse rate and some advocate five years of maintenance therapy to maintain a remission.

Complications of disease and therapy

Immunosuppressive therapy for ANCA associated kidney disease is associated with elevated risks of malignancy and infection. The risk of infection is especially increased at times of leukopenia and infection may be bacterial, fungal, or viral. The degree of immunosuppression may lead to opportunistic infections such as *Pneumocystis jirovecii.* Prophylactic treatment with trimethoprim/sulfamethoxazole can reduce this complication and at full treatment dosage has been shown to reduce the incidence of respiratory relapses in WG.

Infection or reactivation of herpes family viruses may complicate therapy and may require suppressive antiviral therapy.

The combination of inflammatory and corticosteroid effects can lead to osteoporosis. Ensuring adequate calcium intake and vitamin D stores is indicated. The role of routine bone density measurements or use of bisphosphonates in pediatric patients being treated for ANCA associated kidney disease has not been defined.

Adults with WG have an increased risk of thromboembolic events and in one pediatric series 16% of patients had a venous thromboembolic event. Some patients with WG may have antiphospholipid antibodies that predispose to thromboembolic events.

The use of prolonged cyclophosphamide can lead to infertility. This effect is age, sex, and dose dependent. Male infertility may occur after 18 weeks of therapy at typical doses. Pubertal and postpubertal males should be informed of risks and offered cryopreservation of sperm when feasible. For females, the critical cumulative dose of cyclophosphamide varies by age. Although ovarian-tissue cryopreservation may be feasible in prepubertal and pubertal girls, at this time it is still considered experimental.

Prolonged cyclophosphamide treatment or cyclophosphamide induced hemorrhagic cystitis are risk factors for bladder cancer. Long-term monitoring by annual urinalysis and cytology is recommended and patients with the development of nonglomerular hematuria should be referred for cystocopy.

Prognosis

The remission rates for adults with WG in series reported over the last decade range from 50–93% and similar remission rates have been reported in patients with MPA. Factors associated with reduced chance of remission include disease chronicity and renal scarring especially interstitial fibrosis. In pediatric series, poor outcomes have been related to severity of renal insufficiency at presentation and chronicity of lesions seen on renal biopsy.

The relapse rate for adult WG ranges from 18–40% at two years with a slightly lower relapse rate in MPA. One recent WG pediatric series reported a relapse rate of 75% with a median time to first relapse of 10.4 months. The median dose of prednisone at first disease relapse was 10 mg.

The factors that have been identified with an increased relapse rate in adults with WG include: decreased amount and duration of cyclophosphamide and steroid in the induction regimen, lack of prophylactic adjunctive trimethoprim/sulfamethoxazole, positive ANCA at diagnosis, creatinine clearance > 60 at diagnosis, and cardiac involvement. Over time, an increasing ANCA titer is often associated with relapse, but cannot be used alone to justify aggressive treatment.

Deaths in recent pediatric series of WG or MPA have ranged from 0–12%. Without immunosuppressive therapy, WG had a mortality of over 90% at two years in adults. With current treatment regimens, outcomes in adults with WG and MPA have similar survival rates at one year (~90%). The five-year survival for WG declines by approximately 10%, but MPA has a much worse survival at five years with only ~50% survival.

CSS is extremely rare in children and most patients have been reported as case reports. In adults, multi-system involvement (neurological, cardiac, chronic kidney disease, proteinuria, and gastrointestinal) is associated with a poor outcome.

Antiglomerular Basement Membrane Disease

This rare disease can be renal limited with hematuria, proteinuria, and azotemia or less often in children may present as a combined pulmonary renal syndrome (Goodpasture syndrome). It often presents with as a fulminate RPGN. It is caused by autoantibodies to alpha 3 type IV collagen but in 10–40% of adult cases also have a positive MPO-ANCA.

Anti-GBM disease is diagnosed by the presence of GN and a renal biopsy with linear IgG staining of the glomerular basement membrane. Demonstration of circulating anti-GBM IgGs supports but does not make the diagnosis since this test is not 100% sensitive or specific. Goodpasture syndrome is diagnosed when there is also pulmonary involvement (hemorrhage).

Plasmapheresis is used routinely in patients with anti-GBM disease to remove the pathologic antibody. In patients with anti-GBM disease with a good response, a shorter duration of maintenance therapy may suffice.

Pediatric outcomes in anti-GBM disease are difficult to ascertain but appear to be similar to adult outcomes. Patients who present without the need for dialysis and are aggressively treated do well whereas patient who present in renal failure usually progress to chronic renal failure.

Suggested Reading

Akikusa JD, Schneider R, Harvey EA, *et al.* (2007) Clinical features and outcome of pediatric Wegener's granulomatosis. *Arthritis Rheum* **57**(5): 837–844.

Carruthers D, Sherlock J. (2009) Evidence-based management of ANCA vasculitis. *Best Pract Res Clin Rheumatol* **23**(3): 367–378.

De Groot K, Rasmussen N, Bacon PA, *et al.* (2005) Randomized trial of cyclophosphamide versus methotrexate for induction of remission in early systemic antineutrophil cytoplasmic antibody-associated vasculitis. *Arthritis Rheum* **52**: 2461–2469.

Eleftheriou D, Brogan PA. (2009) Vasculitis in children. *Best Pract Res Clin Rheumatol* **23**(3): 309–323.

Hattori M, Kurayama H, Koitabashi Y. (2001) Japanese Society for Pediatric Nephrology. Antineutrophil cytoplasmic autoantibody-associated glomerulonephritis in children. *J Am Soc Nephrol* **12**(7): 1493–1500.

Jayne DR, Gaskin G, Rasmussen N, *et al.* (2007) European Vasculitis Study Group. Randomized trial of plasma exchange or high-dosage methylprednisolone as adjunctive therapy for severe renal vasculitis. *J Am Soc Nephrol* **18**: 2180–2188.

Jennette JC, Falk RJ. (2008) New insight into the pathogenesis of vasculitis associated with antineutrophil cytoplasmic autoantibodies. *Curr Opin Rheumatol* **20**(1): 55–60.

Mukhtyar C, Flossmann O, Hellmich B, *et al.* European Vasculitis Study Group (EUVAS). (2008) Outcomes from studies of antineutrophil cytoplasm antibody associated vasculitis: a systematic review by the European League Against Rheumatism systemic vasculitis task force. *Ann Rheum Dis* **67**(7): 1004–1010.

Ozen S, Ruperto N, Dillon MJ, *et al.* (2006) EULAR/PReS endorsed consensus criteria for the classification of childhood vasculitides. *Ann Rheum Dis* **65**(7): 936–941.

Turnbull J, Harper L. (2009) Adverse effects of therapy for ANCA-associated vasculitis. *Best Pract Res Clin Rheumatol* **23**(3): 391–401.

22

Henoch–Schönlein Purpura Glomerulonephritis

David Kershaw

Introduction

Henoch–Schönlein purpura (HSP) is a systemic small vessel vasculitic disease of unclear etiology that predominately affects children. The disease typically involves the skin, gastrointestinal (GI) system, joints and kidneys but other organ systems may also be involved. The course is typically self-limited; however, recurrences are common. Long-term morbidity is chiefly determined by the degree of renal involvement.

Pathogenesis

HSP is more common in the fall, winter, and spring than summer suggesting an infectious trigger. Many infections have been associated with the presentation of HSP, and in some series, over half the patients had a preceding infection. Other triggers have also been suggested including a variety of medications and malignancies. A pathogenic role for immunoglobulin A (IgA) has been suggested by the deposition of IgA in the mesangial region of the glomerulus, IgA deposits in the small vessels with vasculitis, and the presence of circulating immune complexes containing IgA.

An excess of IgA in the serum is not the cause of HSP since most patients have normal levels of IgA and recent research has focused on the role abnormally glycosylated IgA (galactose deficient IgA) in immune complex formation. The abnormalities in IgA found in HSP and the pathology of the kidney lesions strongly resemble that of IgA nephropathy.

Clinical Presentation

HSP classically features a rash of palpable purpura which typically begins over the buttocks and extensor surfaces of the legs. The trunk is usually spared but the rash may involve the arms and face. The rash evolves over time and may be preceded by a nonpurpuric rash (maculopapular, urticarial). Occasionally, bullous lesions may be seen. The lesions may vary in size from petechiae to large confluent papular lesions.

Usually the rash precedes other systemic involvement, but in over a third of cases, the joint or gastrointestinal symptoms appear before the rash. Typically, the rash appears within a week of the onset of other symptoms. The asynchronous nature in some patients may result in a diagnostic dilemma until the classic rash appears. This includes patients without rash who present with symptoms mimicking appendicitis or testicular torsion.

Gastrointestinal involvement presents with colicky abdominal pain and may involve vomiting and GI bleeding. GI involvement is due to bowel wall edema related to vasculitis. Approximately 30% of children will have melenic or grossly bloody stools. Intussusception (usually ileoileal) occurs in fewer than 1 in 20 children with HSP. Pancreatitis, hydrops of the gallbladder or protein losing enteropathy may also occur. Most severe short term complications of HSP relate to the GI involvement.

Joint involvement is present in a majority of patients and can range from joint pain and swelling to decreased range of motion. Joints typically affected are the large joints of the legs (ankles, knees, and hips). Hand, wrist, and elbow joints may also be affected. Overall, the joint symptoms can be severe but do not cause permanent damage.

Renal involvement causes the most concerning long-term morbidity and patients commonly have microscopic hematuria, and/or proteinuria in their course. Overall, approximately a third of patients will have abnormal urinalysis but more severe renal manifestations such as nephrotic syndrome, nephritic syndrome, hypertension, or acute kidney injury (AKI) occur in less than 10% of patients. Most severe renal involvement develops within the first three months of disease and should be monitored.

Nonspecific crankiness is extremely common although definitive neurologic symptoms are rare. These have ranged from subtle mental status changes to seizure or rarely intracerebral bleeding.

Urologic involvement with symptoms of scrotal pain and swelling are fairly common in boys. Symptoms of orchitis may occur and prompt exploration for testicular torsion or infarction. Rarely a stenosing ureteritis occurs in the setting of HSP with colicky flank pain, and passage of blood clots.

Rarely other organ systems may be involved, including pulmonary, cardiac, and ophthalmologic (see Table 1).

Clinical recurrences may occur in up to a third of patients and typically occur within the six months. Recurrences may be multiple and are more common in patients with nephritis.

Diagnosis

HSP is a clinical diagnosis and routine laboratory testing cannot make the diagnosis of HSP, but is useful in excluding other potential diagnoses and assessing for organ involvement. The American College of Rheumatology 1990 criteria for the classification of HSP are shown in Table 2.

Initial laboratory investigations should include a CBC with platelet count, coagulation panel, liver enzyme panel (to rule out other potential

Table 1. Organ system involvement with HSP

	Number and Percent
Purpura	100
Arthritis	82
Abdominal pain	63
Gastrointestinal bleeding	33
Occult bleeding	23
Gross bleeding	10
Nephritis	40
Hematuria	40
Gross hematuria	7
Proteinuria	25
Nephrotic syndrome	3
Miscellaneous	
Orchitis	5 (9% of boys)
Seizures	2
Duodenal obstruction	1
Recurrence of symptoms	33

Clinical features in 100 children with Henoch–Schönlein purpura. [*Source*: Saulsbury FT. (1999) *Medicine* (Baltimore), **78**(6): 395–404.]

Table 2. Clinical diagnostic criteria for HSP

American College of Rheumatology 1990 criteria for the classification of HSP	
Palpable purpura	Slightly raised "palpable" hemorrhagic skin lesions, not related to thrombocytopenia
Age $\leq$ 20 at disease onset	Patient 20 years or younger at onset of first symptoms
Bowel angina	Diffuse abdominal pain, worse after meals, or the diagnosis of bowel ischemia, usually including bloody diarrhoea
Wall granulocytes on biopsy	Histologic changes showing granulocytes in the walls of arterioles or venules

For purposes of classification, a patient shall be said to have Henoch–Schönlein purpura if at least two of these four criteria are present. The presence of any two or more criteria yields a sensitivity of 87.1% and a specificity of 87.7%.

causes of purpura or abdominal pain, and assess for anemia), electrolytes, albumin, cholesterol, urea nitrogen, albumin, creatinine, and urinalysis (to assess for electrolyte status, and determine if renal involvement). Although the serum IgA level may be elevated in approximately half the patients, the predictive power of this test is poor and contributes little to the diagnosis or management.

In patients who present with a preceding infectious illness or drug exposure, evaluation and treatment of the infection, or withdrawal of the potentially offending drug may be indicated.

In patients presenting with GI or urologic symptoms in the absence of purpura or joint involvement, the diagnosis is sometimes made after surgical exploration. In patients with HSP and suspected intussusception, the preferred imaging test is ultrasound. For boys with HSP and acute scrotal pain, rapid evaluation followed by surgical exploration may be required to exclude testicular torsion.

Skin biopsy is not routinely indicated. In children who undergo skin biopsy for an atypical or persistent presentation, a leukocytoclastic vasculitis consisting of a perivascular accumulation of mononuclear cells and polymorphonuclear leukocytes involving the small blood vessels of the dermis is seen. This finding is not diagnostic for HSP and may also be seen in other vasculitis conditions, infections, and drug reactions. On immunofluorescence microscopy, a deposition of IgA in superficial capillaries is present.

In patients with renal involvement beyond microscopic hematuria or low-grade proteinuria, assessment of the complement system (C3, C4), ANCA, and ANA should be considered.

For patients with acute kidney injury, acute nephritic syndrome, or nephrotic syndrome, renal biopsy should be considered. On renal biopsy, HSP can cause a wide variety of glomerular lesions ranging from fairly normal glomeruli with mesangial expansion to severe crescentic glomerulonephritis. Most commonly a focal and segmental proliferative glomerular nephritis is seen on light microscopy. Immunofluorescence usually shows a predominance of granular IgA deposition in the mesangial region along with IgG, C3, and fibrin. C1q and C4 are typically absent. The renal biopsy findings cannot be distinguished from IgA nephropathy and the diagnosis of HSP is dependent on the presence of the nonrenal manifestations.

Treatment

In most patients with HSP, specific treatment is not required for resolution of their disease except for some patients with severe renal, GI or central nervous system involvement. Supportive treatment with analgesics and rest is helpful.

The role of corticosteroids in the treatment of HSP associated GI disease has been extensively studied. A recent meta-analysis of 15 articles on the role of steroid treatment in HSP concluded that steroid therapy increased the likelihood of early (<24 hours) pain resolution and reduced the mean time of abdominal pain resolution, but did not reduce the median time for abdominal pain resolution. The doses of steroid used in the studies varied widely but ranged between 1–2.5 mg/kg/day for approximately 7–30 days.

In severe GI disease with protein losing enteropathy or hemorrhage not controlled by bowel rest and oral steroids, pulse methylprednisolone has been reported to be effective, but controlled trials are lacking.

Joint involvement has been managed with nonsteroidal anti-inflammatory agents in the rheumatologic literature; however, these agents should be used with caution in light of the risks for renal and GI involvement. Moreover, they should be avoided in the setting of significant renal involvement, severe abdominal pain/hemorrhage or concomitant high dose steroid treatment where acetaminophen is recommended. Steroids can lessen the symptoms but are rarely indicated solely for joint involvement.

Most of the major long-term complications of HSP are related to renal involvement. In general, studies have focused on the use of steroids to prevent the development of renal disease in early HSP or the treatment of biopsy proven renal disease.

Several studies have examined the possible prevention of HSP nephritis by treatment with prednisone (typically 1–2 mg/kg/day for 10–14 days) at the onset of HSP symptoms. The most recent and largest (290 patients) trial showed no benefit. Systematic analysis of prospective controlled trials on the use of steroids at onset of disease to reduce persistent renal disease has not shown a benefit. At this time, the evidence does not support the use of a single course of prophylactic steroids in patients with HSP solely for renal indications. As noted above, for patients with HSP and significant GI involvement, steroids may be indicated.

For those patients with established significant renal disease, only two randomized controlled trials are available. One small trial with 19 patients suggested benefit of cyclosporine over methylprednisolone in achieving remission (OR 0.39 95% CI 0.14–1.06) but this was not statistically significant. Another trial of cyclophosphamide versus supportive therapy showed no differences in outcomes. In contrast, noncontrolled case series in severe nephritis have reported success with methylprednisolone ± cyclophosphamide ± plasma exchange. The lack evidence from randomized controlled trials for the efficacy of treatment in acute nephritis is not unique to HSP and most nephrologists would initial treat a severe HSP nephritis with a combination of steroids (prednisone or pulse methylprednisolone) and cyclophosphamide or cyclosporine.

Prognosis

The nonrenal symptoms usually resolve with supportive therapy and significant complications are uncommon.

Approximately 90% of patients who will have urinary abnormalities will demonstrate them by eight 8 weeks into illness. The renal prognosis for patients without significant evidence of renal involvement in the first six months after presentation is excellent.

The prognosis for patients with nephritic or nephrotic syndrome is more guarded. Approximately a 20–40% of patients with nephritic or nephrotic syndrome will go on to have long-term chronic kidney disease (CKD) manifest by elevated creatinine, proteinuria, or hypertension.

Although the presence of nephritis or nephrotic syndrome places patients in a high risk category no other consistent risk factors have been identified in several long-term follow-up retrospective studies of HSP nephritis. A standardized biopsy scoring system developed by the International Study of Kidney Diseases in Children has been used in many studies but has not been shown to predict those who will develop long-term CKD. This may relate to inconsistent timing of biopsies in the development of disease and lack of consistent treatment.

Patients with HSP nephritis or nephrosis may appear to fully recover (normal urinalysis, blood pressure, and creatinine) but have subclinical renal damage that becomes apparent many years later. Women who have clinically recovered from HSP nephritis or nephrosis have a higher risk of development of proteinuria and/or hypertension during pregnancy and require careful monitoring.

Patients with a history of HSP and renal involvement should be followed regularly until the urinalysis, blood pressure, and creatinine are normal. Those with persistent abnormalities are at risk for progression. The median time to end-stage renal disease progression is greater than ten years and some patients progress to end-stage renal disease 25 years after initial presentation. Those who appear to fully recover should be rechecked every 1–2 years.

In addition, patients who received prolonged treatment with cyclophosphamide, or experienced cyclophosphamide-induced hemorrhagic cystitis have an elevated risk of developing bladder cancer. Long-term monitoring by annual urinalysis and cytology is recommended, and patients with the development of non-glomerular hematuria should be referred for cystoscopy.

Suggested Reading

Butani L, Morgenstern BZ. (2007) Long-term outcome in children after Henoch–Schönlein purpura nephritis. *Clin Pediatr* (Philadelphia) **46**(6): 505–511.

Chartapisak W, Opastirakul S, Hodson EM, *et al.* (2009) Interventions for preventing and treating kidney disease in Henoch–Schönlein Purpura (HSP). *Cochrane Database Syst Rev* (3): CD005128.

Goldstein AR, White RH, Akuse R, Chantler C. (1992) Long-term follow-up of childhood Henoch–Schönlein nephritis. *Lancet* **339**(8788): 280–282.

Lau KK, Suzuki H, Novak J, Wyatt RJ. (2009) Pathogenesis of Henoch–Schönlein purpura nephritis. *Pediatr Nephrol* **25**(1): 19–26.

Mills JA, Michel BA, Bloch DA, *et al.* (1990) The American College of Rheumatology 1990 criteria for the classification of Henoch–Schönlein purpura. *Arthritis Rheum* **33**: 1114–1121.

Narchi H. (2005) Risk of long-term renal impairment and duration of follow up recommended for Henoch–Schönlein purpura with normal or minimal urinary findings: a systematic review. *Arch Dis Child* **90**(9): 916–920.

Ronkainen J, Nuutinen M, Koskimies O. (2004) The adult kidney 24 years after childhood Henoch–Schönlein purpura: a retrospective cohort study. *Lancet* **360**(9334): 666-670.

Saulsbury FT. (1999) Henoch–Schönlein purpura in children. Report of 100 patients and review of the literature. *Medicine* (Baltimore). **78**(6): 395–409.

Tizard EJ, Hamilton-Ayres MJ. (2008) Henoch–Schönlein purpura. *Arch Dis Child Educ Pract Ed* **93**(1): 1–8.

Weiss PF, Feinstein JA, Luan X, *et al.* (2007) Effects of corticosteroid on Henoch–Schönlein purpura: a systematic review. *Pediatr* **120**(5): 1079–1087.

23

Hemolytic Uremic Syndrome

Swasti Chaturvedi and Christoph Licht

Glossary

Atypical HUS: Diarrhea negative (D-) hemolytic uremic syndrome (HUS). This sub-group comprises other infections, genetic causes, drugs, autoimmune diseases like systemic lupus erythematosus (SLE) and posttransplantation HUS. Responsible for 10% of childhood onset HUS.

EHEC: Enterohemorrhagic *E. coli*.

ST/VT: Shiga toxin, verocytotoxin: toxin produced by enterohemorrhagic *E. coli*, the main virulence factor in HUS with cytopathic effect on *Vero* cell line.

STEC/VTEC: Shiga toxin producing *E. coli*/verotoxin producing *E. coil.*

TMA: Thrombotic microangiopathy. Group of diseases characterized by formation of microthrombi in various organ systems caused either by *ADAMTS13* mutation — resulting in thrombotic thrombocytopenic purpura (TTP) — or by alternative complement pathway regulatory defect — resulting in aHUS.

Typical HUS: D+, diarrhea positive hemolytic uremic syndrome. HUS which follows a prodrome of diarrhea and is caused by ST producing bacteria; responsible for 90% of childhood onset HUS.

Introduction

Thrombotic microangiopathy (TMA) is characterized by occlusive microvascular thrombosis. The two classical TMAs are HUS and TTP (see Fig. 1). Both HUS and TTP are characterized by microangiopathic

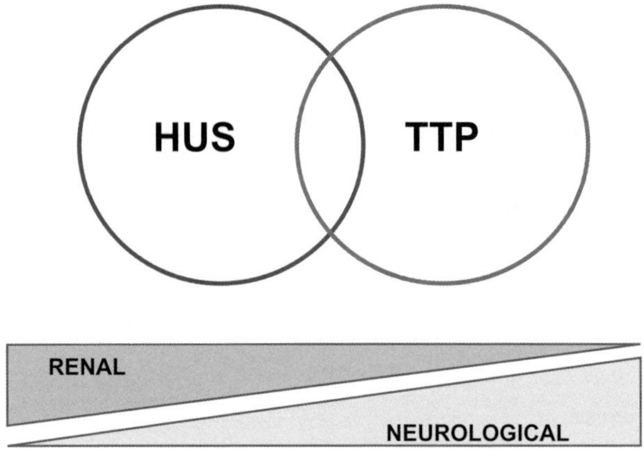

Figure 1. Spectrum of TMAs.

Both HUS and TTP are characterized by microangiopathic hemolytic anemia, thrombocytopenia, and variable signs and symptoms of organ ischemia. HUS has more significant renal involvement whereas TTP has predominant neurological involvement (adapted from Skerka *et al.* (2009) *Mole Immunol* **46**: 2801–2807).

hemolytic anemia (MAHA) and consumptive thrombocytopenia, variable signs and symptoms of organ ischemia. In the past, the two conditions differentiated on clinical grounds with patients being classified as HUS if renal dysfunction predominated or as TTP if neurological features were predominant. In addition, HUS is mainly a childhood disease and TTP is more common in adults. However, the clinical distinction between the two is not always clear and overlap of clinical symptoms of both diseases is common.

In recent years, considerable progress has been made in understanding the etiological basis of these two TMAs, thereby enabling a more informed approach to diagnosis and management. HUS is a triad of MAHA, thrombocytopenia and varying degree of acute kidney injury (AKI). In childhood ~90% of HUS cases are diarrheal (D+; typical) due to Shiga toxin (ST) producing *E. coli* (e.g., O157:H7) and Shigella dysentery. Typical HUS is characterized by a prodrome of bloody diarrhea. It has rapid onset and good prognosis with <5% mortality. Approximately 5–10% children will eventually develop end-stage renal disease (ESRD) requiring renal transplantation. The posttransplant course is favorable with almost no increased risk of disease recurrence.

The remaining 5–10% of HUS cases are labeled diarrhea negative (D-; atypical). Atypical HUS (aHUS) may manifest at any age but is more frequent in adults. aHUS comprises a heterogeneous group with diverse etiology including infections (other than those due to STEC), drugs, genetic causes, autoimmune diseases like SLE, and posttransplantation HUS. This group is characterized by an insidious onset and a progressive course with remissions and relapses. It has a worse prognosis with approximately 50% risk of ESRD and high risk of post kidney transplant recurrence.

TTP is classically described as a pentad of microangiopathic hemolytic anemia, thrombocytopenia, fever, neurologic signs, and renal dysfunction. Both hereditary and acquired forms of TTP are known. Hereditary TTP (Upshaw–Schulman syndrome) is due to inherited deficiency of von Willebrand factor cleaving protease (vWF-CP) known as ADAMTS13 (a disintegrin and metalloproteinase with a thrombospondin type 1 motif, isoform 13). ADAMTS13 (vWF-CP) prevents emergence of large multimers of von Willebrand factor (vWF) by cleaving the multimeric vWF released from endothelial cells and platelets into monomeric units. ADAMTS13 dysfunction leads to accumulation of these unusually large multimers which agglutinate platelets under high shear stress, resulting in clot formation. The acquired form which is more common is the result of the presence of inhibiting antibodies to the vWF-CP.

Shiga Toxin-Associated HUS (Typical or D+ HUS)

Epidemiology

The peak incidence of STEC-associated HUS occurs in childhood, declines with age, but increases again during old age. This pattern is consistent with an age related increase in antibodies associated with anti-ST immunity, followed by decline in such antibodies with old age. Infection is more common in rural versus urban population. In a prospective multicenter study in Germany, the average annual incidence was 0.71/100,000 children <15 years of age. The incidence was higher for children <5 years of age (1.71/100,000). In Canada, the annual incidence was 1.44/100,000 children <15 years of age, and 72% were <5 years of age.

Most *E. coli* infection and HUS cases in the northern hemisphere occur in summer and autumn. The reservoir of ST producing *E. coli* is the intestine of domestic animals. Cattle are considered the main source and vector. The infective dose is 50–100 organisms. In humans, infection is primarily acquired by ingestion of contaminated undercooked meat, unpasteurized milk and milk products, unpasteurized apple cider, fruit, vegetables, and contaminated water. Secondary infection is from person to person transmission which is commonly seen in nursing homes and day care centers. One interesting case of mother to child transmission was described in a seven-day-old child who presented with bloody diarrhea and subsequently developed HUS. STEC are responsible for up to 83% of cases of D+ HUS worldwide. In USA and Europe, 80–86% of these STEC infections are with the *E. coli* serotype O 157:H7. In Australia, most cases are due to non-O157 STEC. *Shigella* dysenteriae type 1 related HUS is described in India, South Africa and Bangladesh.

Histopathology

Endothelial damage is the hallmark of HUS. It causes the adhesion and aggregation of platelets, the formation of thrombi and the impairment of fibrinolysis. Hemolytic anemia is due to damage to red cells as they traverse injured capillaries and small blood vessels with fibrin microthrombi; this results in fragmented red cells (schistocytes). Inflammatory infiltrates in the kidney consist of neutrophils and macrophages. In severe cases, cortical necrosis is a possible complication.

Apart from renal involvement, HUS can affect other organs including the gut, brain, pancreas, liver, and heart. The lesions in the gut consist of small vessel angiopathy in the mucosa and submucosa of the small and large intestines with necrosis and sloughing. Perforation and peritonitis can result. TMA in the brain can result in widespread intracranial hemorrhages, cerebral edema, focal necrosis, spongiosis, and gliosis. In the pancreas, TMA is usually restricted to the region of Langerhans islets resulting in transient or permanent glucose intolerance and diabetes mellitus. The pancreatic acini (pancreatic exocrine function) seem to be less susceptible to TMA. Hepatic lesions are usually comprised of mild focal ischemic damage; hepatic necrosis or fulminant liver failure has not been reported. The most common lesions in the heart are TMA of the small myocardial vessels resulting in small areas of necrosis and occasional infarcts.

STEC virulence factors

STEC virulence factors can be divided into two major classes. Adhesins promote intestinal colonization where toxins are released in the bloodstream, and lead to microvascular injury and disease. STEC virulence factors cause epithelial and endothelial cell damage eventually leading to colitis. ST is picked up by polarized gut cells via the transcellular route and reaches the circulation, a process probably facilitated by transmigration of neutrophils. Neutrophils bind large amounts of ST and may transport the toxin to renal glomerular cells.

ST is a 71-kD protein consisting of a single A subunit (32-kD) linked to five B subunits (7.7-kD). The B subunit helps ST bind to the glycosphingolipid globotriaosylceramide (Gb3) receptor on the target cell. Gb3 receptors are found on cell membranes of monocytes, neutrophils, platelets, glomerular endothelial cells, and tubular epithelial cells. This cell-specific distribution of Gb3 helps to partially explain the organ distribution of the lesions found in HUS. Once inside the cell, the A and B subunits dissociate, and the A subunit translocates to the cytosol. The A subunit is an N-glycosidase which then blocks peptide chain elongation by eliminating one adenine from 28S ribosomal RNA. Additionally, ST also induces endothelial cell apoptosis by inhibiting expression of antiapoptotic Bcl-2 family member, Mcl-1.

Under normal conditions, the endothelium shows an anti-adhesive, anti-inflammatory and thrombo-resistant profile. These hemostatic properties are lost due to ST mediated endothelial dysfunction. The net result is expression of pro-adhesive, pro-thrombotic, and inflammatory genes in endothelial cells. This promotes adhesion and activation of white cells, specifically neutrophils and monocytes. Activated neutrophils and monocytes cause further endothelial damage through release of cytokines, toxic oxygen species, and lipid peroxidation. Cytokines, especially tumor necrosis factor-α (TNF-α) and interleukin 1-β (IL1-β), potentiate toxin action through upregulation of the cellular receptor, Gb3.

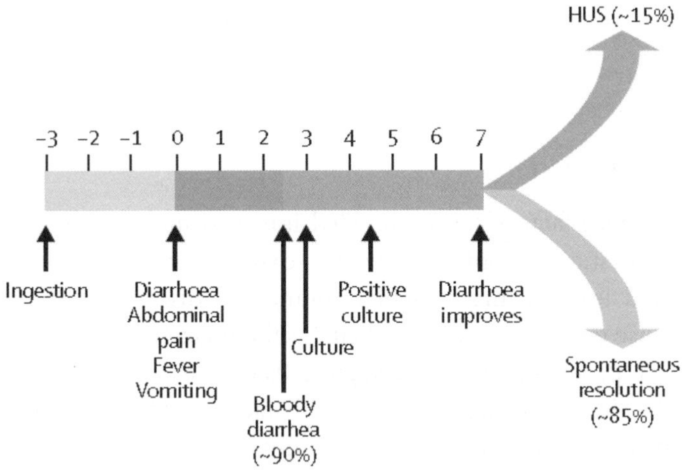

Figure 2. Progression of *E. coli* infection in children.

Patient develops diarrhea, vomiting, abdominal pain and fever about 3 days after ingesting the organism. The diarrhea becomes bloody 1–3 days later. Majority of children (~85%) then undergo spontaneous resolution, however, ~15% develop HUS (with permission from Tarr *et al.* (2005) *Lancet* **365**: 1073–1085).

Clinical features (see Fig. 2)

The mean interval between *E. coli* exposure and onset of illness is 3 days (range 1–8). Affected children exhibit diarrhea in 91% of the cases, which is bloody in 57% of the cases. Vomiting occurs in 30–60% of the cases, and fever in one third of the cases. Of the STEC infected patients, 5–15% progress to HUS after 5–10 days. Renal involvement may manifest as isolated hematuria, proteinuria, or AKI. Renal failure is reported in 55–70% of cases and up to 60% may require dialysis during the acute phase.

Extrarenal involvement

HUS is a systemic disease accompanied by extrarenal manifestations in a variety of organ systems, e.g., central nervous system (CNS) and the gastrointestinal (GI) tract. CNS involvement is common and manifests mainly as irritability, encephalopathy and seizures. In more severe cases focal neurologic deficits and coma may occur. GI tract involvement can occur anywhere from the esophagus to the perianal area and present as hemorrhagic colitis, bowel necrosis, intussusception, perforation, or colonic stricture. Liver involvement manifests as hepatomegaly and elevated transaminases. Pancreatic involvement leading to glucose intolerance is usually limited to the acute phase and occurs in about 10% of patients. Cardiac involvement can lead to congestive heart failure in the acute phase and cardiomyopathy can manifest up to a few months after the first manifestation of HUS.

Diagnosis

The diagnosis of HUS is based on clinical features and lab evidence of Coombs negative MAHA, thrombocytopenia and renal injury. MAHA is evidenced by low hemoglobin, reticulocytosis, elevated LDH and serum unconjugated bilirubin, decreased levels of serum haptoglobin, and schistocytes or fragmented red cells on blood film. Renal involvement manifests as elevated creatinine and urea, and varying degrees of proteinuria, hematuria, and sometimes glucosuria on urine dipstick. Renal biopsy is rarely required for diagnosis.

STEC infections in humans have been identified in many countries. The identification of STEC excretors and STEC strains is requested by Public Health Authorities for the prevention of outbreaks. Children may excrete *E. coli* for more than 3 weeks in their stool but asymptomatic prolonged carriage is unusual. *E. coli* O157:H7, which is the predominant cause of HUS around most of the world, cannot ferment sorbitol. This is best detected by plating of fresh feces on sorbitol-MacConkey agar (SMAC) media. This agar has sorbitol, not lactose, as a carbon source. EHEC O157:H7 therefore produces colorless colonies with overnight incubation on SMAC media.

Direct detection of Shiga toxin or the use of DNA probes for detecting the toxin gene in fecal isolates has the advantage of detecting non O157:H7 *E. coli* as well. However these assays do not detect serotypes of EHEC strains and a stool culture should be done to determine individual strains.

Management

Specific therapy

There is no specific treatment for STEC HUS and management is mainly supportive. Intravenous rehydration with isotonic saline in patients who present early with bloody diarrhea and before development of HUS is recommended. This may provide relative nephroprotection and attenuate renal injury.

Antimotility agents are not recommended as they may potentially prolong recovery time. Antibiotics are generally not recommended for patients with definite or possible STEC diarrhea and should only be used in cases of bacteremia, in which circumstance, they should be initiated early.

ST binding agents may be useful in intervening early and preventing the development of HUS. However, a randomized controlled trial using oral ST binding agent SYNSORB Pk, composed of silicon particles linked to Gb3, failed to show any beneficial effect over placebo in reducing mortality or serious extrarenal or renal events. Plasma therapy, heparin, prostacyclin, fibrinolytics, IVIG and antiplatelet agents have no proven benefit in D+ HUS.

Supportive therapy

Management of AKI

Children with suspected HUS and imminent renal failure need to be transferred early to a pediatric nephrology center that offers renal replacement therapy (RRT) in the form of hemodialysis (HD) or peritoneal dialysis (PD). More than 60% of children show evidence of renal failure in the acute phase. The indications for dialysis in HUS are similar to any other cause of AKI and include volume overload, severe acidosis, electrolyte abnormalities and fluid removal for provision of nutrition. The choice of dialysis modality will depend on each center's expertise and availability.

Hypertension is usually managed with vasodilators. Angiotensin converting enzyme (ACE) inhibitors should be avoided in acute illness as they may exacerbate renal injury. Diuretics can be used to manage volume overload but are unlikely to be effective beyond early HUS. Dialysis is the most effective management of fluid overload and hypertension. In addition nephrotoxic medications should be avoided and drugs dosing adjusted accordingly.

Management of extrarenal involvement

Early identification and management of other organ involvement is important for optimal care. Anemia and thrombocytopenia usually resolve spontaneously and blood product transfusion is rarely indicated. Packed red blood cell transfusion may in fact worsen fluid overload and hyperkalemia in an oliguric patient and should only be given if clinically indicated. Similarly, platelet transfusion is only indicated in case of a surgical procedure or active bleeding. For correction of coagulation abnormalities, fresh frozen plasma (FFP) transfusion may be required.

Other investigations should be tailored to the clinical situation. EEG and MRI/CT should be obtained if a child develops seizures or altered consciousness. An electrocardiogram/echocardiogram should be done if arrhythmia is found or if cardiac involvement is suspected. Upright abdominal film should be done if an ileus or bowel perforation is suspected. Liver enzymes are often elevated and should be monitored serially. Pancreatic involvement may manifest as elevated blood glucose levels. Therefore, they should be carefully monitored and insulin treatment initiated if required. Serum amylase and lipase should be monitored if pancreatitis is suspected. Careful attention should be given to the provision of nutrition and temporary tube feeding or total parenteral nutrition may be required.

Prognosis

Mortality rate during the acute phase is 3–5%. With survival, spontaneous resolution begins 1–2 weeks after the onset of the disease with approximately 25% of survivors having long-term renal sequelae. ESRD occurs in about 5–10% of patients who will ultimately require a kidney transplant.

Kidney transplant is a safe and effective treatment for those patients who progress to ESRD, with <1% risk of recurrence of HUS after transplant.

Potential future therapies

(1) Monoclonal antibodies against A and B subunits of Shiga toxin.
(2) Probiotic bacteria expressing Gb3 trisaccharide on their cell surface. Oral administration of these bacteria to mice protects against virulent STEC by adsorbing and neutralizing the ST.
(3) Synthetic toxin binders STARFISH which binds to all five B-subunits of ST.

(4) Vaccines for humans and cattle. Human vaccines include antitoxin vaccine and antiadhesin vaccines. In previous trials vaccination of cattle with proteins secreted by *E. coli* led to significant reduction in the amount and duration of the bacterial shedding in feces.

Prevention

In the absence of specific therapy, prevention is the most effective strategy. Cattle are the main reservoir of STEC, therefore public health control requires vigilance at all stages of the food chain. Safe food handling and proper cooking of meat will hopefully prevent large outbreaks, and individual illness. In addition, milk and milk product pasteurization, active surveillance with early identification and notification of cases, and removal of contaminated food items will limit the spread of infection.

Non Shiga Toxin-Associated HUS (Atypical or D-HUS)

Atypical HUS (aHUS) or D-HUS (non Stx-HUS) comprises 5–10% of all cases of HUS. It includes HUS due to infections other than Stx-HUS, drugs, genetic causes, etc.

Pneumococcal HUS

Infection caused by *Streptococcus pneumoniae* accounts for 40% of aHUS and 5% of all causes of HUS in children in the USA. The incidence of HUS following invasive pneumococcal infection is 0.4–0.6%. The incidence is expected to decline in the future with the recent introduction of pneumococcal vaccination.

Pathophysiology

The exact pathophysiology has not yet been determined. However, it is thought that neuraminidase released by pneumococci cleaves the N-acetyl neuraminic acid from cell surfaces and exposes the so called Thomsen–Friedenreich (TF) cryptantigen. This antigen is a cell membrane component of RBC, platelets and glomerular endothelial cells. Preformed host IgM antibodies bind to exposed TF antigen and initiate endothelial damage, microvascular injury, hemolytic anemia, and thrombocytopenia characteristic of HUS. Other neuraminidase producing organisms like influenza A virus and *Capnocytophaga canimorsus* have also been reported to cause HUS.

Clinical features

Children with pneumococcal HUS are generally younger and have a more severe course as compared to Stx positive HUS. Approximately 70% of the cases are associated with pneumonia/empyema, 30% with meningitis and 5% with both. They have longer periods of oligo-anuria, more frequent need for acute dialysis (75% vs. 60%), more prolonged hospital stay (33 vs. 16 days), and require more red cell and platelet transfusions as compared to those with typical HUS.

Management

- Critically ill children should be treated with IV vancomycin and a third generation cephalosporin for possible or proven pneumococcal infection.
- Management of complications arising from pneumococcal infection (e.g., chest tube insertion for empyema).
- Supportive management of AKI and hematological abnormalities (e.g., anemia and thrombocytopenia).
- Additional preformed antibody administration via FFP transfusion or unwashed red cells should be avoided as anti-TF IgM antibodies are integral to the pathogenesis.

Prognosis

Acute mortality is approximately 12% and is largely dependent on the site of the infection. Patients with meningitis fare much worse. Another 16% survive with CKD or hypertension. The recurrence risk is very low, and approximately 10% of patients develop ESRD.

Other infections

Infections with HIV, HTLV-1, EBV, *B. pertussis*, *E. histolytica* have all been associated with HUS.

Genetic disorders of complement regulation

The complement system is a part of the immune surveillance system in humans (Fig. 3). It is composed of three activation pathways which terminate in a common lytic pathway. The classical pathway is activated by the binding of C1q to antigen antibody complexes. The lectin pathway is antibody independent and is activated by the binding of mannose binding lectin (MBL) to mannose which is present on the cell surface of many microbes. Different from these, the alternative pathway is antibody independent and constantly active at a low rate. Spontaneously activated C3 (i.e. C3b) binds covalently to the surfaces of the host and of the pathogens as well as "altered self" surfaces. While the classical and lectin pathway are inducible, the alternative pathway has to be constantly down regulated, and a multilayered system of complement regulatory proteins (soluble and membrane anchored) is in place to prevent indiscriminate and continued

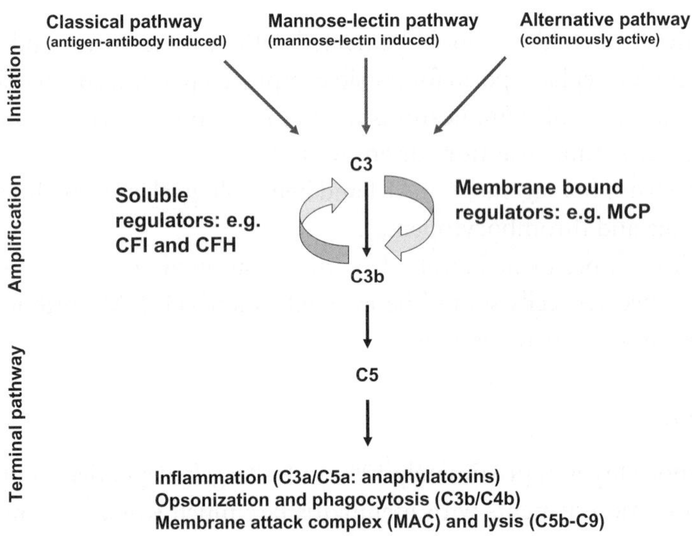

Figure 3. The complement system.

The complement system is a part of immune surveillance system in humans. It is composed of three activation pathways which terminate in a common lytic pathway with formation of membrane attack complex (MAC C5b-C9). While the classical and lectin pathway are inducible, the alternative pathway has to be constantly down regulated. A multilayered system of complement regulatory proteins (soluble and membrane anchored) is in place to prevent indiscriminate and continued activation of alternative pathway.

activation. In principle, there are two classes of alternative complement pathway regulators, (i) soluble or fluid phase regulators [e.g. Factor H (CFH) and complement Factor I (CFI)], and (ii) membrane bound regulators [e.g. decay accelerating factor (DAF; CD55), membrane cofactor protein (MCP; CD46) and complement receptor 1 (CR1)].

Genetic defects in a number of these regulators have been identified in ~60% of the cases of aHUS. Mutations in *CFH* account for 15–30%, mutations in *MCP* for 10% and mutations in *CFI* for 5–12% of aHUS cases. In addition, *CFH* gene conversion, deletion of the complement *CFH*-related genes *CFHR1* and *3* by nonallelic homologous recombination, *CFB* gain of function mutations, *C3* mutations and the presence of CFH autoantibodies have been reported in aHUS patients. The penetrance of the mutations is incomplete and initial presentation or relapses are often triggered by infections. In addition, physiological stressors like pregnancy may trigger aHUS in genetically predisposed individuals. Knowledge of the type of genetic defect has important implication in management and prognosis of these patients.

Factor H (CFH)

CFH is a 150-kD single chain plasma glycoprotein that is considered to be the most important regulator of the alternative complement pathway and has both cofactor and decay accelerating activity (see Fig. 4). CFH serves as a cofactor for the C3b-cleaving enzyme CFI in degradation of newly formed C3b molecules and controls decay, formation and stability of the C3b convertase, C3bBb. CFH serum levels vary considerably (neonates 170–397 μg/ml; adults 242–759 μg/ml). Most children reach adult levels by 1 year of age. The gene encoding for CFH is located on chromosome 1q32. CFH is principally produced in the liver and is composed of 20 homologous units, named short consensus repeats (SCRs) or complement control proteins (CCPs). The N-terminal SCRs1–4 mediate cofactor and decay accelerating activity, and the C-terminal SCRs19–20 form a recognition region, which contains binding sites for C3b, heparin, basement membrane and endothelial cells (polyanions). At present, more than 100 distinct mutations have been reported in aHUS patients. The vast majority of these mutations are heterozygous, are located in the C-terminus (SCR 19–20) and impair CFH binding capability. This in turn leads to

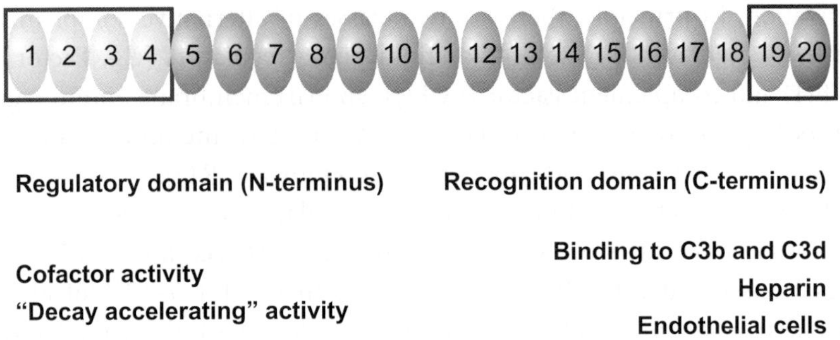

Figure 4. Complement factor H (CFH).

CFH is a single chain plasma glycoprotein and is the most important regulator of the alternate pathway of complement and has both cofactor and decay accelerating activity. It is composed of 20 homologous units, named short consensus repeats (SCRs) or complement control proteins (CCPs). The N-terminal SCRs1–4 mediate cofactor and decay accelerating activity, and the C-terminal SCRs19–20 form a recognition region, which contain binding sites for C3b, heparin, basement membrane and endothelial cells (polyanions). The vast majority of mutations are heterozygous and are located in the C-terminus (SCR 19–20), thus impairing CFH binding capability.

reduction in CFH regulatory activity on e.g., endothelial cells with subsequent cell damage and exposure of subendothelial matrix. Interestingly, CFH auto-antibodies which have been identified in about 10% of aHUS patients with CFHR1/3 deficiency also interfere with the C-terminal recognition function of CFH.

CFH mutations are reported in both sporadic and familial aHUS cases. It is characterized by early onset (<1 year of age), relapsing course and severe disease with 60% patients reaching ESRD or dying within 1 year. The risk of recurrence post-transplant is very high (~80%).

Factor I (CFI)

CFI is an 88kD serine protease with plasma concentration of 35 μg/ml. CFI is also primarily synthesized in the liver. CFI cleaves and thereby inactivates C3b and C4b in the presence of cofactors, i.e. CFH or MCP. CFI is composed of two chains, a heavy and a light chain. The heavy chain has a CFI module, a scavenger receptor module and two low density lipoproteins domains (LDL). The heavy chain is disulfide linked to the light chain. The light chain has serine protease domain. All mutations reported are heterozygous.

CFI mutations have only been reported in sporadic cases. These patients have a similar clinical course as patients with CFH deficiency with 50% incidence of ESRD and ~100% recurrence risk post-transplant.

Membrane cofactor protein (MCP; CD46)

MCP (CD46) is a ~65Kd transmembrane protein that serves as cofactor for CFI mediated cleavage of C3b that is deposited on self tissues. It is composed of four extracellular SCR domains and a transmembranous and cellular domain. Most mutations are heterozygous and cluster in the four extracellular SCRs of MCP. MCP is highly expressed in the kidneys.

Patients with *MCP* mutations present at an older age (median age 4.5 years) and have a much better outcome compared to those with *CFH* or *CFI* mutations. Relapse with complete recovery is common. In those who develop ESRD and undergo renal transplantation, the graft outcome is good with low risk of recurrence as MCP is a transmembrane regulator and a renal allograft will be protected by wild type MCP from the donor kidney.

Treatment (current and future)

(1) *Plasma therapy*: Replacement of defective soluble regulators by plasma exchange (PLEX) or repetitive plasma transfusions is the mainstay of treatment. FFP transfusions replace defective CFH, CFI, CFB and C3. PLEX removes anti-CFH antibodies and antibodies to ADAMTS13. PLEX also prevents volume overload and cardiac failure which may occur if patient receives large amounts of FFP infusions. Since MCP is not a circulating protein, a beneficial effect of plasma therapy is unlikely to be expected in patients with MCP mutation.

Recommendations regarding the time of initiation, dose, frequency and duration of PLEX are empirical, and evidence based research is lacking. Recently published European Pediatric Study Group Guidelines recommend initiating plasma therapy as soon as the diagnosis of aHUS is made. This should be done in parallel with other measures (e.g., dialysis and management of hypertension). PLEX should be first line therapy with exchange of 1.5 plasma volumes per session, replaced by FFP. Plasma transfusions of 10–20 ml/kg should be given if PLEX cannot be performed within 24 hours of presentation. PLEX should be continued daily for five days, then five times a week for two weeks and then three times a week for two weeks. Further frequency of PLEX should be prescribed on an individual basis.

(2) *Specific antibodies (e.g., eculizumab)*: Eculizumab is a recombinant humanized monoclonal anti-C5 antibody that blocks the activation of terminal complement components. It binds specifically to the terminal complement protein C5, inhibiting its cleavage into C5a and C5b, thereby preventing the release of the inflammatory mediator C5a and the formation of the terminal complement membrane attack complex (MAC), C5b-9. Regular eculizumab infusions have been reported to be safe and effective in reducing hemolysis and blood transfusion requirements in patients with paroxysmal nocturnal hemoglobinuria (PNH). Additionally, it has recently been shown to be effective in a child with congenital aHUS and an adult patient with aHUS refractory to plasma therapy. Pharmacodynamic activity is concentration-dependent with a plasma concentration of ≥35 μg/mL resulting in complete inhibition of *in vivo* hemolytic activity.

Treatment side effects are minor and include headache, nasopharyngitis, and upper respiratory tract infections. As terminal complement proteins provide protective immunity against meningococcal infection, eculizumab may increase the risk of infection with *Neisseria meningitides*; therefore vaccination against *Neisseria meningitides* should be provided before starting eculizumab.

(3) *Replacement of missing factors via purified or recombinantly expressed proteins*: A human plasma-derived CFH concentrate is being developed.

(4) *Immunosuppression in case of antibodies*: Corticosteroids and rituximab (anti-CD20 antibody) have been used to prevent production of antibodies after initial therapy with PLEX in patients with antibody mediated aHUS.

(5) *Renal transplantation*: Given the high risk of graft loss due to recurrence, renal transplant is currently not a realistic treatment for patients with identified *CFH* and *CFI* mutations. Kidney transplant is offered in case of *MCP* mutations. Living related donors are discouraged as the risk of disease in the live related donor cannot be ruled out

Table 1. Treatment concepts for aHUS and ADAMTS

Abnormality	Current treatment	Future treatment
Mutations leading to impaired complement control either due to: — Protein deficiency — Functional defect	— Plasma infusion (20 ml/kg/14 days) — Plasma exchange (1–1.5 plasma volume) — Liver transplant — Combined liver and kidney transplant	— Purified CFH — Recombinant CFH — Eculizumab
Autoantibodies to: — Complement regulators — ADAMTS13	— Plasma infusion (20 ml/kg/14 days) — Plasma exchange (1–1.5 plasma volume)	— Rituximab — Eculizumab

with absolute certainty, due to unknown genetic factors possibly shared with the recipient. Bilateral nephrectomy of native kidneys of recipient prior to transplant does not seem to prevent recurrence; neither does the avoidance of calcineurin inhibitors.

(6) *Combined liver and kidney transplantation*: As CFH and CFI are synthesized in the liver, liver transplantation alone or combined liver and kidney transplantation has been proposed as a treatment of severe CFH deficiency and possibly for CFI deficiency. Early results of combined liver–kidney transplantation were disappointing. More recently, however, successful combined liver and kidney transplants have been reported under intensive plasma therapy, to correct complement dysregulation during the perioperative period. A summary of therapeutic options is depicted in Table 1.

Genetic and Acquired Disorders of the von Willebrand Factor Cleaving Protease (vWFCP) ADAMTS13

Hereditary TTP (Upshaw Schulman syndrome) is caused by homozygous or compound heterozygous *ADAMTS13* mutations. Acquired TTP is often but not always associated with severe, autoantibody mediated *ADAMTS13* deficiency.

ADAMTS13, also known as von Willebrand factor-cleaving protease (vWFCP), is a metalloprotease synthesized in the liver and has a plasma half-life of 2–3 days. By cleaving newly generated von Willebrand Factor (vWF) it prevents the formation of ultralarge vWF multimers (ULVWFM) and prevents their accumulation in the circulation. These large multimers are secreted by endothelial cells and are extremely adhesive and have procoagulant properties. ADAMTS13 is encoded by a gene on chromosome 9 and its congenital deficiency is inherited in an autosomal recessive fashion.

Congenital ADAMTS13 deficiency may present in childhood; however, 40–50% remain clinically asymptomatic until adolescence or adulthood, when the first episode may be triggered by infection or pregnancy. Diagnosis is made by detecting ULVWFM in the plasma. In addition ADAMT13 antigen assays can be done. PCR assays can be used to identify genetic mutation. Treatment of affected individuals involves FFP transfusion during acute episodes to achieve remission and prophylactic treatment every 2–3 weeks to prevent relapse in recurrent cases. PLEX is more effective than FFP transfusions in cases of acquired TTP due to ADAMTS autoantibodies. The mortality rate in treated patients is <10%.

Defective Cobalamin Metabolism

A rare form of HUS is seen in infants with an inborn error of cobalamin-C (Cbl-C) metabolism. Cobalamin III is released from its transporter (transcobalamin) in the lysosome. It is then exported into the cytosol and the mitochondrion and undergoes stepwise reduction to cobalamin II and cobalamin I. Cobalamin I initiates synthesis of two coenzymes, adenosyl-Cbl (in the mitochondrion) and methylcobalamin (in the cytosol). Adenosyl-Cbl is coenzyme of methymalonyl-CoA mutase, and methylcobalamin is a coenzyme of the methionine synthase. Defects in synthesis of coenzymes lead to hyperhomocysteinemia and methylmalonic aciduria. Hyperhomocysteinemia is associated with endothelial injury.

Affected infants present with hypotonia, developmental delay and failure to thrive. They rapidly progress to hemolytic anemia, thrombocytopenia, renal, and hepatic failure.

Therapy requires parenteral hydroxocobalamin, betaine (carries synergistic effect with hydroxocobalamin), folic acid (reduces hyperhomocyteinemia), and carnitine supplementation (lowers methyl malonic acid levels).

Autoimmune Disorders

TMA occurs occasionally in SLE and antiphospholipid antibody syndrome and rarely in other autoimmune disorders. The exact pathogenesis of TMA in SLE is unclear but may be the result of a generalized autoimmune process resulting in direct endothelial injury, antiendothelial antibodies and in some cases ADAMTS13 autoantibodies. PLEX, corticosteroids and cyclophosphamide are the most commonly used therapies.

Medications

Many commonly prescribed medications are reported to be associated with TMA. The most commonly reported TMA-associated medications are calcineurin inhibitors (cyclosporine and tacrolimus), antineoplastic agents (mitomycin C, bleomycin, cisplatin), antimalarials (quinine), and antiplatelet agents (ticlopedine and clopidogrel). Endothelial injury due to calcineurin inhibitors is mediated by thromboxane induced vasoconstriction, alterations in prostacyclin synthesis, increased renin-angiotensin activity, increased endothelin secretion, and reduced formation of activated protein C. Treatment is by withdrawal of offending agents, although not all patients will respond.

Transplantation

Posttransplantation TMA may be the result of recurrent disease or a *de novo* process. Recurrent TMA is usually associated with genetic forms of HUS. *De novo* TMA can occur after hematopoietic stem cell transplantation or after solid organ transplantation. An important point to consider in the postkidney transplant setting is differentiating TMA from acute vascular rejection as therapy of these two conditions varies considerably. TMA is a result of primary, nonantibody mediated endothelial injury. On the other hand, acute vascular rejection is due to antibodies to donor endothelium which activates the classical complement pathway, causes deposition of C4d in peritubular capillaries and leads to endovasculitis.

Miscellaneous Causes

These include malignancy, pregnancy, HELLP syndrome (hemolytic anemia, elevated liver enzymes and low platelets), and numerous other triggers.

Summary

HUS and TTP constitute a spectrum of diseases resulting in TMA. Approximately 90% childhood HUS cases are D+ or typical HUS and are caused by ST producing enteric pathogens.

Management of typical HUS is supportive. Extrarenal complications are common and important determinants of morbidity and mortality, and need to be carefully anticipated and managed. Approximately 25% of survivors of typical HUS have long-term renal sequelae, and there is a ~12% risk of ESRD. Thus careful follow-up is required. The rest of 10% of HUS cases are due to other infections, genetically defined defects in alternative complement pathway regulation, medications, malignancies, autoimmune causes, etc., and are labeled atypical or D-HUS.

Genetic disorders of alternative complement pathway regulation account for 50–60% of the cases of aHUS. These cases usually have poor prognosis with a relapsing and remitting course and high risk of ESKD. There is also a ~70–80% risk of disease recurrence post kidney transplant (CFH and CFI deficiency).

TTP is usually an adult onset cause of TMA due to acquired ADAMTS13 antibodies. However, a congenital form due to ADAMTS13 deficiency (Upshaw–Schulman syndrome) is also known.

Plasma therapy (transfusions/exchange) remains mainstay of HUS therapy resulting from complement and ADAMTS13 disorders. Despite much progress in understanding of these diseases, therapeutic options remain limited and newer therapies are desperately needed.

Acknowledgments

The authors gratefully acknowledge the proof-reading of L. Catherine Bishop, RN, BScN.

Suggested Reading

Ake JA, Jelacic S, Ciol MA, *et al.* (2005) Relative nephroprotection during Escherichia coli O157:H7 infections: association with intravenous volume expansion. *Pediatrics* 115: e673–680.

Ariceta G, Besbas N, Johnson S, *et al.* (2009) Guideline for the investigation and initial therapy of diarrhea-negative hemolytic uremic syndrome. *Pediatr Nephrol* **24**: 687–696.

Copelovitch L, Kaplan BS. (2008) Streptococcus pneumoniae-associated hemolytic uremic syndrome. *Pediatr Nepholr* **23**: 1951–1956.

Desch K, Motto D, Desch K, Motto D. (2007) Is there a shared pathophysiology for thrombotic thrombocytopenic purpura and hemolytic-uremic syndrome? *J Am Soc Nephrol* **18**: 2457–2460.

Furlan M, Robles R, Galbusera M, *et al.* (1998) von Willebrand factor-cleaving protease in thrombotic thrombocytopenic purpura and the hemolytic-uremic syndrome. *New Eng J Med* **339**: 1578–1584.

Garg AX, Suri RS, Barrowman N, *et al.* (2003) Long-term renal prognosis of diarrhea-associated hemolytic uremic syndrome: a systematic review, meta-analysis, and meta-regression. *JAMA* **290**: 1360–1370.

Loirat C, Fremeaux-Bacchi V. (2008) Hemolytic uremic syndrome recurrence after renal transplantation. *Pediatr Transpl* **12**: 619–629.

Michael M, Elliott EJ, Ridley GF, *et al.* (2009) Interventions for haemolytic uraemic syndrome and thrombotic thrombocytopenic purpura. Cochrane Database of Systematic Reviews: CD003595.

Moake JL, Rudy CK, Troll JH, *et al.* (1982) Unusually large plasma factor VIII: von Willebrand factor multimers in chronic relapsing thrombotic thrombocytopenic purpura. *New Eng J Med* **307**: 1432–1435.

Noris M, Remuzzi G, Noris M, Remuzzi G. (2005) Hemolytic uremic syndrome. *J Am Soc Nephr* **16**: 1035–1050.

Nurnberger J, Witzke O, Saez AO, *et al.* (2009) Eculizumab for atypical hemolytic-uremic syndrome. *New Eng J Med* **360**: 542–544.

Ruggenenti P, Noris M, Remuzzi G. (2001) Thrombotic microangiopathy, hemolytic uremic syndrome, and thrombotic thrombocytopenic purpura. *Kidney Int* **60**: 831–846.

Sellier-Leclerc AL, Fremeaux-Bacchi V, Dragon-Durey MA, *et al.* (2007) Differential impact of complement mutations on clinical characteristics in atypical hemolytic uremic syndrome. *J Am Soc Nephrol* **18**: 2392–2400.

Spika JS, Parsons JE, Nordenberg D, *et al.* (1986) Hemolytic uremic syndrome and diarrhea associated with Escherichia coli 0157:H7 in a day care center. *J Pediatr* **109**: 287–291.

Tsai HM, Lian EC. (1998) Antibodies to von Willebrand factor-cleaving protease in acute thrombotic thrombocytopenic purpura. *New Eng J Med* **339**: 1585–1594.

Part VII

Tubular Disorders

24

Renal Tubular Acidosis

Rasheed A. Gbadegesin and John W. Foreman

Introduction

Arterial pH is maintained within the narrow range of 7.35–7.45 by pulmonary regulation of arterial partial pressure of carbon dioxide and by the renal alteration of acid base metabolism. Renal tubular acidosis (RTA), which is due to decreased filtered bicarbonate reabsorption or decreased titratable acid and ammonium excretion, is characterized by a normal anion gap, hyperchloremic metabolic acidosis.

Classification of RTA

Four types of RTA exist — each with distinct pathophysiology and clinical characteristics.

Type 1 RTA

Distal renal tubular acidosis (DRTA) is due to impaired hydrogen (H^+) ion and ammonium secretion in the distal tubule.

Pathophysiology

DRTA commonly results from decreased apical proton pump H^+-ATPase activity resulting in decreased H^+ secretion and inability to produce a urine with a pH <5.5. Other mechanisms include increased luminal permeability and back leak of H^+ as seen in amphotericin nephrotoxicity, and reduced sodium reabsorption in the cortical collecting duct. Impaired H^+ excretion leads to decreased ammonium and titratable acid excretion and increased HCO_3^- excretion. Hypokalemia occurs frequently in DRTA resulting from reduced H^+ secretion in the distal tubule and compensatory increased potassium excretion to maintain electroneutrality with sodium reabsorption. Hypokalemia also results from impaired HCO_3^- reabsorption in the distal nephron, inducing kaliuresis. Rickets in children and osteomalacia in adults are associated with DRTA due to H^+ buffering by bone causing impaired mineralization. Other features of DRTA are nephrocalcinosis and kidney stones from hypocitraturia and hypercalciuria.

Etiology

Etiologies of DRTA are listed in Table 1 and include inherited forms: autosomal recessive forms are due to mutations in various subunits of H^+-ATPase; while the dominant form is due to mutations in the electroneutral anion exchanger AE1 (Cl^-/HCO_3^-). Associated phenotypes are summarized in Table 1.

Diagnostic criteria type 1 RTA

- Hyperchloremic metabolic acidosis
- Inability to achieve urine pH <5.5 in systemic acidosis
- Failure to thrive, persistent vomiting
- Hypokalemia

Incomplete DRTA may present with persistently high urine pH, but normal plasma HCO_3^-. Failure to thrive and nephrocalcinosis is common in this variant, which is identified by inability to lower urinary pH <5.5 after acid loading.

Type 2 RTA

Proximal renal tubular acidosis (PRTA) results from impaired ability of the proximal tubule to normally reabsorb filtered bicarbonate and is characterized by hyperchloremic metabolic acidosis with normal or low serum potassium.

Pathophysiology

The proximal tubules normally reabsorb 60–80% of the filtered load of bicarbonate. In normal proximal tubules, water and carbon dioxide are

Table 1. Causes of type 1 RTA (distal RTA)

1. Inherited

Genes/Protein	Locus/Mode of Inheritance	Phenotype
ATP6V0A4 H^+/ATPase A4	7q/AR	Complete or incomplete DRTA Presentation in childhood Late onset deafness
ATP6V1B1/H^+/ATPase A4	2p/AR	DRTA Progressive deafness
SLC4/AE1	17q/AR	Mainly seen in South East Asia DRTA Associated with ovalocytosis
SLC4A1/AE1	17q/AD	Complete or incomplete DRTA Hypercalciuria/Nephrocalcinosis/ nephrolithiasis Hypokalemia Short stature/Osteomalacia/rickets

2. Secondary

Sjogren syndrome	Amphotericin B	Medullary cystic kidney disease
Hypercalciuria	Liver cirrhosis	Obstructive uropathy
Rheumatoid arthritis	SLE	Postrenal transplantation
Hyperglobulinemia	Sickle Cell anemia	Lithium carbonate therapy
Ifosfamide	Ehlers–Danlos syndrome	

combined and cleaved to H^+ and HCO_3^-, a reaction catalyzed by carbonic anhydrase type 2 (CA II). H^+ is secreted into the lumen through the apical Na^+/H^+ exchanger and HCO_3^- is transported through the basolateral Na^+/HCO_3^- (NCB1) cotransporter into the blood. Some H^+, pumped into the tubular lumen by the H^+-ATPase, reacts with filtered HCO_3^- to form H_2CO_3 which is converted to H_2O and CO_2 by carbonic anhydrase type IV (CA IV) present in proximal tubule luminal membrane. The newly generated CO_2 diffuses into the proximal tubule cell to repeat the process. The net result of these reactions is movement (reabsorption) of filtered HCO_3^- into the blood. Proximal RTA occurs when this process is disrupted (see Table 2). Impairment in bicarbonate reabsorption in PRTA is not complete; patients with PRTA are not able to reabsorb 60–80% of the filtered load but can reabsorb a lesser fraction of HCO_3^-. Typically, these patients

Table 2. Causes of type 2 RTA (proximal RTA)

1. Primary/Inherited PRTA

Genes/Protein	Locus/Mode of Inheritance	Phenotype
SLC4A4/NBC1	4q/AR	PRTA Ocular abnormalities: Glaucoma, cataracts, keratopathy Others: Short stature, dental enamel defects, mental retardation, pancreatitis, basal ganglia calcification
CA2/CA(11)	8q/AR	PRTA, mental retardation, cerebral calcification and osteopetrosis
Unknown	AD	PRTA, short stature and osteomalacia

2. Secondary

- Fanconi syndrome
  - Primary/idiopathic
  - Genetic: Cystinosis, Fanconi–Bickel syndrome, galactosemia, fructosemia, Tyrosinemia, Lowe syndrome, Dent disease, Wilson disease
  - Secondary: aminoglycosides, outdated tetracycline, ifosfamide, postrenal transplant, interstitial nephritis
- Hyperparathyroidism
- Vitamin D deficiency
- Metachromatic dystrophy
- Osteopetrosis
- Lowe syndrome
- Leigh syndrome and other mitochondrial disorders
- Tyrosinemia
- Drugs: ifosfamide, carbonic anhydrase inhibitors
- Heavy metal exposure: lead, mercury, cadmium, copper
- Fallot's tetralogy and other cyanotic congenital heart disease
- Cystic kidney disease
- Postrenal transplant
- Nephrotic syndrome
- Hereditary nephritis

will have a low serum HCO_3^- but stabilizes because the filtered load is reduced and the tubule can reabsorb nearly all of this reduced load, with resultant urine pH <5.5. The serum HCO_3^- level at which these patients begin to "spill" HCO_3^- (pH >6.0), is called the bicarbonate threshold.

PRTA is often part of a more global proximal tubular disorder such as Fanconi syndrome, characterized by PRTA, glucosuria, aminoaciduria, and hyperphosphaturia. Fanconi syndrome may be primary or idiopathic, hereditary/genetic or secondary to drug toxicity and other systemic illnesses (see Table 2).

Diagnostic criteria type 2 RTA (PRTA)

- Low serum HCO_3^-
- Fractional excretion of HCO_3^- >15% and normal serum HCO_3^-
- Hypokalemia: Potassium wasting secondary to hyperaldosteronism
- Urine pH <5.5

Type IV RTA

Aldosterone insufficiency or aldosterone receptor insensitivity is the most common type of RTA caused by many renal and extra renal disorders, and characterized by *hyperkalemic* metabolic acidosis.

Pathophysiology

It is due to either aldosterone receptor insensitivity (pseudohypoaldosteronism) or absolute aldosterone deficiency, which causes hyperkalemia since aldosterone is the principal hormone involved in distal tubule, and collecting duct potassium secretion. The resulting hyperkalemia decreases proximal tubule ammonia production and competes with NH_4^+ for the $Na^+/2Cl^-/K^+$ transporter in the ascending loop of Henle, reducing medullary ammonium gradient. Hyperkalemia also impairs NH_4^+ entry into the medullary collecting tubules (MCT) cell from the interstitium via the K^+ secretory site on the basolateral Na^+/K^+-ATPase, resulting in net NH_4^+ and acid excretion. Aldosterone deficiency or resistance decreases H^+ secretion in the collecting duct by decreasing the number and function of H^+-ATPase pumps. Aldosterone is also important for increasing the negativity of the lumen of the cortical collecting tubules (CCT) by enhancing Na^+ absorption via the apical epithelial sodium channel (ENaC) and the basolateral Na^+/K^+-ATPase. Increased lumen negativity facilitates H^+ secretion into the lumen of CCT. These processes are impaired in aldosterone deficiency or receptor insensitivity leading to hyponatremic, hyperkalemic metabolic acidosis, characteristic of type 4 RTA. Impaired ENaC function (pseudohypoaldosteronism) or medications inhibiting ENaC function and hyperkalemia regardless of etiology can cause type IV RTA.

Etiology

Type 4 RTA may be caused by autosomal recessive disorders of adrenal steroidogenesis leading to aldosterone deficiency (see Table 3). Receptor

Table 3. Causes of type 4 RTA

1. Inherited type 4 RTA

Genes/Protein	Locus/Mode of Inheritance	Phenotype
βENaC/ENaC[a]	16p/AR	Pseudohypoaldosteronism type 1 (PHA I) Salt-wasting type 4 RTA Elevated renin and aldosterone Respiratory distress because of impaired water and sodium reabsorption from the alveoli
[b]WNK1 and WNK4	12p and 17q/AD	Pseudohypoaldosteronism type II (PHA II Gordon syndrome) Type 4 RTA with volume expansion and hyperkalemia Hypertension

[a] ENaC: Amiloride sensitive epithelial sodium channel.
[b] Lysine deficient protein kinase.

2. Primary
   Primary adrenal insufficiency
   Congenital adrenal hyperplasia especially 21-hydroxylase deficiency
   Isolated aldosterone synthase deficiency
   Heparin therapy
3. Hyporeninemic hypoaldosteronism
   Drugs: NSAID, ACEI, cyclosporine
   HIV infection
   Diabetic nephropathy
4. Aldosterone resistance/Pseudohypoaldosteronism
   Obstructive uropathy
   Pyelonephritis
   Interstitial nephritis
   Drugs: High-dose trimethoprim, amiloride, spironolactone, triamterene, pentamidine

insensitivity or autosomal dominant pseudohypoaldosteronism 1 (PHA 1) is due to mutation in the collecting tubule mineralocorticoid receptor. Autosomal recessive forms of PHA 1 are due to defective ENaC. Both disorders lead to decreased ENaC activity, hyperkalemia and type IV RTA. Autosomal recessive PHA 1 presents in infancy with severe, life threatening hyperkalemia, salt wasting, metabolic acidosis, and hypotension.

PHA II (Gordon syndrome), an autosomal dominant condition, results from mutation in the WNK1 and WNK4 genes (Lysine deficient protein kinase genes). These patients present with hypertension, hyperkalemia, hyporeninemia, hypoaldosteronism, metabolic acidosis, and volume expansion, often responsive to thiazide diuretics.

Diagnostic criteria type 4 RTA

- Metabolic acidosis
- Hyperkalemia
- Hyponatremia
- Volume depletion or volume expansion
- Hypotension or/hypertension
- Low or high renin and aldosterone

Type III RTA

After the description of types I and II RTA, some infants and young children presented with a mixed picture: Inability to acidify urine in the face of severe acidosis and significant urinary bicarbonate losses, approximately 5–10% of the filtered load. Some infants had fractional bicarbonate loss as high as 15%, which decreased after five years of age. This combined pattern suggested both proximal and distal tubular dysfunction, termed type III RTA. Whether this is due to solely distal tubular dysfunction or is a combination of proximal and distal tubule dysfunction is still unclear. More recently, an autosomal recessive disorder characterized by mental retardation, cerebral calcifications (marble brain disease), acidosis, and osteopetrosis has been described due to CA II deficiency, which impairs both bicarbonate reclamation in the proximal tubule and distal tubule acidification, causing a combination types I and 2 RTA or type III. Decreased CA II activity in the osteoclast impairs H^+ secretion necessary for bone remodeling.

Diagnostic Evaluation

The presence of metabolic acidosis, demonstrated by a low arterial blood pH, low serum HCO_3^-, and a low pCO_2 should be confirmed. Next, the anion gap should be calculated and determined to be normal with an elevated serum chloride. Nonrenal causes of hyperchloremic metabolic acidosis can usually be excluded by good history and physical examination and include gastrointestinal (GI) HCO_3^- loss or acidosis from an organic acid, such as toluene, whose anion is rapidly excreted renally (see Table 4).

Once RTA is established, differentiation between DRTA (type 1), PRTA (type 2) and type 4 RTA is based on diagnostic tools:

Urinalysis

Urinary pH is >5.5 in type 1 RTA in the presence of metabolic acidosis. The presence of glucosuria, aminoaciduria, and phosphaturia are indicative of Fanconi syndrome and type 2 RTA.

Urine electrolytes and the urine anion gap

Urine anion gap = $Na^+ + K^+ - Cl^-$. When $Na^+ + K^+ < Cl^-$, another cation, ammonium, is present. Thus, a negative urine anion gap is indicative of ammonium excretion in nonrenal causes of metabolic acidosis.

Table 4. Extrarenal causes of non anion gap metabolic acidosis

Gastrointestinal loss of bicarbonate
Diarrhea
Small bowel drainage
Intestinal fistula
Pancreatic drainage
Biliary drainage
Ureteroenterostomy
Ureterosigmoidostomy
Medications
Cholestyramine
Magnesium sulfate
Calcium chloride
Excessive infusion of normal saline

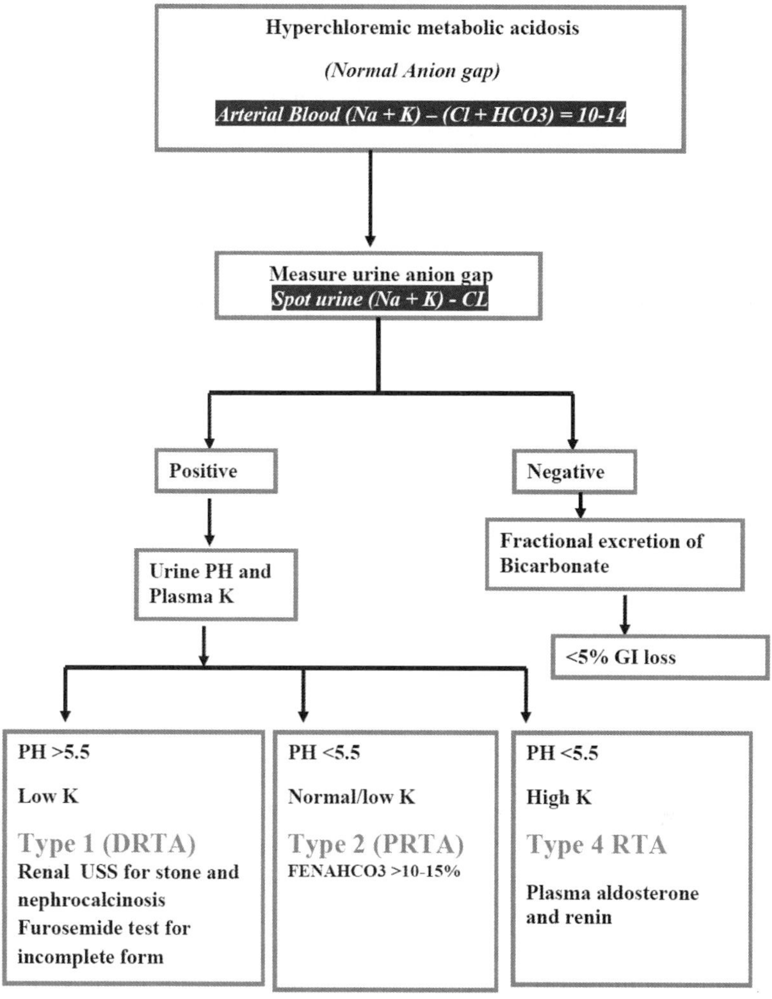

Figure 1. Algorithm for diagnosis of renal tubular acidosis.

Conversely, a positive anion gap indicates a renal cause of metabolic acidosis, such as RTA (see Fig. 1).

Ammonium chloride loading test

An acid load can be used to test the renal tubules' ability to increase titratable acid and ammonium excretion, and lower urine pH. It is often used in patients with suspected RTA, but without frank acidosis, such as incomplete type 1 RTA. The patient ingests a dose of ammonium chloride and the urine pH and excretion of urinary titratable acid and ammonium are measured after achieving a mild acidosis. This test is rarely used in clinical practice due to poor ammonium chloride tolerance and has been replaced by the furosemide + fludrocortisone test.

Furosemide test

The rationale for the test is that furosemide increases distal sodium delivery, leading to increased sodium reabsorption, increased lumen negativity, and subsequent increased H^+ secretion. Giving fludrocortisone with furosemide improves consistency and sensitivity. Normal patients will lower their urine pH to <5.3 following oral administration of furosemide and fludrocortisone, whereas patients with distal RTA will be unable to lower urine pH <5.3.

Fractional Excretion of Bicarbonate ($FE_{HCO_3^-}$)

To test tubular ability to reclaim the filtered load of HCO_3^-, $FE_{HCO_3^-}$ can be determined after normalization of serum HCO_3^- (22–25 meq/L):

$$FE_{HCO_3^-} = \frac{U_{HCO_3^-}/S_{HCO_3^-}}{U_{creatinine}/S_{creatinine}} \times 100\%$$

Blood and urine should be evaluated simultaneously and normal is <5%. With PRTA, the $FE_{HCO_3^-}$ is >15%. Urine HCO_3^- is calculated by measuring the urine pH and PCO_2 on a standard blood gas analyzer

$$HCO_3^- = 10^{(pH-pK)} \times 0.03 \times pCO_2$$

pK approximates 6.1.

Urine–blood pCO2

Urine pCO_2 in alkaline urine can test the distal nephron's ability to secrete H^+. By testing under alkaline conditions, the tubule doesn't secrete H^+ against a gradient. In the distal tubule lumen, H^+ combines with HCO_3^- and resulting H_2CO_3 decomposes slowly into H_2O and CO_2 since CA is not present on the luminal membrane as in the proximal tubule. This slow decomposition means that CO_2 is formed in the lower urinary tract where the volume to surface area favors slow dissipation of the CO_2 gradient. The countercurrent system in the medulla also maintains a high urine pCO_2. To perform the test, the urine pH and HCO_3^- concentration are raised to >7.5 and 85 meq/L, respectively by infusing HCO_3^- or administering acetazolamide, 17 mg/kg, and measuring pCO_2. A normal response is urine pCO_2 > blood pCO_2 by 30 mmHg. If this difference is less than 30 mmHg, then distal H^+ pumping is defective, suggesting DRTA.

Renal ultrasound

This may be a useful adjunct since nephrocalcinosis and/or kidney stones are often found in DRTA. Also, obstructive uropathy is a common cause of type 4 RTA. The algorithm for evaluation of metabolic acidosis of renal origin is shown in Fig. 1.

Treatment

The goal of treatment is to identify the underlying etiology to guide therapy. Often the cause is not directly treatable, so supplemental alkali therapy is given to correct acidosis and improve growth and bone mineralization.

Type 1 RTA

DRTA is an acidification defect, therefore alkali therapy is required to neutralize daily acid production. Most patients will achieve normal plasma bicarbonate with 1–3 meq/kg/day of bicarbonate. Due to increased endogenous acid production in younger children, they often require larger doses of bicarbonate. Patients typically have significant hypokalemia upon presentation, often requiring treatment before acidosis correction. Enough alkali should be provided to normalize urine citrate to prevent stones and nephrocalcinosis.

Type 2 RTA

Unlike DRTA, urinary bicarbonate wasting increases with bicarbonate replacement as the filtered load increases. Individuals with PRTA usually require to 4–20 meq/kg/day of sodium bicarbonate, divided in multiple daily doses, to maintain near normal plasma bicarbonate and satisfactory growth. Kaliuresis increases with alkali supplementation; therefore some replacement alkali should be given as potassium citrate.

Type 4 RTA

Identification of underlying cause is vital to treatment. Drug-induced type IV RTA is treated with discontinuation of the offending medication. In cases due to pseudohypoaldosteronism from obstructive uropathy, adequate urinary tract drainage with normal saline infusion and sodium bicarbonate therapy will correct acidosis. Aldosterone deficiency should be treated with mineralocorticoid replacement. Children with type 4 RTA due to PHA I require salt supplementation and potassium restriction. PHA II is treated with thiazide diuretics and salt restriction. Patients with other causes of hyperkalemia and type IV RTA may respond to symptomatic management of hyperkalemia with dietary restriction. A loop diuretic and/or a cation exchange resin may be required in some cases.

Suggested Reading

Batlle DC. (1986) Segmental characterization of defects in collecting tubule acidification. *Kidney Int* **30**: 546–554.

Borthwick KJ, Kandemir N, Topaloglu R, *et al.* (2003) A phenocopy of CAII deficiency: a novel genetic explanation for inherited infantile osteopetrosis with distal renal tubular acidosis. *J Med Genet* **40**: 115–121.

Bruce LJ, Cope DL, Jones GK, *et al.* (1997) Familial distal renal tubular acidosis is associated with muatations in the red cell anion exchanger (Band 3, AE1) gene. *J Clin Invest* **100**: 1693–1707.

Geller DS, Rodriguez Soriano J, Vallo Boado A, *et al.* (1998) Mutations in the mineralocorticoid receptor gene cause autosomal pseudohypoaldosteronism type 1. *Nat Genet* **19**: 279.

Karet FE, Gainza FJ, Gyory AZ, *et al.* (1997) Mutations in the chloride-bicarbonate exchanger gene AE1 cause autosomal dominant but not recessive distal renal tubular acidosis. *Proc Natl ACAD Sci USA* **95**: 6337–6342.

Karet FE, Finberg KE, Nelson RD, *et al.* (1999) Mutations in the gene encoding B1 subunit of the H^+-ATPase cause renal tubular acidosis with sensorineural deafness. *Nat Genet* **21**: 8–90.

Kurtzman NA. (1990) Disorders of distal acidification. *Kidney Int* **38**: 720.

Laing CM, Toye AM, Capasso G, Unwin RJ. (2005) Renal tubular acidosis: developments in our understanding of the molecular basis. *Int J Biochem Cell Biol* **37**: 1151–1161.

Walsh SB, Shirley DG, Wrong OM, Unwin RJ. (2007) Urinary acidification assessed by simultaneous furosemide and fludrocortisones treatment: an alternative to ammonium chloride. *Kidney Int* **71**: 1310 –1316.

Wilson FH, Disse-Nicoderm S, Choate KA, *et al.* (2001) Human hypertension caused by mutations in WNK kinases. *Science* **293**: 1107–1111.

25

Bartter Syndrome

Scott J. Schurman

Introduction

In 1962, Bartter *et al.* described two African American children with hypokalemia, metabolic alkalosis, and normotension. The children eventually developed renal failure and expired. Careful studies in these patients led the authors to deduce the primary abnormality in what would become known as Bartter Syndrome (BS) was a subnormal vasopressor response to angiotensin II, leading to excessive juxtaglomerular renin production (including pathology showing hypertrophy and hyperplasia of the juxtaglomerular complex), and hyperaldosteronism. Subsequent studies demonstrated markedly elevated urinary prostaglandin production, at least partial dependence of hyperreninemia on excessive renal prostaglandin production, and improvement in polyuria and hypokalemia after treatment with indomethacin. Prostaglandin overproduction was proposed as the proximate cause of BS. However, other studies showed a prostaglandin-independent defect in distal chloride reabsorption, leading to the hypothesis that a defect in distal tubular sodium and chloride reabsorption was the proximal defect in BS. Indeed, molecular genetic studies in the 1990s confirmed abnormalities in electrolyte transporters located in the ascending limb of Henle.

Renal Tubular Physiology

Sodium and its major anions, chloride and bicarbonate, are the main determinants of the extracellular fluid volume, and are regulated by the kidneys. After glomerular filtration, this regulation begins in the proximal tubule with active and passive reabsorption of 50–70% of filtered sodium, driven largely by Na^+/K^+-ATPase and Na^+-H^+ exchanger activity. Regulation

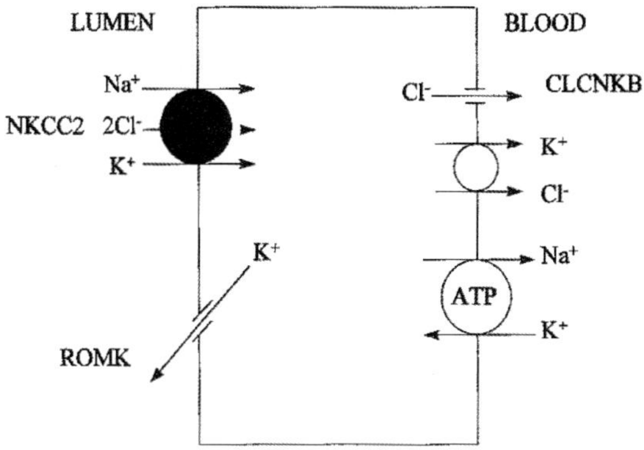

Figure 1. Schematic diagram of NaCl reabsorption in the thick ascending limb of the loop of Henle. NaCl enters the cell from the lumen via the Na-K-2Cl cotransporter (NKCC2). Low intracellular Na^+ and Cl^- concentrations generated by the activity of basolateral Na-K-ATPase, the voltage-gated chloride channel encoded by the gene CLCNKB, and a K-Cl transporter permit proper NKCC2 activity. NKCC2 activity is also rate limited by the availability of potassium in the tubular lumen, and potassium recycling from cell to lumen occurs via the potassium channel ROMK. [From Schurman SJ, Shoemaker LR. (2000) Bartter and Gitelman Syndromes. *Adv Pediatr* **47**: 223–248, with permission].

of these transporter functions is complex and includes angiotensin II, which increases proximal tubular sodium reabsorption.

Subsequent to the proximal tubule, 30% of filtered sodium and chloride are reabsorbed in the thick ascending limb of the loop of Henle (see Fig. 1). Sodium and chloride enter the tubular cell via the apical Na^+-K^+-$2Cl^-$ cotransporter. Na^+-K^+-$2Cl^-$ activity is made possible by the low intracellular sodium and chloride concentrations generated by the activity of basolateral Na^+/K^+-ATPase and chloride channels, including ClC-Kb. Na^+-K^+-$2Cl^-$ activity, however, is rate limited by the availability of potassium in the tubular lumen. Thus, potassium recycling from the cell to lumen via the potassium channel ROMK is essential for normal sodium and chloride reabsorption. In turn, sodium and chloride reabsorption in the thick ascending limb are required to maintain hypertonicity of the renal medullary interstitium, and failure to maintain this environment significantly reduces urinary concentrating capacity.

Beyond the loop of Henle, approximately 5% of filtered sodium and chloride are reabsorbed in the distal tubule via the apical thiazide-sensitive

Na^+-Cl^- cotransporter. Final processing of the glomerular filtrate occurs in the collecting tubule, which generally reabsorbs 5–7% of filtered sodium and chloride, via luminal ion-specific sodium channels, creating negative voltage within the collecting duct lumen that promotes potassium and hydrogen ion secretion. The energy for this and other resorptive processes in the kidney is provided by basolateral Na^+/K^+-ATPase; and the number and activity of Na^+/K^+-ATPase, and apical sodium channels increase with aldosterone stimulation.

Pathophysiology

Mutation analyses have confirmed autosomal recessive inheritance resulting in a defect in thick ascending limb sodium and chloride transport as the cause of BS. All patients described to date have defects in *SLC12A*, the gene for the Na^+-K^+-$2Cl^-$ cotransporter, or genes that encode thick ascending limb proteins which are essential for normal Na^+-K^+-$2Cl^-$ activity: *KCNJ1* (ROMK), *CLCNKB* (ClC-Kb), and *BSND* (barttin). Barttin is an accessory subunit of all ClC-K chloride channels, which are expressed in the vestibular labyrinth of the ear as well as in the kidney. These findings indicate that there is no significant compensatory mechanism to ROMK function for potassium recycling in the thick ascending limb and that ClC-Kb is most likely the dominant basolateral chloride channel responsible for lowering thick ascending limb intracellular chloride concentration and allowing proper Na^+-K^+-$2Cl^-$ function. In contrast, other ClC-K channels are more important to middle ear function and thus patients with *BSND* mutations demonstrate sensorineural hearing loss but patients with *CLCNKB* mutations do not.

Loss of Na^+-K^+-$2Cl^-$ cotransporter function (directly or indirectly) in the thick ascending limb dramatically increases salt delivery to the distal tubule. Distal tubular sodium and chloride reabsorption mechanisms are unable to compensate for this dysfunction resulting in extracellular volume depletion and marked elevation in plasma renin and aldosterone. Aldosterone and increased sodium delivery to the collecting ducts leads to an increase in potassium and hydrogen ion excretion, resulting in hypokalemia and metabolic alkalosis. Blood pressure is normal despite elevated angiotensin II given reduced intravascular volume and vascular hyporeactivity. The latter phenomenon is likely the result of activation of

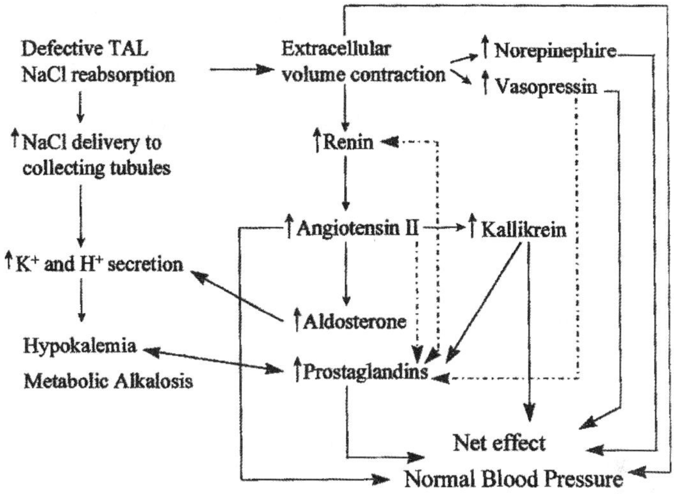

Figure 2. A complex scheme of the pathophysiologic events in Bartter syndrome. Defective NaCl reabsorption in the thick ascending limb (TAL) of the loop of Henle is the proximate event. Activation of multiple secondary mediators, particularly prostaglandins, amplifies the basic pathophysiologic processes. [From Schurman SJ, Shoemaker LR. (2000) Bartter and Gitelman Syndromes. *Adv Pediatr* 47: 223–248, with permission.]

secondary mediators, most notably increased prostaglandin synthesis. Elevations in urinary and systemic prostaglandins have been described in patients with BS and normalize with volume expansion and correction of hypokalemia. This effect may be direct or mediated through elevated angiotensin II, kallikrein, and vasopressin. In turn, prostaglandins increase renin production, reduce sodium and chloride reabsorption in the collecting duct, and decrease vascular reactivity through prostacyclin and perhaps other prostaglandin metabolites. Thus, though prostaglandin synthesis inhibitors (i.e. indomethacin) do not address the cause of BS, they blunt the effects of the maladaptive pathophysiologic circle created by these secondary mediators (see Fig. 2).

Clinical Manifestations

Before the availability of mutation analyses, BS was generally classified as "neonatal" (NBS) or "classic" (CBS). More recently, a classification scheme based upon mutation analysis has been proposed, such that patient with mutations in *SLC12A* have BS type 1, those with mutations in *KCNJ1* have

Table 1. Clinical and laboratory features of neonatal Bartter syndrome, "classic" Bartter syndrome, and Gitelman syndrome

	Neonatal Bartter Syndrome	"Classic" Bartter Syndrome	Gitelman Syndrome
Polyhydramnios/prematurity	+++	++	ϕ
Presentation in adolescence	ϕ	ϕ	+++
Impaired urinary concentration	+++	+++	ϕ
Polyuria/polydipsia	+++	+++	ϕ
Hyperrenin/hyperaldosteronism	+++	+++	+
Elevated prostaglandins	+++	+++	ϕ
Hypokalemia	+++	+++	+++
Metabolic alkalosis	+++	+++	++
Hypercalciuria	+++	++	ϕ
Hypocalciuria	ϕ	ϕ	+++
Nephrocalcinosis	+++	ϕ	ϕ
Hypomagnesemia	+	+	+++
Growth retardation	+++	+++	ϕ

Abbreviations: +++, severe or almost always present; ++, moderate or frequently present; +, mild or occasionally present; ϕ, absent.

BS type 2, those with mutations in *CLCNKB* have BS type 3, and those with mutations in *BSND* have BS type 4. No classification scheme is ideal as there is not perfect phenotype–genotype correlation. However, patients with mutations in a particular gene are more likely to have certain clinical characteristics (Table 1).

Infants classified with NBS have marked polyhydramnios, as a result of intrauterine polyuria, which is noted before 30 weeks gestation. (Removal of fluid amniocentesis) is sometimes required and premature birth is the rule. Polyuria continues postnatally in the range of 12–50 mL/kg per hour. Given massive sodium losses these infants usually have hyponatremia, but generally do not demonstrate hypokalemia or metabolic alkalosis until 1–3 months of life. Delay in these hallmark manifestations is thought to be the result of immaturity of Na^+/K^+-ATPase expression in the distal tubule. In fact, some infants will manifest with hyperkalemia in the first 1–2 weeks of life, sometimes with metabolic acidosis. In the context of elevated plasma concentrations of renin and aldosterone, these infants are often initially diagnosed with pseudohypoaldosteronism type I. Phenotype-genotype correlation studies by Brochard *et al.* showed hyperkalemia at diagnosis in 12 of 19 infants with *KCNJ1* mutations but not in patients with mutations in one of the other BS genes. ROMK likely is important in distal tubular potassium secretion in neonates; however, after maturation of Na^+/K^+-ATPase, these patients transition to hypokalemia.

Multiple reports attempting to correlate genotype and phenotype have demonstrated that patients with mutations in *SLC12A*, *KCNJ1*, or *BSND* present, with only rare exception, with typical clinical features. In addition, infants with mutations in *SLC12A* or *KCNJ1* demonstrate marked hypercalciuria from birth and uniformly have nephrocalcinosis, with renal ultrasounds showing dense, hyperechoic medullary pyramids. In contrast, patients with *BSND* mutation have only modestly elevated urinary calcium excretion and will only occasionally develop nephrocalcinosis; nephrocalcinosis is rarely seen in patients with a *CLCNKB* mutation. Etiology of elevated urinary calcium excretion is multifactorial and includes impaired calcium reabsorption in the thick ascending limb, as 25% of reabsorption of filtered calcium is coupled to Na^+-K^+-$2Cl^-$ activity. However, marked bone reabsorption has also been demonstrated which does not abate with indomethacin. A heparin-like glycosaminoglycan complex to basic fibroblast growth factor has been implicated and may represent another secondary mediator. Osteopenia often develops.

After the neonatal period, patients almost uniformly develop failure to thrive and growth retardation, though severity varies greatly and is likely dependent, at least in part, upon response to therapy. Without treatment, severe polyuria continues. Volume depletion is aggravated in the setting of coexisting acute viral illnesses. Low or low–normal serum magnesium is often seen (in contrast to the marked hypomagnesemia with Gitelman syndrome). Much of the magnesium reabsorption is coupled to Na^+-K^+-$2Cl^-$ function, but compensatory reabsorption in the distal tubule may prevent more severe magnesium depletion. As noted above, patients with *BSND* mutations have sensorineural hearing loss, diagnosed with newborn screening, or apparent later in the first year of life.

Chronic kidney disease (CKD) can develop. In the past, CKD in these patients was attributed to nephrocalcinosis, and in fact, parenchymal calcification may contribute to reduced glomerular filtration rate in an occasional patient. However, CKD is rare in patients with *SLC12A* or *KCNJ1* mutations despite invariable dense nephrocalcinosis. Jeck *et al.* found that only 1 of 60 BS patients with a *SLC12A* or *KCNJ1* mutation had a glomerular filtration rate less than 60 mL/min/1.73m^2, compared to all eight patients with a *BSND* mutation.

Infants with *CLCNKB* mutations may present with polyhydramnios/prematurity and neonatal polyuria and be labeled as having NBS. However, most of these patients demonstrate polyuria that is not as severe as in patients with other mutations, and in fact, they often present later in the first year of life (and rarely later), usually in the context of dehydration with hypokalemia and metabolic alkalosis. Though the polyuria may not be as severe, patients with *CLCNKB* mutations have hypokalemia and metabolic alkalosis as or more severe as seen in other patients, with serum potassium concentrations uniformly below 3 mEq/L. Urinary calcium excretion is often modestly elevated, and nephrocalcinosis is unusual. Progression to CKD has been reported and clearly is not the result of nephrocalcinosis. Renal pathology in these patients has revealed tubulointerstitial inflammation with eventual fibrosis. Other features, such as borderline low serum magnesium and growth retardation, are similar to seen in patients with other mutations.

Diagnosis

The diagnosis of Bartter syndrome in infants with massive polyuria born prematurely with polyhydramnios should be straightforward. As noted above, some patients with a *KCNJ1* defect will present with hyperkalemia and metabolic acidosis, and may be initially diagnosed with pseudohypoaldosteronism type I. Infants with this disorder also may have polyhydramnios, prematurity, hypercalciuria, and nephrocalcinosis, though rarely to the severity seen in BS. Eventually, hypokalemia and metabolic alkalosis develop, and the BS diagnosis becomes apparent. Similarly, complications of prematurity that result in acute kidney injury such as systemic infection or necrotizing enterocolitis may delay diagnosis.

Toddlers generally present with hypokalemia and metabolic alkalosis in association with acute dehydration. Failure to thrive is often present. After rehydration, diagnostic testing begins with urine chloride and blood pressure measurement. Detectable urine chloride essentially excludes cystic fibrosis and gastrointestinal loss of chloride as etiologies. Normal blood pressure makes any form of primary or secondary hyperaldosteronism unlikely. Plasma renin activity and aldosterone concentration should be measured and diuretic abuse excluded, if clinically relevant to the patient presentation.

Other testing is less diagnostic, instead searching for associated features of disease. Urinary calcium excretion and serum magnesium should be measured and renal ultrasound obtained to evaluate for nephrocalcinosis. Hearing testing should be done, if not performed as part of newborn screening. In the past, urine collections to assess excretion of prostaglandins, and to carefully assess sodium and chloride handling may have been recommended. However, such testing is not necessary to make the BS diagnosis. Similarly, genotyping of the patient and parents is generally available. This information may provide some prognostic information, such as increased risk of CKD in patients with a *BSND* mutation or increased risk of osteopenia in patients with a *SLC12A* or *KCNJ1* mutation. However, these risks can generally be inferred from available clinical data and thus mutation analysis is not absolutely necessary.

Treatment

Newborns with massive polyuria require intravenous replacement of salt and fluid. Proesmans has demonstrated that renin, aldosterone, and prostaglandin production will improve and even normalize with fluid and electrolyte therapy to maintain euvolemia and normal serum potassium. Prostaglandin inhibition does not address the cause of BS but does neutralize the amplifying effect of prostaglandins. The major potential complication of such therapy is gastrointestinal bleeding, and premature newborns are particularly vulnerable. Thus, prostaglandin inhibition is not started immediately, but rather after an infant's clinical status has been consistently stable, usually at 1–2 months of age. Indomethacin is still generally chosen as it is longer acting than other alternatives, beginning at a dose of 1 mg/kg/day divided three times daily. Eventually, an indomethacin dose of 2–3 mg/kg/day may be necessary to allow euvolemia with enteral feedings alone. Given the risk of gastrointestinal bleeding, stools should be periodically checked for occult blood.

Similarly, infants or older children diagnosed with BS, who will benefit from prostaglandin inhibition and indomethacin, should be started after the diagnosis is established. Other treatment includes supplementation with potassium chloride. Such therapy is generally necessary to keep the serum potassium above 3.5 mEq/L and successful treatment of hypokalemia will blunt elevation in prostaglandins and other secondary mediators. Ideally, potassium chloride is provided in multiple daily doses, three or four times daily, and there is significant patient variability in the total daily dose necessary. Some patients, particularly those traditionally labeled as CBS (and most likely with a *CLCNKB* defect), require very large potassium chloride doses, 6–10 mEq/kg/day or more. Prostaglandin inhibition therapy should be maximized, and if potassium chloride doses cannot be moderated or if gastroinstestinal distress coincident with the dose delivered, alternative therapy should be considered.

Potassium-sparing diuretics, usually spironolactone, and angiotensin-converting enzyme inhibitors will likely increase the serum potassium concentration, but will potentially increase sodium losses and volume depletion causing hypotension. In this circumstance, concurrent sodium chloride supplementation may be necessary. In fact, some patients require sodium chloride supplementation to prevent hyponatremia and volume depletion. Again, such supplements should be provided in multiple daily doses. Similarly, other therapy depends upon the individual clinical circumstance. Patients with hypomagnesemia may require magnesium supplementation, though the need for such therapy is unusual. Growth and weight gain are difficult, even in the best of circumstances. Addition of multiple medications doses throughout the day can exacerbate feeding issues. Some patients will therefore benefit from gastrostomy tube placement to allow more efficient medication delivery and supplemental feeding.

Treatment of hypercalciuria is problematic. Thiazide diuretic therapy will lower urinary calcium excretion but exacerbate hypokalemia and volume depletion. Bisphosphonate therapy will decrease bone resorption and urinary calcium excretion, though routine therapy is not recommended. Patients with recurrent urolithiasis can be considered for such treatment. In addition, as children age periodic bone densitometry testing should be considered for at-risk patients (those with massive hypercalciuria and nephrocalcinosis), and antiresorptive therapy should be considered in the presence of osteoporosis and/or recurrent fractures.

Suggested Reading

Bartter FC, Pronove P, Gill JR Jr, *et al.* (1962) Hyperplasia of juxtaglomerular complex with hyperaldosteronism and hypokalemic alkalosis. *Am J Med* 33: 811–828.

Brochard K, Boyer O, Blanchard A, *et al.* (2009) Phenotype-genotype correlation in antenatal and neonatal variants of Bartter syndrome. *Nephrol Dial Transplant* **24**: 1455–1464.

Jeck N, Reinalter SC, Henne T, *et al.* (2001) Hypokalemic salt-losing tubulopathy with chronic renal failure and sensorineural deafness. *Pediatr* **108**: E5.

Proesmans W. (1997) Bartter syndrome and its neonatal variant. *Eur J Pediatr* **156**: 669–679.

Rodriguez-Soriano J. (1998) Bartter and related syndromes: the puzzle is almost solved. *Pediatr Nephrol* **12**: 315–327.

Sutton RA, Mavichak V, Halabe A, *et al.* (1992) Bartter's syndrome: evidence suggesting a distal tubular defect in a hypocalciuric variant of the syndrome. *Min Electrol Metab* **18**: 43–51.

26

Gitelman Syndrome

Scott J. Schurman

Introduction

In 1966, Gitelman *et al.* reported three adult patients with hypokalemia and metabolic alkalosis noted after presenting with muscle weakness and tetany. These index patients had marked hypomagnesemia without history of polyuria or growth retardation; the authors correctly surmised that these patients had a disorder distinct from the children described by Bartter *et al.*, and subsequent studies demonstrated subnormal natriuretic response to thiazide diuretic, but normal response to furosemide. Decades later, Simon *et al.* would describe loss of function mutations of *SLC12A3*, the gene encoding the distal convoluted tubule thiazide-sensitive sodium-chloride cotransporter, confirming autosomal recessive inheritance of the disorder. Mutations are relatively common, at least in certain populations, with a prevalence of heterozygotes of 1% in Swedish and Italian populations.

Loss of this cotransporter function increases salt delivery to the collecting tubules producing extracellular volume depletion. This is modest compared to Bartter syndrome (BS) and thus, the degree of activation of the renin-angiotensin-aldosterone axis is less pronounced, and prostaglandin and other secondary mediators are not activated. However, increased sodium delivery to the collecting tubules and elevated aldosterone lead to increased potassium and hydrogen ion secretion, producing hypokalemia and metabolic alkalosis. Pathophysiology of hypomagnesemia remains speculative. The thiazide-sensitive cotransporter does not participate directly in divalent ion (magnesium or calcium) transport and only 5–10% of filtered magnesium is reabsorbed in the distal convoluted tubule. Increased aldosterone may increase expression of a distal tubule epithelial sodium channel leading to increased paracellular magnesium secretion.

Clinical Manifestations and Diagnosis

Patients with Gitelman syndrome are born at term and growth and development are normal (Table 1). As noted above, patients have modest volume contraction, but given the ability to generate an appropriately hypertonic medullary interstitium, maximal urinary concentration is only modestly decreased and polyuria is mild or absent. Patients may be prone to dehydration and may present in this manner with characteristic hypokalemia and metabolic alkalosis. Interestingly, this mode of presentation is seen in the minority of patients and is unusual in infants and young children. Instead, most patients present as adolescents or young adults with episodes of tetany and weakness. Evaluation reveals hypomagnesemia with serum magnesium concentration usually less than 1.0 mg/dL. Hypomagnesemia reduces parathyroid secretion and impairs bone resorbing activity. Metabolic alkalosis further decreases ionized calcium concentrations predisposing to tetany and seizure. Urinary calcium

Table 1. Clinical and laboratory features of neonatal Bartter syndrome, "classic" Bartter syndrome, and Gitelman syndrome

	Neonatal Bartter Syndrome	"Classic" Bartter Syndrome	Gitelman Syndrome
Polyhydramnios/prematurity	+++	++	ϕ
Presentation in adolescence	ϕ	ϕ	+++
Impaired urinary concentration	+++	+++	ϕ
Polyuria/polydipsia	+++	+++	ϕ
Hyperrenin/hyperaldosteronism	+++	+++	+
Elevated prostaglandins	+++	+++	ϕ
Hypokalemia	+++	+++	+++
Metabolic alkalosis	+++	+++	++
Hypercalciuria	+++	++	ϕ
Hypocalciuria	ϕ	ϕ	+++
Nephrocalcinosis	+++	ϕ	ϕ
Hypomagnesemia	+	+	+++
Growth retardation	+++	+++	ϕ

Abbreviations: +++, severe or almost always present; ++, moderate or frequently present; +, mild or occasionally present; ϕ, absent.

excretion is invariably low with random urine calcium/creatinine less than 0.04 mg/mg. As with hypomagnesemia, the etiology of reduced urinary calcium excretion is, at best, speculative.

The diagnosis of Gitelman syndrome should be considered in a child presenting with dehydration and found to have hypokalemia and metabolic alkalosis, particularly if the illness associated with the episode seems mild compared to the degree of laboratory derangement. If hypomagnesemic, these patients should be monitored after recovery from the illness. Otherwise, diagnosis is made after serum magnesium and electrolytes checked in a patient with tetany. History may reveal muscle weakness. Blood pressure and renal function will be normal.

Diagnostic alternatives with these clinical contexts are few. Patients with Gitelman syndrome have at times been diagnosed with "mild" BS. However, differentiation should be possible without measurement of natriuretic response to furosemide and thiazide diuretic. Hypomagnesemia in BS is generally mild and even patients with *CLCNKB* defects have high normal or modestly elevated urinary calcium excretion.

Treatment

Magnesium supplementation will improve hypomagnesemia, weakness and prevent or minimize tetany episodes. Unfortunately, supplements generally are best given in doses divided three or four times daily and large doses can produce diarrhea. Multiple magnesium salts have been tried, though most adolescent patients tolerate magnesium oxide well, usually starting at 400 mg three times daily, increasing, as needed, based upon both the laboratory and clinical response. Most patients also require potassium supplementation. Potassium-sparing diuretic therapy may also prove desirable to moderate the dose of potassium needed and spironolactone may also reduce urinary magnesium losses.

Suggested Reading

Bettinelli A, Bianchetti MG, Girardin E, *et al.* (1992) Use of calcium excretion values to distinguish two forms of primary renal tubular hypokalemic alkalosis: Bartter and Gitelman syndromes. *J Pediatr* **120**: 38–43.

Colussi G, Macaluso M, Brunati C, *et al.* (1994) Calcium metabolism and calciotropic hormone levels in Gitelman's syndrome. *Min Electrol Metab* **20**: 294–301.

Schurman SJ, Shoemaker LR. Bartter and Gitelman Syndromes. (2000) *Adv Pediatr* **47**: 223–248.

Simon DB, Nelson-Williams C, Johnson Bia M, *et al.* (1996) Gitelman's variant of Bartter's syndrome, inherited hypokalaemic alkalosis, is caused by mutations in the thiazide-sensitive Na-Cl cotransporter. *Nat Genet* **12**: 24–30.

27

Tubulointerstitial Nephritis

Kevin D. McBryde

Introduction

Interstitial nephritis refers to inflammation of the renal interstitium and tubular cells accompanied by interstitial edema or fibrosis, and varying degrees of tubular atrophy. More accurately, interstitial nephritis is termed tubulointerstitial nephritis (TIN). Acute tubulointerstitial nephritis (ATIN) refers to sudden onset and rapid decline in renal function, whereas chronic tubulointerstitial nephritis (CTIN) describes a more insidious decline in renal function. In ATIN, acute inflammation of the renal interstitium, interstitial edema, and tubular epithelial cell damage dominates. In CTIN, the histopathology includes tubular epithelial damage, interstitial fibrosis, and tubular atrophy.

Epidemiology

The true prevalence of ATIN in children is unknown. According to the 2008 North American Pediatric Renal Transplant Cooperative Study Annual Report, CTIN and pyelonephritis approximate 1.4% of primary diagnoses of chronic kidney disease (CKD) and 1.5% of all causes of end-stage renal disease (ESRD). In a single pediatric center experience, TIN was reported in 7% of biopsy samples obtained in a three-year period, equaling 2.1 cases annually.

Pathogenesis

T cell and B cell mechanisms are involved in the development of TIN. Immunohistochemical staining of kidney tissue in TIN may demonstrate antitubular basement membrane antibodies, and IgG and complement deposition along tubular basement membranes (TBM). Potential antigens include TBM, Tamm–Horsfall protein, and Heymann nephritis antigen, which may be internalized, processed, and presented by renal tubular epithelial cells with MHC class II antigens to T helper cells, thereby activating cytotoxic T cells or B cells. Alternatively, these antigens may be internalized by extrarenal circulating antigen presenting cells (APC), stimulating immune activation. Finally, an extrarenal antigen may cross-react with a component of the renal tubulointerstitium, inducing antibody response.

In contrast to B cell mediated causes, T cell mechanisms predominate in human TIN. In the syndrome of tubulointerstitial nephritis with uveitis (TINU), T cells infiltrate the tubulointerstitium in the absence of demonstrable antibody deposition. T cell immune response may be mediated by CD8+ T cells recognizing antigens associated with MHC class I antigens. This direct cytotoxic effect of CD8+ T cells may explain tubular cell damage found in TIN. A second mechanism is through delayed-type hypersensitivity, in which CD4+ T cells activate macrophages, which are responsible for the lesions. In a delayed-type hypersensitivity reaction, inflammatory cells contain a mixture of CD8+ T cells, CD4+ T cells, natural killer cells, B cells, and macrophages. A final mechanism of T cell mediated TIN is formation of antibody-dependent immune responses, which is the proposed mechanism of drug-induced TIN in which a drug metabolite binds to TBM, forming a hapten complex, and thereby stimulating production of anti-TBM antibodies.

Clinical Presentation

The clinical presentation of TIN consists of nonspecific constitutional symptoms, including fever, abdominal pain, nausea, vomiting, anorexia, weight loss, polydipsia, polyuria, hypertension, headaches, and skin rash. Seasonal predilection has been described in children, most commonly occurring between December and June. ATIN, regardless of etiology, presents with acute renal dysfunction, including fluid, electrolyte, or acid–base disturbances. The traditional triad of fever, rash, and eosinophilia occurs in $<30\%$ of patients diagnosed with TIN, yielding low sensitivity. Another misconception is drug-related TIN presents 2–3 weeks following administration of the offending agent and prior exposure to the medication without reaction is exclusionary.

Differential Diagnosis

Differential diagnosis of TIN includes acute tubular necrosis (ATN), systemic disorders (i.e., systemic lupus erythematosus, sarcoidosis, etc.), and infectious nephritis (i.e., acute pyelonephritis). Clinical laboratory studies (see Table 1) are useful in discriminating between TIN and other etiologies.

Diagnostic Evaluation

Laboratory findings consistent with TIN are depicted in Table 2. Sterile pyuria, specifically eosinophiluria (>5% of the total urine leukocyte

Table 1.

	Prerenal AKI	Acute GN	ATIN
Serum Creatinine	↑	↔ or ↑	↑
Serum Potassium	↑	↔ or ↑	↓
Serum HCO_3^-	↓	↓ or ↔ or ↑	↓
Proteinuria	None	>2 gm/24 hrs (U_{pr}/U_{cr} >2.0)	<1 gm/24 hrs (U_{pr}/U_{cr} <1.0)
Hematuria	None	↔ or ↑	↔ or ↑
Pyuria	None	↔ or ↑	↔ or ↑
Urine Sediment	Hyaline casts	RBC, WBC, granular, hyaline casts	Granular, hyaline, RBC or WBC casts
FE_{Na}	<1%	<2%	>2%

AKI = Acute kidney injury; GN = Glomerulonephritis; ATIN = Acute tubulointerstitial nephritis; ↓ = decreased; ↔ = normal; ↑ = increased; U_{pr}/U_{cr} = urine protein:urine creatinine ratio; FE_{Na} = fractional excretion of sodium; RBC = red blood cells; WBC = white blood cells.

Table 2.

CBC	Chemistry	Immunology	Urinalysis
Anemia	Acute kidney injury[a]	Elevated ESR[b]	FE_{Na}[c] > 2%
Leukocytosis	Hypoalbuminemia	Elevated IgG	Proteinuria
Eosinophilia		Hypocomplementemia	Hematuria
		Elevated antistreptolysin O and antihyaluronidase titers	Leukocyturia
		Increased anti-DNase titer	Glycosuria
			Granular casts

[a] Acute Kidney Injury (serum creatinine >2 times baseline or calculated glomerular filtration rate <50 mL/min/1.73 m²); [b] ESR = erythrocyte sedimentation rate; [c] FE_{Na} = fractional excretion of sodium.

count), is strongly associated with ATIN. While eosinophiluria may be present in the setting of infection of the upper or lower urinary tract, it may be seen in up to 25% of cases of TIN. Though still nonspecific and nonsensitive, the Hansel's stain as compared to Wright's stain, improves the positive predictive value to 50% from 25%, respectively; and increases sensitivity to 63% from 25%, respectively.

Proteinuria is common, though it is often less than nephrotic-range (<2 gm/24 hours or urine protein:creatinine <2.0), though a hallmark of nonsteroidal anti-inflammatory drugs (NSAIDs)-induced ATIN is nephrosis. Different segments of the nephron may be involved in TIN, manifesting as Fanconi syndrome (proximal tubule) or distal renal tubular acidosis (distal convoluted tubule).

Renal ultrasound is utilized to image the kidneys in cases of AKI. In ATIN, the kidneys often appear enlarged in width, depth, and length, and are echogenic compared to the liver and spleen, with increased echogenicity in the renal cortices. In contrast, chronic TIN is characterized ultrasonographically by small renal size and diffusely increased echogenicity.

Kidney biopsy remains the diagnostic "gold standard" and may provide prognostic information. In one study, greater than 50% of pediatric patients diagnosed with TIN by kidney biopsy were not thought to have TIN based on clinical and laboratory evaluation. Use of a tubulointerstitial score at the time of biopsy is useful in predicting response to therapy and long-term renal function. Once TIN is established by kidney biopsy, the underlying etiology must be defined (see Table 3).

Clinical Course

The clinical course varies based on etiology. In antimicrobial induced ATIN, the onset of AKI is rapid and occurs in a hospitalized patient. Acute TIN due to infection generally develops after the acute infectious illness has presented.

Treatment

Treatment remains primarily supportive in nature. Potentially offending medications should be discontinued if possible, and used with caution if use is necessary. If the etiology is infectious, prompt treatment with appropriate

Table 3. Etiologies of acute interstitial nephritis

Infections	Drug Reactions	Immune Mediated	Other
Bacterial	***Antibiotics***	***Anti-TBM Antibodies***	***Metabolic***
i. β-Hemolytic Streptococcus	i. Penicillins	i. Primary anti-TBM nephritis	i. Oxalate nephropathy
ii. Corynebacterium	ii. Cephalosporins	ii. Secondary anti-TBM nephritis	ii. Hypercalcemic nephropathy
iii. Brucella sp.	iii. Sulfonamides	a. Anti-GBM disease	iii. Urate nephropathy
iv. Legionella penumophilia	iv. Rifampin	b. Membranous nephropathy	iv. Cystine nephropathy
v. Campylobacter jejuni	v. Ethambutal	***Immune-Complex Deposits***	***Heavy Metal***
vi. Mycoplasma sp.	vi. Azithromycin	i. Primary immune complex nephritis	i. Lead
vii. Salmonella sp.	vii. Ciprofloxacin	ii. Secondary immune complex nephritis	ii. Cadmium
iii. Yersinia pseudotuberculosis	viii. Tetracycline	a. Lupus nephritis	iii. Mercury
Viruses	ix. Vancomycin	b. Sjogren syndrome	***Hereditary***
i. Rubeola	x. Erythromycin	c. Membranoproliferative glomerulonephritis	i. Alport's syndrome
ii. Epstein-Barr Virus	xi. Aminoglycosides	d. Membranous nephropathy	ii. Nephrolithiasis-medullary cystic kidney
iii. HIV	***Anti-inflammatory Drugs***	e. Mixed Cryoglobulinemia	***Miscellaneous***
iv. Hepatitis viruses	i. Ibuprofen	***T Cell Mediated***	i. Chinese herb nephropathy
v. Cytomegalovirus	ii. Indomethacin	i. Tubulointerstitial nephritis with uveitis syndrome	ii. Radiation nephritis
vi. Polyomavirus (BK)	***Diuretics***	ii. Sarcoidosis	iii. Ischemic nephropathy
vii. Hantavirus	i. Furosemide	iii. Granulomatous tubulointerstitial nephritis	iv. Balkan endemic nephropathy
iii. Adenovirus	ii. Thiazides		

(*Continued*)

Table 3. (*Continued*)

Infections	Drug Reactions	Immune Mediated	Other
Fungi	***Other Medications***		
i. Candida sp.	i. Cimetidine		
ii. Aspergillus sp	ii. Omeprazole		
iii. Cryptococcus neoformans	iii. Captopril		
iv. Histoplasma capsulatum	iv. Carbamazepine		
v. Coccidioides immitis	v. Phenobarbital		
vi. Blastomyces dermatitidis	vi. Cyclosporine		
vii. Mucormycosis	vii. Lithium		
Parasites	viii. Gold		
i. Plasmodium sp.	ix. Aspirin		
ii. Schistosoma sp.	x. Azathioprine		
iii. Filariasis			

TBM = Tubular basement membrane; GBM = Glomerular basement membrane; MPGN = Membranoproliferative glomerulonephropathy.

antibiotics, antifungals, or antiviral medications should be initiated. If ATIN is secondary to primary glomerular disorder or systemic illness, treatment should be dictated by treatment of the underlying disorder.

For patients presenting with AKI, with indications for dialytic therapies, renal replacement therapy should be provided until renal function recovers.

Corticosteroids can be used in those unresponsive to drug discontinuation in cases of suspected medication-induced TIN or treatment of suspected infection (see Fig. 1). Several uncontrolled adult studies have

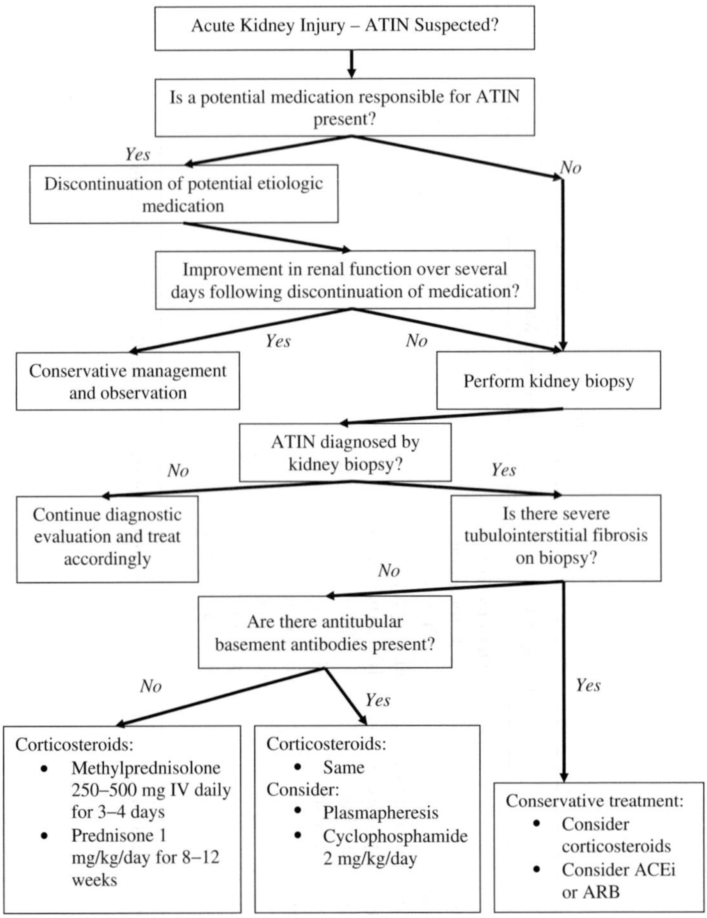

Figure 1.

ATIN = Acute tubulointerstitial nephritis; ACEi = Angiotensin converting enzyme inhibitor; ARB = Angiotensin II receptor blocker.

demonstrated a quicker renal recovery among those receiving corticosteroids compared to those not treated with corticosteroids. Data suggests the longer the delay in the initiation of corticosteroid therapy, the greater the risk of CKD. Given the absence of randomized, controlled prospective studies, treatment with corticosteroids appears to be beneficial. Initial therapy includes methylprednisolone (250–1000 mg intravenously daily for 1–5 doses), followed by oral prednisone (1 mg/kg/day (maximum 60 mg/day)) as a single dose or divided doses. In general, corticosteroids should be continued for at least four weeks, but discontinued if no improvement in seen. However, if the patient demonstrates an improvement in renal function, then corticosteroids should be continued for eight weeks, then tapered. In ATIN associated with antitubular basement membrane antibodies, corticosteroids and cyclophosphamide (2 mg/kg/day) should be given. Ideally, cyclophosphamide should be initiated within 2 weeks of beginning corticosteroids.

In animal models, both enalaprilat and losartan have shown to attenuate tubulointerstitial fibrosis. Recently, mycophenolate mofetil (MMF) has been reported to successfully treat an adult cohort of steroid-resistant, biopsy-proven ATIN. Alternative therapies currently under investigation in animal models of TIN include recombinant human erythropoietin, tumor necrosis factor-alpha inhibitors, colchicine, pravastatin, and flaxseed. However, no human data exists to support their use in treatment of TIN.

Prognosis

The overall prognosis of TIN in children remains good. Greising *et al.* reported that 6 of 7 patients with TIN had complete renal recovery following supportive therapy and corticosteroid therapy in five patients, even though 3 of the 7 patients required temporary hemodialysis. All 13 patients described by Ellis *et al.* had normal renal function 1.5 to 10 years after presentation, with mean time to renal recovery of 69.5 ± 34.7 days. Only 2 of 13 patients required corticosteroids and cyclophosphamide to induce renal recovery and one patient required temporary peritoneal dialysis.

The prognosis for tubulointerstitial nephritis and uveitis in children has a similarly good long-term prognosis. Vohra *et al.* reported 35 patients who all had complete renal recovery, including 26 patients who received corticosteroids.

Suggested Reading

Appel GB. (2001) *Immunologic Renal Diseases*, 2nd ed., Lippincott Williams and Wilkins, Philadelphia. pp. 1269–1281.

Cavallo T. (1998) Tubulointerstitial nephritis. In: *Heptinstall's Pathology of the Kidney*, Jeanette JC, Olson LL, Schwartz MM, Silva FG (eds.), 5th ed., Lippincott-Raven Publishers, Philadelphia. pp. 667–723.

Corwin HL, Bray RA, Haber MH. (1989) The detection and interpretation of urinary eosinophils. *Arch Pathol Lab Med* **113**(11): 1256–1258.

Dell KM, Kaplan BS, Meyers CM. (1999) Tubulointerstitial nephritis. In: *Pediatric Nephrology*, Barratt TM, Avner ED, Harmon WE. (eds.), 4th ed., Lippincott Williams and Wilkins, Baltimore. pp. 823–834.

Ellis D, Fried WA, Yunis EJ, Blau EB. (1981) Acute interstitial nephritis in children: a report of 13 cases and review of the literature. *Pediatrics* **67**(6): 862–870.

González E, Gutiérrez E, Galeano C, *et al.* (2008) Early steroid treatment improves the recovery of renal function in patients with drug-induced acute interstitial nephritis. *Kidney Int* **73**(8): 940–1046.

Greising J, Trachtman H, Gauthier B, Valderrama E. (1990) Acute interstitial nephritis in adolescents and young adults. *Child Nephrol Urol* **10**: 189–195.

Hawkins EP, Berry PL, Silva FG. (1989) Acute tubulointerstitial nephritis in children: clinical, morphologic, and lectin studies. A report of the southwestern pediatric nephrology study group. *Am J Kidney Dis* **14**(6): 466–471.

Jones CL, Eddy AA. (1992) Tubulointerstitial nephritis. *Pediatr Nephrol* **6**(6): 572–586.

Michel DM, Kelly CJ. (1998) Acute intersitial nephritis. *J Am Soc Nephrol* **9**: 506–515.

Vohra S, Eddy A, Levin AV, *et al.* (1999) Tubulointerstitial nephritis and uveitis in children and adolescents. Four new cases and a review of the literature. *Pediatr Nephrol* **13**: 426–432.

Part VIII

Urinary Tract Infections

28

Acute Cystitis

Larisa G. Kovacevic and Tej K. Mattoo

Introduction

Cystitis is inflammation of the urinary bladder that can be caused by various infectious agents, chemicals and drugs, or in association with systemic diseases (Table 1). It is an uncommon diagnosis in children less than 2 years of age and occurs frequently in sexually active teenage girls.

- *Uncomplicated cystitis* is limited to the bladder and occurs in children older than 2 years or adolescents with a normal urinary tract.
- *Complicated cystitis* is associated with pyelonephritis and implies a predisposing or underlying medical condition, such as malignancy, diabetes, anatomic or physiologic abnormalities, indwelling bladder catheter, urodynamic dysfunction, neurogenic bladder, or incomplete bladder emptying.

Risk Factors

- Female sex
- Sexual activity
- Abnormalities of the urinary system
- Associated medical conditions (diabetes, bladder stones, immunodeficiency, sickle-cell anemia, dysfunctional elimination syndrome/fecal impaction, paraplegia and other neurologic conditions, or history of kidney transplant)
- Bladder catheter or recent urethral instrumentation
- Other: tight underwear/clothing, chemicals in soaps, douches

Table 1. Causative agents

Infectious	Bacteria	Viruses	Fungi	Parasites
	Gram + cocci	Herpes	Candida	Schistosoma haematobium
	Streptococcus group B	Adenovirus	Trichosporon	Trichomonas vaginalis
	Streptococcus group D	Polyomaviruses	Aspergillus	Chlamydia
	Staphylococcus aureus	BK virus	Microsporidia	
	Staphylococcus epidermis	JC virus	Blastomyces	
	Staphylococcus saprophyticus	SV 40 virus	Histoplasma	
	Enterococcus	CMV		
	Gram – cocci			
	Neisseria gonorrhoeae			
	Gram – bacilli			
	Escherichia coli			
	Pseudomonas aeruginosa			
	Klebsiella spp.			
	Enterobacter cloacae			
	Enterobacter aerogenes			
	Proteus mirabilis			

Noninfectious	Chemical	Interstitial	Drugs
	Bath products	Behcet's disease	Cetirizine
	Sanitary napkins	Sjogren's syndrome	Ticarcillin
	Tampons	Systemic lupus erythematosus	Doxorubicin
	Deodorants	Rheumathoid arthritis	Methotrexate
	Spermicide	Crohn disease	Cyclophosphamide
		Ulcerative colitis	

Clinical Presentation

Presenting history depends on patient's age.

- Infants less than 90 days of age may have vague and nonspecific symptoms, such as failure to thrive, diarrhea, vomiting, irritability, malodorous urine, jaundice, and fever. Clinical distinction between lower and upper urinary tract infection in this age group is difficult; a positive urine culture with high fever should indicate upper tract infection.
- Infants older than 90 days and young children (<5 years of age) with cystitis who have not yet achieved urine control often present with low-grade fever (usually less than 38°C [100.4°F]), discomfort or crying with urination, mild behavior change and, at times, foul-smelling urine.
- Older children (>5 years of age) typically present with dysuria, urinary frequency, urgency, hesitancy, incontinence, abdominal/suprapubic pain, and/or hematuria. Fever >38.5°C, chills, or flank pain are suggestive of upper tract infection rather than acute cystitis. Symptoms of dysuria or frequency are often absent in patients with neurogenic bladder. Thus, a change in urinary sediment and/or odor helps to differentiate between acute cystitis and chronic bacteriuria due to colonization.

Physical Examination

- Documentation of blood pressure, temperature and growth parameters
- Abdominal examination for tenderness or mass (e.g., enlarged bladder or enlarged kidney secondary to urinary obstruction)
- Assessment of suprapubic and costovertebral tenderness
- Evaluation of the lower back for signs of occult myelodysplasia (e.g., midline pigmentation, lipoma, vascular lesion, sinus, tuft of hair), which may be associated with a neurogenic bladder
- Examination of the external genitalia for anatomic abnormalities (e.g., phimosis or labial adhesions), vulvovaginitis, urethritis (urethral discharge), epididymitis (scrotal pain), vaginal foreign body
- Pelvic examination in a sexually active adolescent female

Diagnosis

1) History and physical examination
2) Urinary findings

   - Significant bacteriuria (defined as at least 100,000 colonies/mL from a clean-catch specimen, 50,000 colonies/mL or more from a catheterized specimen, and any number of uropathogenic bacteria from a suprapubic aspirate) obtained prior to antibiotic initiation
   - Pyuria on dipstick or microscopic examination
   - Viral cultures should be obtained in the setting of hemorrhagic cystitis and in immunocompromised patients when a bacterial pathogen has not been isolated.

3) Renal imaging: Radiological evaluation of urinary tract by ultrasonography or voiding cystourethrogram is not routinely necessary, particularly in older children and adolescents with uncomplicated cystitis. Imaging may be indicated for patients with recurrent cystitis, or cystitis due to an unusual pathogen.

Treatment

Uncomplicated cystitis

Oral first-line agents include trimethoprim-sulfamethoxazole, amoxicillin-clavulanate, and second- and third-generation cephalosporins for a minimum of 3–5 days, with many practitioners treating for 10 days. Amoxicillin should be avoided because approximately 50% of *E. coli* are resistant, unless indicated based on sensitivities.

Complicated cystitis

In an acutely ill child, an immunocompromised patient, or an infant younger than 2 months of age, this should be treated with parenteral antimicrobial therapy. Acceptable initial regimens include the combination of ampicillin or cefazolin plus gentamicin or third-generation cephalosporin for 7–14 days. Parenteral treatment is maintained until the child is clinically stable and afebrile for 48–72 hours, at which point coverage may be changed to an oral agent, based on sensitivities from the urine culture.

Asymptomatic candiduria

This rarely requires antifungal therapy, unless it occurs in the setting of neutropenia, low birth-weight neonates, or urinary tract manipulation. Patients with an indwelling bladder catheter may need removal/replacement.

Symptomatic candiduria

This should always be treated based on identified candida species and whether localized or disseminated infection is present.

Viral cystitis

This requires supportive treatment. Reduction of immunosuppressive medications may be helpful. For viral hemorrhagic cystitis, antiviral therapy (*ribavirin* or *cidofavir*) has been tried with variable results.

Clinical response should be seen within 24–48 hours. If not, repeated urine culture should be ordered. Imaging of the urinary tract may be necessary to evaluate the presence of upper tract infection, renal abscess, urinary calculi, or surgically correctable anatomic abnormalities or obstruction.

Prognosis

- *Uncomplicated cystitis* has excellent prognosis with no long-term sequelae and little risk of recurrence.
- *Complicated cystitis* can lead to chronic bacteriuria, recurrent cystitis, or progression to upper urinary tract disease. The risk for dissemination and multiorgan system infection, which are associated with increased mortality, is greatest in immunocompromised patients.

Suggested Reading

Abrahamsson K, Hansson S, Larsson P, Jodal U. (2002) Antibiotic treatment for five days is effective in children with acute cystitis. *Acta Paediatr* **91**(1): 55–58.

Bensman A, Ulinski T. (2009) Pharmacotherapy of lower urinary tract infections and pyelonephritis in children. *Expert Opin Pharmacother* **10**(13): 2075–2080.

Elliott SP, Villar R, Duncan B. (2005) Bacteriuria management and urological evaluation of patients with spina bifida and neurogenic bladder: a multicenter survey. *J Urol* **173**: 217–220.

Faraci M, Cuzzubbo D, Lanino E, *et al.* (2009) Low dosage cidofovir without probenecid as treatment for BK virus hemorrhagic cystitis after hemopoietic stem cell transplant. *Pediatr Infect Dis J* **28**: 55–57.

Hooton TM, Scholes D, Hughes JP, *et al.* (1996) A prospective study of risk factors for symptomatic urinary tract infection in young women. *N Engl J Med* **335**: 468–474.

Langley JM, Hanakowski M, Leblanc JC. (2001) Unique epidemiology of nosocomial urinary tract infection in children. *Am J Infect Control* **29**: 94–98.

Mehr SS, Powell CV, Curtis N. (2004) Cephalosporin resistant urinary tract infections in young children. *J Paediatr Child Health* **40**: 48.

Pappas PG, Kauffman CA, Andes D, *et al.* (2009) Clinical practice guidelines for the management of candidiasis: 2009 update by the Infectious Diseases Society of America. *Clin Infect Dis* **48**: 503–535.

Tran D, Muchant DG, Aronoff SC. (2001) Short-course versus conventional length antimicrobial therapy for uncomplicated lower urinary tract infections in children: a meta-analysis of 1279 patients. *J Pediatr* **139**: 93–99.

29

Acute Pyelonephritis

Larisa G. Kovacevic and Tej K. Mattoo

Introduction

Acute pyelonephritis results from bacterial seeding of renal parenchyma either via the hematogenous route or the ascending route from the lower urinary tract.

Risk Factors

- Microbial virulence factors include P-fimbriae, protectins, toxins and siderophores. P-fimbriae *E. coli* adheres to uroepithelium in a lock and key fashion impeding the normal flushing action of urine flow, predisposing to pyelonephritis.
- Factors such as age, gender, race, circumcision status, immune status, genitourinary abnormalities, presence of renal calculi, or vesicoureteral reflux (VUR) predispose to pyelonephritis.

Etiology

The most common organism is *E. coli*, accounting for up to 70% of infections. Other common urinary pathogens include *Pseudomonas* (abnormal urinary tract, frequent catheterization, hospitalized children), *Klebsiella*, *Proteus* (renal calculi), *Enterococcus* species, Group B streptococci (neonates), and *Staphylococcus aureus* (hematogenous spread, renal abscess). Fungal UTI can be caused by *Candida* species (associated with instrumentation of urinary tract).

Diagnosis

Acute pyelonephritis is a clinical diagnosis, suggested by the triad of fever, systemic symptoms, and costovertebral angle tenderness; and confirmed by the presence of pyuria and positive urine culture.

History and physical examination

- *Infants less than 90 days of age* may have nonspecific symptoms, such as fever, hypothermia, vomiting, diarrhea, dehydration, jaundice, feeding difficulty, irritability, or failure to thrive. Bacteremia and urosepsis should be considered.
- *Infants older than 90 days and children <5 years of age* can present with high-grade fever >38°C (100.4°F) without a clear source of infection, or with gastrointestinal symptoms (vomiting, abdominal pain, diarrhea).
- *Older children (>5 years of age)* present with fever >38.5°C, chills, and flank pain.

Urinalysis and urine culture

- Positive dipstick findings for leukocyte esterase and the presence of white cells or bacteria on urine microscopy in an appropriately collected urine sample is highly indicative of infection. Pyuria (≥10 WBC/high power field) alone is a nonspecific finding that can occur in the absence of infection. The detection of leukocyte esterase and/or nitrites and may be falsely negative in neonates and infants. Urinary nitrites are negative in infections with gram-positive organisms.
- The gold standard to make the diagnosis is the urine culture obtained by suprapubic aspiration or urethral catheterization in non-toilet–trained children and by mid-stream "clean catch" in toilet-trained children. The number of colony forming units (CFU) required for the diagnosis depends on the method of collection (at least 100,000 CFU/mL from a clean-catch specimen, 50,000 CFU/mL or more from a catheterized specimen and any amount from suprapubic aspirate). Urine gram stain may be helpful for rapid preliminary diagnostic purposes and for guiding the choice of empiric therapy pending culture results.

Supportive evidence

When present, elevated peripheral white blood cell, erythrocyte sedimentation rate, C-reactive protein, and procalcitonin may be helpful in diagnosing acute pyelonephritis, but absence does not exclude it. Blood culture should be obtained in infants less than two months of age.

Renal Imaging

In patients with first acute febrile UTI, renal ultrasonography (RUS), and contrast voiding cystourethrography (VCUG) should be performed.

- RUS is useful in detecting hydronephrosis, congenital renal and urinary tract anomalies (such as renal dysplasia, ectopic kidney, duplex collecting system, ureteropelvic junction obstruction, and ureterocele), and renal abscess. It is not reliable for detecting VUR or renal scarring.
- Contrast VCUG is the gold standard for diagnosing the presence and severity of VUR. It also evaluates the lower genitourinary (GU) anatomy. The procedure involves catheterization to fill the bladder with a radio opaque or radioactive liquid and recording of VUR during voiding. It should be obtained as soon as the infected urine has become sterile or when the child has completed the full antibiotic course.
- Renal scintigraphy using dimercaptosuccinic acid (DMSA) can be used in selected case to detect acute pyelonephritis and renal scarring. DMSA is injected intravenously, and uptake by the kidney is measured 2–4 hours later. Areas of decreased uptake represent pyelonephritis or scarring. DMSA renal scan should not be used routinely, since most of the children with acute pyelonephritis have DMSA defects that resolve on follow-up.

Treatment

Treatment is based on the age and severity of symptoms. Initial treatment includes supportive care and initiation of empiric antibiotic therapy. The choice of antibiotic should be based on the pathogen resistance patterns in the hospital and community, and gram staining of the urine. The ultimate choice of antimicrobial therapy is based upon the sensitivities of the patient's urine culture isolate. Duration of treatment is typically 10–14 days.

In-hospital management is indicated in:

- Infants under three months of age
- Toxic appearing infant or child
- Significant dehydration or the inability to take oral fluids and medication
- Chronic diseases such as sickle cell disease, diabetes mellitus, cystic fibrosis
- Immunocompromised patients
- Complicated urinary tract abnormalities
- Patients with urinary stents or other urinary foreign bodies
- Failure to respond to outpatient therapy, noncompliant patient

Parenteral treatment regimens include:

- Third- or fourth-generation cephalosporin (cefepime, cefotaxime, ceftriaxone) alone
- Combination of ampicillin and gentamicin
- Combination of ampicillin and cefotaxime
- Gentamicin alone
- Ampicillin should be added if enterococcal UTI is suspected

Consider changing to oral therapy in accordance to pathogen sensitivity following clinical response (no fever for 48 hours) to complete 10–14 days of treatment.

Outpatient management is safe and effective for patients who appear non toxic and can be stabilized with oral hydration and antibiotics; an initial dose of intravenous antibiotic can be given and then the patient can be discharged on oral antibiotics with close follow-up within 48 hours.

Oral treatment

- Second- or third-generation cephalosporin (e.g. cefuroxime axetil, cefixime, cefdinir, ceftibuten, cefprozil, and cefpodoxime) are first-line oral agents
- Amoxicillin and ampicillin are not routinely recommended for empiric therapy due to resistance

- Amoxicillin-clavulanate, first-generation cephalosporins (e.g. cephalexin), and trimethoprim sulfamethoxazole (TMP-SMX) should be used with caution because of the increasing rates of resistance to these drugs
- Ciprofloxacin is generally reserved for severe, complicated cases

Antibiotic prophylaxis

Children awaiting VCUG should be assumed to have VUR and should be started on prophylactic antibiotics (amoxicillin in infants younger than 2 months); trimethoprim sulfamethoxazole (TMP-SMX) nitroturantoin can be after the completion of the 10–14 days treatment.

Response to therapy

Most patients improve within 24–72 hours of initiation of appropriate antimicrobial therapy. If not, broadening antimicrobial therapy may be indicated if the culture and sensitivity results are not yet available. In such patients, repeat renal ultrasonography or computed tomography may be necessary to diagnose renal abscess, urinary calculi, or surgically correctable anatomic abnormalities or obstruction.

Complications of acute pyelonephritis include:

- Sepsis
- Abscess formation (renal cortical abscess, renal corticomedullary abscess, or perinephric abscess)
- Acute kidney injury
- Papillary necrosis
- Renal scarring that can lead to hypertension, proteinuria, and chronic kidney disease

Suggested Reading

Chang SL, Shortliffe LD. (2006) Pediatric urinary tract infections. *Pediatr Clin North Am* **53**: 379.

Committee on Infectious Diseases. (2006) The use of systemic fluoroquinolones. *Pediatr* **118**(3): 1287–1292.

Garin EH, Olavarria F, Araya C, *et al.* (2007) Diagnostic significance of clinical and laboratory findings to localize site of urinary infection. *Pediatr Nephrol* **22**(7): 1002–1006.

Hoberman A, Charron M, Hickey RW, *et al.* (2003) Imaging studies after a first febrile urinary tract infection in young children. *N Engl J Med* **348**(3): 195–202.

Hodson EM, Willis NS, Craig JC. (2007) Antibiotics for acute pyelonephritis in children. *Cochrane Database Syst Rev* (4): CD003772.

Johansen TE. (2004) The role of imaging in urinary tract infections. *World J Urol* **22**(5): 392–398.

Jones ME, Karlowsky JA, Draghi DC, *et al.* (2004) Rates of antimicrobial resistance among common bacterial pathogens causing respiratory, blood, urine, and skin and soft tissue infections in pediatric patients. *Eur J Clin Microbiol Infect Dis* **23**: 445.

Lin KY, Chiu NT, Chen MJ, *et al.* (2003) Acute pyelonephritis and sequelae of renal scar in pediatric first febrile urinary tract infection. *Pediatr Nephrol* **18**(4): 362–365.

Pecile P, Miorin E, Romanello C, *et al.* (2004) Procalcitonin: a marker of severity of acute pyelonephritis among children. *Pediatr* **114**(2): 249–254.

Shaikh N, Morone NE, Bost JE, Farrell MH. (2008) Prevalence of Urinary Tract Infection in Childhood: A Meta-Analysis. *Pediatr Infect Dis J* **27**: 302–308.

Zorc JJ, Kiddoo DA, Shaw KN. (2005) Diagnosis and management of pediatric urinary tract infections. *Clin Microbiol Rev* **18**: 417.

30

Vesicoureteral Reflux

Larisa G. Kovacevic and Tej K. Mattoo

Introduction

Vesicoureteral reflux (VUR) is the retrograde flow of urine from the bladder into the upper urinary tract. It is believed that the reflux of infected bladder urine into the kidneys increases the risk of acute pyelonephritis and renal scarring, which is also called reflux nephropathy. Most cases of VUR are diagnosed after urinary tract infection (UTI). However, VUR may be diagnosed in the absence of UTI in certain circumstances such as during follow-up of antenatal hydronephrosis or as a result of screening.

Incidence

The incidence of children diagnosed with VUR following a febrile UTI varies based on age. It is highest in children younger than one year of age (60%), decreases significantly by 2–3 years of age (30%) and by adulthood is decreased to 5%. The incidence of VUR diagnosed during evaluation of hydronephrosis and sibling screening is about 30%.

Etiology

VUR occurs as a result of an anatomical or functional abnormality of the normally competent ureterovesical junction (UVJ). Primary VUR is due to shortening of the intravesical ureter that causes inadequate closure of the UVJ; secondary VUR is caused by an abnormally high pressure in the bladder that results in failure of the closure of the UVJ during bladder contraction. It is important to note VUR is congenital in nature.

Associated Conditions

VUR can be associated with various urologic conditions such as unilateral multicystic dysplastic kidney, unilateral or bilateral cystic dysplasia, unilateral renal agenesis, and renal or ureteral ectopia.

Classification of VUR

The International Reflux Study Group (IRSG) developed a system to grade the severity of VUR based upon the degree of retrograde filling and dilation of the renal collecting system as demonstrated by voiding cystourethrogram (VCUG). The grading of VUR correlates with the potential for spontaneous resolution as well as the potential for renal scarring.

- Grade I — Reflux into a nondilated ureter
- Grade II — Reflux into a nondilated ureter and renal pelvis
- Grade III — Mild dilatation of the ureter and renal pelvis with mild blunting of the calyces
- Grade IV — Moderate tortuosity of the ureter and dilatation of the renal pelvis and calyces
- Grade V — Gross dilatation of the renal pelvis and calyces with significant ureteral tortuosity

Generally, grades I and II are considered mild, grade III is moderate, and grades IV and V are severe.

Diagnosis and Evaluation

The diagnosis of VUR is based upon the demonstration of reflux of urine from the bladder to the upper urinary tract by either contrast VCUG or radionuclide cystogram (RNC). Contrast VCUG is preferable, particularly as the initial study in both boys and girls because it also evaluates the lower genitourinary tract anatomy; RNC can be used for follow-up in both genders.

Renal scan (DMSA) can help in the evaluation of patients with VUR because it can quantify differential function of the kidneys and assess for cortical defects, reflecting scarring. It should be deferred for 4–6 months after acute pyelonephritis to avoid confusion regarding acute, reversible vs. chronic, permanent lesions.

Management

Medical management of VUR includes long-term prophylactic antibiotics. Antimicrobial agents most appropriate for prophylaxis include trimethoprim-sulfamethoxazole (TMP-SMZ), trimethoprim alone, nitrofurantoin, or cephalexin. The dose for prophylaxis is one quarter to one half of the therapeutic dose for acute infection. Amoxicillin should be used in infants less than two months of age due to risk of kernicterus associated with TMP-SMZ in this age group. The duration of antibiotic prophylaxis and the potential need for surgical correction depends on the age of the patient, the severity of the VUR, the frequency of UTI, patient tolerance and compliance, and presence and the severity of renal scarring. The potential limitations with antibiotic prophylaxis include drug resistance, gastrointestinal symptoms, hepatotoxicity, and skin rashes.

Surgical management is appropriate for patients who fail medical management, have a low chance of resolution (severe VUR), and have demonstrated a worsening of renal scarring during follow-up. Surgical interventions include minimally invasive procedures, such as endoscopic injection of a bulking agents (Deflux®), or ureteral reimplantation.

Management includes routine follow-up of patients with VUR with an emphasis on early diagnosis and treatment of acute UTI; changing of antibiotic prophylaxis if the patient has recurrent breakthrough UTIs; and periodic VCUG studies. The timing for follow-up VCUG varies from once every 1–3 years, depending on the severity of VUR and presence of renal scarring.

Complications of VUR

In many patients, VUR is associated with reflux nephropathy, which may be congenital or acquired. Congenital reflux nephropathy is seen mostly in boys with severe congenital antenatal VUR and renal injury occurring independent of UTI. In contrast, acquired reflux nephropathy is seen mostly in girls before the age of five years with severe (grade IV and V) VUR and recurrent UTI. Complications of reflux nephropathy include hypertension, proteinuria, pregnancy-related complications, and end-stage renal disease (ESRD). Rarely, patients may present with nephrotic-range proteinuria due to secondary focal segmental glomerulosclerosis (FSGS).

Prognosis

VUR, particularly if low grade (grade I–III) is more likely to resolve spontaneously over time. Grades I–III VUR resolve at a rate of 13% per year for the first five years of follow-up, and 3.5% per year during subsequent years, whereas grades IV and V VUR resolve at a rate of 5% per year. The goal is to minimize infections, and obviate/minimize reflux nephropathy. If these goals are accomplished, the prognosis of VUR remains good.

Suggested Reading

Chertin B, Puri P. (2003) Familial vesicoureteral reflux. *J Urol* **169**: 1804.

Fanos V, Cataldi L. (2004) Antibiotics or surgery for vesicoureteric reflux in children. *Lancet* **364**: 1720.

Hoberman A, Charron M, Hickey RW, *et al.* (2003) Imaging studies after a first febrile urinary tract infection in young children. *N Engl J Med* **348**: 195.

Mattoo TK, Mathews R. (2009) Vesicoureteral reflux and renal scarring. In: Avner E, Harmon W, Niaudet P, Yoshikawa N (eds.), *Pediatric Nephrology* (6th ed.) Springer-Verlag, Berlin. pp. 1311–1336.

Medical versus surgical treatment of primary vesicoureteral reflux: report of the International Reflux Study Committee. *Pediatr* (1981) **67**: 392.

Morita M, Yoshiara S, White RH, *et al.* (1990) The glomerular changes in children with reflux nephropathy. *J Pathol* **162**(3): 245–253.

Schwab CW, Jr, Wu HY, Selman H, *et al.* (2002) Spontaneous resolution of vesicoureteral reflux: a 15-year perspective. *J Urol* **168**(6): 2594–2599.

Silva JM, Santos Diniz JS, Marino VS, *et al.* (2006) Clinical course of 735 children and adolescents with primary vesicoureteral reflux. *Pediatr Nephrol* **21**(7): 981–988.

Thompson M, Simon SD, Sharma V, *et al.* (2005) Timing of follow-up voiding cystourethrogram in children with primary vesicoureteral reflux: development and application of a clinical algorithm. *Pediatr* **115**(2): 426–434.

van Eerde AM, Meutgeert MH, de Jong TP, *et al.* (2007) Vesico-ureteral reflux in children with prenatally detected hydronephrosis: a systematic review. *Ultrasound Obstet Gynecol* **29**: 463.

Part IX

Hypertension

31

Hypertension in Children

Daniel Feig

Introduction

Hypertension is the most common disease in the world, with nearly 130 million adults in the United States, and >1 billion people worldwide affected. Hypertension is the leading risk factor for cardiovascular (CV) disease and the second most important risk factor for renal disease, following diabetes, in adults. It contributes to death in over 1 million Americans a year. Large longitudinal epidemiologic studies have identified blood pressure (BP) ranges associated with CV risk and have resulted in definitions from the Joint National Commission VII (JNC7) of optimal BP <125/75, prehypertension >130/80 and hypertension >140/90. Despite tremendous public health impact, hypertension screening is lacking, and even when detected and treated, control rarely reaches 50%.

In children, the definition of hypertension is not so straightforward. Because hypertension associated myocardial infarction, stroke or renal failure is exceedingly rare, definitions based on CV risk assessment are not useful. This does not imply that hypertension does not confer CV risk on children but rather that relative lack of concomitant conventional risk factors or disease of sufficient duration results in CV events not occurring in children. Consequently, hypertension in children is defined statistically. Normative BP tables derived from the National Health and Nutrition Examination Survey III (NHANES III) have been updated, most recently in 2004. BP normally increases with age and height so tables are stratified by sex, age, and height percentile. Consensus guidelines define normal BP in children as < 90th percentile for sex, age, and height. Prehypertension is defined as BP between 90th and 95th percentile. Stage 1 hypertension is BP that ranges from 95th percentile to 5 mm Hg above the 99th percentile; stage

2 hypertension is BP that is > 5 mm Hg above the 99th percentile (Table 1). To diagnose hypertension, a child must have BP > 95th on three consecutive provider encounters over two weeks minimum. Isolated increase in systolic blood pressure (SBP), or diastolic blood pressure (DBP), or combined hypertension meets criteria. Populations at particular risk, including children with structural heart disease, renal disease, or diabetes are considered hypertensive when blood pressures exceed the 90th percentile. In screening populations, such as the NHANES cohort and the Houston Independent School District, hypertension prevalence approximates 3–4%.

Why Worry about Hypertension in Children?

Hypertension is far from benign in children. Various types of observed hypertensive target organ damage are listed in Table 2. Left ventricular hypertrophy (LVH) and elevated left ventricular mass index (LVMI) are associated with significant CV risk in adults. Other experts prefer subjective estimates of wall thickness that incorporate three-dimensional geometry rather than cross-sectional geometry of LVMI measurements. This variability results in disparate estimates of LVH prevalence in children. Regardless of definition used, adequate BP control generally results in LVH improvement within 3–6 months.

The prevalence of other target organ damage in children is uncertain but not insignificant. Trials have demonstrated conventional CV risk factors, particularly hypertension, are associated with atherosclerotic, coronary, and aortic disease in adolescents. Incidence of hypertensive renal injury in children is 10–15% at the time of initial diagnosis. Retinal vascular injury due to hypertension is relatively common. Assessment of vessels by retinal photography indicates the mean cross-sectional retinal vessel diameter to be 2 μm narrower than normotensive children. Most concerning is cognitive impairment associated with hypertension. In a posthoc assessment of cognitive tests, children with BP in excess of the 90th percentile performed poorly in mathematical and geometric reasoning scores compared to normotensive children. Hypertension is associated with decreased verbal and mathematical skills. It is unknown if observed deficits are reversible with good BP control.

In addition to target organ damage, hypertensive children have increased symptom complaints including frequent (>once/week) headaches, chest or abdominal pain, and sleep disturbances.

Table 1. Portion of normative BP tables for children

Age	BP percentile	SBP							DBP						
		Ht%							Ht%						
11-year-old boy		5	10	25	50	75	90	95	5	10	25	50	75	90	95
	50	99	100	102	104	105	107	107	59	59	60	61	62	63	63
	90	113	114	115	117	119	120	121	74	74	75	76	77	78	78
	95	117	118	119	121	123	124	125	78	78	79	880	81	82	82
	99	124	125	127	129	130	132	132	86	86	87	88	89	90	90
14-year-old girl		5	10	25	50	75	90	95	5	10	25	50	75	90	95
	50	106	106	107	109	110	111	112	63	63	63	64	65	66	66
	90	119	120	121	122	124	125	125	77	77	77	78	79	80	80
	95	123	123	125	126	127	129	129	81	81	81	82	883	84	84
	99	130	131	132	133	135	136	136	88	88	89	90	90	91	92

Tables are modified from the 4th Task Force report in 2004. An 11-year-old boy who is 25th height for age is considered to have prehypertension >115/75, stage 1 hypertension >119/79 and stage 2 hypertension >132/92. A 14-year-old girl who is 90th percentile for height is considered to have prehypertension >125/80, stage 1 hypertension >129/84 and stage 2 hypertension >141/96. A hypertensive child is one who meets either systolic, or diastolic, or both criteria on three consecutive encounters.

Table 2. Target organ damage in children with hypertension

Target organ damage	Significance	Technique to measure
Left ventricular hypertrophy	40% of newly diagnosed children	Echocardiography, M-mode left ventricular mass index >38.6gm/ (height in m)
Nephrosclerosis	15–20% of newly diagnosed children	Proteinuria, urinary protein/ creatine ratio
Retinopathy	Retinal vessel diameter is inversely related to blood pressure	Dilated fundoscopic exam/ retinal photographs
Cognitive impairment	Reduced mean scores	Posthoc analysis of NHANES III data, comparison of performance on Wechsler Intelligence Scale and Wide-range Achievement Tests
Accelerated atherosclerosis	General severity or prevalence unknown	Autopsy of accident victims, comparison of those known to have prior hypertension versus those know to have been normotensive
Subjective symptoms	Reported rates in newly Diagnosed hypertension	Questionnaire administered in referral clinic at time of initial evaluation of hypertension. Frequency of the symptoms are 3–6 times greater than in normotensive controls
Headache	42%	
Chest pain	14%	
Abdominal pain	10%	
Sleep latency	27%	
Daytime tiredenss	26%	

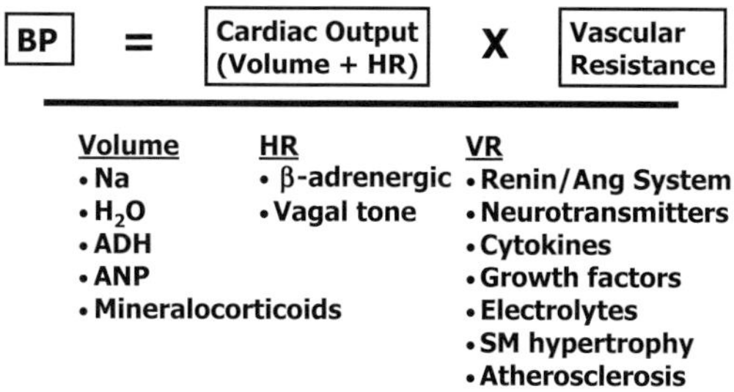

Figure 1. The basic physiology of blood pressure BP = CO × SVR, CO = HR × SV. Physiological changes causing sustained increases intravascular volume status, heart rate, or systemic vascular resistance will increase blood pressure. This figure depicts several common mechanisms for elevating BP. In children, most BP variability is based vascular tone regulation, especially due to the renin-angiotensin system and sympathetic nervous system.

Treatment results in improvement in symptoms and end organ damage, therefore, screening and evaluation of hypertension is imperative. Further, hypertensive children become hypertensive adults, reiterating the need for aggressive therapy (Fig. 1).

How Should BP Be Measured in Children?

Consensus guidelines for on whom, when and how BP should be measured in children are detailed in the 4th Task Force Report published in 2004. All children over age three should have BP measured at all medical encounters. Children less than 3 years of age with special circumstances that increase their risk for hypertension require BP checks at an earlier time point. These circumstances include: prematurity, prolonged NICU care, congenital renal, urologic or cardiac disease (even if repaired), solid organ transplant, increased intracranial pressure, family history of congenital renal malformations, family history of monogenetic hypertension, recurrent urinary tract infections (UTI), history of malignancy or bone marrow transplantation, medications associated with hypertension, or genetic syndrome associated with high BP (e.g., Neurofibromatosis (NF), Tuberous Sclerosis (TS), William syndrome, etc.).

As normative tables for BP assessment in children are auscultatory based using mercury and aneroid sphygmomanometers, these devices are preferred for measurements. In many physician offices, hospitals, and emergency rooms, oscillometric devices are employed for ease, efficiency, and reduction of observer variability. Oscillometric devices measure mean arterial pressure, then use algorithms to calculate both SBP and DBP. Consequently, different devices, or even different models from the same manufacturer can vary. BP obtained at a vital sign station using an oscillometric device compared to exam room use of aneroid monitor after the child has been sitting quietly for five minutes revealed an average difference of 12 and 9 mm Hg for systolic and diastolic blood pressures, respectively. However, due to simplicity and efficiency of oscillometric devices and general use of vitals sign stations, a practical approach is required. Initial screening revealing a BP > 90th percentile, should be confirmed in a quiet exam room, using an auscultatory monitor, with the child seated with feet on the floor and back supported for at least five minutes. When ausculatory BP is measured, the initiation of audible tapping, the first Korotkov sound, is SBP and the disappearance of sound, the fifth Korotkov sound, is DBP. In some children, audible sound is present until the cuff deflates completely in which instance, the pressure on the stethoscope bell should be reduced and the measurement repeated or the muffling of tapping, the fourth Korotkov sound, should be used to define DBP.

BP cuff size is critical to accurate measurement in order to minimize inaccuracies. The width of the inflatable bladder should cover at least 40% of the arm circumference halfway between the acromion and the olecrenon; and be of sufficient length to cover 80–100% of the circumference of the upper arm at its midpoint. Many commercial BP cuffs have less than a 2:1 length to width ratio required by convention and some patients, particularly morbidly obese children, may have arms for which above criteria cannot be met. The practical approach is to have an aneroid monitor with at least five cuff sizes, preferably seven and round upward on cuff size to minimize overestimation errors.

An alternative method to measure BP is ambulatory blood pressure montitoring (ABPM). ABPM involves wearing a portable oscillometric monitor for 24–72 hours. Blood pressure is measured 2–4 times an hour through the day during regular activities and sleep. Most commonly, ABPM is used in children is to diagnose white coat hypertension (WCH), (BP > 95th percentile in a physician's office but consistently normal at home). ABPM can also help assess target organ injury risk, therapy efficacy, and episodic patterns. Absence of nocturnal dipping, the normal physiologic fall of BP during sleep periods, is associated with secondary hypertension and target organ damage.

ABPM results in absolute BP values are not comparable to the Task Force Tables applied to auscultatory measurements. Alternative normative data have been established with the most common device. ABPM requires specialized equipment and training and may not be available at all centers. Use of ABPM in clinical studies has led to the discovery of masked hypertension, in which children have normal BP in casual, office based measurements but have hypertension by mean BP or load criteria on ABPM. Children with masked hypertension have increased risk for progression to sustained hypertension with more target organ damage than a normotensive cohort suggesting that this is a prehypertensive state. No recommendations currently exist regarding screening for masked hypertension as this would require ABPM in an apparently normotensive population.

How Should a Child with Hypertension Be Evaluated?

Hypertension in childhood is tremendously under-diagnosed. Reasons for this include lack of regular preventive care; not having BP measured at physician or nurses visits; and elevated BP not recorded, recognized or evaluated even when obtained. A cohort study of children in primary care offices between 1999 and 2006 of >14,000 children who had ≥3 BPs documented over seven years showed 3.6% met criteria for hypertension. Only 26% of those children had documented hypertension or recommended evaluation. In the same cohort, prehypertension prevalence was 3.4%, of whom only 11% received recommended evaluation or management. In short, less than 1 in 5 children with abnormal BP are evaluated, much less receive appropriate care.

Hypertension evaluation is directed at confirmation, distinction of essential hypertension, secondary hypertension, WCH, and detection of target organ damage. Because secondary hypertension is more common in children, evaluation for secondary causes should be comprehensive as it guides therapy. An exhaustive evaluation of a patient with BPs in the pre or stage 1 hypertension range should not be undertaken until hypertension is confirmed with at least three separate encounters. Stage 2 hypertension or hypertensive crises should be evaluated more promptly. If WCH is suspected, ABPM or home monitoring is reasonable in advance of detailed studies.

Patient history is critical and guides the evaluation, with particular attention to when elevated BP was first noted and when the child was normotensive. Chronic, insidious hypertension is often different from acute severe hypertension with the later likely associated with glomerulonephritis or acute illness. Preexisting illnesses and comorbid conditions that modify risk should be noted including history of UTIs, vesicoureteral reflux (VUR), or fevers of unknown origin resulting in renal scars. Pregnancy and birth history are important as low birth weight and prematurity confer increased risk of secondary (renal) and essential hypertension as do pregnancy complications such as preecclampsia, pregnancy associated hypertension and gestational diabetes. Family history of hypertension is a risk factor for essential hypertension but may also be associated with fibromuscular dysplasia, autosomal dominant polycystic kidney disease (ADPKD), Alport Syndrome or other genetic diseases. Dietary history including portion size, caloric intake, sodium and fat intake, and caffeine consumption is useful in planning lifestyle modification. Sleep disordered breathing and sleep apnea are associated with hypertension and a detailed history can identify patients requiring polysomnography.

Physical exam is frequently normal but attention to several specific aspects can direct evaluation: vitals signs, height, weight, and body mass index (BMI) should be measured and overweight/obese children (> 90th percentile BMI) should be further evaluated for obesity related comorbidities. Tachycardia, irregular heart rate, or murmur can suggest secondary cardiovascular hypertension. Fundoscopic exam can reveal papilledema resulting from increased intracranial pressure and CNS hypertension or retinal vascular changes of target organ damage. Abdominal mass may represent urinary tract obstruction, tumor mediated hypertension, or ADPKD and an abdominal vascular bruit suggests renal artery stenosis. Skin exam may suggest genetic syndromes, particularly NF, TS and obesity comorbidities (i.e. acanthosis nigricans) [Table 3].

Recommended laboratory tests are aimed at diagnosing secondary hypertension and target organ damage and include urinalysis to detect glomerulonephrits, chronic kidney injury or hypertensive nephrosclerosis. Bloodwork includes serum BUN and creatinine screening for decreased renal function. Serum electrolytes, particularly potassium (K^+), are quite useful. Hypokalemia can be observed in renin-dominant hypertension,

Table 3. Causes of hypertension by age group

Age group	Cause of hypertension
Infants <12 months	Congenital renal and urinary tract abnormalities Renal parenchymal injury Renovascular Coarctation Cardiac Endocrine Genetic Tumor (Wilm's, neuroblastoma)
Young children 1–5 years	Renal parenchymal Renovascular Coarctation Essential and obesity Cardiac Endocrine Genetic Tumor (Wilm's, neuroblastoma)
School age 6–11 years	Renal parenchymal Essential and obesity Renovascular Medications, drugs Cardiac Endocrine Genetic Tumor (pheochromocytoma)
Adolescents 12–18 years	Essential and obesity Renal parenchymal Medications, drugs Renovascular Cardiac Coarctation Genetic Tumor (pheochromocytoma)

Modified from Bartosh SM, Aronson AJ. (1999) Childhood hypertension. An update on etiology, diagnosis, and treatment. *Pediatr Clin North Am* **46**: 235–252.

hyperaldosteronism, adrenal hypertension, and low renin monogenetic hypertension such as Liddle syndrome. Hyperkalemia suggests impaired renal clearance or Gordon syndrome. If drug abuse is suspected, a urine and/or serum drug screen is needed. In obese or diabetic children, lipid profile, serum insulin, glucose and hemoglobin A1c should be obtained to guide management. Serum uric acid may be useful diagnostically as elevation has been linked to newly diagnosed essential hypertension, and in select patients, urate lowering therapy may reduce BP (Table 3).

In younger children with stage 1 hypertension or older children with stage 2 hypertension, further laboratory testing including renin and aldosterone profiling, thyroid and adrenal screening and genetic screening for monongenetic hypertension should be performed. Interpretation of renin and aldosterone values can be complicated. Both direct renin measurement of enzyme quantity; and peripheral renin activity values are commercially available. The later varies somewhat depending on patient position immediately before and during phlebotomy and values can vary significantly based on lab. No specific value rules out or establishes renin-mediated hypertension; however, patients with very elevated values are generally more responsive to angiotensin converting enzyme inhibitor (ACEi) and angiotensin receptor blocker (ARB) type drugs whereas those with very low values tend to be respond to calcium channel blocker (CCB) or diuretics. Plasma aldosterone >35 ng/dl, particularly with low renin is suggestive of primary hyperaldosteronism. If symptoms are compelling (palpitations, diaphoresis, weight loss, anxiety, abdominal pain), measurement of plasma metanephrines for pheochromocytoma may be useful (Table 4).

All children with confirmed hypertension should have renal ultrasound (US) to detect congenital anomalies of the urinary tract, obstruction, hydronephrosis suggestive of VUR and renal asymmetry suggesting parenchymal scarring or vascular insufficiency. An echocardiogram should be obtained to detect coarctation of the aorta, or hypertensive target organ damage, the presence of which necessitates immediate pharmacologic therapy. The echocardiogram can detect structural heart disease, particularly hypertrophic cardiomyopathy that can cause sudden cardiac death during athletic participation.

In children under eight years of age and older children with stage 2 hypertension, renal perfusion scintigraphy can detect parenchymal scars. Static renal scans using Tc labeled DMSA (dimercaptosuccinic acid) or dynamic scans using DTPA (diethylenetriamine pentaacetic acid) are highly sensitive for scars. To diagnose renal artery stenosis, renal US, even with Doppler, has variable sensitivity, especially for branch stenosis so if this is suspected, CT angiography or MR angiography should be performed. In experienced hands, CT and MR have similar sensitivity for

Table 4. Evaluation of stage 1 hypertension

	Tests
History	History of present illness General medical history Pregnancy, birth, neonatal history Current and former medications and or drug use Family history Dietary history (including caffeine intake) Sleep history Cognitive development or school performance Prior blood pressure measurements
Physical exam	Vital signs Weight, height, BMI Fundoscopic Thyroid Cardiac Abdominal Skin
BP monitoring	Casual, in clinic, at least three measurements Consider ABPM Consider home monitoring
Laboratory tests	Urinalysis CBC Chemistries (Na, K, Cl, HCO3, BUN, Cr, Glu) Uric acid Lipid profile, glucose, insulin, HbA1c (if obese or diabetic) Drug screen (if indicated by history or exam) Thyroid or adrenal screening (if indicated by history or exam)
Imaging	Renal ultrasound Echocardiogram Renal scintigraphy (under age eight) Renal artery imaging (under age eight)

primary and branch stenoses; however CT angiography is quicker and generally less expensive, while MR takes longer and may require anesthesia, but lacks radiation exposure (Table 5).

Several other imaging tests are frequently ordered, but add little value. Chest X-ray is often ordered, but a child with confirmed hypertension should have an echocardiogram. Chest X-ray is indicated in the presence of respiratory symptoms. Electrocardiogram (ECG) is frequently used for LVH screening but has poor sensitivity for mild changes and should be

Table 5. Evaluation of stage 2 hypertension

	Tests
History	Same as stage 1
Physical exam	Same as stage 1
BP monitoring	Confirm BP with auscultatory measurement
Laboratory tests	Same as Stage 1
	Particular attention to urinalysis and renal function
	Renin and aldosterone profiling
	Thyroid function tests
	Plasma metanephrines
	Consider 24-hr urinary catecholamines
	Drug screen
	Consider screening for monogenetic hypertension
Imaging	Renal ultrasound
	Echocardiogram
	Renal scintigraphy
	Renal artery imaging
	Consider CNS imaging (CT or MRI)

reserved for hypertensive children in whom arrhythmia is suspected. Due to concern of death during athletics, exercise tolerance testing and cardiac stress tests are often obtained, but neither test has sound normative data in children so interpretation is difficult.

How Should Childhood Hypertension Be Treated?

Treatment should be tailored to specific etiology. A general schematic for a treatment algorithm is shown in Fig. 2. This approach is different from that used for adults, in whom a thiazide diuretic may be started empirically with little or no evaluation.

For most children with stage 1 essential hypertension, initial therapy involves nonpharmacologic lifestyle modification, particularly in overweight/obese children. Sodium reduction to no added sodium or 3 gm/day and caffeine avoidance/reduction are recommended. Some experts recommend increasing K^+ intake but a diet high in fruits and vegetables will likely accomplish this without other specific recommendations. Fructose loading acutely increases BP so reduction in refined sugars (sucrose, high fructose corn syrup) may be helpful but has not been formally tested in children. The most effective dietary intervention in adults is the DASH (Dietary

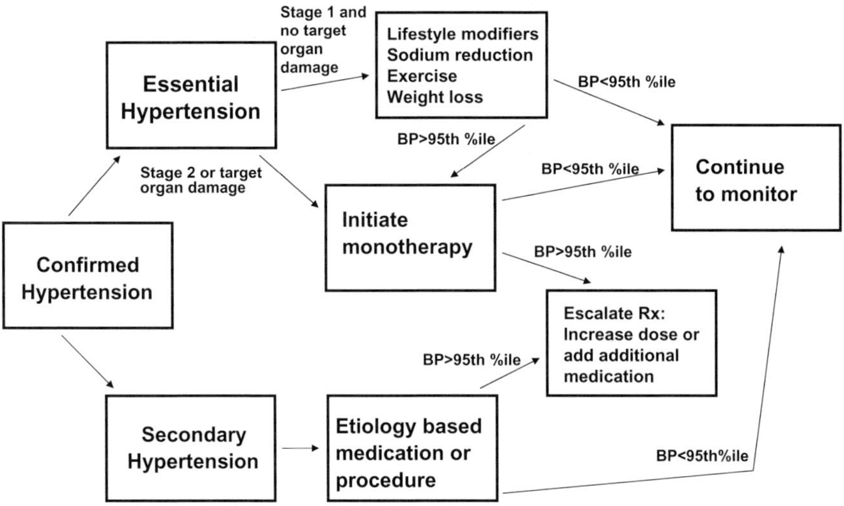

Figure 2. Algorithm for the treatment of hypertension in children. The management scheme shown in this diagram can be initiated only after sustained hypertension has been confirmed and etiology assessed.

Approaches to Stop Hypertension) diet but only small short term studies exist in adolescents. Proximity to and frequency of visits to fast food establishments correlate with weight gain and BP so reduction is likely to be helpful. For sedentary children, >30 minutes of vigorous, endurance exercise at least four times a week is recommended. For some, these recommendations represent a dramatic change and significant resistance and/or nonadherence is often encountered. Successful lifestyle modification requires significant commitment from the patient and family, so educational reinforcement and gauging adherence at regular intervals is critical to success. If there is no improvement either in BP or weight management is seen in 3–6 months, pharmacologic therapy should be initiated.

Obesity represents a specific challenge in childhood and adolescent hypertension. Ample evidence indicates BP rise and fall parallels weight: weight reduction is critical and often sufficient to manage obesity related hypertension. The myriad of obesity related comorbidities including diabetes, nonalcoholic steato-hepatitis (NASH), obstructive sleep apnea, orthopedic complications, exercise intolerance, lipid abnormalities, metabolic syndrome, and depression can have significant impact on implementation and success of therapy and these issues need to be managed to effectively treat BP. Unfortunately, successful weight reduction is the exception not the rule as abnormal body image is prevalent and must be rectified before families are likely to embrace realistic goals. Exercise is a critical adjunct to obesity management and strategies for gradual endurance development, injury prevention and low impact exercises are necessary. Consultation with an exercise therapist can be invaluable.

The question of athletic participation is one of the first that is often asked during the office visit. It is important because exercise is a critical component of nonpharmacologic therapy of essential hypertension, with or without obesity. Sudden death during athletics is a very rare but tragic occurrence and has been studied in detail. Most causes of death in young athletes are related to congenital or acquired cardiac and coronary anomalies with *commotio cordis* from chest trauma, drug abuse, and hyperthermia being potential confounders. The prevalence of unexpected cardiac arrhythmias cannot be assessed with confidence, however. Current recommendations regarding athletic participation of hypertensive patients are that in the absence of structural heart disease (following echocardiography evaluation), children with pre or stage 1 hypertension should not have their activity restricted, children with stage 2 hypertension should be treated and exercise allowed once BP has reached stage 1 or better. Because exercise is integral to treatment, most hypertensive children should not be restricted from athletic participation.

Antihypertensive medications are indicated for all stage 2 hypertension, all secondary hypertension, and stage 1 essential hypertension with target organ damage, high risk comorbidities, or lack of improvement with lifestyle modification therapy. In children with essential hypertension, most classes of antihypertensives are safe and effective (see Table 6) so the decision on agent is often predicated on physician comfort, third party payer formulary, and side effect profile. Diuretics, particularly thiazides, are first-line medications in adult essential hypertension and are safe and effective in children. They can be useful in obesity related hypertension and acute glomerulonephritis, but side effects including hypokalemia, volume depletion, hypomagnesemia,

Table 6. Medications for the treatment of hypertension in children

Class	Drugs	Dosing Range	Notes on Class
Angiotensin Converting Enzyme inhibitors (ACEi)	Benzapril	0.2–0.6 mg/kg/d, max 40 mg	Severe fetal toxicity
	Captopril	0.3–0.6 mg/kg/dose, tid	Renoprotective in diabetes, proteinuria
	Enalapril	0.05–0.1 mg/kg, qd or bid, max 20 mg	Cough less common with newer drugs
	Fosinopril	5–40 mg/d, children >50 kg	Rare angioedema
	Lisinopril	2.5–40 mg/d	Monitor renal function and K^+
	Quinapril	5–80 mg/d	
Angiotensin receptor blockers (ARB)	Candesartan	4–32 mg/d	Severe fetal toxicity
	Irbesartan	75–300 mg/d, tested >6 years	Renoprotective in diabetes, proteinuria
	Losartan	0.7–1.4 mg/kg/d, max 100 mg	Monitor renal function and K^+
Calcium channel blockers (CCB)	Amlodipine	2.5–20 mg/d, suspension	Common side effects: tachycardia and edema
	Felodipine	0.1–0.4 mg/kg/d	Amlodipine, isradipine and nicardipine can be prepared as a stable suspension
	Isradipine	2.5–10 mg/d	Short acting and extended release forms of felodipine and nifedipine may be confused by pharmacies
	Nicardipine	0.15–0.8 mg/kg/d, max 20mg	
	Nifedipine extended release	0.1–3 mg/kg, max 120 mg/d	

(*Continued*)

Table 6. (*Continued*)

Class	Drugs	Dosing Range	Notes on Class
Beta-blockers	Atenolol	0.25–2 mg/kg qd-bid	Common side effects: bradycardia, impaired athletic performance, fatigue, weight gain, erectile dysfunction
	Carvedilol	0.05– 0.4 mg/kg bid, max 25 mg	Relatively contraindicated in diabetes, worsens insulin resistance
	Metoprolol	1–6 mg/kg/d, max 200 mg	Heart failure and asthma are contraindicated in less specific agents
	Propranolol	1–4 mg/kg bid-tid, max 640 mg/d	
Alpha-blockers, central	Clonidine	0.1–0.3 mg/d transdermal patch	Common side effects: dry mouth, sedation
			Rebound hypertension with acute cessation
			Oral formulation requires dosing 2–4 times a day and is more frequently limited by sedation
Vasodilators, pure	Hydralazine	0.2–2 mg/kg/dose qid	Common side effects: tachycardia, edema, hypertrichosis (with minoxidil)
	Minoxidil	5–50 mg/d, max 100 mg	Minoxidil reserved for severe, resistant hypertension

(*Continued*)

Table 6. (*Continued*)

Class	Drugs	Dosing Range	Notes on Class
Diuretics	Furosemide	0.5–2 mg/kg/d, qd-bid	Electrolyte monitoring is required
	Hydrocholorothiazide	1–3 mg/kg/d, max 50 mg	K^+ sparing diuretics may cause hyperkalemia when administered with ACEi, ARB or beta-blockers
	Spironolactone	1–3 mg/kg/d, qd-bid	
	Triamterene	1–4 mg/kg/d, max 300 mg	
Newer agents	Aliskiren	75–300 mg/d	Renin inhibitor
	Epleronone	25–100 mg/d	Specific aldosterone receptor blocker
			Neither of these agents is currently approved for children, but both were being studied at the time of writing

Modified from The fourth report on the diagnosis, evaluation, and treatment of high blood pressure in children and adolescents. *Pediatr* **114:** 555–576, 2004.

hypercalcemia, decreased glucose tolerance, and hyperlipidemia are not insignificant.

ACEi and ARB medications are extremely well-tolerated and often used as first-line medications. As they inhibit the renin-angiotensin system, they can be less potent in low-renin hypertension but are very effective for most essential and renal hypertension. They are first line medications for diabetics due to inhibition of progressive diabetic nephropathy. ACEi cough is most common with lisinopril and is only rarely a limiting factor. Angioedema is very rare but potentially serious. Hyperkalemia, decreased renal function, elevated transaminases and anemia can be seen and periodic laboratory screening is necessary. The most serious complication is fetal toxicity and girls and young women must be consistently and repeatedly counseled. While most fetal injury occurs late in pregnancy, even first trimester exposure is associated with risk of birth defects. Aliskiren is a new oral renin inhibitor has been approved for use in hypertensive adults but has not yet completed clinical trials in children.

Calcium channel blockers (CCBs) and beta blockers are also effective agents. Dihydropyridine CCBs such as amlodipine, isradipine, nicardipine, and nifedipine are far more often used in children than the nondihydropyrindine drugs like diltiazem and verapamil, as the latter are typically used for coronary artery spasm and angina in the context of hypertension. Most children have good response and tolerance to CCBs. They can be less effective in pure renin mediated hypertension, but generally do not cause decrease in renal function occasionally seen with ACEi or ARBs. CCBs are most often complicated by peripheral edema, especially if sodium restriction is suboptimal and occasionally cause increased serum transaminases. Beta-blocker use can induce fatigue, weight gain, exacerbate insulin resistance, worsen depression and are consequently not first-line agents for obesity-related hypertension.

Central alpha-blockers and pure vasodilators are very useful second- and third-line agents. Transdermal clonidine patches enhance adherence as they are applied once weekly and provide efficacy and while some complain of dry mouth and or sedation, they are less common than with oral clonidine. Clonidine has little or no effect on GFR so is useful and children with CKD. The major drawback is rebound hypertension if the patch falls off or is not changed on time. In some patients, especially if significant diaphoresis is present, efficacy may be optimized by changing the patch more frequently. Minoxidil is extremely effective for multidrug resistant hypertension, but use is significantly limited by hypertrichosis, edema, and tachycardia.

The approach to medication initiation should be monotherapy followed by dose escalation. Contrary to adults, most hypertensive children can be controlled with an appropriately dosed single medication. Gradual titration minimizes side effects due to abrupt BP changes, such as headache, nausea and syncope which impair long-term adherence. If BP cannot be controlled to <95% after single agent maximization, a second should be started. Thiazide diuretics are particularly useful adjuncts as sodium and fluid retention can be caused by most CCB, ACEi, ARB or beta blocker. When adding an additional agent, medications of different classes should be selected for synergy. "Combo pills" that contain multiple antihypertensive medications in fixed dose combinations, including ACEi/CCB, ACEi/HCTZ, ARB/HCTZ, are convenient due to once daily dosing.

Hypertensive emergencies is defined as SBP or DBP is at least 20–30mm Hg > 99th percentile, with impending or current life- or organ-threatening symptoms, such as seizures, pulmonary edema, stroke, heart failure, or myocardial infarction. Treatment goal is to reduce BP sufficiently to eliminate dangerous symptoms and reduce risk without impairing tissue perfusion. In general, 20–25% total BP reduction, or a reduction of 50% of the difference between starting BP to the 95th percentile over 8–12 hrs is both safe and sufficient; and allows safe, gradual BP normalization over two days. Occasionally, symptoms persist and greater initial BP reduction is necessary. If available, titratable antihypertensive medication infusions are preferred (see Table 7). In emergencies, this allows rapid, controlled BP reduction with the ability to retract quickly if target reductions are exceeded. For less symptomatic or emergent, "hypertensive urgencies" IV bolus medications or rapid onset oral medication are reasonable alternatives. Rapid onset oral agents or IM hydralazine administration are good alternatives if timely IV access cannot be established.

Table 7. Medications for the treatment of hypertensive crisis in children

Medication	Mechanism	Dose Range	Titration Increment	Notes
Continuous Infusions				
Esmolol	β-blocker	100–500 mcg/kg/min	50 mcg/kg	Very short acting, bradycardia common
Fenoldopam	Dopamine agonist	0.2–0.8 mcg/kg/min	0.1 mcg/kg	May be less effective in children than adults
Furosemide	Loop diuretic	0.5–3 mg/kg/hr	1 mg/kg	For volume overload in nonanuric patient
Labetalol	α and β-blocker	0.5–3 mg/kg/hr	0.5 mg/kg	Safe in renal failure, avoid in asthma, CHF
Nesiritide	Natriuretic peptide	10–40 ng/kg/min	5 mcg/kg	Useful in CHF
Nicardipine	CCB	0.5–4 mcg/kg/min	0.5 mcg/kg	Reflex tachycardia common
Sodium Nitroprusside	Vasodilator	1–10 mcg/kg/min	1 mcg/kg	Risk of cyanide toxicity in renal failure patients
Intravenous Bolus				
Enalaprilat	ACEi	5–100 mcg/kg q4–6 hr	5 mcg/kg	Best for pure renin mediated hypertension Hypotension in renal failure and neonates
Furosemide	Loop diuretic	0.5–2 mg/kg q6–12 hr	1mg/kg	For volume overload in nonanuric patient
Hydralazine	Vasodilator	0.2 mg/kg q4–6 hr	Frequency	Variable response
Labetolol	α and β-blocker	0.2–1 mg/kg q2–6 hr	Frequency	Safe in renal failure, avoid in asthma, CHF
Nicardipine	CCB	30 mcg/kg q4–6 hr	10 mcg/kg	Reflex tachycardia common
Phentolamine	α-blocker	1–5 mg q2–6 hr	1mg	For known or suspected pheochromocytoma
Oral Administration				
Clonidine	Central α agonist	0.05–0.0.8 mg q2–6 hr	0.1 mg	Dry mouth and drowsiness are common
Hydralazine	Vasodilator	0.25–0.4 mg/kg q6–8 hr	0.1 mg/kg	Variable response, onset 20-30min
Isradipine	CCB	0.05–0.1 mg/kg	Max 5 mg	Slower onset, long acting
Minoxidil	Vasodilator	0.1–0.2 mg/kg	Max 10 mg	Slow onset, long acting, powerful vasodilator
Nicardipine	CCB	0.4–0.5 mg/kg	Max 20 mg	Suspension has shorter half life and more rapid onset, risk of hypotension

Modified from Flynn JT, Tullus K. (2009) Severe hypertension in children and adolescents: pathophysiology and treatment. *Pediatr Nephrol* **24**(6): 1101–1112.

Suggested Reading

Cardiovascular disease statistics. (2008) [URL http://www.americanheart.org] American Heart Association.

Chen X, Wang Y. (2008) Tracking of blood pressure from childhood to adulthood: a systematic review and meta-regression analysis. *Circulation* **117**: 3171–3180.

Chobanian AV, Bakris GL, Black HR, *et al.* (2003) The seventh report of the Joint National Committee on prevention, detection, evaluation, and treatment of high blood pressure: the JNC 7 report. *Jama* **289**: 2560–2572.

Croix B, Feig DI. (2006) Childhood hypertension is not a silent disease. *Pediatr Nephrol* **21**: 527–532.

Feig DI, Soletsky B, Johnson RJ. (2008) Effect of allopurinol on blood pressure of adolescents with newly diagnosed essential hypertension: a randomized trial. *JAMA* **300**: 924–932.

Feld LG, Waz WR. (1997) Pharmacologic therapy of hyperntension. In: *hypertension in Children.* Feld LG. (ed.), Butterworth-Heineman, Boston pp. 133–178.

Feld LG, Corey H. (2007) Hypertension in childhood. *Pediatr Rev* **28**: 283–298.

Flynn JT, Tullus K. (2009) Severe hypertension in children and adolescents: pathophysiology and treatment. *Pediatr Nephrol* **24**(6): 1101–1112.

The fourth report on the diagnosis, evaluation, and treatment of high blood pressure in children and adolescents. *Pediatr* **114**: 555–576, 2004.

Urbina E, Alpert B, Flynn J, *et al.* (2008) Ambulatory blood pressure monitoring in children and adolescents: recommendations for standard assessment: a scientific statement from the American Heart Association Atherosclerosis, Hypertension, and Obesity in Youth Committee of the council on cardiovascular disease in the young and the council for high blood pressure research. *Hypertension* **52**: 433–451.

Part X

Urologic Disorders

32

Voiding Dysfunction

Marlo A. Eldridge and Yegappan Lakshmanan

Introduction

Voiding dysfunction is an abnormality in one or both phases of the voiding (micturition) cycle. During a normal voiding cycle, the bladder stretches when it fills with urine and then contracts during the voiding phase. This is characterized by a relatively low internal bladder pressure to allow for developmentally appropriate filling, followed by a coordinated relaxation of the external urethral sphincter, during bladder contraction. Thus, uninterrupted urine flow through the urethra occurs, resulting in complete bladder emptying. Premature contractions of the bladder (i.e. detrusor contractions during filling) or increased pressure (over 40 cm H_2O) suggest the possibility of voiding dysfunction. An interrupted or intermittent flow of urine with incomplete bladder emptying is a hallmark of dysfunctional voiding. In addition to the normal anatomy and physiology of voiding, this chapter will focus on dysfunctional voiding and voiding disorders.

Normal Anatomy and Physiology of Voiding

In children, the bladder is located in the pelvic cavity and is a muscular viscus. The bladder wall is lined, from the inside out, by the mucosa, the detrusor muscle, and the adventitia. The detrusor consists of a meshwork of smooth muscle fibers arranged into a functioning unit with an ability to elicit nearly maximum active tension over a wide range of lengths. This allows the bladder to fill with urine from the upper tracts at low pressures. The ability of the bladder to store urine is determined by the activity or inactivity of both the detrusor muscle and the bladder outlet, consisting of the bladder neck and the proximal urethra. In addition, it is directly supported by the musculature of the pelvic floor.

During the filling and storage phase, the bladder is continuously filled with urine draining from the ureters. During filling, the detrusor remains relaxed in order to maintain low intravesical pressure, and the sphincter contracts to prevent urine from leaking. The voiding phase consists of volitional relaxation of the pelvic floor which triggers reflex bladder emptying, with relaxation of the sphincter and contraction of the bladder detrusor. When all of this occurs in simpatico, the effect is a normal coordinated void.

The bladder detrusor and sphincter are innervated by sacral parasympathetic, thoracolumbar sympathetic, and sacral somatic nerves. The neurologic control of normal micturition occurs at different levels, from the "sacral micturition center" in the spinal cord to the "pontine micturition center" within the brainstem to the cerebellum, the basal ganglia, the limbic system, the thalamus, the hypothalamus, and the cerebellar cortex. Within the spinal cord, information from bladder efferent is integrated with that from other viscera and somatic sources and projected to the brain stem centers that coordinate the micturition cycle.

It was formerly accepted that micturition in newborns and young infants was driven by a simple spinal cord reflex to a full bladder and occurred frequently throughout sleep–wake cycles. More recently studies have indicated that micturition is modulated by higher centers, even in full term fetuses and newborns. Ohel *et al.* showed that intrauterine micturition almost exclusively occurs while the fetus is awake rather than randomly distributed over various behavioral (sleep/arousal) states. Further modulation then occurs in the postnatal period. During the first 2–3 years of life, there is progression from an indiscriminate infantile voiding pattern to a voluntary and conscious (adult type), micturition. Achievement of this requires an intact neurologic system and also requires an increase in functional bladder storage capacity, development of volitional control over the bladder and sphincter so that the child can voluntarily initiate or inhibit the micturition reflex, and maturation of voluntary control over the urethral striated muscle sphincter. In addition to bladder storage capacity, progressive maturation of micturition from infantile to adult type voiding involves a decrease in voiding frequency, increase in voided volume, improved emptying efficiency, and the achievement of decreased detrusor pressure during voiding.

Pathogenesis of Voiding Dysfunction

Pathogenesis occurs when the detrusor begins to contract, and rather than relaxing, the pelvic floor and anal sphincter also contract, thus working in opposition to the detrusor, rather than in sync. There are neurologic causes of dysfunctional voiding which involve some abnormality of the brain or spinal cord, diminishing the neural control over the bladder and urinary sphincter. However, it is far more often an acquired dysfunction resulting from long term urine holding behavior. This both stretches the bladder and causes the child to increase the contraction/tension in the pelvic floor in order to attempt to maintain continence. Over time, children lose the ability to fully relax the urethral sphincter due to this constant isometric contraction. Thus, they harbor large postvoid residual volumes which in turn contribute to urinary tract infection (UTI), incontinence, increased bladder pressures and deterioration of the upper tract (including renal function). There are a multitude of scenarios which precipitate urine holding. Some are volitional or learned, for instance, the young child who doesn't want to be distracted from playing, the child who has experienced dysuria due to a UTI, or a child with a history of painful elimination due to constipation.

In addition to bladder sphincter dyssynergia/dyscoordination, other etiologies of voiding dysfunction include neurologic conditions, untreated constipation, and in some cases toileting fears resulting from issues surrounding negative toilet experiences.

Voiding dysfunction can be further classified as detrusor overactivity (overactive bladder), stress incontinence, giggle incontinence, postvoid dribbling, dysfunctional voiding, infrequent voiding (underactive bladder), and nonneurogenic neurogenic bladder (Hinman syndrome). This nomenclature is often confusing even among urology professionals, and in 1997 the International Children's Continence Society (ICCS) recommended a standardized terminology (see Fig. 1). It is important to note however that since 1997, the understanding of the significance of constipation in voiding disorders has evolved, resulting in the emergence of an important and prolific category/diagnosis of Dysfunctional Elimination Syndrome (DES) that was not included in the ICCS 1997 nomenclature.

DES is defined as an abnormal pattern of elimination of unknown cause, categorized by both bladder and bowel incontinence, occurring in

	Clinical Features	Urodynamic Findings	Management
Transient detrusor-sphinter discoordination	• Age of <2 • Interrupted Voiding • May present with complications such as urinary tract infection	• Detrusor-sphinter discoordination • Interrupted voiding • High voiding pressures • Good bladder emptying	• Transient phenomena • Resolves with toilet training
Detrusor overactivity (overactive bladder)	• Urinary frequency • Urgency • Urge incontinence	• Unstable detrusor contrations during filling	• Anticholinergic drugs • Standard urotherapy • Neuromodulation
Stress Incontinence	• Associated with increased intravesical pressure during laughing, running, coughing, and so on	• May be normal • May elicit leakage when the patient is asked to strain or cough during procedure	• Standard urotherapy • Pelvic floor rehabilitation
Giggle Incontinence	• Usually found in girls • Associates with laughing and giggling • May amount to complete bladder emptying	• May be normal • May elicit leakage when the patient is asked to giggle	• Standard urotherapy • Pelvic floor rehabilitation
Postvoid Dribbling	• Usually found in toilet-trained girls • Leakage after voiding and on standing	• Usually normal	• Vesicovaginal reflux may be demonstrated with a micturating cystourethrogram • Advise on toilet posture (i.e., sitting with legs apart)
Dysfunctional Voiding	• May manifest as daytime urinary symptoms	• Staccato or fractionated voiding • Pelvic floor activity during voiding • Voiding commences with a drop in abdominal pressure	• Standard urotherapy • Biofeedback and pelvic floor rehabilitation
Infrequent voider/ underactive bladder	• Infrequent voiding as a result of diminished urge sensation • Refuses to void when engaged in play • Overflow incontinence • Urinary tract infection	• Poor detrusor contractility • Poor bladder emptying • Abdominal straining • High compliance	• Standard urotherapy, including timed voiding and scheduled drinking training
Non-neurogenic, neurogenic bladder (Hinman syndrome)	• May present as urinary tract infection • Poor bladder emptying • Incontinence • No neurologic pathway identified • May involve bowel dysfunction	• Sphincteric overactivity • Increased pelvic floor activity	• Same as for neurogenic bladders • May require clean intermittent catheterization

Figure 1. Summary of functional voiding disorders in children.

previously toilet-trained children without anatomic or neurologic abnormalities. It is important to note that DES is a quickly growing category of patients and is often misdiagnosed as a straightforward voiding disorder. It has become increasingly clear that patients with constipation issues as well as urinary symptoms will rarely achieve success from a urinary perspective, if constipation is not appropriately and aggressively managed.

It is important to recognize that it is difficult to completely separate and categorize voiding disorders as there is a great deal of overlap of symptoms among different diagnoses. This fact makes treatment via an algorithm difficult, and the child must be treated holistically to achieve optimal and long-term resolution of symptoms.

The scope of these problems is vast, accounting for nearly 30% of patients presenting to pediatric urology practices. Approximately 7% of all female children and 3% of all male children will experience problems with voiding dysfunction or DES during childhood.

Clinical Presentation

These children represent a challenge, often presenting to general pediatrics as well as to pediatric nephrology when dysfunction has led to renal sequelae. Typical presentations include recurrent UTIs, persistent daytime incontinence, urinary dribbling, urinary urgency, urinary frequency, encopresis, or urine holding behaviors. Children will often present with multiple symptoms which have progressively worsened over several months to years. Subtle manifestations, as a response to voiding dysfunction or DES, include renal calculi, VUR subsequent to recurrent UTIs, and hematuria secondary to urine holding. Unfortunately, initial presenting symptoms are sometimes viewed as a "nuisance" by parents, school officials, and at times medical professionals. Thus, early diagnosis and intervention are not always achieved and by the time a child presents to specialty practice, damage to the bladder has frequently been exacerbated by the repetition of the dysfunctional patterns they have adopted.

It is not unusual to see children with voiding dysfunction who have associated attention deficit issues, academic difficulties, and socialization challenges due to their outward symptoms. This is especially true if the child's symptoms include diurnal enuresis, or severe urinary frequency, as both symptoms tend to bring a great deal of negative attention to the child. Some parents elect to home school in an attempt to spare the child the ramification of such negative social stigma. In short, it is imperative that medical providers understand the far-reaching ramifications of this diagnosis and approach it by mobilizing mental health support and behavioral intervention specialists as appropriate.

Diagnosis

The diagnosis of voiding dysfunction and DES can be made only *via* thorough and appropriate evaluation. The most important diagnostic tool is a voiding diary, a simple chart kept by the child and family for approximately 2 weeks documenting frequency of voids, attempted voids, bowel movements, urine leakage, water intake, and encopretic episodes (including consistency and size of the bowel movement). An invaluable tool in obtaining objective stool data is the Bristol Stool Form Scale (Fig. 2). The family should be provided written instructions as to how to record voids, stools, etc. and a copy of the Bristol Stool Form Scale should be provided to the family for reference during recording. All members of the medical team treating the patient should also be extremely familiar with the scale. In addition, it is helpful if the family can be provided with a measuring device so that average voided volumes, as well as functional bladder capacity (the largest voided volume other than the first void of the day) can be documented. Although low tech in a medically complex system, these tools should not be underestimated and are of paramount importance in making a correct diagnosis of voiding dysfunction or DES. A "normal" voiding diary should illustrate between 4–8 voids per day, daily bowel movements of Bristol type 4 or 5. A voiding diary indicating greater than nine voids per day, fewer than four voids per day or no bowel movement for three or more days is indicative of an elimination disorder.

In addition to the voiding diary, an evaluation should include a physical exam looking for abdominal masses or gross abnormalities, perineal neurologic exam; and urinalysis and urine culture to assess possible underlying infectious processes. A comprehensive past medical history should be obtained, as well as a detailed history of the progression of presenting symptoms (obtained from the child whenever possible). It is important to note age at toilet training, difficulties with toilet training, confirmed or suspected abuse, negative connotations with the toilet, and toileting fears. Additional questions should include observed holding behaviors, parent–child conflicts regarding the toilet, urgency, frequency, crossed legs dance (often referred to by parents as the "pee dance"), Vincent's Curtsy, and heel-sitting behaviors. Initial radiologic exams should include a KUB to assess the quantity and location of stool in the colon, renal ultrasound to assess for hydronephrosis, and a pre- and postvoid ultrasound of the bladder to assess for bladder wall thickening, incomplete bladder emptying, and spinning top/funnel shaped urethral outlet. A voiding cystourethrogram may also be ordered to rule out vesicoureteral reflux and outflow obstruction. Additional imaging studies may

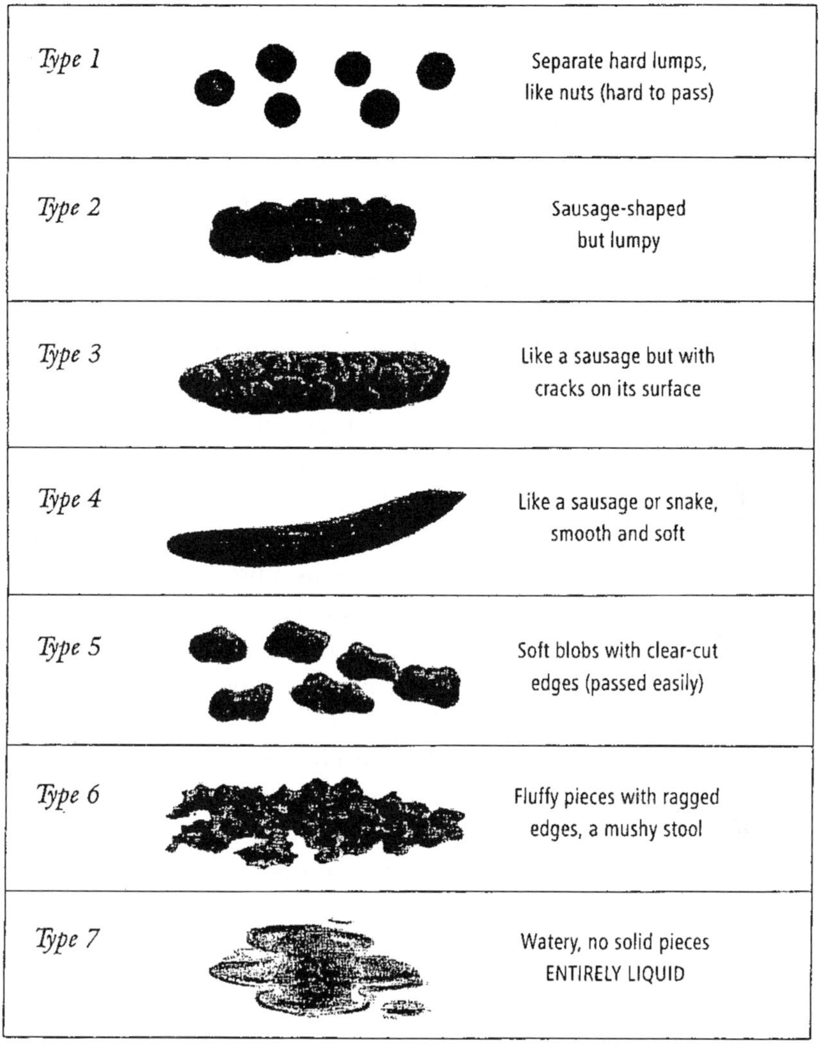

Figure 2. The Bristol Stool Form Scale.

Reproduced by kind permission of Dr KW Heaton, Reader in Medicine at the University of Bristol. ©2000 produced by Norgine Limited, manufacturer of Movicol®.

include a plain radiograph of the spine to assess for neurogenic causes of the dysfunction, such as spina bifida or spina bifida occulta. In cases where a child has developed secondary bladder and bowel incontinence after achieving full continence, (defined as a period of six or more months of having achieved reliable and consistent continence), a spinal MRI may be indicated to rule out a tethered spinal cord.

Urodynamic studies are a valuable tool in assessing dysfunction but the invasive nature, expense, and sometimes lack of availability are often barriers. In addition, urodynamics are often not necessary in the evaluation of voiding dysfunction. However, if conservative management fails for unidentifiable reasons, then urodynamic studies can be an important tool in more detailed assessment and diagnosis of voiding dysfunction and should certainly be considered.

Uroflowmetry can be performed separate from a urodynamic study and is also a useful and noninvasive tool in proper diagnosis of voiding dysfunction. Flow rates in children are of less importance than the flow curve pattern and attention should focus on those patterns. Patterns vary greatly from patient to patient but can be generally defined by the five following descriptions. A *bell-shaped flow pattern* with a progressive and smooth increase in flow to a peak followed by a progressive and smooth decrease in flow rate back to baseline is indicative of a normal voiding pattern. An *interrupted flow pattern* is often seen in underactive bladder and those with high compliance. A *staccato pattern* occurs in patients with spincter overactivity or constipation in which they must push to expel small amounts of urine repeatedly (see Fig. 3). An *inverted V pattern* (sometime referred to as a Tower-shaped pattern) is seen both in children with overactive bladders and high pressure voiding. And finally a *low plateau pattern* can illustrate either outlet obstruction or low bladder/detrusor contractility.

Management

Management of voiding dysfunction should occur in an interdisciplinary setting including medicine, nursing, behavioral psychology, and nutrition as indicated. Single treatment modalities are rarely successful long term and management should include a multimodal approach, including bowel management, timed voiding, hydration management, improved fiber intake, behavioral management, biofeedback when appropriate, and drug therapy when necessary.

When the diagnosis of voiding dysfunction/DES has been made, initial therapy should focus on constipation management. This should

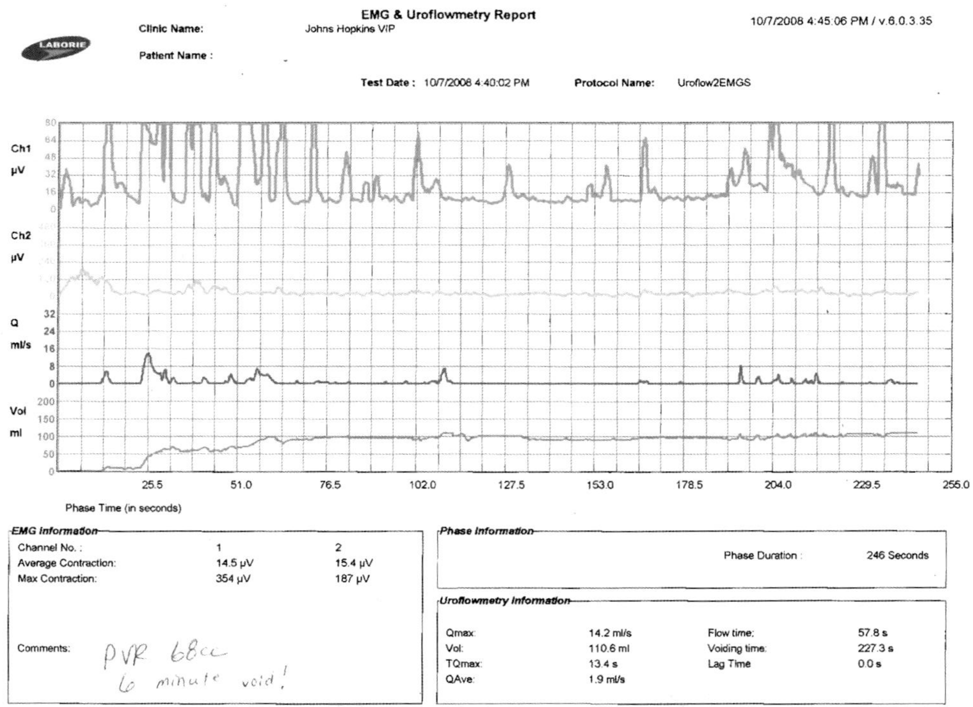

Figure 3. An Electromyogram (EMG) and Uroflowmetry tracing to demonstrate the "staccato voiding" pattern. Channel 1 is the pelvic floor EMG, and Channel 2 indicates abdominal wall EMG, both recorded by surface electrodes. "Q" indicates urine flow in ml/sec, which is sporadic in this case, occurring only when the pelvic muscles relax. "Vol" represents the amount of voided urine.

begin with an initial bowel clean out with oral laxatives and possibly enemas depending on the degree of fecal load. Subsequently, further management should be consistent and requires thorough education of the patient and family, with an appropriate description of the physiologic implications of constipation on bladder function and the necessity for good medication compliance. It is important that families understand that constipation occurs slowly over time and that the focus should be on long-term management, not only on short-term resolution of outward symptoms. Without receiving this important information, families tend to comply with medications recommendations only until they feel bowel symptoms improve and then discontinue laxatives or stool softeners. Then both patient and provider find themselves starting over with regard to bowel progress. Successful management may be achieved with the use of stool softeners, but the majority of patients require laxatives. Although stimulant laxatives may be necessary initially, an optimal choice for daily therapy is an osmotic laxative as it does not carry the long-term tolerance risks that stimulant laxatives do. One issue that should not be overlooked is the need to integrate fluid and fiber education into the long-term management plan. Not only should increased fiber be emphasized, but parents should be counseled that fruits and vegetables as well as whole grains are the best sources of fiber, and limiting processed foods is important. Fiber supplementation with powders and even some food additives is reasonable as adjunct therapy. When families are faced with a picky eater they tend to abandon attempts at whole food intake of fiber and simply provide fiber in the form of massive supplementation, usually with quick dissolving powders in the child's fluid. A more helpful strategy to share with parents is to aim for the AAP recommendations for fiber intake (26 grams per day for young girls 9–11 years old and 31 grams per day for boys the same age) and to then utilize supplementation in the dinner drink only when they have not achieved their whole food fiber intake for that particular day. This decreases supplementation and stresses to families that the focus should remain on whole, minimally processed food sources of fiber.

In addition to aggressive bowel management, timed voiding should be part of the initial management of voiding dysfunction and DES. Many children harbor urine-holding behaviors for so long that they develop significantly diminished sensitivity bladder sensation, and will not achieve success without a stringent timed voiding regimen. Initiating a void prior to the bladder being overfilled achieves more complete emptying. Timed voids are also essential in the establishment of positive voiding habits. It should be stressed that voiding on a strict two-hour schedule should be done "by the clock" and not at approximate times. This should be conveyed to the child's school in writing, with specific detail to verbal reminders, follow up and documentation. Vibrating and alarm watches can be helpful tools for children to receive reminders but it should be well-understood by parents and school officials that a child cannot be given a watch and then expected to be independent. Children respond well to these tools but will begin to ignore the alarms very quickly without adult supervision. This is especially true of children with attention issues. In addition, having schools keep voiding charts during school hours promotes long-term compliance and provides objective feedback regarding progress between appointments (see Fig. 4).

When conservative measures fail to produce the desired outcomes, the provider must determine whether the lack of progress is due to noncompliance, behavioral issues, recalcitrant pelvic floor dysfunction, or a combination of these. When noncompliance and behavioral issues stand out, reinitiating the aforementioned conservative measures under the direction of pediatric behavioral psychology can be effective.

Drug therapy with anticholinergics may be useful in reducing uninhibited bladder contractions, allowing increased functional bladder capacity, reduced urge incontinence and improved long term growth in low capacity bladders. However, the side effect profiles of these drugs must be considered. Many cause or further exacerbate constipation, which is already a major challenge in many of these children. As non-drug therapies become more readily available, the focus should be on making long-term, permanent improvements in pelvic floor function and bladder emptying rather than only short-term symptom resolution via drugs. Therefore, drug therapy for voiding dysfunction, is for the most part, secondary.

When appropriate, biofeedback therapy is an important tool in the treatment of voiding dysfunction and DES. Biofeedback is a noninvasive method of teaching a child to properly utilize (both contract and relax)

Voiding Tracking Sheet for_____________

Dear School Staff, We feel that it is medically necessary for _______ to adhere to the following voiding regimen.

1. Please prompt _______ to TRY to void every _______ hours. Please allow her to use the bathroom in the nurses office.
2. Please prompt ______ to drink 3–4 ounces of water after each voiding attempt every _____ hours.
3. Please send the data sheet to _________'s parent at the end of each week or to us via fax: _____________
4. Please do not hesitate to call us if you are in need of further clarification of our recommendations.

____

Medical Provider signature

	Date/Time	Able to void	Urine color	AMOUNT OF URINE	WATER 3–4 OUNCES	STOOL PRODUCED BRISTOL TYPE
Monday						
		Y / N	Light Dark		Y/N	No Yes: Type 1 2 3 4 5 6 7
		Y / N	Light Dark		Y/N	No Yes: Type 1 2 3 4 5 6 7
		Y / N	Light Dark		Y/N	No Yes: Type 1 2 3 4 5 6 7
		Y / N	Light Dark		Y/N	No Yes: Type 1 2 3 4 5 6 7
Tuesday						
		Y / N	Light Dark		Y/N	No Yes: Type 1 2 3 4 5 6 7
		Y / N	Light Dark		Y/N	No Yes: Type 1 2 3 4 5 6 7
		Y / N	Light Dark		Y/N	No Yes: Type 1 2 3 4 5 6 7
		Y / N	Light Dark		Y/N	No Yes: Type 1 2 3 4 5 6 7
Wednesday						
		Y / N	Light Dark		Y/N	No Yes: Type 1 2 3 4 5 6 7
		Y / N	Light Dark		Y/N	No Yes: Type 1 2 3 4 5 6 7
		Y / N	Light Dark		Y/N	No Yes: Type 1 2 3 4 5 6 7
		Y / N	Light Dark		Y/N	No Yes: Type 1 2 3 4 5 6 7
Thursday						
		Y / N	Light Dark		Y/N	No Yes: Type 1 2 3 4 5 6 7
		Y / N	Light Dark		Y/N	No Yes: Type 1 2 3 4 5 6 7
		Y / N	Light Dark		Y/N	No Yes: Type 1 2 3 4 5 6 7
Friday						
		Y / N	Light Dark		Y/N	No Yes: Type 1 2 3 4 5 6 7
		Y / N	Light Dark		Y/N	No Yes: Type 1 2 3 4 5 6 7
		Y / N	Light Dark		Y/N	No Yes: Type 1 2 3 4 5 6 7
		Y / N	Light Dark		Y/N	No Yes: Type 1 2 3 4 5 6 7

Figure 4. A typical form sent with the child to school to track their voiding as well as bowel habits during the day, to assess progress over time.

their pelvic floor muscles, at appropriate times. External sensors are held in place with adhesive, then transmit data regarding muscle function to a computer device that in turn provides either auditory or visual feedback to the child when the child achieves a preset goal. Through watching urine flow rates, pelvic floor EMG, or detrusor pressures in real time, children can learn to relax the pelvic floor during voiding. Recent reports have demonstrated the efficacy of this process clinically and by pre and post-treatment urodynamic studies. Generally, biofeedback is most useful for children with incontinence and/or staccato voiding. This translates into children with weak pelvic floors (usually occurring secondary to

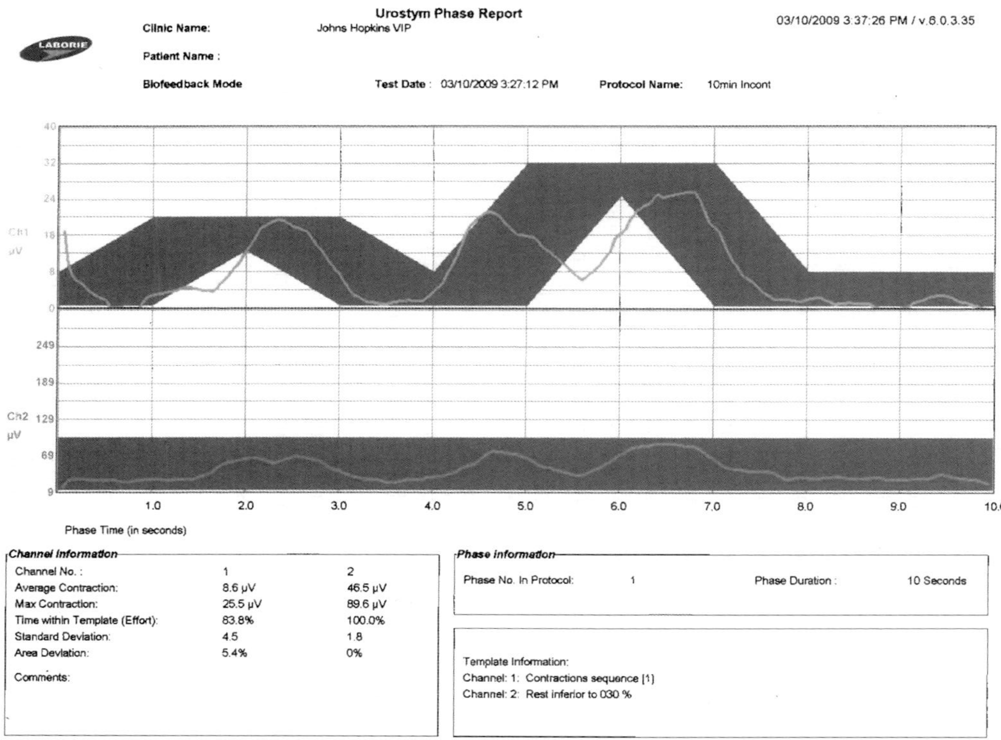

Figure 5. A biofeedback tracing with the shaded areas indicating the goals established for sequential pelvic muscle contraction, and the lines within indicating the child's attempt to achieve them. Ch1 and 2 indicate pelvic floor and abdominal wall muscle EMG, respectively.

longstanding uninhibited bladder contractions), or hyperreflexic pelvic floors. Children with low-capacity bladders are typically less likely to respond to biofeedback in isolation. However, for this subset of children, success may be achieved with anticholinergics followed by biofeedback to address changes incurred from uninhibited bladder contractions. The fact that biofeedback is so versatile and applicable to a variety of voiding disorders makes it both appropriate and effective for straightforward voiding dysfunction; but also for those in which there is overlap of several dysfunctional elements. Biofeedback comes in many forms, including auditory and visual feedback systems. Biofeedback can be as simple as a child having bladder scans done pre- and postvoid to visually illustrate incomplete emptying. More traditional biofeedback focuses on giving a child a target goal for muscle conditioning, whether it is contraction or relaxation and then provides an auditory or visual reinforcement when the child achieves said goal (see Fig. 5). Most modern equipment utilizes visual and auditory feedback and many centers of pediatric urology offer animation biofeedback in which children master muscle function by essentially playing video games. This method is engaging for young children, as well as adolescents. It focuses not only on contraction and relaxation of the muscles, but fosters a higher level of muscle control depending on the gaming options available to the individual system. Additionally, the "reward" of being allowed to play video games during clinic visits can also be utilized as a motivator for regular home pelvic muscle exercises. One additional benefit of animation biofeedback is that it is an effective and engaging option for children with autistic spectrum disorders as they tend to be visual learners.

Conclusion

Voiding dysfunction and DES are challenging diagnoses, often presenting with multiple and overlapping symptoms. They are disorders which have not been well understood until recent years and are wrought with additional challenges due to negative social implications. Initiating treatment early, and employing an interdisciplinary, multipronged approach is paramount in limiting bladder and renal damage, and ensuring positive long-term outcomes. Thus early recognition and intervention is important.

Suggested Reading

de Groat WC. (1993) Anatomy and physiology of the lower urinary tract. *Urol Clin North Am* **20**: 383–401.

Harrison SCW, Abrams P. (1994) Bladder function. In Sant GR (ed.) *Pathosphysiologic Principle of Urology*, Blackwell Scientific Publications, London. pp. 93–121.

Mattiasson A. (1994) Bladder and urethral physiology and pathophysiology. In Krane RJ, Siroky MB, Fitzpatrick JM. (eds.) *Clinical Urology*, JB Lippincott, Philadelphia. pp. 536–557.

Nelson JD, Cooper S, Boyt MA, *et al.* (2004) Improved uroflow parameters and postvoid residual following biofeedback therapy in pediatric patients with dysfunctional voiding does not correspond to outcome. *J Urol* **172**: 1653–1656.

Norgaard JP, van Gool JD, Hjalmas K, *et al.* (1998) Standardization and definitions in lower urinary tract dysfunction in children. *Br J Urol* **81**: 1–16.

Ohel G, Haddad S, Samueloff A. (1995) Fetal urine production and micturition and fetal behavioral state. *Am J Perinatal* **12**: 91–92.

Yagci S, Kibar Y, Akay O, *et al.* (2005) The effect of biofeedback treatment on voiding and urodynamic parameters in children with voiding dysfunction. *J Urol* **174**: 1994–1997.

33

Neuropathic Bladder and Spinal Dysraphism

Sanjeev Kaul and Yegappan Lakshmanan

Introduction

Nearly 25% of clinical problems seen in pediatric urology are related to neurologic lesions that affect lower urinary tract function. In the normal state, the lower urinary tract functions through a balanced state of reflexes modulated by higher cortical control. Normal bladder function involves a coordinated activity of the detrusor, and both intrinsic and extrinsic periurethral sphincter to provide low pressure storage of urine and voluntary micturition with complete emptying of bladder. Neurologic processes, both congenital and acquired, that disturb this equilibrium result in a "neuropathic bladder," which becomes a source of common clinical problems with the potential to damage renal function. The challenge to pediatric urologists centers on preventing hydronephrosis, development of vesicoureteral reflux (VUR) and deterioration of upper tracts, and to provide for urinary continence.

Etiology and Classification

The most common cause of neuropathic bladder in children is abnormal development of the spinal canal and the spinal cord (spinal dysraphism, myelomeningocele, spina bifida, myelodysplasia). The lumbosacral region of the spinal cord is the most involved (see Table 1). It affects 1 in 1000 children in the United States and 95% of those affected have abnormal innervation of the bladder. Consequently, they are at high risk for urinary incontinence, high bladder pressures, VUR, recurrent urinary tract infections (UTIs), and renal failure.

Myelodysplasia/spinal dysraphism is a term used to denote all abnormal conditions of the vertebral column that affect spinal cord function.

Table 1. Incidence of spinal dysraphism according to spinal level of involvement

Location of Defect	Incidence (%)
Cervical — high thoracic	2
Low thoracic	5
Lumbar	26
Lumbosacral	47
Sacral	20

Table 2. Classification of spinal dysraphism

1. **Cystic**: Posterior protrusion of spinal elements through spinal defect
   a. *Meningocele*: meninges and CSF
   b. *Myelomeningocele*: meninges, spinal cord, nerve roots, CSF
   c. *Lipomyelomeningocele*: all above and fat
   d. *Myeloschisis*: open neural plate or cleft spinal cord
   e. *Rachischisis*: cleft spinal cord and vertebral column
2. **Noncystic/Occult**: No protrusion of spinal elements. Presence of dimple, hair tuft, lipoma, cutaneous hemangioma
   a. *Anterior*: anterior herniation of spinal elements
   b. *Cauda equina tumor*: causes cord compression
   c. *Dermoid cyst*: cord compression from epidermal invagination cyst
   d. *Diastematomyelia*: bony spicule/fibrous band splitting spinal cord
   e. *Intradural lipoma*: fatty infiltration of spinal cord
   f. *Syringomyelia*: cystic degeneration of spinal cord
   g. *Sacral agenesis*: non development of sacral bone
   h. *Tethered cord*: congenital fixation of distal spinal cord or acquired from postoperative adhesions

Meningocele, myelomeningocele, and lipomyelomeningocele indicate progressively severe malformation with meninges, spinal nerve roots and fatty tissue and cord respectively that herniate through the defect in the skin and vertebral column. The classification of spinal dysraphism reflects the affected internal and external anatomy (see Table 2).

The etiology is uncertain and multifactorial. Epidemiologic data implicate environmental factors because the birth prevalence has varied over geographic locations. Genetic factors have been suggested by studies showing female preponderance, ethnic variability and familial tendencies. Neural tube defects are associated with trisomy 13 and 18, Meckel syndrome, and cloacal exstrophy. Several teratogens have been implicated, including alcohol, zinc, and valproic acid. There is strong evidence that folate deficiency can lead to spina bifida and the CDC recommended in 2004 that women of childbearing age ingest at least 400 micrograms of folate daily; this has decreased the incidence of spinal dysraphism by 50%. Family history of spina bifida increases the risk of development of the condition in siblings from 0.1% to 2–5% and the risk doubles to 10% if more than one member of the family is affected. The Medical Research Council Vitamin Study Group recommends that women of child bearing age with a family history of spina bifida take 4 mg of folic acid per day starting two months prior to planning pregnancy. These recommendations along with intensive prenatal screening have decreased the incidence of neonates born with neural tube defects in the United States.

Pathogenesis

Formation of the spinal cord and vertebral column begins at the 18th day of gestation and is completed by the 35th day in a cranio-caudal fashion. The exact mechanism of closure has not been elucidated. Herniation of the meninges, nerve roots, and spinal cord are associated with abnormal innervation of pelvic organs in 95% cases. In 85% of affected children, there is associated herniation of the cerebellar tonsils through the foramen magnum obstructing the fourth ventricle, and causing hydrocephalus (Arnold Chiari malformation). The neurologic lesion is extremely variable and depends to some extent on the type of lesion (cystic vs. noncystic) and also on the contents within the herniated sac (nerve roots vs. spinal cord). It is important to remember that the level of bony abnormality has no relation to the neurologic level of lesion and that no two children will have exactly the same neurologic defect. The bony level may vary by up to three vertebral levels in either direction from the level of neurologic lesion. Generally, the higher the vertebral lesion, the worse the neurologic sequelae; however, children with a high thoracic lesion may have a normal sacral spinal cord and normal sacral reflexes. Differential growth of the bone and spinal cord may cause fixation of the nerve roots, and/or spinal cord, and create a dynamic component to the neurologic defect as a child grows — 24% children will develop a new onset upper motor neuron lesion over time. In addition, the Arnold Chiari malformation, if present, can affect cerebral control of micturation and the pontine micturation center and further complicate an already nebulous situation. The fact that mere clinical examination of the sacral area and the lower limbs does not predict the status of urinary function makes it necessary for these children to undergo a comprehensive clinical, urodynamic, and radiologic evaluation as soon as possible after birth.

Clinical Presentation and Diagnostic Assessment

Newborn assessment

As a result of prenatal ultrasound screening, a diagnosis of spinal dysraphism may be made antenatally and these fetuses are delivered in a tertiary care hospital with multispecialty care. The diagnosis of spinal dysraphism may be obvious with a meningocele or occult with no or minimal external evidence such as a gluteal dimple, aberrant gluteal cleft (sacral agenesis), tuft of hair, cutaneous hemangioma, or a small lipoma. Ideally, one would like to perform urodynamic assessment prior to closure of the spinal defect; however, this is neither practical nor feasible. Therefore, renal ultrasound and measurement of postvoid residual urine should be performed as early as possible after birth, either before or following spinal surgery. The normal bladder capacity at birth is 15–20 ml and a postvoid residual volume >5 ml is considered abnormal. If the neonate cannot void spontaneously, clean intermittent catheterization (CIC) should be initiated, even before urodynamic assessment. Once the spinal closure has healed sufficiently, a voiding cystourethrogram (VCUG), and urodynamic study should be performed.

The goals of these studies are:

1. To provide baseline information about the radiologic appearance of the upper and lower urinary tracts
2. To facilitate comparison with future examinations, so that deterioration of urinary tract function or neurologic function can be detected early
3. To provide prognostic information by identifying children who are at risk for upper tract damage, such as those with Detrusor Sphincter Dyssynergia (DSD), poor compliance, or overactive bladder
4. To guide individualized treatment for patients based on their unique situation

Childhood assessment

Not infrequently, urologists are called upon to evaluate older children with known or suspected neurovesical dysfunction. The child's medical and developmental history should be reviewed to determine if the dysfunctional pattern is acute, chronic, stable or progressive, and primary or secondary to a period of normal urinary control. One should also evaluate for associated symptoms such as changes in bowel patterns (constipation and encopresis), recurrent febrile UTIs, gait disturbances, perform a complete neurologic evaluation, and review prior medical and surgical history. These children are prone to allergies, especially to latex, and precautions are recommended. The most frequent symptom at presentation is incontinence of urine. This should be further characterized as continuous dribbling or occasional leakage, stress or urge incontinence, prevoid or postvoid, and diurnal or nocturnal. Sensation of bladder filing if present points to intact sacral innervation. Some children present with recurrent urinary tract infections, both febrile and nonfebrile. Infrequently, the presenting picture may be one of end-stage renal disease due to progressive upper tract damage. Attention should also be directed to a social history, including motivation and the nature of family support. It should be emphasized that the neurologic lesion and urinary dysfunction is a dynamic process in which changes occur throughout childhood, especially in early infancy and puberty when growth spurts occur. Periodic assessments are therefore mandatory to detect changes at an early stage.

Physical examination

A complete physical examination should include assessment of blood pressure, gait, balance, muscular symmetry, and general neurologic status. Reflexes should be tested for symmetry and the back should be examined for signs of spinal dysraphism — these are present in 90% patients with occult spina bifida. The abdomen is examined for palpable kidneys, bladder, or colon filled with feces. The ability to express urine by suprapubic pressure should be noted. The genitalia are examined for skin excoriation (as a result of urine incontinence), hypospadias, presence of foreskin, cryptorchidism, and labial or introital anomalies. Rectal examination should assess anal tone and perianal sensation, presence of hard stool, and presence of normal sacrum. A positive bulbocavernous reflex points to an intact sacral reflex arc.

Laboratory assessment

Urinalysis is an important part of the initial examination of all children with suspected urinary tract disease. In the infant, a bag specimen is acceptable; however, a catheterized sample must be obtained if UTI is suspected. An abnormal urinalysis should be plated for culture and antibiotic sensitivity.

Once neuropathic bladder has been documented, a serum creatinine and cystatin C should be measured, and if necessary, glomerular filtration rate (GFR) determined by creatinine clearance. Serum electrolytes are also measured if GFR is low.

Radiologic examination

Radiologic assessment of the upper and lower urinary tract is an integral part of the evaluation of children with neurovesical dysfunction since abnormal bladder function is known to cause upper urinary tract deterioration from hydronephrosis and VUR.

The initial investigation is frequently an ultrasound of the kidneys and bladder. Renal size and symmetry are assessed, and presence or absence of hydronephrosis is noted (10–15% patients will demonstrate abnormal ultrasound findings at initial ultrasound). The bladder is assessed for wall thickness and residual urine is estimated. Ultrasound may also be used to image the spinal cord effectively in first few months of life in patients with low suspicion for occult spinal dysraphism. It is possible to evaluate the level of termination of the cord (L1) and also recognize the filum terminale, and determine tethering of the cord.

VCUG is performed after ultrasound examination to evaluate bladder contour (Christmas tree appearance in thickened trabeculated bladder) and bladder neck configuration (open bladder neck in sacral cord lesions and closed bladder neck or external sphincter in DSD). Vesicoureteral reflux may be demonstrated and should be graded for future comparison.

MRI is indicated if occult spinal dysraphism is strongly suspected for anatomical delineation of vertebral column, spinal cord, and cauda equina. It is the investigation of choice in older children and those with change in symptoms and/or worsening of radiologic findings.

Urodynamic examination

This remains perhaps the most important test to characterize the urinary tract function and determine treatment strategy in the neonate period. Invasive urodynamics requires urethral catheterization and rectal catheter placement to measure abdominal pressure; and needle electrodes for sphincter EMG. This process carries the risk of pain, hematuria, infection, and possible urinary retention. Pretest family and patient education helps to reduce anxiety. Testing is initiated with the patient in a supine position on a table that may accommodate fluoroscopic imaging during the evaluation. Rectal tone is assessed, and a rectal balloon catheter is inserted. Most often a dual-lumen transurethral catheter is placed. Electromyography electrodes, in the form of a surface gel pad, wires, or a needle, are placed on or in the perineum. The surface gel pad has the advantage of providing little discomfort to the patient, but its accuracy is limited and represents all perineal activity. The wire or needle electrodes are more specific for external sphincter activity but do cause momentary pain with placement; regardless, either device provides for perineal sensory assessment. Bladder dynamics and function are recorded in cystometry. The bladder is filled with either an isotonic solution or a contrast medium at room or body temperature. Typically, the bladder is filled at a rate that does not exceed 10% per minute of the patient's predicted bladder capacity. A rectal balloon catheter is used to measure the pressure of the abdominal cavity, P_{abd}. The urethral catheter measures the total pressure inside the bladder, P_{ves}. A child who is moving, coughing, or crying will indirectly affect the bladder pressure; therefore, a corrected detrusor pressure (P_{det}) is generated to account for this artifact. The P_{det} is calculated with the formula P_{ves} minus P_{abd}. Additionally, abdominal pressure recording is useful during the voiding phase to identify straining, or the Valsalva maneuver as a technique to eliminate urine. Measurements of perineal EMG occur simultaneously with the evaluation of synergy or dyssynergy.

Using a combination of detrusor pressure during filling, and external sphincter activity, patients may be placed in 1 of 3 categories of lower urinary tract dynamics:

1. *Synergic* (26%): Where the sphincter contracts and relaxes coordinating with bladder filing and emptying respectively providing low pressures within the bladder
2. *Dyssynergic with/without poor detrusor compliance* (37%): When external sphincter contracts during detrusor contraction causing high intravesical pressures during voiding
3. *Denervated* (36%): When no bioelectric potentials are seen in the region of the external sphincter in response to voiding

This classification best predicts those at risk for upper tract deterioration, who need proactive treatment, and helps determine the ideal monitoring interval. In the first three years of life, 71% of patients in group 2 developed deterioration of urinary tract, compared to 17% of group 1 and 23% of group 3. Increased outflow resistance and detrusor pressure greater than 40 cm H_2O are predictors of progressive upper tract damage.

Management

Prenatal

Tests, including serum α-fetoprotein (AFP), triple, quad and penta screen, may be performed in patients at high risk for neural tube defects (e.g. advanced maternal age and family history). An elevated AFP greater than three standard deviations above normal prior to 24 weeks gestation is suspicious for open neural tube defects. However, false positive rates as high as 80% have been reported limiting widespread utility. Prenatal ultrasound in conjunction with the above blood tests increases the sensitivity and specificity of diagnosing spina bifida to 80% and 99%, respectively.

Several centers in the United States have evaluated prenatal closure of defects between 19 and 25 weeks of gestation in an effort to prevent or mitigate the neurologic defects after birth. No change in severity of neurologic defect was noted; however, patients who were closed prenatally had a significantly lower incidence of hydrocephalus.

It is prudent that delivery occur in a tertiary care hospital to facilitate multispecialty postnatal care by a team including neonatologists, neurosurgeons, urologists, orthopedic surgeons, experienced nurses and ICU staff, physical therapists, and social service personnel. Controversy exists as to whether cesarean section is better than vaginal delivery to prevent rupture of the herniated sac.

Postnatal treatment

Immediate newborn management includes covering the area with sterile precautions and urgent closure of the defect. A ventriculo–peritoneal shunt is also created if indicated. Once the urologic evaluation is complete, prophylactic treatment is instituted in children based on the urodynamic findings:

a. *Synergic sphincter, normal bladder*: Expectant management. Surveillance should be instituted per Table 3.
b. *Dyssynergic sphincter*: These children are at the highest risk for progressive damage and CIC should be instituted before discharge. When started in the newborn period, CIC is easy for parents to master and for children to accept as they grow older. Complications, including epididymitis, meatitis, and urethral injury, are uncommon and UTIs occur in 30% of patients. Asymptomatic bacteriuria is seen in over

Table 3. Surveillance in patients with spinal dysraphism

Sphincter activity	Recommended tests	Frequency
Intact and synergic	Postvoid residual volume	q 4 mth
	Renal bladder ultrasound	q 12 mth
	Urodynamics	q 12 mth
Intact and dyssynergic	Renal bladder ultrasound	q 6 mth
	Urodynamics	q 12 mth
	VCUG	q 12 mth
Partial denervation	Postvoid residual volume	q 4 mth
	Renal Bladder Ultrasound	q 12 mth
	Urodynamics	q 12 mth
	VCUG	q 12 mth
Complete denervation	Postvoid residual volume	q 6 mth
	Renal bladder ultrasound	q 12 mth

70% and does not require any treatment in absence of symptoms. Crede maneuver has fallen into disrepute owing to the fact that it is nonphysiologic, difficult to perform and raises the intravesical pressure. Again, periodic surveillance must be continued as in Table 3.

c. *High detrusor pressure*: When detrusor pressure exceeds 40 cm water or voiding pressure exceeds 80–100 cm water, anticholinergics must be added to prevent upper tract deterioration. Oxybutynin is administered in a dose of 1 mg per year of age q 12 hourly. In neonates and infants, a dose of 0.1 mg/kg may be used. This dose has been shown to be safe in neonates with minimal side effects.

Management of reflux

VUR occurs in 3–5% of newborns with spinal dysraphism and neurogenic bladder. It is usually associated with dyssynergic voiding and/or overactive bladder. If untreated, 30–40% patients will exhibit reflux by age of five years. Reflux can also occur later during childhood if the bladder function changes from synergic/denervated to dyssynergic as a result of tethered cord, and hence reflux should always be ruled out if the child's symptoms change, or if there is worsening of renal function during surveillance. Anticholinergic medications with timed voiding may prevent the development of reflux in children at risk.

Low-grade VUR (grades I–III)

Antibiotic prophylaxis should be instituted to prevent infections. This may be all that is required for children who can void to completion and do not have poor bladder compliance/overactive bladder. In the presence of the latter conditions or outflow obstruction, CIC should be added to facilitate bladder emptying. Treatment will lead to resolution of VUR in up to 50% patients. Crede maneuver is contraindicated in patients with VUR, especially in the presence of dyssyngeric voiding as this can cause development of high bladder pressures and worsen reflux and kidney function.

High-grade VUR (grade IV and V)

These patients are more likely to require surgical measures in addition to the medical treatment. Persistent breakthrough UTIs, persistent hydronephrosis, and worsening reflux despite medical management are indications for surgical management. Patients who are candidates for augmentation cystoplasty may also undergo ureteral reimplantation at the same surgery. Surgical options in these patients include vesicostomy in infants to promote effective emptying of the bladder and decrease bladder pressures, subureteric injection of dextranomer microspheres (Deflux) to increase the resistance at the ureterovesical junction, and finally traditional surgical ureteroneocystostomy, either open or minimally invasive. Postoperative complications such as anastomotic strictures tend to be higher in patients with neuropathic bladder and success is centered upon ensuring complete bladder emptying with or without CIC.

Incontinence management

Urinary incontinence

Urinary incontinence is a result of a combination of low urethral sphincter function and high detrusor pressures. Treatment of urinary incontinence is important as these children attend school with their peers and attempt to integrate into society. It has been shown that children who are continent have greater self-confidence and better social acceptance than incontinent children. Treatment is based on urodynamic findings. Those with low bladder compliance or overactive bladder should be initially managed with anticholinergics and CIC. Treatment should be started with a single drug at the lowest possible dose to ensure a dry interval of 3–4 hours between catheterizations. If patients continue to be wet, the dose may be increased before adding a second drug. Oxybutynin, tolterodine and the recently introduced trospium are all safe and effective in children. Other options include long acting forms of oxybutynin and tolterodine, transdermal patches, and intravesical instillation of oxybutynin. Intravesical injection of botulinum toxin A has been shown to be efficacious in paralyzing the detrusor muscle for up to 6–12 months although repeated injections may be required. If medical and endourologic options fail, surgery may be a viable option, although this is usually delayed at least until 5 years of age and the child is ready to start school. A persistently poorly compliant or overactive detrusor may be treated with augmentation cystoplasty, in which the detrusor muscle is split and a detubularized patch of either small or large intestine is inserted to increase bladder capacity and disrupt detrusor contractions. Common complications include electrolyte disturbances from exchange of urinary electrolytes across the bowel mucosa, pyelonephritis, and urinary stones. The stomach segment is especially suitable in children with renal failure because it secretes acid. The ileocecal segment should not be used in children with spinal dysraphism because this may impair fecal continence. Other options include augmentation with ureteral segments from hydronephrotic or nonfunctioning renal units.

If bladder neck or urethral resistance is poor, several bladder neck reconstruction procedures can increase the resistance at the bladder neck by increasing intravesical urethral length and providing a "wrap" of tissue around the bladder neck. These are formidable surgical endeavors and newer techniques include placement of periurethral or bladder neck slings, artificial urinary sphincters, and injection of bulking agents at the bladder neck or proximal urethra. It is important to confirm that the bladder can be emptied completely postoperatively and if not, CIC may be required.

Urinary diversion is the last resort for management of intractable incontinence. This may include closure of the bladder neck and a continent catheterizable stoma creation (Mitrofanoff) through which the patient/family member may catheterize to empty the bladder at periodic intervals. For a nonurethral catheterizable channel, the Mitrofanoff procedure is favored due to its ease of use for patients and caregivers, and low complication rates. Either the appendix or a reconfigured ileal segment (Monti) may be used.

Bowel incontinence and constipation

Disorders of defecation, both constipation and fecal incontinence are common in patients with neurogenic bladder secondary to spina bifida, as the same nerves that innervate the urinary sphincter also innervate the anal sphincter. Abnormal intestinal motility delays transit of fecal material through the colon. Regulation of bowel emptying is important to prevent urinary infections. Treatment usually begins just before the children are due to attend school. Initial management includes use of fiber, suppositories, and enemas to promote rectal emptying. If diet and medications fail to regulate fecal emptying, a MACE procedure (Malone Antegrade Colonic Enema) is performed. This involves creating a conduit from the abdominal wall to the appendix or a segment of ileum. Daily enemas are administered through the stoma to evacuate the colon. Complete fecal continence is achieved in 89% children. Further, older children are able to manage this independently, greatly improving sociability and self-esteem.

Prognosis

With modern proactive management in a multidisciplinary clinic setting, the outlook has greatly improved for children born with myelomeningocele. A vast majority currently survive well into adulthood, and with a better quality of life due to prevention of UTIs and achievement of bowel and urinary continence.

Suggested Reading

Bauer S. (2003) The management of the myelodysplastic child: a paradigm shift. *BJU Int* **92**(Suppl 1): 23–8.

Bauer SB. (2002) Voiding dysfunction in children: neurogenic and non-neurogenic. In: Walsh PC, Wein AJ, Retick AB, Vaughn ED. (eds.) *Campbell's Urology* (8th ed.), WB Saunders, pp. 2231–2261.

Bellinger MF. (1996) Myelomeningocele and neuropathic bladder. In: Gillenwater JY, Howard SS, Grayhack JT. (eds.) *Adult and Pediatric Urology* (3rd ed.), Mosby Year Book, pp. 2489–2528.

Ellsworth PGE, Cendron M. (1999) Urodynamic testing in the pediatric patient. AUA.

MacLellan DL. (2009) Management of pediatric neurogenic bladder. *Curr Opin Urol* **19**(4): 407–411.

Malone PS, Wheeler RA, Williams JE. (1994) Continence in patients with spina bifida: long-term results. *Arch Dis Child* **70**(2): 107–110.

Mingin GC, Baskin LS. (2003) Surgical management of the neurogenic bladder and bowel. *Int Braz J Urol* **29**(1): 53–61.

Novak TE, Salmasi AH, Mathews RI, *et al.* (2008) Complications of complex lower urinary tract reconstruction in patients with neurogenic versus nonneurogenic bladder — is there a difference? *J Urol* **180**(6): 2629–2634; discussion 34–35.

Pham-Huy A, Leonard M, Lepage N, *et al.* (2003) Measuring glomerular filtration rate with cystatin C and beta-trace protein in children with spina bifida. *J Urol* **169**(6): 2312–2315.

Shipstone DP, Thomas DG, Darwent G, Morcos SK. (2002) Magnetic resonance urography in patients with neurogenic bladder dysfunction and spinal dysraphism. *BJU Int* **89**(7): 658–664.

34

Urolithiasis

Vimal Chadha and Uri S. Alon

Introduction

Urolithiasis can cause significant morbidity due to severe pain, and associated complications, including urinary tract obstruction, infection, and potentially renal failure. Urolithiasis is much less common in children (approximately one-tenth to one-fiftieth) than in adults, but recent reports suggest increasing incidence in children, likely as a result of lifestyle changes. Urolithiasis is likely underdiagnosed in children because they often present with vague abdominal symptoms, or may present as an incidental finding during imaging studies performed for unrelated issues. Nonetheless, urolithiasis affects all pediatric age groups with a male preponderance, and occurs more commonly in Caucasians than in African Americans.

Incidence of urolithiasis and underlying etiological factors vary around the world, reflecting differences in geographic, genetic and socioeconomic backgrounds. Overall, urolithiasis incidence is higher in the western hemisphere (5–9% in Europe, 12% in Canada, 13–15% in USA) than in the eastern hemisphere (1–5%), while some Middle Eastern countries, such as Saudi Arabia, have very high rates (20.1%) of stone development. In North America, urolithiasis is most prevalent in the southeastern region, and the states of Virginia, North Carolina, Georgia, Tennessee, and Kentucky have been collectively described as the North American "stone belt." The incidence of urolithiasis is higher in warmer climates and stone recurrence is higher in summer and fall than in winter and spring. Over time, stone composition has changed substantially, with a progressive increase in calcium oxalate and calcium phosphate stones. Recent worldwide epidemiology studies report calcium oxalate accounts for 40–60% of stones in children, followed by calcium phosphate (10–25%), magnesium ammonium phosphate (struvite) (17–30%), uric acid (2–10%), cystine (6–10%), and mixed or miscellaneous (4%).

In developed countries, most stones are intrarenal, and ureteral stones usually originate in the kidneys; in contrast to urinary bladder stones endemic in some underdeveloped and developing countries. Dietary factors likely influence this difference in primary site of origin of stones. A diet with a high content of whole-grain cereal and/or oxalate-rich vegetables combined with low calcium, phosphate, and animal protein is associated with bladder calculi.

Clinical Presentation

Renal colic characterized by excruciating migrating pain from flank to inguinal region associated with hematuria is pathognomonic of urolithiasis in older children and adults, but is uncommon in young children, who present with nonspecific abdominal pain. Urolithiasis is often diagnosed during evaluation of hematuria (gross or microscopic), urinary tract infection (UTI), or frequency/dysuria. Uroliths may be incidentally noted by radiograph during unrelated evaluation.

Management of Acute Episode

The immediate management goals for renal colic and suspected urolithiasis are pain relief, control of nausea/vomiting, and volume repletion (see Fig. 1). Apart from detailed history and physical examination, initial evaluation should include:

- Basic serum chemistries to assess electrolyte disorders and renal function
- Complete blood count with differential
- Urinalysis with microscopic examination and culture
- Imaging studies to confirm presence, size and site of stone, and rule out obstruction

Pain

Effective pain control can be achieved with intravenous (IV) narcotics or nonsteroidal anti-inflammatory drugs (NSAIDs). Morphine sulfate

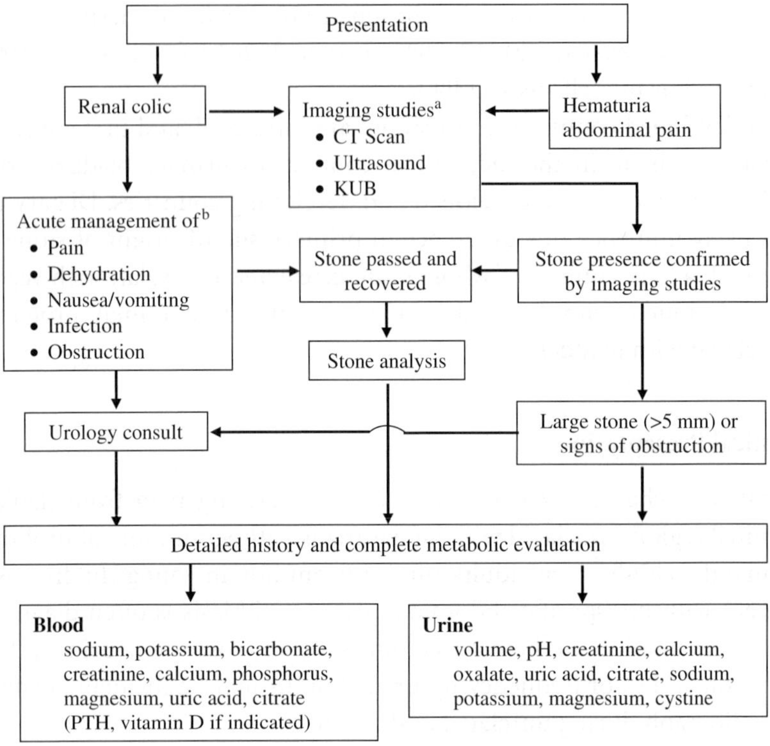

Figure 1. Algorithm for urolithiasis evaluation.

[a] For patients presenting with renal colic, the imaging modality of choice is the spiral CT scan; patients with abdominal pain or hematuria who are suspected to have urolithiasis can be first screened with renal ultrasound, a CT scan can be obtained if no stone is visualized on renal ultrasound but there is still a strong suspicion of stone.

[b] Immediate urology consult should be obtained if both obstruction and infection are present.

(0.1–0.2 mg/kg; maximum dose 15 mg given every 4–6 hrs) is the narcotic analgesic of choice. ketorolac tromethamine (0.5 mg /kg I.V.; maximum dose 15 mg, or 1 mg/kg I.M., maximum dose 30 mg) is the only I.V. NSAID approved in United States. While effective for pain management, ketorolac can precipitate acute kidney injury in volume depletion; therefore, the patient should be well hydrated before receiving this medication. If oral intake is tolerated, the combination of narcotic agents, such as codeine, oxycodone, or hydrocodone with acetaminophen, and antiemetic agents can be used.

Nausea/vomiting

Metoclopramide hydrochloride or prochlorperazine are effective antiemetic agents for controlling nausea/vomiting, however, ondansetron is preferred in children due to favorable side effect profile.

Dehydration

While volume repletion via intravenous fluid administration is mainstay, the role of overhydration to facilitate stone passage remains controversial. Currently, rehydration to a euvolemic state is recommended.

Obstruction and infection

Isolated obstruction or infection should be managed with analgesics and antibiotics, respectively, and urology consult requested. Concurrent infection and obstruction requires prompt antibiotic administration in addition to urgent urologic consultation for decompression.

Medical expulsive therapy

In adults, several medical interventions such as combined usage of antispasmodic agents, calcium channel blockers, and alpha blockers have been tried to enhance ureteral stone passage. Experience with these agents is very limited in children and no current recommendations exist.

Indications for hospitalization

In those whose pain alleviates in the emergency department, further management should occur in an outpatient situation; however, hospitalization is recommended in the case of:

- Dehydration requiring prolonged IV fluids
- Need for parenteral analgesics
- Ureteral obstruction in a solitary or transplanted kidney
- Ureteral obstruction in the presence of UTI, fever, or sepsis
- Large stones unlikely to pass spontaneously requiring surgical intervention

Imaging Studies

Imaging studies are most useful to confirm the presence of, and determine the number, size and location of stones. These studies also provide useful information regarding associated urinary tract anomalies and acute obstruction. Noncontrast computerized tomography (CT), renal ultrasound (US), and abdominal radiograph of kidney, ureter, and bladder (KUB) are the most commonly used imaging modalities. Importantly, the presence of a renal stone may be a "red herring"; therefore, imaging studies should be carefully planned to evaluate other intra-abdominal emergencies such as acute appendicitis.

In patients with acute renal colic, the best initial imaging is noncontrast helical (spiral) CT (see Fig. 2), which can detect stones as small as 1 mm, in addition to cystine and uric acid calculi, which are radiolucent on KUB. Contrast agent should be avoided initially as it can mask stones; however, if initial images suggest obstruction or renal anomalies, postcontrast images can identify anatomical abnormalities.

While helical CT can be performed rapidly (in a single breath hold), and can diagnose abdominal pathologies such as appendicitis, it is costly and exposes the patient to radiation. However, current technology can significantly reduce radiation doses by adjusting scanning parameters to the size of the child while maintaining imaging quality. Despite high sensitivity, precise identification of small distal stones is occasionally difficult, and indinavir stones are not visible on CT.

Renal ultrasound is easy, safe, inexpensive, effective, and avoids radiation (see Fig. 3). Radiolucent uric acid and cystine stones can be visualized, and it is the only modality capable of detecting indinavir calculi. Ureteral stones (especially distal ureter), stones <5 mm, and papillary/calyceal stones can be missed. Sensitivity and accuracy depends in large part on user expertise.

Once confirmed by CT, a KUB can delineate the size, shape, and relative position of the calculus (see Fig. 4) as it is superior to CT because the X-ray beam of the CT may not cross the stone at its widest point. The "scout" reconstruction of the CT is less sensitive than a true KUB in detecting calculi. Additionally, subsequent KUBs can track calculus progression through the urinary system, avoiding the need for repeat CT. KUB is not a good initial study for stone detection due to low sensitivity and specificity.

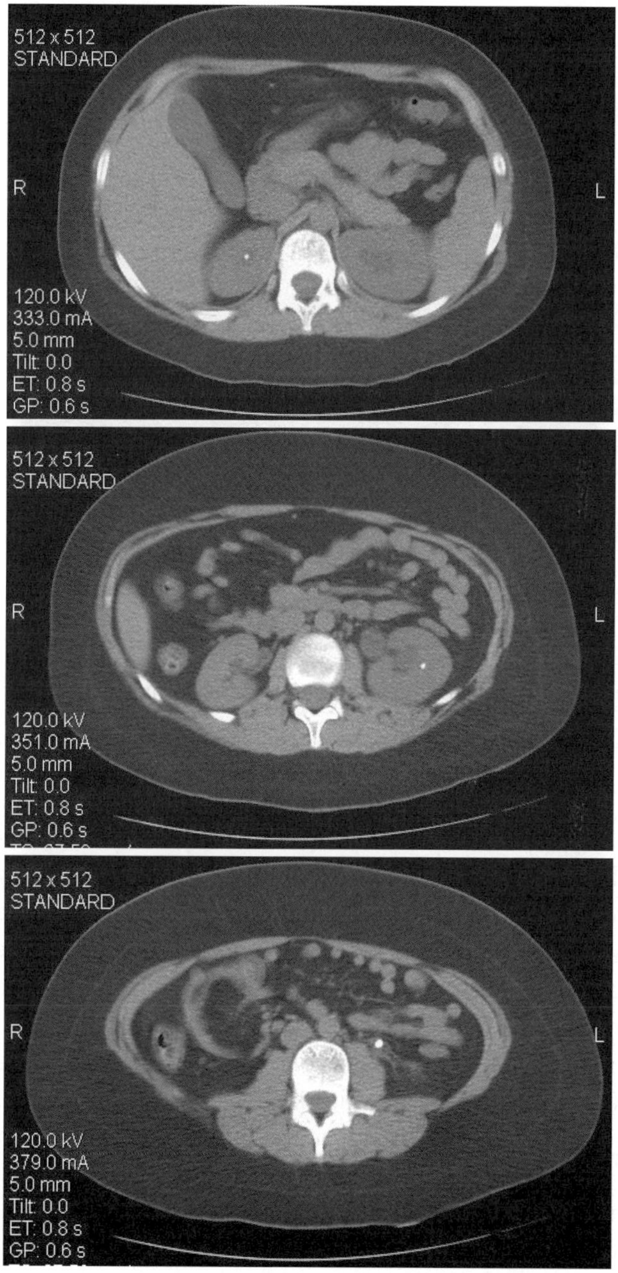

Figure 2. Noncontrast CT scan showing bilateral small calculi and 5 mm stone in the left proximal ureter.

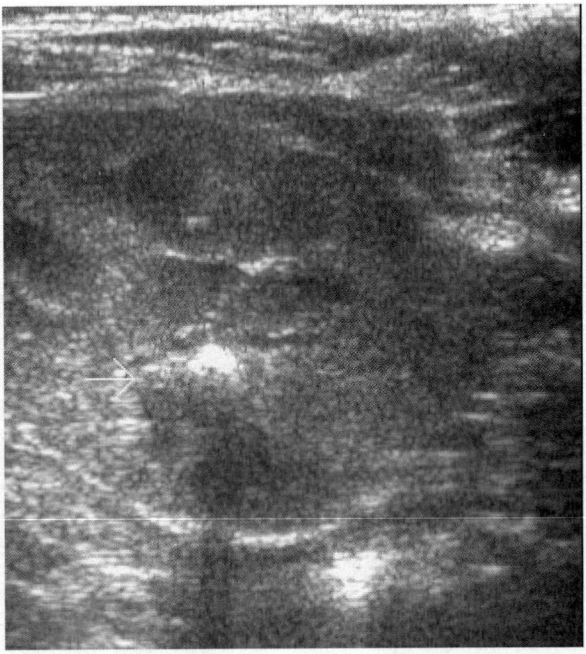

Figure 3. US showing a stone with acoustic shadowing in the left kidney.

Uric acid, cystine, and indinavir-induced stones are relatively radiolucent; small radio-opaque stones, those that overlay bony structures, or are obscured by overlying gas/ stool, can also be easily missed. Many calcifications observed on KUB could be phleboliths, vascular calcifications, calcified lymph nodes, or even bowel contents, all of which can be confused with urinary tract calculi. As such, KUB is usually a confirmatory test or used when CT or ultrasound is not readily available.

In summary, patients with renal colic should be imaged by noncontrast CT, followed by contrast series if initial images show obstruction or other abnormalities. Hematuria or nonacute abdominal pain can be initially evaluated by renal ultrasound, but if stone is not detected and clinical suspicion remains high, noncontrast CT can be obtained. KUB is not recommended as an initial study but may be used as an adjuvant following CT or ultrasound to track the course of stone. In some cases, a stone may pass before the definitive imaging procedure has been completed. Residual inflammation and edema may cause transient or diminishing

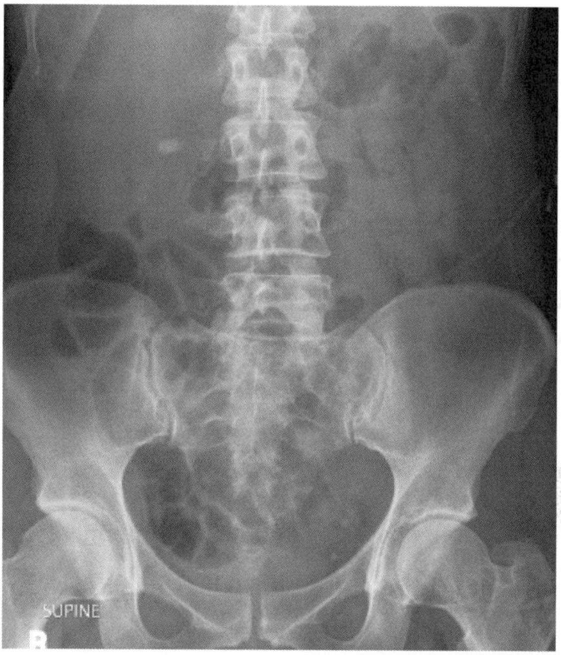

Figure 4. KUB showing radio-opaque calculus in the right renal pelvis.

obstruction and pain even in the absence of stone identification. Magnetic resonance imaging (MRI) has virtually no role in the current evaluation of acute renal colic as most stones are not detectable.

Spontaneous Stone Passage

Smaller stones most often pass spontaneously, but passage also depends on stone shape and location and upper urinary tract anatomy. For example, the presence of ureteropelvic junction (UPJ) obstruction or ureteral stricture can preclude passage of very small stones. If the stone is <4 mm, it will eventually pass in 90% of cases; stones 5–7 mm generally pass spontaneously in 50%; and those >7 mm are unlikely to pass unassisted. Predictions regarding passage are difficult to make during the management of renal colic. All patients with urolithiasis should strain the urine as stone analysis can help determine the underlying metabolic disorder and plan treatment strategies to prevent recurrence.

Stone Analysis

Qualitative stone analysis is important to provide information regarding the underlying metabolic disorder. All recovered fragments should be sent for analysis as most liths are heterogeneous in composition. Infrared spectroscopy and X-ray diffraction are used for analysis, while chemical methods are prone to errors and have become obsolete. With current methods, stone fragments of <1 mg can be accurately analyzed. Recurrent stones should be analyzed with each passage as stone composition may have changed.

Subsequent Outpatient Evaluation

History

A detailed history should cover the following components:

- Severity, site, and nature of pain including any past episodes
- Symptoms of frequency, dysuria, hematuria
- History of UTIs
- History of passing stone/gravel and stone analysis, if performed
- History of known renal anomaly (i.e. UPJ obstruction, hydronephrosis, horseshoe kidney, solitary kidney, kidney transplant)
- History of extreme prematurity
- History of immobilization
- History of chronic bowel diseases (i.e. Crohn disease, bowel resection, cystic fibrosis)
- Dietary history including fluid intake, salt intake, animal protein intake, special diets (i.e. ketogenic diet)
- Drug history: vitamin D, corticosteroids, loop diuretics, anti-HIV medications, carbonic anhydrase inhibitors, cephalosporins, aminoglycosides
- Family history of urolithiasis (present in up to 40%)

Urinalysis

Persistently acidic urine can be associated with uric acid stones, while persistently alkaline urine may signify infection with a urea-splitting organism, such as *Proteus*, *Pseudomonas*, or *Klebsiella*. During microscopic examination, presence or absence of leukocytes, crystals, and bacteria should be noted. Urinary crystals of calcium oxalate, uric acid, or cystine may be found on microscopic evaluation (see Fig. 5).

Predisposition to stone formation

Unlike adults, 75% of children likely have a predisposition for stone formation, such as metabolic disorders, structural urinary tract anomalies, or UTIs. Of these, metabolic risk factors account for >50%. Evaluation for underlying risk factors should be comprehensive and thorough.

Metabolic work-up

All children with urolithiasis (except those with struvite stones who should to be evaluated for infections and structural urological abnormalities) should undergo complete metabolic evaluation. Serum chemistries include sodium, potassium, bicarbonate, calcium, phosphorus, magnesium, uric acid, and alkaline phosphatase. Parathyroid hormone and vitamin D studies should be considered. Twenty-four hour urine measurement should include total volume, pH, calcium, oxalate, uric acid, citrate, sodium, potassium, magnesium, phosphorus, and cystine. For infants and young children, or cases in which timed urine collection is not reliable, random urinary solute to creatinine ratios can be measured, but interpreted with caution as normal values vary by age, time of day, and prandial state (see Tables 1 and 2). Urine evaluation should be conducted while the patient receives his/her usual diet, fluid intake, and with normal activity. Urine evaluation should be delayed for at least one month after acute UTI or stone passage because urinary excretion of calcium, oxalate, or uric acid may be falsely low as they may be absorbed by the stone. Similarly, recent stone fragmentation procedure may cause erroneous results.

Specific metabolic abnormalities and management

Common metabolic abnormalities include chemical excess such as calcium, oxalate, uric acid, or rarely cystine, or lack of inhibitors, such as citrate. While these are often idiopathic, a careful search for secondary

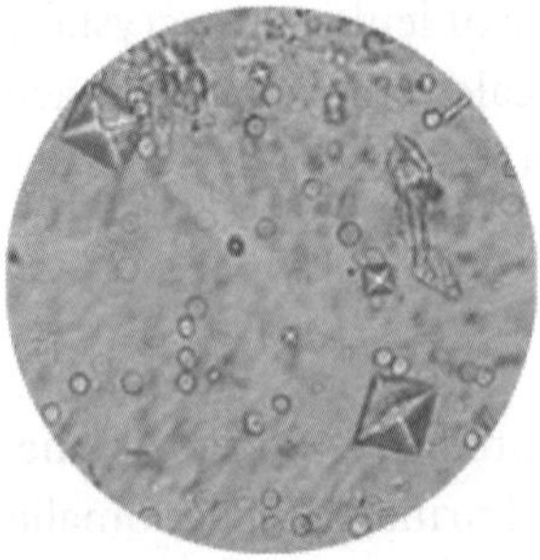

Envelope-shaped calcium oxalate dihydrate crystals

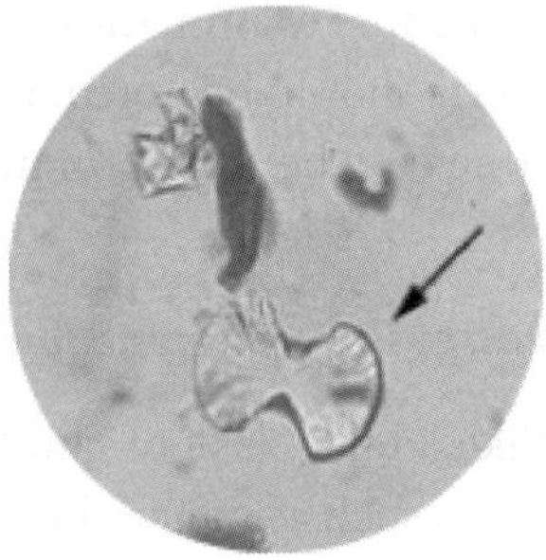

Dumbbell-shaped calcium oxalate monohydrate crystal

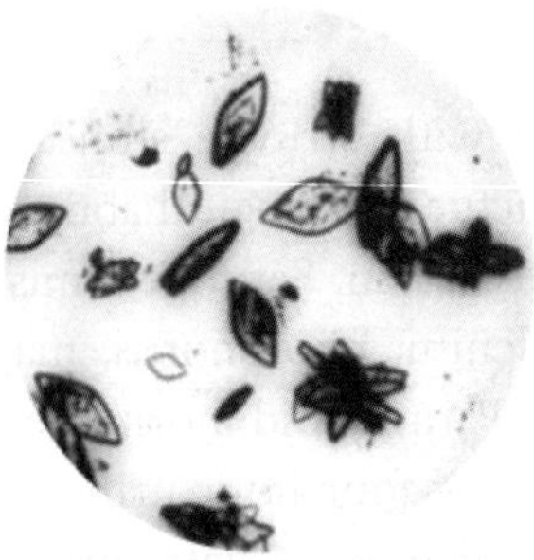

Pleomorphic (rhombic plates or rosettes) uric acid crystals that are seen only in an acidic urine

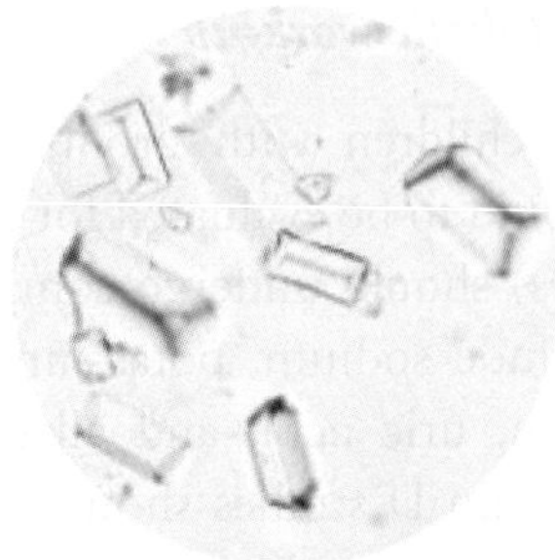

Coffin-lid shaped magnesium ammonium phosphate crystals that are seen only in an alkaline urine

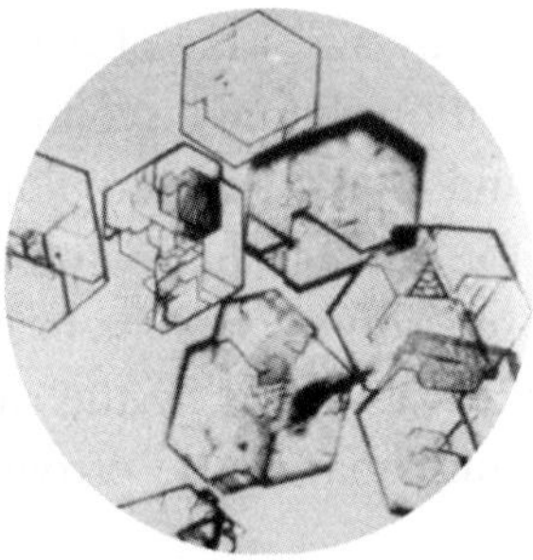

Hexagonal cystine crystals are essentially pathognomonic of cystinuria

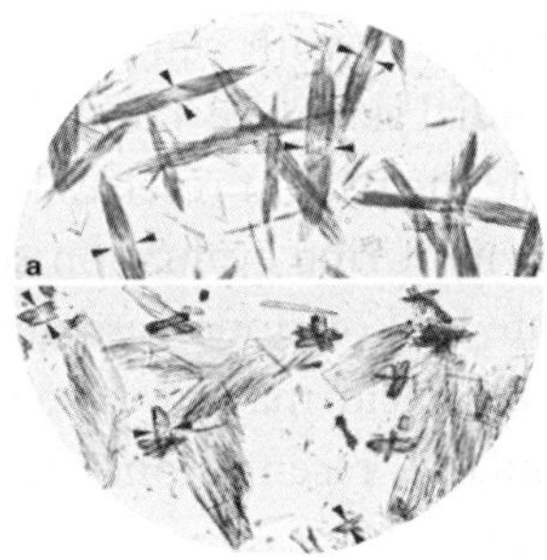

Needles, plates and rosette-shaped indinavir crystals

Figure 5. Urine microscopic appearance of crystals.

Table 1. Normal 24-hour urinary excretion rates of various metabolites

Constituent	Age/Sex group	Rate per 24-hr
Calcium		<4 mg/kg
Sodium		<3 mEq/kg
Potassium		>3 mEq/kg
Magnesium		>88 mg/1.73 m^2
Oxalate	≥2 years	<50 mg/1.73 m^2
		<2 mg/kg
Uric acid	≥1 year	<815 mg/1.73 m^2
		<35 mg/kg
Citrate		>180 mg/g creatinine
Cystine	<10 years	<13 mg/1.73 m^2
	>10 years	<48 mg/1.73 m^2
	Adults	<60 mg/1.73 m^2
Glycolate		0.19 ± 0.07 mmol

Note: Completeness of urine collection can be verified by checking the creatinine excretion (15–20 mg/kg/day in adolescent males, 12–15 mg/kg/day in adolescent females). 24-hour urine chemistry findings may be within the reference range in active stone formers but urinary supersatuartion is achieved because of low urinary volume, or extreme pH values.

Table 2. Normal urine excretion rates in random urine samples

Constituent	Age/Sex group	Ratio
Calcium/creatinine (mg/mg)	0–6 months	<0.8
	7–12 months	<0.6
	1–3 years	<0.53
	3–5 years	<0.39
	5–7 years	<0.28
	>7 years	<0.21
Sodium/potassium (mEq/mEq)		<2.5
Magnesium/creatinine (mg/mg)	>2 years	>0.12
Oxalate/creatinine (mmol/mmol)	<1 year	0.15–0.26
	1–5 years	0.11–0.12
	5–12 years	0.006–0.15
	>12 years	0.002–0.083
Uric acid/creatinine (mg/mg)	10–14 years	<0.65
	14–17 years	<0.60
Uric acid/GFR (mg/dL)[a]	>3 years	<0.56

(*Continued*)

Table 2. (*Continued*)

Constituent	Age/Sex Group	Ratio
Citrate/creatinine (mg/mg)	Children Adult males Adult females	>0.18 >0.14 >0.30
Cystine/creatinine (mg/mg)		<0.075
Glycolate/creatinine (mmol/mmol) L-glycerate/creatinine (μmol/mmol)	Excretion of glycolate and glycerate is highly age dependent and varies with the testing method. One should refer to the normal values provided by the testing laboratory.	

[a] A correction for the amount of uric acid excreted per GFR is needed to assess the upper limit for uric acid excretion in children older than 2 years (uric acid/GFR = $U_{\text{uric acid}} \times S_{\text{creatinine}}/U_{\text{creatinine}}$).

causes and specific disorders should be conducted to optimize therapy (see Table 3).

Hypercalciuria

Hypercalciuria, urinary calcium excretion of >4 mg/kg/day is the most common metabolic abnormality detected in urolithiasis, present in up to 4% of healthy children. Prior to calculus development, clinical presentation may include urinary frequency-dysuria syndrome, with or without microscopic or gross hematuria. Hypercalciuria is most often idiopathic with 4–17% risk of stone development over 1–11 years subsequently. A strong direct correlation between urinary sodium and calcium excretion suggests a detrimental role of dietary sodium in idiopathic hypercalciuria. Conversely, dietary potassium decreases urinary calcium excretion. When hypercalciuria is secondary to corticosteroid or loop diuretic administration or prolonged immobilization, correction of the primary cause is necessary for successful treatment. Less common causes include distal renal tubular acidosis (type I RTA), Dent disease, Bartter syndrome, renal tubular phosphate leak, and familial hypomagnesemia with hypercalciuria (FHH). Most children have normal serum calcium levels; however, if hypercalcemia should prompt evaluation for hyperparathyroidism, hypervitaminosis D, osteolytic metastasis, sarcoidosis, and mutations in calcium sensing receptor.

Idiopathic hypercalciuria can often be managed with dietary modification, specifically, a sodium-restricted (<2000–3000 mg/day), potassium-rich

Table 3. Metabolic abnormalities associated with urolithiasis

	Idiopathic	Secondary	Renal tubule transport disorder or inborn error of metabolism
Hypercalciuria	Inherited Sporadic	Dietary salt excess Dietary calcium excess Vitamin D excess Ketogenic diet Corticosteroids Loop diuretics Immobilization Metabolic acidosis Phosphate depletion Prematurity Hypercalcemia Hyperparathyroidism Hyper- or hypothyroidism	Dent disease RTA Familial hypomagnesemia, hypercalciuria Calcium-sensing receptor mutations
Hyperoxaluria	Mild, associated with idiopathic stone disease	Dietary oxalate excess Enteric hyperoxaluria Parenteral nutrition in premature infants	Primary hyperoxaluria I and II
Cystinuria			Cystinuria

(*Continued*)

Table 3. (*Continued*)

	Idiopathic	Secondary	Renal tubule transport disorder or inborn error of metabolism
Hyperuricosuria	Mild, associated with idiopathic stone disease Familial forms	High protein diet Ketogenic diet High-dose pancreatic enzyme therapy Diabetes Tumor lysis Myeloproliferative disorders SIADH Salicylates Sulfinpyrazone Phenylbutazone	HPRT deficiency, complete (Lesch–Nyhan syndrome) or partial
Hypocitraturia	Mild, associated with idiopathic stone disease	Metabolic acidosis Ketogenic diet Hypokalemia Bacteriuria	Distal RTA

RTA: renal tubular acidosis; HPRT: hypoxanthine phosphoribosytransferase; SIADH: syndrome of inappropriate secretion of antidiuretic hormone
Source: Milliner DS. (2004) Urolithiasis. In: *Pediatric Nephrology*, p. 1094, Lippincott, Williams and Wilkins, Philadelphia; with permission.

(3000–3500 mg/day) diet should be prescribed. Dietary compliance can be assessed by measuring urine sodium to potassium ratio which should be <2.5. Dietary calcium restriction is not recommended as increases the risk of negative calcium balance and poor bone mineralization in growing children. Additionally, a low-calcium diet may increase urinary oxalate excretion from increased gastrointestinal (GI) oxalate absorption. Accordingly, daily recommended allowance of calcium is advisable while excessive calcium intake should be avoided. If hypercalciuria persists after 4–6 weeks of dietary changes, treatment with potassium citrate (0.5–2 mEq/kg of potassium) is recommended. If this is not tolerated or hypercalciuria persists, thiazide diuretics (chlorothiazide 10–20 mg/kg/day or hydrochlorothiazide 1–2 mg/kg/day) can be used. Children receiving long-term thiazide therapy should be monitored for electrolyte abnormalities, hyperlipidemia, and hyperglycemia. Amiloride (0.1–0.2 mg/kg/day) can help maintain serum potassium level and augment the anticalciuric effect of thiazides. In children with RTA, potassium citrate corrects both hypercalciuria and hypocitraturia.

Hyperoxaluria

It is important to differentiate if oxaluria is absorptive or genetic. Mild idiopathic hyperoxaluria may be seen in conjunction with hypercalciuria. Under normal circumstances, most urinary oxalate results from endogenous production, almost equally from ascorbic acid and glyoxylate metabolism. Dietary contribution is low as <10% of ingested oxalate is absorbed from the GI tract. However, in circumstances of malabsorption, inflammatory bowel disease, bowel resection or loss of colonization with *Oxalobacter formigenes*, GI oxalate absorption increases especially with an oxalate rich diet (see Table 4). Increased GI oxalate absorption is termed *enteric hyperoxaluria*, in which undigested fatty acids complex with calcium that otherwise bind with oxalate in the intestines; leading to increased absorption of unbound oxalate. Increased luminal bile salts damage colonic epithelium, also increasing oxalate absorption. The degree of enteric hyperoxaluria is highly diet dependent and varies from mild to severe resulting in recurrent urolithiasis due to low urinary solubility of oxalate. Treatment includes dietary oxalate reduction, calcium supplement administration to bind oxalate in the GI tract, increased fluid intake, low-fat diet and possibly bile sequestering agents. In the presence of low urinary citrate levels, addition of potassium citrate may be helpful.

Table 4. Oxalate content of foods

Food group	Low or no oxalate, eat as desired	Moderate oxalate, limit intake	High oxalate, avoid intake
Beverages	Apple juice Pineapple juice Grapefruit juice Orange juice	Cranberry juice Grape juice	Juices containing berries Lemonade Tomato juice Ovaltine Tea, cocoa
Dairy products	Milk, yogurt, cheese		
Meat	Lean lamb, beef, pork, poultry, seafood	Sardines	
Fruits and Vegetables	Asparagus Avocado Cauliflower Cabbage Mushrooms Onions Potatoes Sweet corn Bananas Cherries (Bing) Grapefruits Grapes (white) Mangoes Melons Nectarines Pears Pineapple	Broccoli Cucumber Green peas Lettuce Tomato (1 small) Turnips Eggplant Apples Apricots Peach Plum (red) Prunes Squash	Beans Beets Carrots Celery Chives Collards Dandelion greens Kale Okra Berries Sweet potato Tangerines
Breads, pasta, and cereal	Macaroni Noodles Rice Spaghetti White bread	Cornflakes Sponge cake Bran cereal	Soybean crackers Wheat germ
Miscellaneous	Mayonnaise Vegetable oils Butter	Fruit cake	French fries Nuts Pretzels Chocolate

Primary hyperoxaluria (types I and II) are rare and serious causes of nephrolithiasis. Primary hyperoxaluria (oxalosis), an autosomal recessive disorder caused by defects in hepatic enzymes, results in marked oxalate overproduction. In type I, the more prevalent form, mutation of alanine glyoxylate aminotransferase, results in increased urinary excretion of oxalate, glyoxalic acid, and glycolic acid. In type II, a defect in D-glycerate dehydrogenase, results in increased urinary excretion of oxalate and L-glycerate. Due to severe hyperoxaluria and presence since birth, primary hyperoxaluria is characterized by aggressive stone formation and sometimes nephrocalcinosis, which may impair renal function. Once the glomerular filtration rate is <30 ml/min/1.73m^2, plasma oxalate concentration increases rapidly, with resulting deposition of calcium oxalate in multiple organs (oxalosis). Patients with type I primary hyperoxaluria, homozygous for G630A mutation, benefit from pharmacological doses of pyridoxine, reducing oxalate excretion. Apart from increased fluid intake, patients with primary hyperoxaluria should receive neutral phosphate therapy to reduce urinary supersaturation of calcium oxalate. Once renal failure develops, aggressive hemodialysis with subsequent combined kidney–liver transplantation is required.

Hyperuricosuria

Uric acid stones are radiolucent and occur in <5% of children with metabolic stones. Uric acid is a weak acid that exists in a relatively insoluble nonionized form and propensity for stone formation increases significantly in acidic urine. Uric acid crystals may precipitate calcium oxalate excretion. Idiopathic hyperuricosuria is often familial and coexists with hypercalciuria. Secondary hyperuricosuria may result from:

- *Overproduction*: Tumor lysis syndrome, lymphoproliferative or myeloproliferative disorders
- *Dietary*: High protein (purine rich) intake
- *Renal hypouricemia*: Hypouricemia secondary to hyperuricosuria due to defective renal tubular urate absorption
- *Medications*: Probenecid, phenylbutazone, salicylates, and pancreatic extract therapy
- *Inborn errors of metabolism*: Complete (Lesch–Nyhan syndrome) or partial deficiencies of hypoxanthine phosphoribosyltransferase (HGPRT) enzyme activity

Most patients with uric acid stones have hyperuricosuria; however, uric acid excretion may be normal in states of acidic urine. Uric acid crystals are poorly soluble in acidic urine and precipitate easily as seen in children receiving ketogenic diets for intractable seizures or in obese patients with metabolic syndrome. The low urine pH results from deficient ammonia production.

Treatment for uric acid stones includes high fluid intake and alkalinization of urine to pH of 6.5–7.0 with potassium citrate or sodium bicarbonate. The former is preferred as citrate decreases the risk of crystallization, while the latter increases sodium load potentially exacerbating hypercalciuria. A low purine diet is advisable: Restriction of red meat, fish, fowl, coffee, cocoa, chocolate, and cakes with high yeast content. Patients with inborn errors of metabolism or overproduction (e.g. tumor lysis or myeloproliferative disorders) may require allopurinol in addition to standard treatment. Allopurinol should be used with care as long-term usage can lead to xanthine and oxypurinol calculi.

Hypocitraturia

Citrate is a naturally occurring inhibitor of calcium oxalate and calcium phosphate crystallization. Hypocitraturia may contribute to stone formation in a subset of patients, and is significant in children with hypercalciuria and stones than in nonstone forming hypercalciuric children and controls. Calcium to citrate ratio of <0.326 (mg/mg) is likely to protect against stone formation. Hypocitraturia can result from systemic acidosis or hypokalemia which are believed to impair citrate synthesis and increase renal resorption, resulting in hypocitraturia. Thus, renal tubular acidosis should be considered in those with hypocitraturia. A subtle renal acidification defect can occur secondary to renal tubular injury from chronic hypercalciuria and urolithiasis. Potassium citrate is the drug of choice to treat children with hypocitraturia and hypercalciuria.

Cystinuria

Cystinuria, an autosomal-recessive disorder of renal tubular cystine and other dibasic amino acids ornithine, arginine, and lysine transport, can cause lifelong recurrent stones, especially in homozygous individuals. Normal individuals excrete <60 mg of cystine/1.73 m^2/day, whereas homozygous patients have excretion rates >400 mg/1.73 m^2/day. Patients with nonspecific proximal renal tubular aminoaciduria may excrete up to 200 mg cystine/1.73 m^2/day. At usual urine volumes and pH, cystine excretion rates exceed solubility, which is limited to 240 mg/L (1000 μmol/L). Cystine stones have been identified in 2–7% of children with metabolic stones.

Management of cystinuria includes high fluid intake to maintain a low urinary cystine concentration and alkalization of urine to pH of 7.0–7.5, preferably using potassium citrate. If potassium citrate is intolerable, acetazolamide can be added at nighttime (noting that carbonic anhydrase inhibitors potentially may increase stone formation). Urine pH >7.5 should be avoided due to risk of calcium precipitation. Alkalization should be suspended in the presence of UTI. Urinary cystine excretion has been linked to dietary sodium intake: A low-sodium diet is recommended. In children in whom hydration, decreased salt intake, and urinary alkalization have failed, D-penicillamine or α-mercaptopropionyl glycine, sulfhydryls that cleave cystine into two cysteine moieties to form mixed disulphides 50 times more soluble than cystine can be prescribed. D-penicillamine (20–50 mg/kg/d) is administered in divided doses, with half of the daily dose taken at bedtime, as urinary cystine concentration is at its maximum during the night. The dose for α-mercaptopropionyl glycine is 15 mg/kg/d. The therapy should be supplemented with pyridoxine hydrochloride (vitamin B6) 25–50 mg/d, because of the antipyridoxine effect of the drug. Adverse effects of D-penicillamine include skin rash, fever, lymphadenopathy, and loss of taste. Proteinuria may develop after several months of treatment and may progress to nephrosis, which improves upon discontinuation. Due to potential toxicity associated with long-term use, discontinuation or dose reduction (prophylactic administration of bedtime dose) should occur when calculi resolve. Captopril, which is a sulfhydryl agent, has been used with mixed results in cystinuria.

Struvite stones

Struvite, (infection related stones) have decreased significantly in developed countries as a result of improved management of obstructive uropathy and UTIs, but are still commonly seen in Third World countries, most commonly in young girls with history of multiple UTIs. Struvite stones are composed of magnesium ammonium phosphate and form in alkaline urine provided by breakdown of urea by urease producing bacteria such as *Proteus, Staphylococcus aureus, Klebsiella, Serratia, Pseudomonas,* and *Staphylococcus epidermis*. Genitourinary tract abnormalities, especially obstruction, predispose to formation of infected stones. Therefore, careful urologic evaluation of children with infected stones is mandatory. Infection with these organisms may produce a soft radiolucent mucoid substance called a "matrix concretion," which calcifies rapidly into a radio-opaque struvite stone (see Fig. 6). These stones can completely fill and form a cast of the pelvocalyceal system, known as "staghorn calculi," which can cause severe urinary obstruction, pyelonephritis, and urosepsis. Patients with surgically augmented urinary bladders are at risk for struvite stones.

Struvite stones are challenging: eradication of infection without stone removal is difficult because antibiotics do not penetrate well within the interstices of the stone where bacteria reside. Less than 50% of patients with staghorn calculi are rendered stone-free with extracorporeal shock wave lithotripsy (ESWL); and combination with percutaneous nephrostolithotomy (PCNL) is often needed as retained stone fragments can serve as a nidus for early recurrence; rarely, nephrectomy may be required.

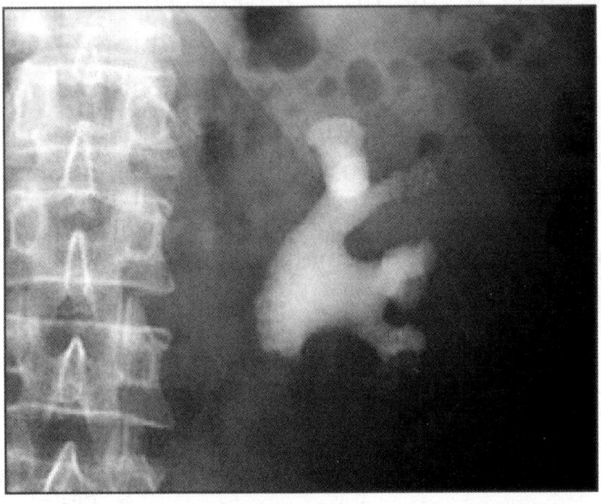

Figure 6. Staghorn calculus in the left kidney.

Surgical management

Primary indications for surgical intervention include pain, infection, and obstruction. The vast majority of urinary tract stones are now managed with noninvasive or minimally invasive techniques, while open surgical excision (lithotomy) is rare. ESWL, ureteroscopy, and PCNL are most commonly used, and selection is based on the size of the stone, location and composition, and urinary tract anatomy.

ESWL is least invasive and is safely used in children with high success rates and little variability amongst lithotriptors. Success in part depends on the chemical composition of stone. Uric acid and calcium oxalate dihydrate stones fragment easily, but calcium oxalate monohydrate and struvite stones are more difficult to fragment, and cystine calculi are relatively resistant. ESWL may be limited by the size and location of calculus. Multiple stone fragments resulting from large stones (>2 cm) located in the lower pole of the kidney may fail to pass because of their dependent position. In addition, results may be suboptimal in large patients, especially if skin-to-stone distance exceeds 10 cm; and in children with anatomically abnormal urinary tracts. Common side effects of ESWL include renal or perinephric hematoma, posttreatment flank pain, gross hematuria, and trauma to extrarenal tissues in the blast path, such as skin bruising, pulmonary infiltrates, pulmonary contusion, and hemoptysis. Although renal blood flow is reduced transiently following ESWL, no significant long-term consequences are reported.

In patients with mid or distal ureteral calculi, usually 5–8 mm in diameter, ureteroscopic manipulation is preferred. The stone can be directly extracted using a basket or grasping forceps, or broken into small pieces by using various lithotrites, such as laser, ultrasonic, electrohydraulic or ballistic.

For patients with renal stones >2 cm in diameter, PCNL is preferred. PCNL can be used alone or in combination with other surgical techniques and is especially useful in children with a large stone burden, orthopedic rods for spine stabilization, or history of renal surgery. Percutaneous access to the renal pelvis is established, and a rigid or flexible nephroscope is used to manipulate the calculi. Available nephroscopes can accommodate laser, electrohydraulic or ultrasonic probes, grasping forceps, and basket extractors. Calculi can then be broken and extracted. Potential complications include significant blood loss and urosepsis.

Open surgery is required for calculi not amenable to ESWL, PCNL, or endoscopic techniques. In children with severe stone burden, complex urinary anatomy, or previous surgical procedures, these techniques may be used in combination or succession. Large bladder calculi are best managed by open cystolithotomy. Rarely, children with large stones in a nonfunctioning kidney may require nephrectomy.

Medical management

Patients with idiopathic urolithiasis and normal urine chemistries or mild hypercalciuria may be managed initially with increased fluid intake and dietary modification. A 24-hour urinalysis should be repeated two months after dietary changes and/or institution of medical therapy to assess patient compliance and adequacy of metabolic response. If control is inadequate, addition of potassium citrate therapy — or, for those with hypercalciuria, therapy with a thiazide diuretic, is the next step. At times a combination of the two medications is required. Treatment of metabolic factors should be directed specifically to the abnormalities found (see Fig. 7). If existing stones increase in size, or new stone formation occurs despite medical treatment, a more intensive regimen should be implemented and additional studies for unusual causes pursued.

Children with urolithiasis should receive long-term follow-up with periodic assessment of stone forming activity as urolithiasis is a recurrent

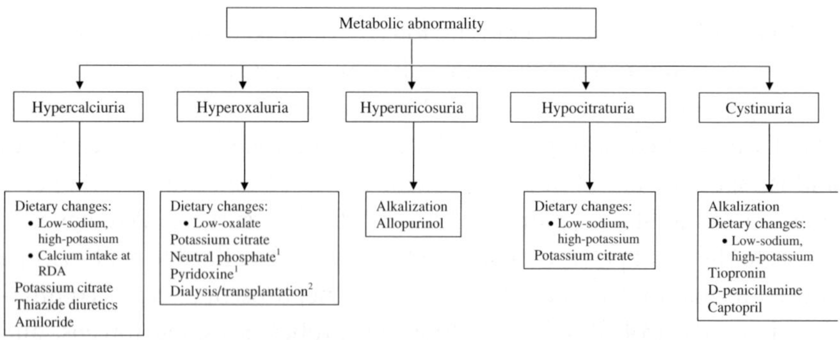

* RDA – Recommended daily allowance; 1 – Initial therapy for primary hyperoxaluria; 2 – Needed with the onset of renal failure

Figure 7. Algorithm of suggested therapies for specific metabolic abnormalities.

disease, especially in those with metabolic abnormality. The frequency of renal imaging depends on the type and number of stones and the severity of the metabolic abnormalities detected. In asymptomatic, infection free children, annual or every other year imaging with renal US is sufficient, but may be required more frequently in primary hyperoxaluria, cystinuria, or marked hypercalciuria. Acute symptoms suggestive of stone should prompt immediate reevaluation.

Suggested Reading

Alon U, Costanzo LS, Chan JCM. (1984) Additive Hypocalciuric effects of amiloride and hydrochlorothiazide in patients treated with calcitriol. *Miner Electrolyte Metab* **10**: 379–386.

Assimos DG, Holmes RP. (2000) Role of diet in the therapy of urolithiasis. *Urol Clin North Am* **27**: 255–268.

Curhan GC, Willett WC, Rimm EB, Stampfer MJ. (1997) Family history and risk of kidney stones. *J Am Soc Nephrol* **8**: 1568–1573.

Defoor W, Asplin J, Jackson E, *et al.* (2005) Results of a prospective trial to compare normal urine supersaturation in children and adults. *J Urol* **174**: 1708–1710.

Durkee CT, Balcon A. (2006) Surgical management of urolithiasis. *Pediatr Clin North Am* **53**(3): 465–477.

Kaufman DW, Kelly JP, Curhan GC, *et al.* (2008) Oxalobacter formigenes may reduce the risk of calcium oxalate kidney stones. *J Am Soc Nephrol* **19**: 1197–1203.

López M, Hoppe B. (2010) History, epidemiology and regional diversities of urolithiasis. *Pediatr Nephrol* **25**(1): 49–59.

Musulumanoglu AY, Tefekli A, Sarilar O, *et al.* (2003) Extracorporeal shockwave lithotripsy as first-line treatment alternative for urinary tract stones in children: a large scale retrospective analysis. *J Urol* **170**: 2405–2408.

Osorio A, Alon US. (1997) The relationship between urinary calcium, sodium, and potassium excretion and the role of potassium in treating idiopathic hypercalciuria. *Pediatrics* **100**: 675–681.

Palmer JS, Donaher ER, O'Riordan MA, Dell KM. (2005) Diagnosis of pediatric urolithiasis: role of ultrasound and computerized tomography. *J Urol* **174**: 1413–1416.

Part XI

Acute Kidney Injury (AKI)

35

Acute Kidney Injury (AKI)

Prasad Devarajan

Introduction

Acute kidney injury (AKI) refers to a complex syndrome that comprises multiple causative factors and occurs in a variety of settings with varied clinical manifestations ranging from a minimal elevation in serum creatinine to anuric renal failure. AKI is characterized functionally by a rapid (within hours to days) decline in the glomerular filtration rate (GFR), and biochemically by the accumulation of nitrogenous wastes, such as blood urea nitrogen (BUN), and creatinine. The term AKI has largely replaced acute renal failure (ARF), the terminology historically used for this condition, since the latter designation overemphasizes the failure of kidney function, and fails to account for the diverse spectrum of molecular, biochemical, and structural processes that characterize the AKI syndrome. AKI is a common clinical condition, afflicting all ages in both hospital and community settings, and associated with potentially serious consequences and treatment options that are largely supportive in nature. The etiology of AKI varies widely according to age, geographic region, and clinical setting. The prerenal forms of AKI associated with dehydration are usually fully reversible with timely therapy. The prognosis remains guarded for subjects with the intrinsic forms of AKI often encountered in the intensive care setting as a result of sepsis, multiorgan failure, nephrotoxins or prolonged ischemia. Intrinsic AKI in the critically ill patient is one of the most important risk factors for mortality, with an estimated death rate of greater than 50%, which has not appreciably changed in the past three decades. However, the cellular and molecular tools of modern science are rapidly providing critical new insights into the pathogenetic pathways and early biomarkers of AKI. Novel strategies that modulate these pathways in a timely manner hold considerable promise for the prevention and treatment of AKI.

Classification and Definitions

AKI may be classified according to the urine output, as being *nonoliguric*, *oliguric* (urine output <1 ml/kg/h in infants, <0.5 ml/kg/h in children, or <400 ml/day in adults), or *anuric*. Measurement of urine output is especially useful in the critical care setting, since the degree of oliguria reflects severity of the kidney injury, has important implications for volume and electrolyte imbalances, and provides prognostic information. However, even moderately severe forms of AKI due to nephrotoxins, and a majority of AKI seen in neonatal intensive care, are typically nonoliguric. Also, pharmacologic conversion of an oliguric AKI to a nonoliguric form (i.e. by the use of diuretics) does not necessarily improve the long-term prognosis, although it can facilitate the acute supportive care.

The traditional classification of AKI, based on the anatomic location of the initial injury, remains useful for the purposes of understanding the pathophysiology, making a diagnosis, and outlining a management plan. *Prerenal azotemia* or *volume-responsive AKI* is an appropriate physiologic response of structurally normal kidneys to hypoperfusion. It is the most common form of AKI, and is usually associated with dehydration, sepsis, or other causes of transient hypotension. There is a reduction in GFR, but the renal tubules remain intact and avidly conserve salt and water in the face of sensed renal hypoperfusion, leading to oliguria. When normal renal perfusion is restored, urine flow and GFR return to normal. Because the reduction in GFR represents a self-protection mechanism to preserve tubule integrity, and the oliguria embodies a renal mechanism for preserving intravascular volume, this syndrome has also been referred to as "*acute renal success*." On the other hand, *intrinsic* or *intrarenal AKI* is characterized by structural damage to the renal parenchyma, most commonly from prolonged ischemia, sepsis, nephrotoxins, or severe glomerular diseases. Prerenal and intrinsic AKI are parts of a spectrum of consequences of renal hypoperfusion that often coexist, and there may be significant overlap in the clinical and biochemical manifestations of these two forms of AKI. Indeed, the most common factor leading to the development of intrinsic AKI is prolonged or untreated prerenal AKI. Finally, *postrenal* or *obstructive AKI* is characterized by acute obstruction of the urinary tract at extra-renal anatomic sites. This is distinct from the acute intra-tubular obstruction at the single nephron level commonly seen in intrinsic AKI. Postrenal AKI is typically the result of *congenital* or acquired anatomic obstructions to the lower urinary tract.

AKI may also be classified according to the circumstances in which it occurs. *Community-acquired AKI* is more likely to be associated with a single predominant insult. The medical approach is often conservative and expectant, including discontinuing the insult, supportive fluid and electrolyte management, and awaiting spontaneous recovery of renal function. In contrast, *hospital-acquired AKI*, especially in the critical care setting, is frequently multifactorial, and often part of more extensive multiorgan failure. Management is usually more aggressive with early initiation of renal replacement therapies to optimize the overall care of the severely compromised patient.

In the past, there have been over 35 definitions of AKI that have been used in clinical studies. This lack of a consensus definition has led to a myriad of quoted epidemiology, morbidity and mortality rates in the AKI literature. Recently, a group of adult and pediatric nephrologists and intensivists founded the Acute Dialysis Quality Initiative, and proposed a consensus definition called the *RIFLE classification of AKI* that has been increasingly employed. This diagnostic classification scheme is based on changes in serum creatinine and urine output, and includes three levels of renal dysfunction of increasing severity, and two outcome categories (see Fig. 1). Several studies in adult patients have now established that worsening AKI severity by RIFLE classification has direct associations with increased mortality and morbidity. A modification of this classification for use in children has recently been published (see Fig. 2). AKI defined by these criteria has emerged as an independent risk factor for mortality and length of hospitalization in critically ill children. Adoption of these promising multidimensional definitions is anticipated to dramatically improve our understanding of the epidemiology and outcomes of AKI.

Epidemiology

Large epidemiologic studies in adults have established that AKI occurs in about 3–7% of all hospitalized patients. Over the past two decades, this incidence has progressively increased by about 11% annually. The precise

Stage	Serum Creatinine Criteria	GFR Criteria	Urine Output Criteria
R = Risk for renal dysfunction	Increase in serum creatinine ≥ 1.5x baseline	Decrease in GFR ≥ 25%	< 0.5 mL/kg/hr for 6 h
I = Injury to the kidney	Increase in serum creatinine ≥ 2.0 x baseline	Decrease in GFR ≥ 50%	< 0.5 mL/kg/hr for 12h
F = Failure of kidney function	Increase in serum creatinine ≥ 3.0x baseline OR serum creatinine ≥ 4.0 mg/dL in the setting of an acute rise ≥ 0.5 mg/dL	Decrease in GFR ≥ 75%	< 0.3 mL/kg/hr for 24 hr or anuria for 12 hr
L = Loss of kidney function	Persistent failure > 4 weeks		
E = End-stage renal disease (ESRD)	Persistent failure > 3 months		

Figure 1. RIFLE classification of AKI.

Stage	Estimated Creatinine Clearance (eCCL)	Urine Output
R = Risk for renal dysfunction	eCCl decrease by 25%	< 0.5 mL/kg/hr for 8 h
I = Injury to the kidney	eCCl decrease by 50%	< 0.5 mL/kg/hr for 16 h
F = Failure of kidney function	eCCl decrease by 75% or eCCl < 35 mL/min/1.73m^2	< 0.3 mL/kg/hr for 24 hr or anuria for 12 hr
L = Loss of kidney function	Persistent failure > 4 weeks	
E = End-stage renal disease (ESRD)	Persistent failure > 3 months	

Figure 2. Pediatric RIFLE classification of AKI. Estimated creatinine clearance is calculated using the Schwartz formula.

incidence of pediatric AKI is not known, largely due to the lack of a consensus definition in published studies, but also appears to be common and rising at an alarming rate. For example, AKI defined by a serum creatinine level of >1.5 mg/dL complicates 25% of all neonatal intensive care unit admissions, and is present in 30% of all preterm infants and in more than

60% of neonates with asphyxia. AKI defined as a doubling of serum creatinine is present in about 5% of all patients admitted to a pediatric intensive care unit. This incidence jumps to 82% if only children receiving mechanical ventilation and vasopressors are included. AKI defined by the RIFLE criteria is encountered in about 30% of infants and children undergoing cardiac surgery, and 10% of children administered contrast agents.

The etiology of pediatric AKI is greatly influenced by the clinical setting and geographic location. In developed countries, the epidemiology of pediatric AKI has shifted during the past two decades from primary glomerular diseases to a hospital-acquired disease resulting from other systemic illnesses. The most prevalent causes now include sepsis, congenital heart disease, nephrotoxins, and renal ischemia in critically ill children with multiorgan failure. Reports from the Indian subcontinent identify glomerular diseases such as hemolytic uremic syndrome, acute glomerulonephritis, and acute gastroenteritis as predominant causes, although the pattern in urban areas resembles that seen in more developed nations. Studies from Africa reveal malaria, gastroenteritis, and HIV nephropathy as common etiologies, and hemolytic uremic syndrome remains the predominant cause in South America.

Pathophysiology of Prerenal AKI

Table 1 lists the common causes of prerenal AKI, based on mechanistic considerations. Any decrease in circulatory volume, either due to true volume depletion, or effective hypovolemia (decreased cardiac output, peripheral vasodilatation) evokes a primal systemic response (see Fig. 3). Stimulation of baroreceptors in the carotid sinus and aortic arch activate the sympathetic nervous system and renin-angiotensin axis, leading to the

Table 1. Common causes of prerenal AKI

Mechanism	Etiology
Volume depletion	Dehydration, hemorrhage, diuretics, burns, shock, nephrotic syndrome, diabetes
Decreased cardiac output	Cardiac failure, arrythmias
Peripheral vasodilatation	Sepsis, anaphylaxis, antihypertensives
Renal vasoconstriction	Sepsis, nonsteroidal anti-inflammatory drugs, ACE inhibitors

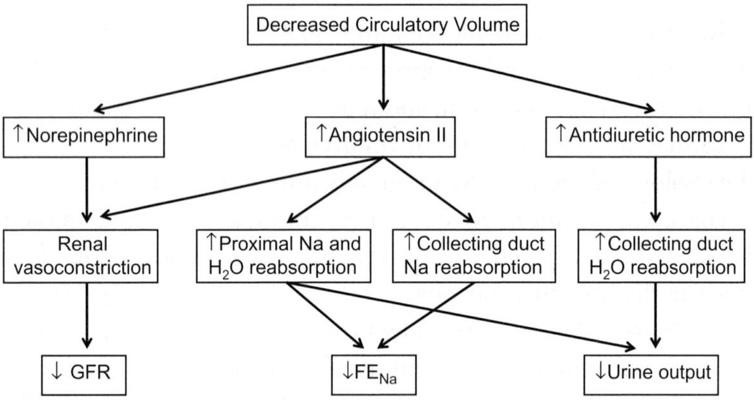

Figure 3. Pathophysiology of prerenal AKI.

systemic release of angiotensin II, norepinephrine, and antidiuretic hormone (ADH). These systems help maintain perfusion to the brain and heart by normalizing intravascular volume and blood pressure, but at the potential expense of GFR. Both angiotensin II and norepinephrine are powerful renal vasoconstrictors, and diminish renal perfusion with a resultant reduction in GFR. Fortunately, several intrarenal compensatory mechanisms are brought into play in response to renal hypoperfusion, and these help maintain GFR during the initial phases (see Fig. 4). The most effective response involves the increased intrarenal generation of vasodilatory prostaglandins. During normal physiologic states, the cyclooxygenase (COX-1 and COX-2) enzyme systems catalyze the intrarenal production of prostaglandin (PG) E_2 and PGI_2, both important afferent arteriolar vasodilators. Volume depletion dramatically induces this system, primarily by the upregulation of COX-2 expression in the *macula densa* and medullary interstitial cells. Nonsteroidal anti-inflammatory drugs inhibit this response and can therefore precipitate AKI, especially when used in the setting of renal hypoperfusion. Two common scenarios in which this occurs are (a) following the use of indomethacin for closure of a patent ductus arteriosus in neonates, and (b) following the use of ibuprofen in febrile children with a dehydrating illness.

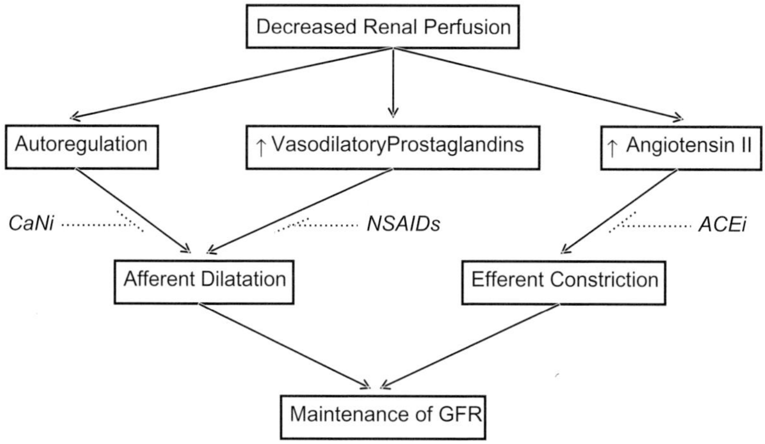

Figure 4. Renal compensatory mechanisms that maintain GFR in prerenal AKI are illustrated by arrows. Iatrogenic interference with these mechanisms can precipitate a reduction in GFR, as shown by dashed lines. CaNi, calcineurin inhibitors; NSAIDs, nonsteroidal anti-inflammatory drugs; ACEi, angiotensin converting enzyme inhibitors.

A second mechanism for maintenance of normal GFR involves the differential effect of intrarenal angiotensin II on the afferent and efferent arterioles. The renin-angiotensin system (RAS) has been traditionally viewed as a systemic cascade that regulates blood pressure. The classic pathway begins with angiotensinogen, which is secreted into the systemic circulation by the liver. It is cleaved by renin, a protease produced by the juxtaglomerular cells of the kidney, to form angiotensin I, an inactive decapeptide. This is further cleaved by angiotensin converting enzyme (ACE), a metalloprotease produced by the pulmonary endothelium, to form angiotensin II, a highly active octapeptide. Angiotensin II induces vascular smooth muscle constriction, proximal tubular reabsorption of sodium and water, reabsorption of sodium in the collecting duct via stimulation of aldosterone release, and reabsorption of water in the collecting duct via stimulation of ADH release. Collectively, these mechanisms account for the increase in intravascular volume and blood pressure that are typically associated with this system. In addition to the classical circulating RAS, there exist robust and complete RAS pathways in the kidney and heart. The intrarenal RAS consists of angiotensinogen expressed by proximal tubular cells, renin released by the juxtaglomerular apparatus, ACE expressed by glomerular endothelial cells and proximal tubule cells, and widespread expression of angiotensin receptors on the afferent and efferent arterioles, mesangial cells and tubular epithelial cells. The intrarenal RAS regulates glomerular hemodynamics in normal, as well as hypoperfused states. A decrease in renal perfusion results in a reduction in solute delivery to the distal tubule by several mechanisms. The decrease in luminal chloride ion concentration is sensed by the *macula densa* cells, which stimulate the release of renin from the juxtaglomerular cells. Angiotensin II tends to constrict both the afferent and efferent arteriole. However, this effect is more marked in the efferent arteriole, leading to increased hydrostatic pressure across the glomerulus and maintenance of GFR. An interference with this compensatory mechanism can occur following angiotensin-converting enzyme inhibitor therapy.

Myogenic autoregulation refers to the unique ability of the afferent arterioles to rapidly vasodilate in response to a decrease in lateral stretch caused by hypoperfusion. Calcineurin inhibitors commonly used for immunosuppression following kidney transplants are known to interfere with myogenic autoregulatory mechanisms. The role of this response in volume-depleted states in humans has recently been challenged, and several investigators have suggested a more important role for autoregulation in maintaining intraglomerular pressure during systemic hypertension.

In spite of these compensatory mechanisms that help maintain GFR in volume-depleted states, prolonged reduction in renal perfusion pressure can overwhelm these pathways, lead to persistent vasoconstriction, and precipitate intrinsic AKI.

Pathophysiology of Intrinsic AKI

Table 2 lists the common causes of intrinsic AKI. The most common underlying mechanism relates to prolonged renal hypoperfusion.

Table 2. Common causes of intrinsic AKI

Mechanism	Etiology
Tubular injury (acute tubular necrosis)	Prolonged ischemia, nephrotoxins
Renal vascular diseases	Hemolytic uremic syndrome, vasculitis
Interstitial diseases	Interstitial nephritis, infections, infiltrations
Glomerulonephritides	Postinfectious, crescentic

However, intrinsic AKI in the critical care setting is frequently multifactorial in etiology, with ischemic, nephrotoxic, and septic components that interplay with and amplify each other. Pathologically, this form of AKI is associated with *acute tubular necrosis (ATN)*, and it is common clinical practice to use the terms intrinsic AKI and ATN interchangeably. However, ATN is a misnomer, since frank tubular cell necrosis is rarely found in human AKI. Instead, there is effacement and loss of proximal tubule brush border, patchy loss of tubule cells, focal proximal tubular dilatation and distal tubular casts, and areas of cellular regeneration. Necrotic cell death is restricted to the outer medullary regions (S3 segment of the proximal tubule and medullary thick ascending limb of Henle's loop). On the other hand, apoptosis is frequently encountered in both distal and proximal tubules, in both ischemic and nephrotoxic forms of human AKI. In addition, an intense inflammatory response is often apparent, especially in the later phases of intrinsic AKI. The molecular, biochemical, and cellular mechanisms underlying these morphologic changes have been subjects of intense contemporary research, and are yielding novel therapeutic approaches, as detailed below.

Intrinsic AKI is characterized by an intense and persistent renal vasoconstriction (see Fig. 5). This has been attributed to endothelial damage,

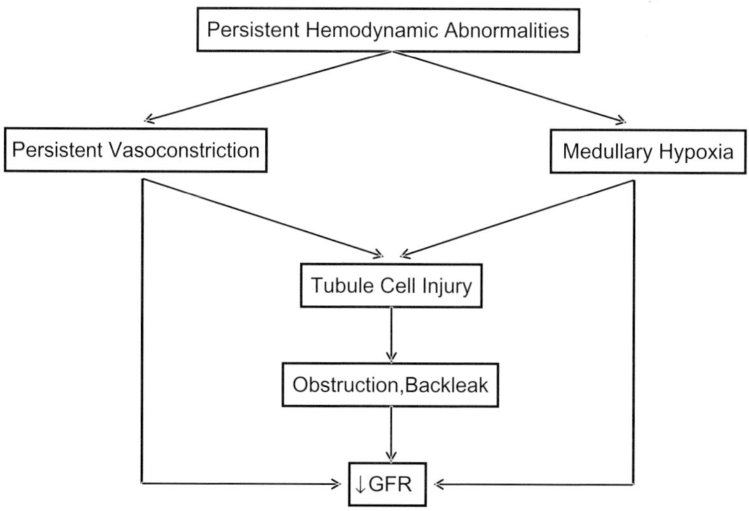

Figure 5. Pathophysiology of intrinsic AKI.

leading to enhanced release of vasoconstrictor endothelin and decreased release of vasodilatory endothelium-derived nitric oxide. In addition, there are regional alterations in renal blood flow, with marked congestion of the outer medullary region. This region normally subsists under low oxygen tensions although paradoxically containing tubule segments with high energy requirements (namely, the S3 segment of the proximal tubule, and the medullary thick ascending limb). The medullary congestion worsens the relative hypoxia, leading to prolongation of the injury, and necrotic tubule cell death. Desquamated tubule cells and brush border membranes combine with Tamm–Horsfall mucoprotein that is normally secreted by the cells of the thick ascending limb, leading to intraluminal cast formation, tubular obstruction, and movement of the glomerular filtrate back into the circulation. However, trials of vasodilators such as dopamine or forced diuresis with furosemide or mannitol have not improved survival or renal recovery in humans with established AKI.

The biochemical consequences of intrinsic AKI due to ischemia-reperfusion injury have been investigated extensively (see Fig. 6). A profound reduction in intracellular ATP content occurs early after ischemic renal

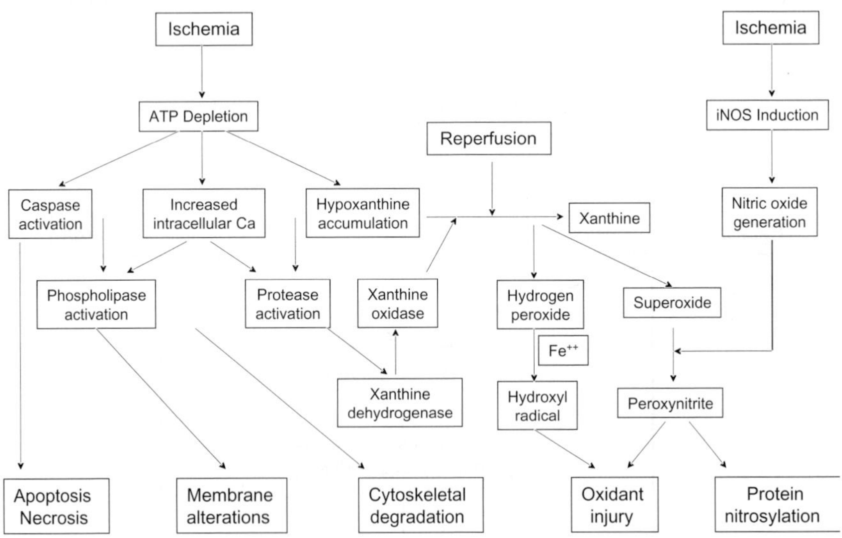

Figure 6. Biochemical consequences of acute ischemia and reperfusion injury to kidney tubule cells; inhibition of these pathways may provide novel therapeutic approaches to AKI.

injury, which triggers several metabolic consequences in tubule cells. Intracellular oxygen deprivation leads to a rapid degradation of ATP to AMP and to hypoxanthine. These metabolites are freely diffusible, and their intracellular depletion precludes re-synthesis of ATP. An increase in free intracellular calcium has also been documented, leading to activation of proteases and phospholipases. Calcium channel blockers may provide some protection from renal injury in the transplant setting, but evidence for their efficacy in other forms of AKI is lacking. During reperfusion, the conversion of accumulated hypoxanthine to xanthine generates hydrogen peroxide and superoxide. In the presence of iron, a molecule that is especially abundant in the kidney after AKI, hydrogen peroxide forms the highly reactive hydroxyl radical. Concomitantly, ischemia induces nitric oxide synthase in tubule cells, and the nitric oxide generated interacts with superoxide to form peroxynitrate, which results in cell damage via oxidant injury, as well as protein nitrosylation. Several antioxidants protect against ischemic and nephrotoxic AKI in animals, but human studies have been inconclusive. Also, the iron scavenger deferoxamine ameliorates AKI in animal models, but the associated toxicity precludes its clinical in humans. Major advances have recently emerged in the area of iron chelation, yielding safer alternatives that hold promise for the treatment of human AKI.

The biologic response of the tubule cell to ischemia is multifaceted, and includes loss of cell polarity and brush borders, cell death, de-differentiation of viable cells, proliferation, and restitution of normal epithelium (see Fig. 7). Ischemia results in a rapid disruption of the apical actin cytoskeleton and redistribution of actin from the apical domain and microvilli into the cytoplasm. This results in loss of brush border membranes, which contribute to cast formation and obstruction. Disruption of the apical cytoskeleton also results in loss of tight junctions and occludens junctions. This accounts for some of the back-leak of glomerular filtrate. Ischemia also results in the early disruption of at least two basolaterally polarized proteins, namely Na^+/K^+-ATPase and integrins. The Na^+/K^+-ATPase is normally tethered to the spectrin-based cytoskeleton at the basolateral domain via the adapter protein ankyrin. This provides the driving force for the normal reabsorption of salt and water by the proximal tubule. Ischemia leads to reversible cytoplasmic accumulation of Na^+/K^+-ATPase, ankyrin, and spectrin in viable cells. The physiological consequence is impaired proximal tubular sodium reabsorption (and therefore high

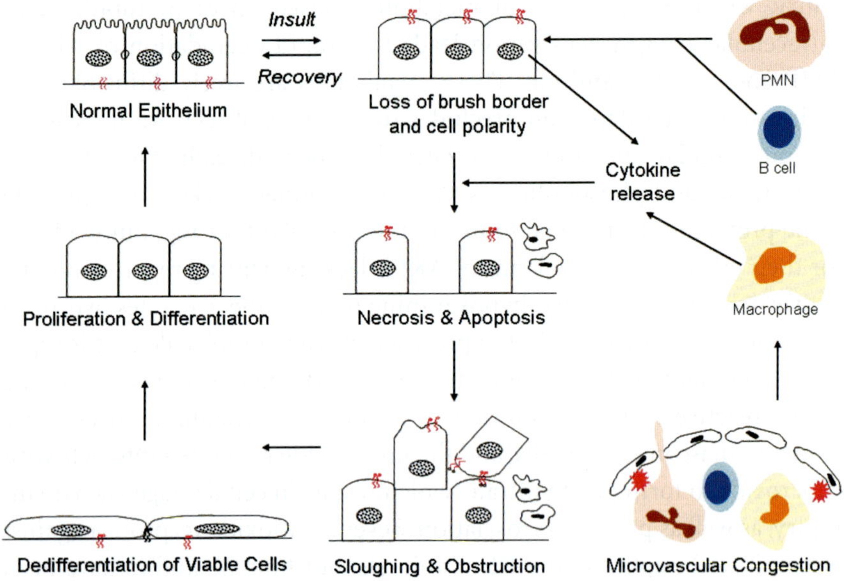

Figure 7. Morphology of intrinsic AKI. The structural consequences of AKI to kidney tubule cells, as well as the accompanying inflammatory response, are shown. Novel therapeutic approaches in AKI have targeted prevention of cell death, acceleration of the endogenous recovery process, and anti-inflammatory agents.

fractional excretion of sodium) that is characteristic of intrinsic AKI. The $\beta 1$ integrins are normally polarized to the basal domain, where they mediate cell-substratum adhesions. Ischemic injury leads to redistribution of integrins to the apical membrane, with consequential detachment of viable cells from the basement membrane. There is good evidence for abnormal adhesion between these exfoliated cells within the tubular lumen, mediated by an interaction between apical integrin and the Arg-Gly-Asp (RGD) motif of integrin receptors. Administration of synthetic RGD compounds attenuates tubular obstruction and renal impairment in animal models of ischemic AKI.

AKI leads to tubule cell death by at least two mechanisms. Necrosis is characterized by loss of membrane integrity, cytoplasmic swelling, nuclear pyknosis, cellular fragmentation, and an inflammatory response. Apoptosis is characterized by cytoplasmic and nuclear shrinkage, DNA fragmentation, and breakdown of the cell into apoptotic bodies that are rapidly removed by phagocytosis. These two forms of cell death frequently coexist, and are two extremes of a continuum. Following AKI, the mode of cell death depends primarily on the severity of the insult and resistance of the cell type. Necrosis occurs following more severe injury and in more susceptible proximal tubules, whereas apoptosis predominates after less severe injury and especially in the relatively resistant distal nephron segments. Mounting evidence now indicates that apoptosis is a major mechanism of early tubule cell death in human AKI. Considerable attention has recently been directed towards unraveling the molecular pathways involved in renal tubule cell apoptosis. Inhibition of apoptotic pathways holds promise; however, current inhibitory maneuvers have only been investigated in animals, provide only partial functional protection, and are most effective when administered before the injury.

Renal tubule cells possess a remarkable ability to regenerate and repair after AKI. Morphologically, repair is heralded by the appearance of de-differentiated tubule cells. In the next phase, the cells upregulate genes encoding for a variety of growth factors such as insulin growth factor 1 (IGF-1), hepatocyte growth factor (HGF), and fibroblast growth factor (FGF), and undergo marked proliferation. In the final phase, cells undergo re-differentiation until the normal fully polarized epithelium is restored. Understanding the molecular mechanisms of repair may provide clues towards accelerating the recovery process. The potential use of growth factors, progenitor cells and stem cells as exciting therapeutic strategies in AKI is currently under investigation.

There is now increasing evidence for a role of inflammation in the pathogenesis of AKI (see Fig. 7). The major components of this response include endothelial injury, leukocyte recruitment, and production of inflammatory mediators by injured tubule cells. Endothelial injury is manifested by endothelial swelling, narrowing of blood vessels, abnormal retrograde blood flow upon reperfusion, and the induction of adhesion molecules such as ICAM-1 and P-selectin that promote endothelial-leukocyte interactions. Morphologically, both neutrophils and T cells have been shown to aggregate in peritubular capillaries following AKI in humans. The sublethally injured proximal tubular epithelium can generate mediators including cytokines such as TNF-α, IL-6, IL-1β, and chemotactic cytokines (MCP-1, IL-8, RANTES) that potentiate the inflammatory response. Strategies that modulate the inflammatory response may provide significant beneficial effects in human AKI.

Pathophysiology of Postrenal AKI

Postrenal AKI is a result of obstruction to the outflow tract on both sides, and is uncommon beyond the neonatal period. Postrenal AKI is usually reversed by relief of the obstruction, but is accompanied by a significant postobstructive diuresis. The common causes of postrenal AKI are listed in Table 3. The pathophysiology and management of the obstructive uropathy syndrome that can result from congenital obstruction are detailed elsewhere in this Manual.

Clinical Manifestations

AKI most commonly presents with progressive accumulation of fluid and/or nitrogenous wastes, in a predisposed patient who has been exposed to one or more of the factors outlined in Tables 1–3. Less frequently, one encounters an increase in BUN and creatinine which is not readily explained. The evaluation requires a complete history, physical examination, laboratory evaluation, renal imaging, and rarely a kidney biopsy. A detailed history of all drugs and medications ingested is especially important, even when another cause for AKI is evident. The initial approach to a patient with known or suspected AKI should be directed towards (a) identifying the underlying cause, (b) distinguishing between prerenal and intrinsic AKI, (c) discriminating between AKI and chronic kidney disease (CKD), (d) determining the severity of AKI, and (e) considering a diagnostic fluid challenge.

Identifying the underlying cause

The initial history should be directed towards uncovering an obvious risk factor (Tables 1–3). Additional relevant aspects of the history and physical examination are shown in Tables 4 and 5, respectively. These, in

Table 3. Common causes of postrenal ARF

Mechanism	Etiology
Congenital	Posterior urethral valves, uroteropelvic junction obstruction
Acquired	Calculi, clots, neurogenic bladder, drugs that cause urinary retention

Table 4. History taking in patients with suspected AKI

- Fluid loss
  - Diarrhea, vomiting
  - Burns
  - Surgery
  - Shock
- Nephrotoxic agents
  - Nonsteroidal anti-inflammatory drugs
  - Aminoglycosides
  - Contrast agents
- Glomerular disease
  - Streptococcal infection (*Poststreptococcal glomerulonephritis*)
  - Bloody diarrhea (Hemolytic-uremic syndrome)
  - Fever, joint complaints, rash (Systemic lupus erythematosus)
- Obstruction
  - Complete anuria
  - Poor urinary stream

Table 5. Physical findings in AKI

- Signs of intravascular volume depletion
- Signs of fluid overload (edema, hypertension)
- Signs of underlying renal disease
  - Butterfly rash, joint swelling (Systemic lupus erythematosus)
  - Purpuric rash (Henoch–Schönlein purpura)
  - Fever, macular rash (Interstitial nephritis)
  - Palpably enlarged kidneys (Polycystic/multicystic kidney disease, renal vein thrombosis)
- Signs of obstruction
  - Poor urinary stream
  - Palpably enlarged bladder
  - Therapeutic catheterization

combination with urinalysis including microscopy, will yield the etiology of AKI in the majority of cases. Typically, the urine in prerenal AKI contains only a few hyaline and fine granular casts, with little protein or blood. In contrast, proteinuria and hematuria are prominent in intrinsic AKI.

A heme positive urine by dipstick in the absence of RBCs suggests hemolysis or rhabdomyolysis. Urine microscopy reveals dysmorphic RBCs in primary glomerular diseases, and WBCs in pyelonephritis or interstitial nephritis. Broad brown granular casts are typically encountered in ischemic or toxic AKI, whereas RBC casts are characteristic of acute glomerulonephritis and WBC casts indicate interstitial nephritis or pyelonephritis.

Distinguishing between prerenal and intrinsic AKI

This determination is important because (a) treatment and prognosis are different, and (b) prompt identification and management of prerenal AKI can prevent progression to intrinsic AKI. The distinction is based on the principle that prerenal AKI is associated with maximal reabsorption of solutes and water by the intact proximal tubule, whereas the tubule cell damage typical of intrinsic AKI results in impaired reabsorptive capacity of the proximal tubule. Urinary indices based on this principle are shown in Table 6.

The fractional excretion of sodium (FE_{Na}) is a convenient bed-side measurement for making this distinction. It is calculated from measured concentrations of sodium (Na) and creatinine (Cr) in the urine (U) and plasma (P), as follows:

$$FE_{Na} = ([U/P]Na)/([U/P]Cr) \times 100$$

Interpretation of these indices must take into account any previous fluid administration, or any abnormal substances in the urine such as protein, glucose, mannitol, contrast agents, and diuretics. The FE_{Na} can be low (<1%) in conditions such as congestive heart failure, nephrotic

Table 6. Urinary indices in AKI

Measurement	Prerenal AKI	Intrinsic AKI
Urine specific gravity	>1,020	<1,012
Urine/plasma creatinine	>40	<20
Urine Na (mEq/L)	<20	>40
FE_{Na}	<1%	>2%
FE_{Urea}	<35%	>50%

syndrome, contrast nephropathy, or pigment nephropathy. The fractional excretion of urea (FE_{Urea}) has been proposed as a more accurate determinant of prerenal AKI, especially in patients receiving diuretics.

By the same principle of increased proximal tubular solute reabsorption, the BUN/creatinine ratio in the serum is markedly elevated (>20) in prerenal AKI. This is because the proximal tubule can avidly reabsorb urea but is impermeable to creatinine. However, increases in BUN without AKI can be encountered in patients receiving steroids or total parenteral nutrition, in catabolic states, and those with gastrointestinal bleeding.

Distinguishing between AKI and CKD

Kidney and bladder ultrasound is a sensitive, widely available, noninvasive modality that can differentiate not only between AKI and CKD, but can also rule out postrenal causes. Typically, the kidneys in AKI are normal in size or enlarged (due to inflammation or edema), with increased echogenicity, whereas those in CKD are frequently small and shrunken. Other distinguishing features are shown in Table 7.

Determining the severity of AKI

Estimating the baseline pre-illness serum creatinine can determine the severity of AKI, and allow for classification based on the RIFLE criteria. This is best achieved when a previously drawn serum creatinine level is available. If not, the baseline kidney function in children can be estimated using the Schwartz formula:

$$\text{Estimated creatinine clearance in ml/min} = kL/Pcr$$

Table 7. Differentiating AKI from CKD

Acute Kidney Injury	Chronic Kidney Disease
Progressive rise in BUN and Cr	Stable elevated BUN and Cr
History of ARF etiology	History of chronic hypertension
Normal growth	Stunted growth
Normal bones	Renal osteodystrophy
No broad urinary casts	Broad waxy urinary casts
Anemia usually mild	Anemia usually severe
Normal or enlarged kidney size	Small shrunken kidneys

where L = height (cm), Pcr = plasma creatinine in mg/dl, and k = proportionality constant, the value of which is 0.45 in the first year of life, 0.55 in children and adolescent girls, and 0.70 in adolescent boys. Recent investigations have allowed for a simplification of this formula, and have indicated that a single uniform k value of 0.413 provides a good approximation of GFR in children of all ages and both genders.

Another important index of AKI severity is the degree of fluid overload. Extent of fluid overload during a hospitalization period can be estimated by the following formula:

$$\%\ \text{Fluid} = \frac{[\text{Total fluid in (Liters)} - \text{Total fluid out (Liters)}]}{\text{Admission weight in kg} \times 100}$$

Additional estimates of the degree of fluid overload may be obtained by determining total in-hospital weight gain, amount of peripheral edema, degree of pulmonary edema by imaging studies, and serial measures of central venous pressure. Routine laboratory evaluation for the presence of metabolic complications can also assist in establishing AKI severity.

Considering a diagnostic fluid challenge

A common clinical scenario is one where a patient presents with an increase in BUN and serum creatinine, history and physical findings are consistent with a prerenal etiology, but the duration of the prerenal insult is unknown. Another common diagnostic dilemma occurs when a subject presents with an increase in serum creatinine but the cause is unclear. In both these cases, a fluid challenge may be diagnostic as well as therapeutic. Typically, fluid challenges in children consist of normal saline in the dose of 10–20 ml/kg/hr, repeated once or twice until urine output improves. A reduction in BUN and serum creatinine would indicate a pre-renal etiology, whereas an absence of improvement in these parameters (and/or the development of fluid overload) would confirm the diagnosis of intrinsic AKI.

Problems with serum creatinine measurements in AKI

A progressive increase in serum creatinine (1–2 mg/dL/day) is a hallmark of intrinsic AKI, and has served as a biomarker of AKI for several decades. However, serum creatinine concentration is a poor AKI biomarker for several reasons: (a) it does not differentiate the nature, type and timing of the renal insult; (b) changes in creatinine lag behind changes in GFR until steady state has been reached; which can take several days; (c) dialysis clears serum creatinine, rendering this marker useless in assessing improvement in renal function once dialysis has begun; and (d) normal serum creatinine can vary widely with age, gender, diet, muscle mass, nutrition status, medications, and hydration status. Thus, serum creatinine is an imperfect and delayed marker of AKI. In the acute setting, it is estimated greater than 50% of kidney function must be lost before serum creatinine begins to rise. However, animal studies have shown that while AKI can be prevented and/or treated by several maneuvers, these measures must be instituted very early after the insult, well before the serum creatinine rises. The lack of early biomarkers of AKI in humans has impaired the ability to launch potentially effective therapies in a timely manner.

Fortunately, the genomic and proteomic tools of modern science have identified novel markers of early structural injury to the kidney, which appear in the urine or plasma before a rise in serum creatinine is detected. Many are presently being developed and validated as early noninvasive biomarkers for the prediction of AKI and its clinical outcomes in humans. This is a rapidly evolving field, and the current status of the most promising examples is shown in Tables 8 and 9.

Complications

AKI is associated with a number of life-threatening complications, which the clinician must diligently monitor (see Table 10).

Hyponatremia is a common laboratory finding and usually dilutional (secondary to fluid retention and administration of hypotonic fluids). Less common causes of hyponatremia include sodium depletion (hyponatremic dehydration) and hyperglycemia (serum sodium concentration decreases by 1.6 mEq/L for every 100 mg/dL increase in serum glucose above 100 mg/dL). Hypernatremia in AKI is usually a result of excessive sodium administration (inappropriate fluid therapy or overzealous sodium bicarbonate administration).

Hyperkalemia is due to the reduction in GFR, reduction in tubular secretion of potassium, increased catabolism, and metabolic acidosis

Table 8. Novel urinary biomarkers for the early diagnosis of AKI

Biomarker	Cardiopulmonary bypass (CPB)	Contrast-induced nephropathy	Kidney tsransplant (Tx)	ICU or emergency room
NGAL	2 hrs post-CPB 2 days pre-AKI	2 hrs post contrast 1–2 days pre-AKI	6 hrs post-Tx 2–3 days pre-DGF	On admission 2 days pre-AKI
IL-18	12 hrs post-CPB 1–2 days pre-AKI	Not increased	12 hrs post-Tx 2–3 days pre DGF	2 days pre-AKI
KIM-1	12 hrs post-CPB 1–2 days pre-AKI	Not tested	Not tested in acute setting	Not tested in acute setting

NGAL, neutrophil gelatinase-associated lipocalin. IL-18, interleukin 18. KIM-1, kidney injury molecule 1. AKI, defined as a 50% or greater increase in serum creatinine from baseline. DGF, defined as dialysis requirement within the first week after transplant. Times shown are the earliest time points when the biomarker becomes significantly increased from baseline.

Table 9. Novel urinary biomarkers for the prediction of AKI outcomes

Biomarker name	Cardiopulmonary bypass (CPB)	Kidney transplant	ICU or emergency room
NGAL	Predicts AKI duration, severity, dialysis, death	Predicts AKI duration	Predicts AKI duration, severity, and dialysis
IL-18	Predicts AKI duration	Predicts AKI duration	Predicts death
KIM-1	Not tested	Predicts long term graft loss	Predicts dialysis and death

NGAL, neutrophil gelatinase-associated lipocalin. IL-18, interleukin 18. KIM-1, kidney injury molecule 1. AKI, defined as a 50% or greater increase in serum creatinine from baseline.

Table 10. Major complications of AKI

Metabolic	Cardiovascular	Gastrointestinal	Neurologic	Hematologic	Infectious
Hyperkalemia	Fluid overload	Nausea, vomiting, anorexia	Altered mental status	Anemia	Pneumonia
Metabolic acidosis	Arrythmias	Malnutrition	Irritability	Bleeding	Sepsis
Hyponatremia	Pericarditis	Gastritis	Seizures		
Hypocalcemia	Hypertension	GI Bleeding	Somnolence		
Hyperphosphatemia		GI Ulcers	Coma		

(each 0.1 unit reduction in arterial pH raises serum potassium by 0.3 mEq/L). Hyperkalemia is most pronounced in patients with excessive endogenous production (rhabdomyolysis, hemolysis, and tumor lysis syndrome). Symptoms are nonspecific and may include malaise, nausea, and muscle weakness. EKG should be evaluated for tall peaked T waves, prolonged PR interval, flattened P waves, widened QRS complex, ventricular tachycardia, and fibrillation.

A high anion gap metabolic acidosis is common, and is secondary to the impaired renal excretion of acid and the impaired reabsorption and regeneration of bicarbonate. Acidosis is most severe in shock, sepsis, or impaired respiratory compensation.

Hypocalcemia is commonly encountered in AKI, and is due to increased serum phosphate and impaired renal conversion of vitamin D to the active form. Hypocalcemia is most pronounced in patients with rhabdomyolysis. Metabolic acidosis increases the fraction of ionized calcium (the active form). Therefore, overzealous bicarbonate therapy can decrease the concentration of ionized calcium and precipitate symptoms of hypocalcemia, including tetany, seizures and cardiac arrythmias. Hyperphosphatemia in AKI is primarily due to impaired renal excretion, and can aggravate hypocalcemia.

The accumulation of incompletely identified "uremic toxins" is postulated to play a major role in the cardiac, gastrointestinal, and neuropsychiatric disturbances. The degree of fluid overload has emerged as an independent predictor of mortality in children and adults with AKI. On the other hand, during recovery from AKI, the vigorous diuretic phase may be accompanied by significant volume depletion, hypernatremia, hypokalemia, and hypophosphatemia.

Management

Fluids, electrolytes, and nutrition

Normalization of intravascular volume, blood pressure and cardiovascular function are the cornerstones of initial AKI management. AKI associated with intravascular volume depletion requires prompt and vigorous fluid resuscitation with normal saline (20 ml/kg over 30–60 minutes, repeat twice if necessary). This should result in urine output within 4–6 hours; if not, the bladder should be catheterized to confirm anuria. Potassium is contraindicated until urine flow is well established and serum potassium begins to normalize. Patients who are oliguric should be provided fluids to equal insensible water loss plus output replacement. Oliguria with fluid overload is initially managed with fluid and salt restriction, and diuretics. Resistance to diuretics (typical of intrinsic AKI) may necessitate dialysis. Aggressive nutritional support is crucial to enhance recovery. Adequate calories to provide for maintenance requirements and combat excessive catabolism should be administered, by oral, enteral, or parenteral routes as appropriate. If adequate nutrition cannot be achieved because of fluid restriction, early institution of dialysis should be strongly considered.

Table 11. Nondialytic treatment of hyperkalemia

Agent	Mechanism	Dose	Onset of action
Sodium polystyrene sulfonate	Exchanges Na^+ for K^+ across colonic mucosa	1 g/kg PO or PR with sorbitol	1–2 hours
Calcium gluconate	Stabilizes the myocardial membrane potential	1 ml/kg IV over 5–15 min	Immediate
Glucose and insulin	Stimulates cellular uptake of K^+	Glucose 0.5 g/kg, Insulin 0.1 U/kg over 30 min	30 minutes
β-Agonists (albuterol)	Stimulates cellular uptake of K^+	5–10 mg dose by nebulizer	30 minutes
Sodium bicarbonate	Shifts K^+ into cells	1 mEq/kg IV over 10 min	15 minutes

The management of hyperkalemia deserves special mention, and is detailed in Table 11. Mild to moderate hyperkalemia (serum potassium of 5.5–6.5 mEq/L) is treated by eliminating all sources of potassium from the diet or IV fluids, and administration of an ion exchange resin such as sodium polystyrene sulfonate. This therapy requires several hours of contact with the colonic mucosa to be effective. In addition, patients with hyperkalemia who continue to have some urine output may benefit from the kaliuresis induced by intravenous administration of loop diuretics such as furosemide, but fluid depletion and hypotension should be avoided. Emergency treatment is indicated when the serum potassium exceeds 6.5 mEq/L or if ECG changes are present. In addition to ion exchange resin, such patients should emergently receive calcium gluconate to counteract the effects of hyperkalemia on the myocardium. Uptake of potassium by cells can alternatively be stimulated by infusion of glucose and insulin (in the absence of significant fluid overload), the β-agonist albuterol by nebulizer, or intravenous sodium bicarbonate. Use of bicarbonate therapy in AKI can precipitate hypocalcemia and hypernatremia, and bicarbonate administration is currently advocated only in the presence of significant metabolic acidosis. In practice, the definitive therapy for significant hyperkalemia in oliguric AKI is dialysis, and the nondialytic therapy outlined above serves mostly to tide over the crisis.

Medications

Nephrotoxic agents should be avoided in AKI as they may worsen the injury and delay recovery of function. The dose of all medications should be adjusted based on residual renal function. However, patients with AKI in the early phase with a rising creatinine should be assumed to have a GFR of less than 10 ml/min, irrespective of the absolute value of the serum creatinine.

Pharmacologic therapies

Over the past few decades, advances in AKI basic research have identified several therapeutic targets that have been successfully employed in animal models. However, translational research efforts in humans have not yielded encouraging results to date. This may be attributed, at least in part, due to the delay in initiating therapies imposed by the imprecision of currently available AKI biomarkers. As novel early AKI biomarkers are validated and enter mainstream clinical practice, it is likely that many of these therapies may prove efficacious. The current status of these interventions is reviewed below.

"Renal dose" dopamine (1–3 mcg/kg/min) has been shown in healthy humans to increase renal blood flow and GFR. However, this did not prevent or ameliorate the course of ischemic or nephrotoxic AKI in prospective controlled human trials. Dopamine is potentially toxic, and can induce tachyarrythmias and myocardial ischemia. Therefore, its use for the treatment of AKI cannot be recommended at this time. Fenoldopam is a selective postsynaptic dopamine agonist that mediates more powerful renal vasodilatation and natriuresis than dopamine. However, it can induce hypotension by decreasing peripheral vascular resistance. Previous small studies suggested a renoprotective effect of fenoldopam in critically ill adult populations, but subsequent larger randomized controlled trials did not reduce mortality or dialysis requirement in critically ill patients with intrinsic AKI. Selective intrarenal administration of fenoldopam, via specially designed vascular catheters, has recently proven efficacious in treating AKI in pilot studies of critically ill adults.

Atrial natriuretic peptide (ANP) is normally released from myocytes in response to atrial stretch in states of volume overload. Its physiologic role is to dilate the afferent arterioles and increase GFR. A synthetic analogue of ANP (anaritide) showed promise in initial studies but was not efficacious in a large clinical trial of adults with established AKI, since it did not improve clinical outcomes such as dialysis requirement or mortality. However, the two limitations of this study were (a) the dose of anaritide used resulted in hypotension, and (b) anaritide was administered after intrinsic AKI was firmly established (mean serum creatinine was 4.5 mg/dl at enrollment), which is likely too late for any therapy to be effective.

The use of high-dose intravenous loop diuretics such as furosemide in patients with oliguric AKI has recently been questioned. While this approach may increase urine output and counteract fluid overload, there is no evidence that it alters mortality or dialysis requirement in patients with established AKI. In addition, loop diuretics carry the significant risk of irreversible ototoxicity and exacerbation of any prerenal component of the AKI. Their use is therefore best restricted to the conservative management of fluid overload in subjects at risk of developing oliguria, and as an initial approach to the prevention of AKI.

Renal replacement therapy

The common indications for acute renal replacement therapy in AKI include (a) fluid overload that is unresponsive to diuretics or is a hindrance to provision of adequate nutrition and other aspects of standard of care, (b) hyperkalemia that is unresponsive to nondialytic therapy, (c) refractory hypertension, and (d) symptomatic uremia, including pericarditis, pleuritis, and neurologic symptoms. The choices available include hemodialysis (HD), peritoneal dialysis (PD), and continuous renal replacement therapy (CRRT). These modalities are described in detail in other chapters, and only general comments pertaining to AKI are included here. The choice of dialysis modality depends on the clinical status of the patient, the expertise of the physician, and the availability of appropriate resources. Hemodialysis requires central vascular access, specialized equipment and technical personnel, anticoagulation (except in patients with coagulopathy), and the ability to tolerate a large extracorporeal volume. Critically ill patients frequently require additional pressor support for effective hemodialysis. The advantage of acute HD lies in its ability to rapidly correct imbalances in fluid, electrolyte and acid–base status.

The advantages of PD include ease of performance, and no requirement for specialized equipment, personnel, or systemic anticoagulation. Peritoneal dialysis is the therapy of choice in neonates and small infants. CRRT is especially useful in the presence of hemodynamic instability and multiorgan dysfunction, since it allows for gentle, continuous management of fluid overload.

Outcomes and Prognosis

AKI has serious short- and long-term consequences. Severe AKI requiring renal replacement therapy in children and adults has been associated with a mortality rate of about 50%, and this has not changed appreciably over the past three decades. It is now clear that patients die of AKI and its complications, and not simply with AKI. Children who "recover" from AKI secondary to hemolytic-uremic syndrome exhibit a 10–25% rate of progression to CKD or end-stage renal disease (ESRD). Long-term follow-up of premature infants with AKI has shown a 45% rate of CKD. In older children who survived dialysis-requiring AKI, about 60% showed signs of CKD and about 20% progressed to end-stage renal disease at 3–5 year follow up. Collectively, these data strongly suggest that long-term follow-up is warranted for children who survive AKI.

Prevention

Vigorous fluid administration has been successfully employed to prevent AKI in patients at high risk, including cardiac surgery, renal transplantation, hemoglobinuria, myoglobinuria, early tumor lysis syndrome, and administration of nephrotoxic agents, such as radiocontrast, cisplatin, and amphotericin. Adjunctive pharmacologic agents for the prevention of AKI, including diuretics and "renal dose" dopamine, are still widely used in the intensive care setting, even though they have been shown to be ineffective and perhaps even deleterious. The administration of these agents early in the course of AKI does not alter the natural history of the disease, but can potentially convert the syndrome from oliguric to a nonoliguric form and therefore simplify fluid, electrolyte and nutritional therapy. One common and reasonably safe clinical approach is to use high dose furosemide (2–5 mg/kg/dose bolus followed by a continuous infusion of

0.1–0.3 mg/kg/hr) for oliguria of less than 48 hours' duration that has not responded to adequate hydration. Furosemide should be discontinued if bolus doses do not result in diuresis, and care should be taken to avoid hypotension since that can increase the risk of death and nonrecovery of renal function. The use of intravenous sodium bicarbonate and oral antioxidants such as N-acetylcysteine for the prevention of contrast-induced nephropathy has been advocated, but definitive evidence is lacking.

Summary

AKI represents a very significant and potentially devastating problem in pediatric medicine. The precise incidence of pediatric AKI is not known, but appears to be rising. Serious forms of AKI are often a hospital-acquired complication of other systemic illnesses. Despite many improvements in supportive care, AKI in the critical care setting is still associated with an unacceptably high mortality rate. Many advances in basic research have illuminated the pathogenesis of AKI and have paved the way for successful therapeutic approaches in animal models. However, translational efforts in humans have yielded disappointing results. One reason for this is the lack of early markers for AKI, akin to troponins in acute myocardial disease, and hence a delay in initiating therapy. In current clinical practice, AKI is typically diagnosed by measuring serum creatinine, which is an unreliable indicator during acute changes in kidney function. However, animal studies have shown that while AKI can be prevented and/or treated by several maneuvers, these measures must be instituted very early after the insult. The lack of early biomarkers of acute renal injury in humans has crippled our ability to launch potentially effective therapies in a timely manner. Indeed, human investigations that have now established that the earlier the intervention, the better the chance of ameliorating the renal dysfunction. Conversely, the longer the duration of AKI, the greater the mortality. Fortunately, several potential candidates are currently being developed and tested as early biomarkers of AKI. Examples include NGAL, KIM-1, IL-18, and cystatin C. It is likely that not any one biomarker but a collection of strategically selected proteins may provide the "AKI panel" to predict AKI and its clinical outcomes. Such a tool would be indispensable for the timely institution of potentially effective therapies in human AKI, a common clinical condition still associated with a dismal prognosis where early intervention is desperately needed.

Suggested Reading

Akcan-Arikan A, Zappitelli M, Loftis LL, *et al.* (2007) Modified RIFLE criteria in critically ill children with acute kidney injury. *Kidney Int* **71**: 1028–1035.

Askenazi DJ, Feig DI, Graham NM, *et al.* (2006) 3–5 year longitudinal follow up of pediatric patients after acute renal failure. *Kidney Int* **69**: 184–189.

Bellomo R, Ronco C, Kellum JA, *et al.* (2004) Acute renal failure — definition, outcome measures, animal models, fluid therapy and information technology needs: the Second International Consensus Conference of the Acute Dialysis Quality Initiative (ADQI) Group. *Crit Care* **8**: R204–212.

Devarajan P, Goldstein SL. (2007) Acute renal failure. In: Kher KK, Schnaper HW, Makker SP. (eds.), *Clinical Pediatric Nephrology*, (2nd ed.), Informal Healthcare, pp. 363–376.

Devarajan P. (2006) Update on mechanisms of ischemic acute kidney injury. *J Am Soc Nephrol* **17**: 1503–1520.

Devarajan P. (2008) Neutrophil gelatinase-associated lipocalin — an emerging troponin for kidney injury. *Nephrol Dial Transplant* **23**: 3737–3743.

Devarajan P. (2008) The future of pediatric acute kidney injury management — Biomarkers. *Semin Nephrol* **28**: 493–498.

Nguyen MT, Devarajan P. (2008) Biomarkers for the early detection of acute kidney injury. *Pediatr Nephrol* **23**: 2151–2157.

Zappitelli M. (2008) Epidemiology and diagnosis of acute kidney injury. *Semin Nephrol* **28**: 436–446.

Part XII

Dialysis Therapy in AKI

36

Dialysis Therapy in Acute Kidney Injury

Shaunna Lyon, Patrick D. Brophy and Carla M. Nester

Introduction

The treatment of acute kidney injury (AKI) with dialysis in the pediatric population requires special considerations not commonly encountered in the care of adult patients. For example, children with AKI may range in weight from a 1 kg preterm neonate to an obese 200 kg adolescent. In addition, there are disease states in the pediatric population that may require acute renal replacement therapy (RRT) in the absence of significant kidney disease. Postoperative infants with congenital heart defects and infants with inborn errors of metabolism are two such examples.

Indications for initiation of RRT in AKI are extrapolations of those traditionally used for dialysis initiation in end-stage renal disease (ESRD) (see Table 1). In many circumstances, medical management of uremic

Table 1. Indications for dialysis

Acidosis
Electrolyte Abnormalities
Hyperkalemia
Hyperphosphatemia
Intoxications
Lithium
Methyl alcohol
Salicylate
Overload
Fluid overload with pulmonary edema and/or respiratory failure
Oliguria requiring fluid restriction limiting nutritional intake
Uremia with encephalopathy or bleeding
Inborn errors of metabolism
Urea cycle defects

toxins, fluid overload, electrolyte abnormalities, and blood pressure control may be sufficient, but dialysis may become necessary if conservative measures fail.

The two main goals of RRT of pediatric AKI are improved solute clearance and fluid removal (ultrafiltration). There are a variety of dialysis modalities available that will achieve these goals. These modalities include peritoneal dialysis (PD), intermittent hemodialysis (IHD) and continuous renal replacement therapies (CRRT). The continuous renal replacement therapies currently include continuous venovenous hemofiltration (CVVH), continuous venovenous hemodialysis (CVVHD), continuous venovenous hemodiafiltration (CVVHDF), slow continuous ultrafiltration (SCUF), slow low efficiency dialysis (SLED). Choosing an appropriate modality depends on both the clinical status of the individual patient and the specific indication for dialysis. There are several patient characteristics that may influence the modality chosen (see Table 2) including patient age, size, acuity, comorbidities, and extent of other organ system involvement.

Table 2. Factors affecting choice of renal replacement therapy modality

Patient-centered Factors
Age
Size
Illness acuity
Mechanical ventilation
Inotropic support
Presence of comorbidities
Presence/extent of multiorgan system involvement
Presence of pulmonary edema
Cardiac arrhythmias
Mental status
Quantification of urine output
Institution-centered Factors
Resource availability
Type of institution
Type of intensive care unit
Type of provider
Cost of therapy
Provider-centered Factors
Individual physician beliefs
Perceived cost of therapy

The presence and volume of urine are important in determining the patient's ability to handle both fluid and solute load. A comprehensive patient assessment should precede any decision regarding RRT modality choice in order to determine the major issue(s) to be addressed with RRT for each patient. It is also vitally important to consider which modalities might be feasible given the overall clinical status of the patient. For example, a patient with mild fluid overload and no respiratory compromise may not require rapid fluid removal. Such a patient may be best managed with PD. On the contrary, a patient with severe hyperkalemia may be better served by IHD. Institutional factors and individual physician beliefs may also impact modality choice.

While indications for dialysis initiation are well understood, very little data exists regarding the timing of initiation. For example, should dialytic therapy be initiated prior to the onset of symptoms or after symptoms/complications have become apparent? Over the last several years both pediatric and adult data have supported earlier initiation. Because AKI is potentially reversible, it may not be appropriate to delay initiation of dialysis. Ongoing areas of investigation include the impact that timing of initiation has on outcomes.

The last decade has seen changes in the treatment approaches to AKI. There are few studies in children comparing outcomes of AKI based on various renal replacement therapies used. A wide range of mortality rates in children requiring RRT have been reported: from 35–73%. Additionally, there has been the perception that patients who received CRRT had higher mortality rates. In practice however, CRRT has generally been used in pediatric patients who have multiorgan system dysfunction, tend to be hemodynamically unstable and require vasopressor support. Given these patient variables, it is not surprising that the patient population that received RRT had higher mortality rates. Some more recent pediatric data has suggested that using severity of illness scores and earlier intervention may be providing improved care, regardless of modality used.

There is little agreement regarding the timing of therapy discontinuation. Factors that influence discontinuation of therapy, regardless of modality, are urine output, hemodynamic stability, nutritional status, volume status, clinical improvement or deterioration, family wishes, long-term patient needs, and available resources.

The remainder of this chapter will address the use of the following renal replacement modalities for the treatment of pediatric AKI: PD, intermittent hemodialysis, and continuous renal replacement therapy (CVVH, CVVHD, CVVHDF). The basic elements of each of the modalities will be covered. The chapter will also review issues of access, dialysis solutions, the dialysis prescription, the use of anticoagulation and the therapeutic advantages and disadvantages of each modality (see Table 3).

Peritoneal Dialysis

Historically, PD has been the primary RRT modality utilized in children, and it has been used effectively for the management of AKI. Most

Table 3. Comparisons of dialysis modality choices

Variable	PD	IHD	CRRT
Complexity	Low	Intermediate	High
Cost	Low/moderate	Moderate/high	High
Vascular access required	No	Yes	Yes
Anticoagulation	Not required	Not required; usually used at least intermittently	Yes, continuous
Continuous therapy	Yes	No	Yes
Hemodynamic stability	Yes	No	Yes
Ultrafiltration control	Variable	Intermittent	Yes, pump controlled
Metabolic control	Yes	Yes, intermittent	Yes
Optimal nutrition	No	No	Yes
ICU nursing support	Moderate level of support	No	High level of support
Dialysis nursing support	Institution dependent	Yes	Institution dependent
Patient mobility	If intermittent	No	No
Rapid poison removal	No	Yes	Variable, depending on pt size; dose
Continuous toxin removal	Variable, larger toxins not well cleared	No	Yes
Use in inborn errors of metabolism	No	Yes	Yes

clinicians have a relatively greater comfort level with this therapy. The use of PD is critical in the treatment of AKI in facilities and countries where pediatric HD and CRRT are not available.

In PD, dialysate is instilled into the peritoneal cavity where the peritoneal lining, which is a semipermeable membrane, acts as a dialyzer. Solutes filter across the membrane from blood into dialysate via diffusion, moving from an area of high concentration to low concentration. In PD, ultrafiltration (fluid removal) occurs as a consequence of an osmotic gradient between the hyperosmolar dialysate and peritoneal capillary blood.

For PD, access can be safely and easily obtained even in a hemodynamically unstable child. Though PD catheters are often placed in the operating room, some facilities have the capability to place acute PD catheters percutaneously at the bedside, allowing for relatively quick initiation of therapy. Freshly placed catheters are at the greatest risk for infection and leakage. Because of the tendency to leak, dialysis is usually initiated with small dialysate volumes, although this may limit the ability to achieve adequate clearance. Other complications of bedside placement of acute PD catheters include bladder and bowel perforation as well as bleeding. Placement of Tenckhoff catheters in the operating room is recommended when the clinical situation and patient status allow it. Most neonates and small infants generally tolerate the placement of a PD catheter without difficulty.

Once access has been established, little other specialized equipment is required for the successful institution of PD, as compared to other RRT modalities. Continuous PD may be provided with either a gravity dependent manual system or via an automated cycler. Manual PD in infants can be performed utilizing the preassembled Dialy–Nate® system (Utah Medical Products). Manual exchange systems are relatively inexpensive, and are readily available worldwide compared to the equipment required for either IHD or CRRT; however, they can be labor intensive for the bedside nurse. Automated cyclers are also available and low volume cyclers can deliver PD to infants.

Dialysate solution, most often glucose based, is widely available through commercial vendors. Glucose serves as an osmotic agent, creating a gradient that favors net movement of water into the peritoneal cavity. Peritoneal dialysis solutions are available with dextrose concentrations of

Table 4. Complications associated with dialysis modalities

Modality	Complication
All	Volume depletion
	Removal of drugs and nutrients
	Electrolyte imbalance
	Access infection
	Access malfunction (leak, hemorrhage, obstruction, thrombosis)
Peritoneal dialysis	Hyperglycemia
	Hydrothorax
	Infection (exit site, peritonitis)
	Hypothermia
	Hyponatremia
	Drainage failure
	Respiratory compromise
Intermittent hemodialysis	Hypothermia
	Disequilibrium syndrome
	Membrane bioincompatibility
CRRT	Hypothermia
	Membrane bioincompatibility

1.5, 2.5, and 4.25%. It is important to recognize that glucose absorption into blood provides additional calories in patients receiving PD, which may be problematic for patients without adequate insulin release. Peritoneal dialysis solutions also contain physiologic amounts of sodium, calcium, magnesium, and a buffer, usually lactate, which is converted hepatically to bicarbonate. In patients with hepatic dysfunction or lactic acidosis, lactate solutions should be used with caution. Bicarbonate-based dialysis solutions are available outside the United States. Alternatively, in the United States, custom-made bicarbonate-based solutions can be prepared in hospital pharmacies, but needs to be done cautiously to minimize risk of human error in the preparation. Additives to dialysate include heparin to prevent fibrin clot formation; and antibiotics to treat peritonitis. Dialysate solutions should be warmed to body temperature prior to infusion to avoid discomfort and enhance solute transport/clearance.

The components of an acute PD prescription are length of dialysis session, dialysate composition, exchange volume, inflow and outflow (drain) times, dwell time, number of exchanges, and if necessary, dialysate additives. The length of the dialysis session can vary significantly as it depends on the cause and duration of kidney injury. The patient's clinical status and laboratory studies should be closely monitored with periodic adjustments to the dialysis prescription being made based on reassessment. The choice of dextrose concentration, the major determinant of ultrafiltration, depends on the degree of fluid overload and should be individualized. For example, the use of a 1.5% dextrose solution would be appropriate in patients who are hemodynamically unstable or who have mild fluid overload, whereas higher dextrose concentrations may be necessary for greater ultrafiltration. The exchange volume is the amount of dialysate instilled into the peritoneal cavity during a single exchange; and is affected by estimated peritoneal cavity size, presence of pulmonary compromise, presence of hernias, and catheter leakage risk. Initial exchange volumes generally approximate 10 mL/kg and is gradually increased over several days as tolerated to a maximum of approximately 50 ml/kg (not to exceed 2.5 L). The inflow (fill) time, the time required to instill the dialysate into the peritoneal cavity, a process driven by gravity in a manual system, usually takes 10–15 minutes. Factors that influence the fill time include dialysate volume, degree of elevation of the dialysate bag, and the presence of catheter resistance (i.e. kinking, omental obstruction). Keeping fill time to a minimum improves dialysis efficiency. The dwell time (the period for which the exchange volume remains in the peritoneal cavity) will determine solute removal. Generally, 30 minute dwell times are considered optimal, allowing for the most favorable gradients for solute clearance and fluid removal. Dwell times can be lengthened as the need for RRT decreases. Outflow time is the time required to drain the effluent from the abdominal cavity and is comprised of the dialysate, plus an ultrafiltrate volume. Drain time and volume can be manipulated to some extent by adjusting the height of the drainage bag. Incomplete drainage may result in progressive accumulation of dialysate in the peritoneal cavity, leading to respiratory compromise or abdominal discomfort. Drainage problems are usually associated with catheter malfunction due to intestinal omental wrap or fibrin clot induced obstruction, but may be related to constipation as well. The number of exchanges is usually determined by the amount of fluid and solute removal required in a particular patient and may range from 6–24 exchanges in a 24-hour period.

Despite the availability and ease of PD, there are disadvantages that may preclude its use. The gradual nature of the therapy is both an advantage and disadvantage. Because ultrafiltration and solute clearance occur slowly, PD is not optimal in patients with severe volume overload, hyperkalemia, or intoxications who require more rapid ultrafiltration or solute clearance. Ultrafiltration volumes cannot be as precisely controlled as they can be with IHD or CRRT. Patients with respiratory compromise or preload dependent cardiac physiology may not tolerate large volumes of dialysate in the abdomen due to the resulting increased intra-abdominal pressure and impaired diaphragmatic excursion. Patients with preload dependent cardiac physiology may experience instability with the drain phase of a PD exchange. In cases of severe lactic acidosis or hepatic impairment, if a bicarbonate-based solution cannot be prepared, another modality that can utilize a bicarbonate-based dialysate may be preferred. Very few underlying medical conditions preclude the use of PD for treatment of AKI, but there are circumstances that may limit its effective use. A history of extensive abdominal surgeries may be a contraindication due to adhesions which render the peritoneal membrane impermeable. Patients with ventriculoperitoneal shunts have been successfully dialyzed with PD, but do present unique challenges and are at increased risk for complications. The presence of a diaphragmatic hernia is an absolute contraindication to PD as dialysate may leak in to the pleural space, causing a hydrothorax. While the dextrose content of the dialysate can serve as a source of additional calories, it can also lead to hyperglycemia requiring insulin therapy. Peritoneal dialysis can also result in significant protein and immunoglobulin losses, resulting in nutritional challenges and increased susceptibility to infections, including peritonitis. Peritonitis can lead to further protein losses, loss of ultrafiltration capacity and permanent damage to the peritoneum. Ultimately, decisions regarding the use of PD should be made on a case-by-case basis in conjunction with a surgeon.

Intermittent Hemodialysis

Any discussion about the use of IHD for the treatment of pediatric AKI warrants a discussion regarding the basic principles of hemodialysis. Both IHD and CRRT require access to the patient's circulation. During HD, blood passes through an extracorporeal circuit that includes a dialyzer made of a polyurethane capsule which houses hollow fibers serving as a semipermeable membrane. During dialysis, the dialysate bathes the fibers and solute is cleared from the intravascular compartment by diffusive transport. When the patient is connected to the dialysis machine, the patient's blood flows through each of the hollow fibers where it meets the surrounding dialysate that bathes the fibers. Diffusion of solute occurs down a concentration gradient. The patient's blood and the dialysate flow in opposite directions within the dialyzer creating bidirectional flow, which maintains a high concentration gradient, allowing for more efficient solute clearance. According to the laws of diffusion, the larger the molecule the slower the rate of transfer across the membrane. A small molecule such as urea (60 Daltons) is cleared efficiently; however, a larger molecule like creatinine (113 Daltons) is cleared less efficiently. Fluid removal occurs via a hydrostatic pressure gradient across the membrane generated by the hemodialysis machine, the transmembrane pressure (TMP). Ultrafiltration is the filtering of cell-free fluid from the high pressure blood side of the membrane to the low-pressure dialysate side of the membrane.

Vascular access is probably the most important aspect contributing to the successful provision of IHD. This is especially important given the wide range in patient size. Double-lumen IHD catheters can usually be placed expeditiously at the patient's bedside by intensivists or nephrologists. Permanent tunneled catheters should be placed in the operating room by surgeons or interventional radiologists if IHD is anticipated chronically. A variety of catheter types exist to accommodate pediatric patients of all sizes, including small infants. In neonates, umbilical veins may be used if access is urgent and other options do not exist; however, use can be problematic due to difficulty obtaining adequate blood flows. The utilization of neck veins allows for less recirculation and avoids high venous return pressures often associated with groin lines in patients who are not cooperative enough to remain still for the duration of treatment. Complications related to catheter placement include air emboli and hemorrhage. Another important consideration when deciding where to place vascular access for IHD is the impact on future access sites in the event the patient does not have renal recovery. In these circumstances, a cuffed central venous catheter (CVC), or arteriovenous fistula should be considered for chronic use.

Equipment for HD is usually readily available in tertiary care centers; however, personnel capable of performing IHD in smaller children may not be as readily available. Intermittent hemodialysis can also be performed without the use of anticoagulation if indicated, although intermittent heparin or citrate anticoagulation is often used.

The prescription for acute HD has several components including dialyzer to be used and dialysate composition. The choice of dialyzer varies based on patient size, dialyzer surface area, and dialyzer clearances. Because small molecules diffuse across the dialyzer from regions of high concentration to regions of lesser concentration, the composition of the dialysate is designed to produce near normalization of plasma. For example, the sodium concentration of the dialysate is within physiologic range; however, since potassium is often elevated in the blood, the potassium concentration of dialysate is lower than plasma establishing a concentration gradient. Substances to be removed completely from the patient's blood would not be included in the dialysate. Determining an optimal blood flow rate through the dialyzer is dependent on various factors, such as catheter performance, length and location. Venous blood flows are the highest in the superior vena cava and the inferior vena cava, and dialysis catheters must be long enough to reach one of these locations. Femoral venous and right-sided internal jugular catheters provide the best blood flows. Higher blood flows (up to 3–5 mL/min/kg) are necessary during IHD compared to CRRT to provide sufficient solute clearance during the relatively short treatment time. Determination of ultrafiltration volume is dependent on the patient's clinical status. Anticoagulation during IHD can be continuous or in the form of small intermittent boluses.

Compared to PD and CRRT, IHD provides rapid ultrafiltration and solute removal. In addition, IHD is the optimal modality for the treatment of ingestions, drug toxicity, tumor lysis syndrome, severe hyperkalemia, severe fluid overload, and hyperammonemia. Like PD, IHD has the advantage of being able to be performed outside of the intensive care setting for hemodynamically stable patients. Another advantage of IHD is the ability to adjust the composition of dialysis solutions to treat electrolyte abnormalities quickly. Hemodialysis machines can also be adjusted to provide isolated ultrafiltration without solute clearance.

Despite the availability of IHD equipment for the treatment of AKI in the pediatric population, its use does require some technical expertise on the part of the physicians, nurses, and dialysis technicians. For this reason, it is often only available in large secondary and tertiary care centers. Intermittent hemodialysis may not be feasible in small infants, in whom it may be difficult to obtain access adequate enough to achieve high blood flows. A significant disadvantage with IHD is hemodynamic instability that often occurs in patients with more significant illness. Hypotension may lead to early termination of a treatment or even preclude its initiation. Hypotensive patients may also have a limited ability to achieve their goal fluid removal. In these cases, PD or CRRT may be more preferred modality choices given the more gradual ultrafiltration. Another major disadvantage associated with IHD is the need for fluid restriction in patients who are being treated with this modality. While daily hemodialysis treatments may help the volume overload state, it does not usually completely eliminate the need for fluid restriction. Such fluid restrictions usually lead to limitations in the amount of nutritional support that patients may receive during the acute hospitalization.

Patients with AKI being treated with IHD should be closely monitored for two specific complications (see Table 5): dialysis disequilibrium syndrome and membrane bioincompatibility. While rapid solute and fluid removal are clear advantages, they also carry the risk of inducing disequilibrium syndrome. Disequilibrium syndrome occurs as a consequence of rapid osmolar shifts from solute removal, leading to cerebral edema manifesting clinically as mental status changes to seizures and death in the most severe cases. Disequilibrium syndrome can be avoided by limiting initial solute removal with dialysis. The goal of the initial treatment is to lower the BUN levels by approximately 30–40%. This goal can be progressively increased with subsequent IHD sessions as the patient adjusts to IHD. This can be assessed by obtaining pre- and post-treatment BUN levels. Membrane bioincompatibility is problematic as certain dialysis

Table 5. Suggested modality choice in pediatric acute kidney injury

Goal of dialysis	Hemodynamic status	Modality
Ultrafiltration	Normotensive	IHD (with isolated UF)
	Hypotensive	CRRT or PD
Urea clearance	Normotensive	IHD or PD
	Hypotensive	CRRT or PD
Treatment of hyperkalemia	Normotensive	IHD
	Hypotensive	CRRT or PD
Correction of metabolic acidosis	Normotensive	Any
	Hypotensive	CRRT or PD

membranes cause complement activation, leading to cytokine release and other adverse effects that can worsen the patient's overall clinical status, potentially prolonging the AKI. For this reason, it is wise to use only biocompatible membranes such as cellulose acetate.

Continuous Renal Replacement Therapy

Though CRRT in children is still in its relative infancy, it is quickly becoming a favored modality. Issues related to when and how to use these therapies, which patient populations will benefit the most and how to manage the various potential complications are still being studied. Over the last several years, several defining principles of CRRT in infants and children have been established. This work has been led by a pediatric based consortium comprised of 13 US centers and is known as the prospective pediatric CRRT (ppCRRT) consortium. This group has redefined the demographics, outcomes, and anticoagulation strategies in the treatment approach to AKI in children. For example, this consortium has able to establish a relationship between degree of volume overload at initiation of CRRT and outcome. CRRT as a therapy for AKI has seen a steady increase in use over the last several years.

The CRRT treatment can be delivered by continuous venovenous hemofiltration (CVVH), continuous venovenous hemodialysis (CVVHD), or continuous venovenous hemodiafiltration (CVVHDF). Less commonly used techniques include SCUF and continuous arterio-venous hemofiltration (CAVH). CAVH is often preferred when CRRT is performed in concert with extracorporeal membrane oxygenation (ECMO). The basic principles of CRRT are the same as IHD in terms of how diffusion occurs. Hemofiltration, however, uses the principles of convection in which solutes are dragged with solvent removal. This can be performed independent of or in conjunction with the diffusive properties of dialysis. CRRT allows the clinician the option between convective clearance (CVVH), diffusive clearance (CVVHD), or both (CVVHDF). The choice on which modality to use is often based on individual institution standards, the availability of replacement and dialysate solutions, and on the goal of therapy. For example, small molecular weight solute clearance, such as urea, is similar with CVVH and CVVHD. However, larger molecular weight compounds have improved clearance with CVVH due to convective properties.

The use of CRRT requires attention to several pediatric-specific details. Indications for use of CRRT in the pediatric population include acute kidney injury, electrolyte abnormalities, catabolic patients with increased nutritional needs, sepsis, poisoning, inborn errors of metabolism, hypervolemia unresponsive to diuretics, hepatic, or drug induced coma. CRRT can also be used in conjunction with other therapies such as IHD, ECMO, and therapeutic plasma exchange (TPE), and hepatic support therapies.

As with IHD, provision of adequate vascular access is vital to the success of CRRT. The primary goal with access is to have adequate flow to provide optimal therapy with minimal interruptions. A free-flowing catheter allows for more efficient therapy and less tendency for circuit loss secondary to clotting. Like in acute IHD, an acute, noncuffed catheter can be placed at the bedside or a tunneled, cuffed catheter can be placed in the operating room. Prior to the use of citrate for anticoagulation, double-lumen catheters were adequate for sufficient CRRT. With the increasing use of citrate for anticoagulation, an additional central line is sometimes necessary for calcium infusion due to citrate induced hypocalcemia. A separate catheter is preferred over the additional port on the return line of a double-lumen catheter to avoid port clotting particularly in smaller children and infants. Possible access sites are the same as for IHD and the decision is based on surgeon comfort and expertise, patient size, anatomy, and concerns for bleeding. Options generally include the internal jugular and femoral vessels. Many nephrologists prefer to avoid using the subclavian vessels because of the risk of vessel stenosis, complicating the use of these vessels for fistula formation in patients who go on to develop end-stage renal disease. In addition, subtle catheter kinking may occur between the first rib and the clavicle, impacting access pressures and blood flow. The advantage of using internal jugular catheters is that they provide adequate blood flow and minimal resistance. Disadvantages associated with internal jugular catheters include the increased risk of pneumothorax, hemothorax, or carotid artery puncture during placement of the catheter; however, the risk can be minimized with ultrasound-guided placement. Femoral lines are associated with a decreased risk of complications at the time of placement, but are associated with increased risk of infection and increased susceptibility to kinking with resultant flow problems, especially in nonsedate patients. All catheters carry the risk of vessel thrombosis/stenosis.

The type of modality, dialysis (diffusive) or filtration (convective), and anticoagulation to be utilized should be considered when determining what type of solution to use during CRRT. A variety of bicarbonate-based solutions can be used for CRRT. Dialysate and filter replacement fluids are both commercially available. CRRT is usually initiated with blood flow rates of 3–5 mL/kg/min. Dialysate or filter replacement fluid flow rates in isolation or combined, if applicable, should not exceed 2000 mL/1.73 m^2/hr. Ultrafiltration rates can be adjusted based on hourly patient intake and are often initiated at 1–2 mL/kg/hr but are dependent on the patient's clinical status.

Anticoagulation is often necessary for provision of CRRT, but may not be necessary in the setting of excessive bleeding or thrombocytopenia. Activation of the clotting cascade occurs in the circuit due to contact of circulating blood with the artificial surfaces of the circuit. Low blood flow rates, turbulent blood flow and elevated hematocrits may occur in the system and increase the risk for clot formation. There are currently two main options for anticoagulation for CRRT: Heparin and citrate. Pediatric protocols exist for both anticoagulation options. The use of citrate anticoagulation has increased and gained wide acceptance due to its ease of administration and relatively low side effect profile compared to heparin.

Heparin is one option for anticoagulation in the provision of CRRT. Heparin is infused in the circuit prefilter, functionally anticoagulating the system. Heparin anticoagulation is initiated with a heparin bolus of 10–20 units/kg and then infused continuously at 10–20 units/kg/hr. Anticoagulation is monitored by measuring the partial thromboplastin time (PTT) or activated clotting time (ACT) postfilter every 1–4 hours depending on the institution's standard of care. The goal for the PTT and ACT are 1.5–2 times normal and 180–220 seconds, respectively. The main advantage of heparin is its familiarity to medical personnel. The biggest disadvantage of using heparin is systemic anticoagulation resulting in increased risk for bleeding. Heparin can also be associated with heparin-induced thrombocytopenia that further increases the risks for bleeding and thrombosis.

Because of the risks associated with systemic heparin anticoagulation, citrate anticoagulation is being used in pediatric CRRT with increasing frequency. Citrate is infused prefilter allowing for regional anticoagulation of the CRRT system. Because clotting is a calcium-dependent mechanism, citrate provides successful anticoagulation by binding free calcium, inhibiting coagulation and minimizing clot formation in the circuit. Patient hypocalcemia can be obviated by infusing calcium back to the patient via a second central line separate from the CRRT access. When citrate is used for anticoagulation, calcium-free dialysis, and replacement solutions must be used to reduce the risk of coagulation. Complications of citrate anticoagulation include an anion gap metabolic acidosis, metabolic alkalosis, citrate toxicity, hypocalcemia, hypomagnesemia, and hypernatremia. The metabolic acidosis and alkalosis are often related to the rate of citrate metabolism by the liver. One mmol of citrate is metabolized into 3 mmol of bicarbonate by the liver. A unique complication related to the use of citrate anticoagulation is "citrate lock," defined as a rising patient total calcium and decreasing ionized calcium, occurs when the delivery of citrate exceeds the hepatic metabolism and CRRT clearance. "Citrate lock" is easily managed by discontinuing the citrate infusion for 3–4 hours and then restarting it at 70% of the prior rate.

CRRT has a number of distinct advantages in the management of pediatric patients with AKI. Perhaps the most important among these is that it provides continuous solute clearance and ultrafiltration, similar to the functions of the normal kidney. The gradual nature of fluid removal provided by CRRT makes it an ideal dialysis modality for those with cardiovascular instability and hypotension. While PD also provides a gradual, continuous removal of solute and fluid, it cannot be predicted as easily by the prescription. With CRRT, solute clearance is efficient, and ultrafiltration is not only predictable, it is prescribed. Like IHD, ultrafiltration and solute clearance can be addressed independently of one another, allowing greater flexibility as compared with PD. Perhaps an even greater advantage of CRRT is that because fluid is removed on a continuous basis, the need for fluid restriction is minimal, allowing for adequate provision of parenteral or enteral nutrition. In pediatric patients with AKI not receiving dialysis, goal protein intake should approximate 1.5 g/kg/day. In patients receiving dialysis, the recommendation is for 3–4 g/kg/day of protein intake to account for increased amino acid losses which occur through the circuit due to high clearance.

CRRT may also have several specific metabolic advantages compared with other dialysis modalities. Because dialysate and filter replacement fluids electrolyte composition are adjustable, a wide variety of metabolic abnormalities can be corrected with CRRT including severe metabolic acidosis, lactic acidosis and electrolyte abnormalities such as hyperkalemia. However, as with any customized solution, compounding errors are a risk and caution should be observed when homemade solutions are used. CRRT also provides superior control of uremia compared with PD and IHD and can be used to gradually correct hyperosmolar states, decreasing the risk of cerebral edema compared to IHD. CRRT can also be used as a step-down therapy for IHD in the treatment of intoxications or hyperammonemia once the initial hemodialysis session is complete.

An active area of ongoing research in the CRRT arena is the possible benefit of restoring immunohomeostasis via removal of pro- and anti-inflammatory molecules which may contribute to pathogenesis of the sepsis syndrome. These substances appear to be cleared by CRRT likely via convection and/or membrane adsorption.

Currently, one of the greatest disadvantages of CRRT is related to its complexity and expense compared to PD and IHD. Newer equipment for CRRT has resulted in improved safety but greater costs which may be prohibitive in some centers. Furthermore, the equipment is often not made for pediatric patients but rather adapted for use in children. The establishment of CRRT programs requires specialized nursing education, especially in the Intensive Care Unit (ICU), and pharmacy support. While CRRT can be labor intensive for the bedside ICU nurse, compared to the nursing time involved with continuous manual PD, there may be little difference. Dialysis nursing time may actually be less with CRRT compared to IHD in institutions where ICU nurses take over after initiation. There are commercially available dialysate and filter replacement solutions, and this has led to improved safety and less cost compared to local pharmacy compounded solutions.

Infants and children with AKI for whom CRRT is chosen as a treatment modality present a unique challenge. Delivery of CRRT to these patients, particularly those weighing less than 10 kg, requires that a significant portion of their blood volume be pumped through the extracorporeal CRRT circuit, exposing the patient to hemodynamic instability. Therefore, extracorporeal circuits that exceed 10–15% of the patient's blood volume should be primed with whole blood to prevent significant hypotension and anemia. With such blood primes, it is important to remember that because the prime volume is not discarded, the blood should not be reinfused to the patient when the treatment is discontinued for circuit changes or at the completion of therapy to prevent volume overload and hypertension. Larger patients with overwhelming multiorgan system failure and hemodynamic instability may not tolerate the rapid circulation of blood through the CRRT circuit and be at risk for hemodynamic instability.

Another disadvantage of CRRT seen more often in the pediatric population is the development of hypothermia. Infants and small children have large body surface area to weight ratios. This combined with the significant volume of their blood that circulates through the extracorporeal circuit at any given time, places these children at significant risk for developing low body temperatures. Radiant warmers may help ameliorate this but are often not adequate to maintain body temperature. This issue has been addressed by placing line warmers on newer dialysis machines. When line warmers are not available, adaptations have been made in the form of heating pads and nondialysis blood line warmers.

Another complication of CRRT is a bradykinin release phenomenon, which is pH related and occurs when the patient's blood (or blood prime) contacts the filter. It can cause anaphylaxis with refractory hypotension when initiating CRRT in patients who are acidotic or in those smaller pediatric patients. Banked blood is acidotic, has an elevated potassium, low calcium and bioactive components which all increase the risk of developing cardiac instability. The bradykinin release phenomenon can be avoided by normalizing the pH of the patient or the blood prime prior to initiating CRRT. This can be accomplished with prefilter alkalinization with sodium bicarbonate, and using bicarbonate based dialysate or replacement fluid.

Summary

At the present time, the data for dialysis modality choice in the treatment of AKI in the pediatric population is limited but increasing. To date, there have been no randomized clinical trials comparing PD vs. intermittent hemodialysis versus CRRT. The information we have regarding improved outcomes and cost with CRRT is extrapolated from adult studies. Several questions must be addressed when making the decision on which dialysis modality to employ (see Table 5).

- When should dialysis be initiated?
- What are the specific indications for dialysis?
- What is the underlying cause of the AKI?
- What are the goals of dialysis (i.e. solute clearance, ultrafiltration or both)?
- How ill is the patient?
- What modalities are available at a particular institution?
- What is the expertise of the available clinicians?

Standard principles must be developed before comparative studies can be successfully performed to answer these questions, starting with common criteria and definitions for the diagnosis of AKI. The establishment of the pediatric RIFLE criteria and the work being done by ADQI (Acute Dialysis Quality Initiative) and AKIN (Acute Kidney Injury Network) should lead to the long awaited advances in the field of pediatric dialysis.

Suggested Reading

Brophy PD. (2008) Renal supportive therapy for pediatric acute kidney injury in the setting of multiorgan dysfunction syndrome/sepsis. *Semin Nephrol* **28**: 457–469.

Bunchman TE, Brophy PD, Goldstein SL. (2008) Technical considerations for renal replacement therapy in children. *Semin Nephrol* **28**: 488–492.

Fischbach M, Warady BA. (2009) Peritoneal dialysis prescription in children: bedside principles for optimal practice. *Pediatr Nephrol* **24**(9): 1633–1642.

Flynn JT. (2002) Choice of dialysis modality for management of pediatric acute renal failure. *Pediatr Nephrol* **17**: 61–69.

Walters S, Porter C, Brophy PD. (2009) Dialysis and pediatric acute kidney injury: choice of renal support modality. *Pediatr Nephrol* **24**: 37–48.

Part XIII

Chronic Kidney Disease (CKD)

37

Chronic Kidney Disease

John D. Mahan

Introduction

Chronic Kidney Disease (CKD) is defined as persistent, irreversible, abnormalities affecting renal structure and/or function. Historically, chronic renal insufficiency was used to describe glomerular filtration rate (GFR) <75 ml/min/1.73 m^2. Since 2001, the National Kidney Foundation Kidney Disease Outcomes Quality Initiative (NKF-K/DOQI) CKD classification is used for staging renal dysfunction in children >2 years of age and adults and stratifies five stages based on the degree of impairment, irrespective of underlying diagnosis (see Table 1).

CKD in children progresses over time, although some may experience prolonged stability even throughout childhood. Physiologic demands of growth often worsen severity, as impaired kidneys cannot grow sufficiently to meet increased demands incurred with somatic and muscle growth. Rapid renal function decline occurs in children who suffer severe intercurrent illnesses, such as dehydration, infection and/or sepsis, and in children with severe hypertension, recurrent urinary tract infection (UTI), or receiving nephrotoxic medications. Mild CKD may be diagnosed in asymptomatic children, by abnormal urinalysis or serum chemistries, whereas, those with advanced CKD (stages 3 or 4) usually have clinical signs/symptoms. Increasingly, infants are diagnosed by antenatal ultrasound (US) screening.

Important factors contributing to morbidity include age at onset, etiology, calorie-protein malnutrition, metabolic acidosis, anemia, and mineral bone disorder (MBD). Anemia has been associated with poor growth and correction correlates with improved stature. Metabolic acidosis impairs growth, as seen in children with untreated renal tubular acidosis (RTA), by

Table 1. NKF-K/DOQI classification of stages of CKD

Stage	GFR[a] (ml/min per 1.73 m^2)	Description
1	>90	Renal parenchymal disease and or mild kidney damage
2	60–89	Kidney damage with mild decrease in GFR; usually asymptomatic but may develop biochemical abnormalities of CKD
3	30–59	Moderate reduction of GFR; biochemical abnormalities and signs of CKD such as poor appetite and growth
4	15–29	Severe reduction of GFR; biochemical abnormalities and clinical complications more frequent and severe
5	<15 (or dialysis)	Significant kidney failure; renal replacement typically required

[a] GFR ranges apply to children aged 2 years and older.

altering GH–IGF-I axis. MBD may further impair growth by causing various bone disorders (high-turnover bone disease due to secondary hyperparathyroidism, low-turnover osteomalacia, and adynamic bone) that affect height and reduce bone mineral density, increased bone fractures, and bone deformities. Other contributing factors include salt and water losses, and medications, such as corticosteroids and cytotoxic agents.

Growth Impairment

Growth impairment occurs in up to 50% of children with moderate renal dysfunction (CKD 3–5). The etiology is multifactorial, reflecting abnormalities in the growth hormone (GH)–insulin-like growth factor (IGF)-I axis and nutritional and metabolic problems.

Children with congenital renal disorders, in whom impairment is present in the first two years of life, are particularly affected, since 33% of final adult height is attained during this period. Nutrition, which is often inadequate in these children due to anorexia and vomiting, determines growth during infancy; after which, growth is more impacted by endogenous GH. Some children with CKD who experience growth delay in infancy may demonstrate normal growth velocity, but not catch up growth during childhood. Growth is likely to be more impaired during pubertal ages due to the combination of delayed puberty and blunted pubertal growth spurt due to disordered secretion of gonadotropins and altered sex hormone binding globulins. Growth impairment is more likely in severe CKD and is more common in tubulointerstitial disorders than glomerular disorders. Some syndromes associated with CKD are known to independently hinder growth.

The annual report of the North American Pediatric Renal Transplant Cooperative Study (NAPRTCS) provides a comprehensive growth profile in children with CKD, undergoing dialysis, or postrenal transplant. Of 6907 children with CKD and anthropometric data, >33% exhibited significant growth failure at the time of registry entry, defined by a standardized height measurement <33% for age. Patients who entered the NAPRTCS CKD registry at a younger age tended to exhibit substantial height deficits, with significant growth failure reported in 58.3%, 41.2%, 32.5%, and 22.1% of patients aged 0–1 years, 2–5 years, 6–12 years, and >12 years, respectively. A significant correlation exists between severity of renal impairment and growth retardation; however, significant short stature was seen at early CKD stages. Dialysis administration did not improve height SDS, and values worsened after 24 months of dialysis. Growth impairment was evident at the time of renal transplant, with greater deficits in younger children. Among children who received transplants between 1987 and 2007, the mean baseline height SDS was −1.78; mean values of −2.21, −2.26, −2.00, and −1.41 were observed in patients aged 0–1 years, 2–5 years, 6–12 years, and older than 12 years, respectively. Younger children (aged 0–5 years) showed improvement in growth posttransplant, whereas older children (>12 years) did not and many showed worsening several years later.

The impact of growth failure can be substantial. Growth impairment in children requiring dialysis is associated with a nearly threefold increase in mortality and increased hospitalization, primarily for infection. Although limited data in CKD exists, children with growth failure from other causes have impairments in psychosocial development, as well as quality of life (QOL). Short children have an increased incidence of attention deficit hyperactivity disorder, learning disability, and mood disorders. The magnitude of psychopathology correlates with the degree of growth failure and improves with better growth. Children with CKD and poor growth often become very short adults impacting marital status, education, employment, and independence.

Table 2. GH/IGF axis in healthy children and children with CKD

Normal Renal Function	Decreased Renal Function (CKD)
• GH release from pituitary controlled by GHRH and SRIF and GH secretagogues (e.g., ghrelin)	• GH release from pituitary controlled by GHRH and SRIF and GH secretagogues (e.g., ghrelin)
• GHRH and SRIF controlled by serum GH and IGF-I	• GHRH and SRIF controlled by serum GH and IGF-I
• Serum GH binds to GH receptors on many cells	• Serum GH levels are normal to elevated due to diminished renal clearance
• Hepatic GH receptor activation increases IGF-I production and serum IGF-I level • GH receptor activation in cells generates IGF-I independent effects	• Serum GH binds to GH receptors on many cells — cellular GH receptor density is diminished
• Hepatic GH receptor activation increases IGF-I production and serum IGF-I level	• Hepatic GH receptor activation leads to less efficient IGF-I production without increase in serum IGF-I levels
• GH receptor activation in cells generates IGF-I independent effects	• GH receptor activation in cells generates IGF-I independent effects
• Most serum IGF-I bound to IGFBP-3 in ternary complex with ALS • Unbound or free IGF-I activates IGF-I receptors to generate cellular responses: o Longitudinal bone growth o Increased renal plasma flow and GFR	• More serum IGF-I bound to increased levels of IGFBP1, 2, and 4 leading to less IGF-I bound to IGFBP-3 in ternary complex with ALS • Increased proteolysis of ALS further diminishes IGF-I complexed to IGFBP3 and ALS • Less unbound or free IGF-I available to activate IGF-I receptors therefore generating less cellular responses

Pathogenesis

Growth failure results from abnormalities in GH–IGF-I axis (see Table 2). The sum of these physiologic abnormalities may result in delayed pubertal development and suboptimal pubertal growth spurt in adolescents with CKD, and growth impairment in younger children.

Clinical presentation/evaluation

Since growth failure is common, anthropometrics must be obtained routinely and should be considered as a fifth vital sign in addition to head circumference (measured until 3 years of age), height/length, weight and body mass index (BMI); and plotting these values on age and gender appropriate growth charts, including percentiles and standard deviations scores (SDS) identifies trends and can prevent growth failure. In some situations, calculating height velocity SDS score will demonstrate suboptimal growth rate before height becomes abnormal, allowing for corrective treatment.

Since causes of poor growth vary, a thorough evaluation to uncover modifiable factors is critical (see Table 3).

Table 3. Factors impairing growth in children with CKD

Non-modifiable factors	Modifiable factors
Age of onset of CKD	Poor caloric intake
Level of renal function	Excessive salt and water losses
Type of renal disorder	Metabolic acidosis
Corticosteroid therapy	Anemia
	Renal osteodystrophy
	GH/IGF-I resistance
	Gonadotropin abnormalities

Recombinant growth hormone therapy

Treatment of growth failure in children with CKD must be based on a thorough evaluation and therapy directed toward modifiable factors (see Table 4). After correction of nutritional deficiencies, anemia, acidosis or salt/water abnormalities, it may take 4–6 months to detect a favorable growth response. When all other factors have been corrected, therapy with recombinant GH (rGH) should be considered. Both serum phosphorus (P), and parathyroid hormone (PTH) must be controlled to avoid bone deformities. Goal PTH level during GH therapy is iPTH <400 pg/ml in CKD 2–4 and <900 pg/ml in CKD 5.

Exogenous rGH can overcome GH and IGF-1 resistance. Clinical trials have demonstrated safety and efficacy of rGH in promoting linear growth

Table 4. Treatment recommendations for modifiable factors associated with growth failure in children with CKD

Modifiable factor	Recommended treatment
Malnutrition (cachexia)	Provision of 100–120% RDA calories
Salt and water wasting	Supplemental Na/H2O
Metabolic acidosis	Alkali to improve serum HCO_3^- >22
Anemia	Iron and/or erythropoietin to boost Hb >11
CKD — mineral bone disease (renal osteodystrophy)	Dietary phosphate restriction Phosphate binders Vitamin D analog therapy to keep PTH in acceptable range for CKD level
GH/IGF-1 resistance	Exogenous recombinant GH therapy
Gonadotropic hormone abnormalities	Replacement of gonadotropin or sex hormone deficiencies

in children with CKD, on dialysis, or following renal transplant. Long-term GH therapy results in catch-up growth and many patients achieve normal final adult height if treatment is started early enough. Recommendations support long-term rGH therapy in children with CKD because up to 70% of children will experience growth velocity reduction if rGH is discontinued before growth is complete. Compared with untreated children, rGH-treated patients showed no significant increase in malignancy, slipped capital femoral epiphysis (SCFE), avascular necrosis, glucose intolerance, pancreatitis, deterioration of renal function, acute allograft rejection, or fluid retention. No significant increase in benign intracranial hypertension (ICH) was observed among GH recipients.

The algorithm for the evaluation and treatment of growth failure in children with CKD summarizes a logical approach to rGH therapy (see Fig. 1). rGH treatment is contraindicated in patients with active malignancies and should be used cautiously in disorders associated with malignancy risk. Baseline hip and knee X-rays, fundoscopic examination, blood chemistries, PTH levels, and thyroid studies should be performed. GH stimulation tests are not required in children with CKD. With rGH therapy, children must be monitored every 3–4 months for dose modification based on weight gain, response to therapy, adverse events, and complicating factors. Yearly bone age monitoring should be accompanied by hip and knee X-rays if hip or leg pain is present. Higher rGH doses may be required during puberty (up to 0.7 mg/kg/wk) to optimize height

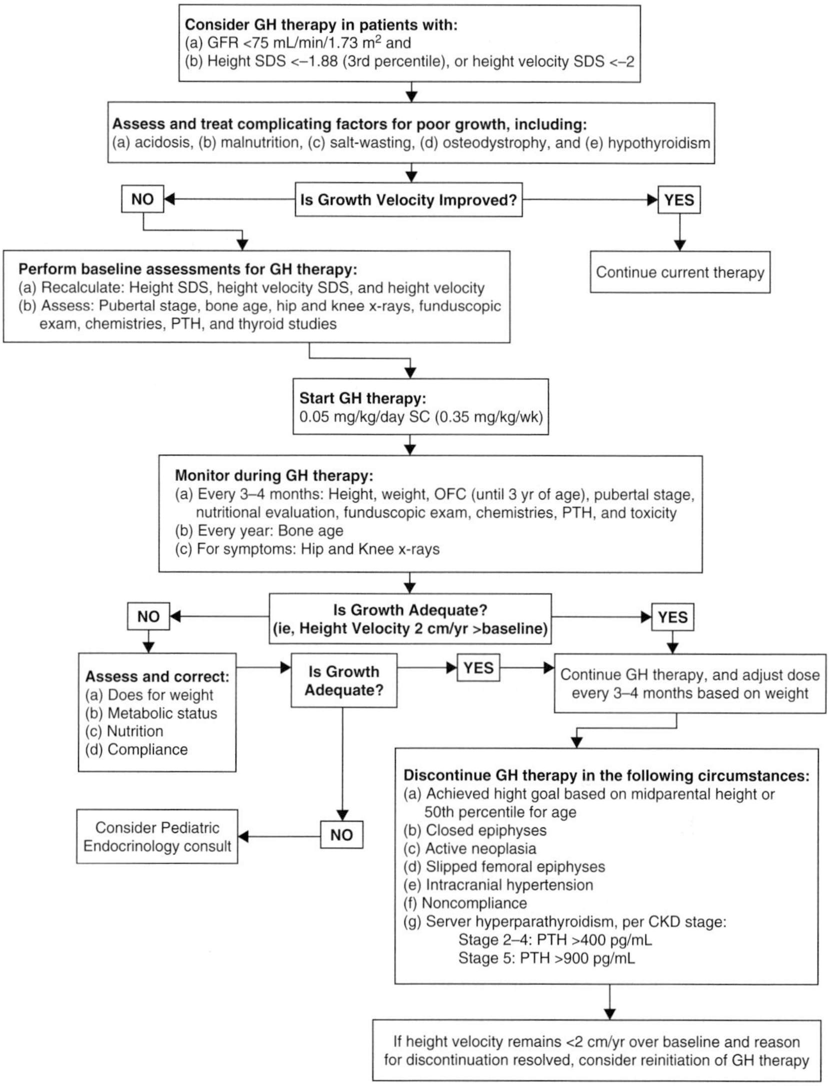

Figure 1. US Consensus 2006 statement algorithm for evaluation and treatment of growth failure in children with CKD.

velocity, and final height. Because GH administration increases plasma IGF-I levels, which mediates growth-promoting effects, a relationship between plasma IGF-I concentrations and catch-up growth has been suggested. Therefore, IGF-I may be used to measure therapeutic efficacy and adherence. rGH therapy may provide other benefits to children with CKD, including improvement in body weight, midarm circumference, improved bone mineral density and better lipid profiles.

Patients with persistent poor growth despite appropriate therapy require referral to a pediatric endocrinologist for further evaluation.

rGH should be discontinued upon epiphyseal closure or attainment of final height goal (based on midparental height or the 50th percentile for age). Temporary discontinuation should occur in the presence of active neoplasia, SCFE, benign ICH, severe hyperparathyroidism, noncompliance, or renal transplant. Continued growth monitoring should occur, since reinitiation may be necessary if height velocity decreases and issues have been resolved.

Anemia

Anemia of CKD is related to insufficient erythropoietin (Epo) production. Over 90% of Epo is synthesized in the kidneys, and deficiency usually becomes apparent during CKD stage 3, when approximately 50% renal function is lost. Anemia is seen in nearly all children with CKD stage 5.

Pathogenesis

Erythropoietin is a glycoprotein (MW 34,000) produced by specialized tubulointerstitial (TI) cells in the renal medulla in response to low oxygen delivery. Due to high oxygen extraction by proximal tubular cells, TI cells respond early to decreased oxygen saturation and delivery by producing and releasing Epo. Epo binds to receptors in colony-forming units-erythroid and erythroblasts in the bone marrow to induce proliferation of red blood cell (RBC) precursors ultimately releasing more RBCs into the circulation, with subsequent increase in RBC in 1–3 days with full effect noted in 7–10 days. Epo is metabolized by the liver. In children with CKD, Epo levels are inappropriately low for the level of anemia. In addition, uremia inhibits the erythroid progenitor cell response to Epo. The extent of Epo deficiency and anemia typically increases as GFR decreases, but onset of detectable anemia varies greatly. Significant anemia usually presents when GFR is <35 ml/min/1.73 m^2. While Epo deficiency is the most prominent cause of anemia in children with CKD a number of other factors may contribute (see Table 5).

Table 5. Causes of anemia in children with CKD

Decreased erythropoietin production	Decrease RBC survival
Iron deficiency	Folate and/or B12 deficiency
Hemolysis	Chronic or acute inflammation
Bone marrow inhibition (uremia)	Osteitis fibrosa (hyperparathyroidism)
Blood loss (GI tract, hemodialysis, menses)	Malnutrition
Medications (ACE inhibitors)	Carnitine deficiency
Aluminum toxicity	

Clinical manifestations

A wide range of clinical manifestations exist (see Table 6). Anemia is associated with increased mortality in children as well adults with CKD, probably through its effects on the cardiovascular (CV) system. Some studies have correlated anemia correction with improved CV parameters, such as left ventricular hypertrophy (LVH).

Anemia has now been linked to growth failure and delayed development in children with CKD. Anemia may decrease appetite; however, studies have not shown reproducible evidence of improved intake or anthropometrics with correction. Improvement of anemia in adults with CKD has been clearly linked to improvement in systemic symptoms; less data is available in children with CKD, but improvements in QOL and exercise tolerance have been seen.

Diagnosis/evaluation

Most anemic children with CKD can be treated empirically, after ensuring adequate iron stores, with an erythropoiesis stimulating agent (ESA), such as recombinant human erythropoietin (rHuEPO) (rHuEPO or darbopoetin-alpha) unless other causative factors exist. Epo deficiency results in a normocytic, normochromic anemia. Macrocytosis suggests B12 or folate deficiency; microcytosis suggests iron deficiency, hemoglobinopathy, or inflammation. In children with a history of aluminum containing phosphate binders, aluminum toxicity should be excluded. If inadequate reticulocytosis is present, sources of blood loss should be explored.

Determination of a complete blood count (CBC), reticulocyte count, serum ferritin and iron, and total iron binding capacity (TIBC) allow calculation of the transferrin saturation (TSAT). Iron deficiency is common in children with CKD due to decreased iron intake, poor GI absorption, and occult GI, and/or menstrual blood loss. The laboratory picture of iron deficiency is low reticulocyte count, low serum ferritin and low TSAT; in some children with CKD and iron deficiency, serum ferritin, a marker of chronic inflammation, may be elevated.

If iron deficiency is not present before initiation of ESA, it often develops as a result of erythropoiesis. CBC should be monitored every 3–6 months in CKD stage 3–4. Children on ESA therapy require CBC at least monthly, with periodic reticulocyte counts and iron monitoring. Acute infection and surgical procedures often cause mild decreases in hemoglobin (Hb) and dampened response to ESA. Some children with CKD may develop functional iron deficiency, with normal ferritin and TSAT, and still respond with erythropoiesis after IV iron administration. An elevated CRP is a good indicator of chronic inflammation; an elevated reticulocyte count in the face of decreasing Hb and/or increasing ESA requirements indicates occult blood loss or hemolysis.

Although a normal or elevated ferritin does not exclude iron deficiency, a low ferritin is diagnostic of iron deficiency. NKF-K/DOQI recommends treating patients with serum ferritin <100 ng/ml and/or TSAT <20% for iron deficiency, although not routinely using IV iron if the serum ferritin is >500 ng/ml. If TSAT is low with serum ferritin >100 ng/ml, indicating functional iron deficiency due to inflammation, erythropoiesis may respond to IV iron.

Treatment

Almost all children with CKD 3–5 require ESA treatment to maintain near normal Hb levels. In addition, almost all patients require oral or IV iron. Other causes of anemia should be sought and treated where indicated. Blood transfusions should be restricted to children with CKD who emergently need repletion for surgery, or who are symptomatic. Optimal target Hb levels remain controversial and are frequently changing; current guidelines for children with CKD from NKF-K/DOQI state:

1. Selection of Hb target and Hb level at which ESA therapy is initiated should include consideration of potential benefits (improved QOL, school attendance/performance, and transfusion avoidance) and potential harms (life-threatening adverse events)
2. With ESA therapy, Hb target should be 11.0–12.0 g/dl

3. With ESA therapy, Hb target should not exceed 13.0 g/dl. Most clinicians start ESA when Hb <10 mg/dl, and although levels 11–12 gm/dl are suggested, some clinical situations require different targets

After initiation of ESA or after dose change, Hb should be monitored every 1–2 weeks. Once stable dosing and Hb levels are attained, monthly Hb in dialysis patients and every 1–2 months in CKD 3–4 are recommended. Subcutaneous (SQ) and intravenous (IV) ESA are effective, with longer half-lives using the SQ route. Dosing is highly variable with higher unit/kg doses expected in children with lower GFR, on hemodialysis, and of younger age. Higher doses are also required with IV route and less frequent dosing regimens. Blood loss, iron deficiency, inflammation, and hyperparathyroidism result in higher ESA doses while residual kidney function may lessen the dose requirement. SQ rHuEPO dosing typically starts at 100 units/kg/week in 1–3 doses with better response seen with thrice weekly dosing. Younger children (<5 years of age) and children receiving IV rHuEPO while on hemodialysis may be started at 150–200 units/kg/week in three doses with adjustments as necessary. Frequent dose adjustments are to be expected and total weekly dose of ESA should be increased by 50% when converting a child from SQ to IV ESA therapy. The goal of therapy is to gradually improve Hb, 1–2 gm/dl/month with incremental ESA dose increases of 25% when still below target. If Hb is above target or increase in Hb is >2 gm/dl/month, then dose reduction by 25% is warranted. If Hb is >1 gm/dl above target, then ESA should be held for 2–4 weeks then resumed at a lower dose. Complications of ESAs include hypertension, particularly with rapid rise in Hb. Antierythropoetin antibodies are a rare complication of therapy and can cause pure red cell aplasia.

Darbopoetin-alpha (Darbo), a genetically derived form of Epo, is effective for anemia correction. Due to longer half-life, less frequent administration is required. RHuEPO and Darbo have similar efficacy and Darbo can be given successfully every 2–4 weeks to maintain normal Hb levels. Typical starting dose is 0.5 mcg/kg/week or the same total dose given every 2 weeks. Although 1 mcg of Darbo is equivalent to 200 units rHuEPO based on protein content, recommended conversion ratio is 0.84 mcg/kg/week of Darbo for every 200 units/kg/week of rHuEPO. Complications are similar to rHuEPO although pain at administration site is more severe with Darbo.

Oral iron therapy is less effective in uremic individuals due to poor GI absorption. Absorption is better when oral iron is given without food. Concurrently administered calcium containing P binders also inhibit oral iron absorption while sevelamer does not appear to affect GI iron absorption. The dose of oral iron is 3–5 mg/kg/day elemental iron (maximum dose 300 mg/day). In patients with poor response to oral iron, and for most hemodialysis patients, IV iron is preferred. Studies show IV iron therapy is associated with correction of iron deficiency, better Hb levels and less ESA usage. Iron gluconate or iron sucrose is effective in restoring iron stores. Higher doses of iron sucrose, to maximum of 200 mg/dose, are safe in children with CKD. Chronic maintenance therapy at 1 mg/kg/week, usually used for children on hemodialysis, can be titrated to keep TSAT and serum ferritin in desired ranges and is associated with lower ESA dose. Complications of IV iron include anaphylactic reactions with the older iron dextran preparations and acute reversible symptoms of abdominal pain, emesis, flushing and hypotension reported with too rapid administration of iron gluconate and iron sucrose. Due to potential side effects, iron gluconate, and iron sucrose maximum single dose limits should be followed. IV iron is often held in acute infection as IV iron may depress immune response.

Metabolic Acidosis in CKD

Acid–base hemostasis is deranged as kidney function declines, especially as GFR <50% of normal. Factors significantly affecting the presence and severity of metabolic acidosis include excessive protein intake (increased acid load), inflammation, and catabolism. As metabolic acidosis worsens, potassium is displaced from cells (chiefly RBCs) that buffer acid resulting in hyperkalemia causing cardiac conduction abnormalities.

Pathogenesis

Causes of metabolic acidosis in children with CKD include inability to filter and excrete acid due to diminished GFR, causing an elevated anion gap. This “uremic” metabolic acidosis may be quite profound as GFR worsens, particularly in those with obstructive uropathy, structural defects, and tubular disorders as component of RTA may be superimposed on "uremic" metabolic acidosis. These may be due to distal tubule acid excretion defects (distal RTA) or combined distal tubular acid, and potassium defects (hyperkalemic or type IV RTA).

Clinical manifestations

Metabolic acidosis may be associated with poor weight and height gain. Increased protein catabolism may contribute to uremic symptoms. Decreased appetite, strength, energy and endurance may all occur. Excessive fatigue may be difficult to ascribe to metabolic acidosis since numerous factors may contribute to this symptom. Increased protein degradation likely explains endurance and muscle weakness issues. Downregulation of GH secretion, decreased expression of GH and IGF-1 receptors in tissue, and decreased serum levels of IGF-1 explain poor longitudinal growth.

Metabolic acidosis may have deleterious effects on bone, including net calcium removal due to bone buffering of acid, inhibition of osteoblast function and activation of osteoclasts. The end result is poor bone mineralization and osteomalacia, causing bone pain, increased fractures, and bone deformities.

Diagnosis/evaluation

Serum chemistries will reveal metabolic acidosis (low HCO_3^-) and provide information on contributory factors such as creatinine, BUN and potassium. Delineation of RTA vs. uremic acidosis is unnecessary as treatment is the same. Children with a RTA component, however, will typically have metabolic acidosis disproportionate to level of uremia and are more likely to demonstrate chronic effects of metabolic acidosis. Metabolic acidosis coinciding with severe uremia (CKD stage 4) may be difficult to control with oral sodium bicarbonate therapy since the extra sodium may contribute to edema and hypertension. In such cases, renal replacement therapy as a means to remove acid, as well as uremic toxins may be indicated. Poor growth and defective bone mineralization often improve with adequate acidosis correction; improvements in more general manifestations, such as fatigue and anorexia, are more difficult to achieve with isolated acidosis correction, consistent with multifactorial causality.

Treatment

Regardless of the cause, appropriate treatment of metabolic acidosis is alkali, in doses sufficient to increase the serum HCO_3^- >22 mg/dl. Therapy with oral $NaHCO_3^-$ or sodium citrate usually starts at 2 mEq/kg/day, divided in 2–4 doses. Doses as high as 12 mg/kg/day have been described in children with profound tubular defects. Similar doses of IV sodium bicarbonate may be needed during acute illness or when the child is unable to tolerate oral therapy; typically this is provided in similar doses to that given by oral route.

Phosphate Control

Maintenance of normal serum P is critical to prevent hyperparathyroidism and MBD. Increased incidence of CV disease in adults and children with CKD related to elevated serum Ca and P values, as well as elevated Ca x P product underscores the importance of strict P control. The major source of phosphate causing hyperphosphatemia, hypocalcemia, and MBD is from dietary intake. With continued positive P balance, chronic complications can develop. The process of P retention and effects on serum calcium, parathyroid, vitamin D status and the skeleton are central to clinical manifestations seen in MBD including poor growth, bone pain, myopathy, skeletal deformities, SCFE, fractures, conjunctivitis, pruritis, joint and skin calcifications, and CV complications (vascular calcifications, coronary artery disease and arrhythmias). Attention to P balance should begin in early stages of CKD. Restriction of P intake and measurement of intact PTH should begin at stage 3, allowing for early treatment to prevent significant clinical manifestations. As a result, periodic monitoring of serum P, calcium and intact PTH, obtained every 3–6 months in CKD 3, is an important. In CKD 4–5, P monitoring should occur at least every three months.

Treatment

Dietary P restriction may be sufficient to control hyperphosphatemia initially. Normal P levels are achieved at the cost of endocrine responses, such as secondary hyperparathyroidism and increased

Table 6. Clinical manifestations of anemia in children with CKD

Cardiovascular	Systemic
Increased left ventricular mass index	Fatigue
LVH	Depression
	Decreased quality of life
	Impaired cognitive function
	Sleep disturbances
	Decreased exercise ability
	Decreased growth
	Loss of appetite

fibroblast growth factor 23, which inhibit tubular phosphate reabsorption. Eventually, these adaptive mechanisms are insufficient and hyperphosphatemia develops, at which point oral P binding agents are required to maintain serum P values <50th percentile of normal for age (see Table 6).

Calcium containing salts effectively bind P in the GI tract. Prolonged hypercalcemia and/or increased Ca × P product (>55) are associated with CV complications and mortality in adults with CKD. This data and evidence of increased vascular calcifications in children with CKD have relegated the use of calcium containing P binders to hypocalcemic children. NKF-K/DOQI guidelines now target Ca × P <55 for adolescents and <65 for younger children and infants, resulting in avoidance of calcium containing P binders. Calcium acetate is more effective in P binding per unit of Ca content than calcium carbonate and is now more widely used. Calcium acetate does have more GI side effects, such as pain, bloating and diarrhea, than calcium carbonate, and may limit usefulness. Calcium containing P binders should only be given with food; without which calcium absorption leads to hypercalcemia.

Aluminum containing P binders are effective in lowering serum P acutely but should only be used for a short duration (maximum 4 weeks) due to the severe side effects including CNS toxicity, osteomalacia/adynamic renal bone disease, and hemolysis. Magnesium (Mg) containing P binders are now being used with some success in adults with CKD and are typically adjuncts to calcium containing P binders and serum Mg must be monitored. Side effects of oral Mg include diarrhea and abdominal pain, possibly hindering use.

Table 7. Phosphate binding agents

Agent	Calcium Content (%)	Calcium Absorption (%)	Phosphate Bound/Gram Agent	Comments
Ca Carbonate	40	25	39 mg	High Ca load, GI side effects
Ca acetate	25	22	45 mg	Less Ca than $CaCO_3$ GI side effects
Mg + Ca carbonate	Variable	25	NA	Less Ca load, more GI side effects
Sevelamer	0	0	NA	Ca and Al free, acidosis, decreased cholesterol
Aluminum binders	0	0	45 mg	Effective, toxic, not recommended

Calcium free P binders are emerging as first-line agents. For children requiring P binder who already have high oral calcium intake, hypercalcemia, reduced PTH (consistent with adynamic bone), and/or soft-tissue calcifications, sevelamer is the agent of choice. This hydrogel binds P in the GI tract without being absorbed. LDL cholesterol is lowered due to binding of bile acids in the GI tract. Although sevelamer is less effective at P binding than calcium containing P binders, absenceof hypercalcemia is an important advantage. Side effects include heartburn, bloating, abdominal pain, nausea, and vomiting. In adult CKD studies, improved survival related to less CV complications has been described but no similar studies are available in children with CKD. Sevelamer powder can be used in smaller children and those with gastrosomy tubes.

Lanthanum carbonate has a greater affinity for P, but its use in children has yet to be defined due to uncertainties about long term tissue load.

Suggested Reading

Boehm M, Riesenhuber A, Winkelmayer WC, *et al.* (2007) Early erythropoietin therapy is associated with improved growth in children with chronic kidney disease. *Pediatr Nephrol* 22: 1189–1193.

Fine RN, Stablein D, Cohen AH, *et al.* (2002) Recombinant human growth hormone postrenal transplantation in children: a randomized controlled study of the NAPRTCS. *Kidney Int* **62**(2): 688–696.

KDOQI Clinical Practice Guideline and Clinical Practice Recommendations for Anemia in Chronic Kidney Disease 2007 *Update of Hemoglobin Target.* [Online] http://www.kidney.org/professionals/KDOQI/guidelines_anemiaUP/index.htm.

Kraut JA, Kurtz I. (2005) Metabolic acidosis of CKD: diagnosis, clinical characteristics, and treatment. *Am J Kidney Dis* **45**: 978–993.

Mahan JD, Warady BA for Consensus Committee. (2006) Assessment and treatment of short stature in pediatric patients with chronic kidney disease: a consensus statement. *Pediatr Nephrol* **21**: 917–930.

Mahesh S, Kaskel F. (2008) Growth hormone axis in chronic kidney disease. *Pediatr Nephrol* **23**: 41–48.

Mehls O, Wuhl E, Tonshoff B, *et al.* (2008) Growth hormone treatment in short children with chronic kidney disease. *Acta Paediatrica* **97**: 1159–1164.

NAPRTCS Annual Report 2008. [Online] https://web.emmes.com/study/ped/annlrept/Annual%20Report%20-2008.pdf.

National Kidney Foundation Kidney Disease Outcomes Quality Initiative. (2002) K/DOQI Clinical Practice Guidelines for Chronic Kidney Disease: Evaluation, Classification, and Stratification. Part 4. *Definition and classification of stages of chronic kidney disease.* NKF. National Kidney Foundation. Accessed June 13, 2009.

National Kidney Foundation Kidney Disease Outcomes Quality Initiative. K/DOQI Clinical Practice Guidelines for Bone Metabolism and Disease in Children with Chronic Kidney Disease. [URL http://www.kidney.org/professionals/Kdoqi/guidelines_pedbone/guide7.htm].

Part XIV

End-Stage Renal Disease (ESRD)

38

Pediatric Hemodialysis

Konggrapun Srisuwan and Denis F. Geary

Introduction

According to the Kidney Disease Outcomes Quality Initiative (KDOQI) guidelines, dialysis initiation should be considered when the GFR falls below 14 ml/min/1.73 m^2 body surface area and is strongly recommended when the GFR is <8 ml/min/1.73 m^2. However, clinical deterioration or symptoms suggestive of increasing uremia, such as increasing lethargy, impaired appetite, or nausea should prompt initiation of dialysis even if the GFR exceeds the values outlined above.

The choice between hemodialysis (HD) versus peritoneal dialysis (PD) is dependent on a number of factors, including the considerations outlined in Table 1. Additionally, the anticipated duration of dialysis should be considered; if transplantation is anticipated in the near future, it is usually not appropriate to disrupt a household and devote weeks to training for home PD, and such patients can easily be maintained on HD for a short period of time.

Vascular Access in Children

The KDOQI guidelines concerning vascular access recommend that 50% of all incident ESRD patients should have an arteriovenous fistula (AVF) before starting hemodialysis (HD). A European expert panel also suggested that AVF is the preferred vascular access for children receiving long-term HD. Despite these suggestions for practice, the North American Pediatric Renal Trials and Collaborative Studies (NAPRTCS) report shows that almost 90% of children are dialyzed using central venous catheters (CVCs). The decision about optimal vascular access for an individual child

Table 1. Initiation of Hemodialysis — Considerations

1. Clinical: Uremic symptoms, fluid overload, hypertension, growth deterioration,weight loss.
2. Metabolic: Elevated potassium, phosphate, urea, acidosis
3. Social: Geographic location, transport, compliance, schooling, home facilities, and support
4. Vascular access: Patient age, surgical referral for fistula, central venous catheter (CVC)

Table 2. Factors to consider for vascular access choice in children

• Patient size
• Surgical expertise
• Interventional radiological expertise
• Anticipated euration of dialysis
• Patient choice (e.g. cosmetic, swimming, pain)

should consider the factors listed in Table 2, the most important of which are certainly patient size and available surgical expertise.

As illustrated in Fig. 1, in centers with the greatest expertise for creation of AVFs, approximately 75% will survive at least two years. However, the incidence of primary failure of AVF is as high as 23–33%, which must be factored into the decision of which access to create for a child. CVCs are the overwhelming choice for children undergoing HD. However, despite their relative ease of insertion, and the fact that they avoid repeated needle sticks, these devices are associated with frequent complications, the most important of which are clotting and infections. The frequency, and description of these complications which necessitated catheter removal, including our own unpublished data, are outlined in Table 3.

The frequency of clotting episodes with CVCs is also well illustrated by Valentini *et al.* who reported on 61 children from 11 centers within the Midwest Pediatric Nephrology Consortium. CVLC dysfunction (defined as reduced blood flows, need for reversed lines, or frequent intradialytic alarms) occurred in 46% of patients in a single one month period. Also, 16 of these patients required treatment with tissue plasminogen activator (TPA) for presumed clots in the same month.

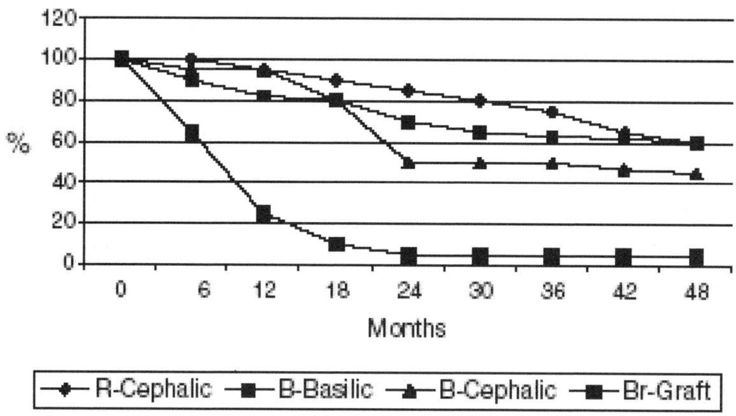

Figure 1. AV Fistulas in Children Long-term Patency. From Bourquelot P *et al.* (2005) Ther Apler Dial 7(6): 498.

Table 3. Central Venous Catheters in Children on HD Removal for Complications

	Boston[a]	Toronto	Glasgow[b]
Inserted	n = 22	n = 147	n = 182
Infection	8	33	30
Thrombosis	1	33	54
Extrusion	0	6	11
Kinking	3	0	0
Other	4	5	5
Total (%)	16(73)	77(52)	100(55)

[a] Goldstein SL, Macierowski CT, Jabs K. (1997) Hemodialysis catheter survival and complications in children and adolescents. *Pediatr Nephrol.* 11(1): 74–77.
[b] Ramage IJ, Bailie A, Tyerman KS, *et al.* (2005) Vascular access survival in children and young adults receiving long-term hemodialysis. *Am J Kidney* Dis **45**(4): 708–714.

The decision which vascular access to choose should certainly favor creation of an AVF where local expertise exists, unless early renal transplant is confidently anticipated. Because there are no data defining the risk of fistula loss in children in the peritransplant period, and because limb vessels must be preserved for future long-term HD access, it is reasonable to initiate HD with a CVC when HD is anticipated to be a short-term treatment. Whereas the United States Renal Data Systems (USRDS) 2008 report illustrates clearly that approximately half of adults listed for renal transplantation will remain on the waiting list at the end of five years, for children the median wait-time for a kidney varies from only 5–12 months depending on race and blood type. Therefore a reasonable argument can be made for short-term dialysis using a CVC in an unsensitized child who is listed for transplantation for the first time. For all other children initiating HD, including those transferring from PD, or starting HD after a failed transplant, creation of AVF is preferred.

Pediatric Hemodialysis Prescription

Optimal provision of hemodialysis must consider a large number of factors, all of which should each be included in a prescriptive order sheet, and include clear instructions related to the following;

- Choice of dialyzer and blood lines — biocompatibility of dialyzer, appropriate volume of blood lines, priming solution
- Estimation of dry weight and ultrafiltration (UF) volume (volume of fluid to be removed during the HD treatment)
- Dialysate composition and flow rate
- Blood flow rate
- Prevention and treatment of hypotension during HD
- Anticoagulation

Further details related to the choice and classification of dialyzers are outlined in Tables 4 and 5, and each of the factors outlined are discussed in more detail.

Typically the dialyzer chosen should be of biocompatible material to minimize acute reactions and reduce long-term inflammation. The blood lines should be long enough to allow space for nursing invterventions, and the total volume of blood lines and dialyzer should not exceed 10% of the patient's blood volume. If this is greater than 10% of the total blood volume (TBV), a circuit prime with 5% albumin or blood (if patient's Hb is <7 g/dL) is recommended. It is important not to retransfuse blood prime postdialysis if the patient is volume overloaded and to avoid a blood prime with AN 69 membranes because of associated cytokine reactions. The TBV is approximately equal to 100 ml/kg in neonate, 80 ml/kg

Table 4. Choice of dialysis membranes

1. Membrane surface area to match body surface area of patient and its influence on priming blood volume requirement
2. Type of membrane: Biocompatibility to decrease complement and coagulation cascade activity
3. Hydraulic Permeability: Estimated from K_{uf} of dialyzer. This is important for HF or HDF procedure, but because of back filtration risk, ultrapure dialysate recommended for high flux membranes
4. Solute Permeability: Estimated from KoA of dialyzer. The goal is to achieve maximum clearance for urea and the other uremic toxins related to potential patient osmotic risk
5. Adsorption capacity on to the membranes (a characteristic of synthetic membranes)
6. Mode of sterilization: reduced allergic reaction with steam sterilization/gamma irradiation compared with ethylene oxide if reuse is applicable
7. Cost

Table 5. Dialyzer classification

Class	Surface area	Kuf (ml/hr/mmHg)	Urea clearance	Beta2M clearance
Conventional	<1.5 m^2	<12	moderate	negligible
High efficiency	>1.5 m^2	>12	high (KoA >600ml/min)	negligible
Mid-flux	Variable	12–30	Variable	moderate
High-flux	Variable	>30	Variable	high (>20 ml/min)

From Clark WR, Ronco C. (2001) Determinants of haemodialyser performance and the potential effect on clinical outcome. *Nephrol Dial Trans* **16**(5): 56–60.

for infant and children up to 16 years of age and 70 ml/kg in older than 16 years of age.

Estimation of dry weight usually requires a careful dietary history, including estimated fluid intake, physical examination for evidence of fluid overload, and a precise estimate of weight and interdialytic weight gain. Ancilliary methods to help with this estimate include chest X-ray to review heart size, changes in plasma hemoglobin and albumin values, and use of a blood volume monitor device during the dialysis session to define the limits of safe ultrafiltration. The net fluid removal should aim to reach dry weight. Although we have successfully removed as much as

9% of dry weight in a three-hour dialysis session, the following is usually recommended.

2 hrs treatment; usually <4% of estimated dry weight
3 hrs treatment; usually <6% of estimated dry weight
4 hrs treatment; usually <7% of estimated dry weight

The dialysate composition should also be considered when prescribing HD. Typical dialysate sodium is 140 mmol/L and can range from 135–145mmol/L. Sodium ramping can be used to maintain intravascular blood volume and help to reduce intradialytic hypotension. There are two methods that can be employed to manipulate the dialysate sodium. The linear method involves a decrease in dialysate Na from 145 to 135 mmol/L linearly throughout dialysis. The step method involves maintenance of dialysate Na 145 mmol/L until the last 30 minutes of the dialysis session, when it is reduced to 135 mmol/L. A schematic of each type of sodium ramping is depicted in Fig. 2.

Dialysate potassium may be prescribed based on a sliding scale as estimated below.

If serum K (mmol/l)	dialysate K
>5	0
4–4.9	1
3.5–3.9	2
2–3.4	3

The usual bicarbonate level of dialysate is 35 mmol/L (range 25–40 mmol/L). The use of acetate as a buffer may cause vasodilatation and intradialytic hypotension. Therefore, it is not used.

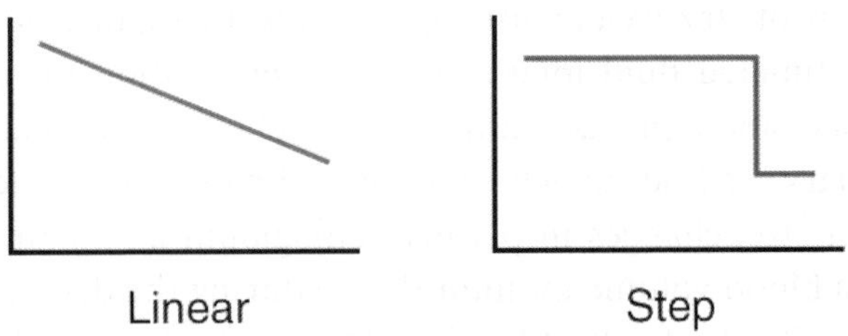

Figure 2. Sodium ramping.

Standard dialysate calcium concentration is 1.25 mmol/L (3.5 mEq/L). Higher dialysate calcium, 1.5–1.75 mmol/L, is useful in hypocalcemic patients and can help to maintain intradialytic blood pressure. However, high dialysate calcium levels may cause hypercalcemia and elevated calcium phosphate product which may predispose to vascular calcification, and also require reduced dosage of calcium containing phosphate binders. Dialysate usually dose not contain phosphate. However, the addition of phosphate is often necessary in patients receiving nocturnal hemodialysis to prevent hypophosphatemia, and may be required in severely malnourished children who develop hypophosphatemia secondary to refeeding syndrome. Typically, the concentration of magnesium in dialysate is 0.5–1 mmol/L (1.0–2.0 mEq/L). Glucose concentration of dialysate usually approximates 6–11 mmol/L (100–200 mg/dl).

Standards for water quality, as outlined in Table 6, vary in different geographic regions. Less pure water may contribute to the chronic inflammation observed in dialysis patients. Ultrapure water should be used for hemodiafiltration. Water quality is monitored at routine intervals, generally monthly, based on federal guidelines.

Potential complications associated with water contamination are shown in Table 7.

Blood flow rate is a major determinant of solute clearance on dialysis and the anticipated fall in plasma urea can be estimated from blood flow

Table 6. Upper limit for bacterial and endotoxin in water and dialysate used for hemodialysis

	Water		Dialysate	
	Bacterial (CFU/ml)	Endotoxin (EU/ml)	Bacteria (CFU/ml)	Endotoxin (EU/ml)
AAMI,RDF 1981	200	NS	2000	NS
AAMI,RD62:2001	200	2	NS	NS
AAMI,proposed	NS	NS	200	2
ERA-EDTA	100	0.25	100	0.25
European pharmacopoeia	100	0.25	NS	NS
Swedish pharmacopoeia	100	0.25	100	0.25
Ultrapure	0.1	0.3	0.1	0.3

From Ward RA. (2004) Ultrapure dialysate. *Semin Dial* 17(6): 489–497.

Table 7. Water contamination and associated complications

Contaminants	Complications
Pesticides, herbicides	No documentation during dialysis
Chloramine, Chlorine compounds	Severe hemolytic anemia
Bacteria	Bacteremia or septicemia Fever, chills, shaking Hypotension and death
Pyrogens	Pyrogenic reaction fever Chills, uncontrollable Shaking, vomiting, hypotension

prescribed in ml/kg/min. The first HD should have a goal of 2 ml/kg/min urea clearance (equivalent to 2 ml/kg/min blood flow for most dialyzers) in a two-hour dialysis session, then increase to 3–4 ml/kg/min urea clearance or increase session length for subsequent treatments. For chronic hemodialysis, blood flow rate should approximate 4–6 ml/kg/min. In infants, this should be a minimum of 20 ml/min to reduce the risk of clotting.

The major barrier to achieving the goal of hemodialysis is the development of hemodynamic instability. This occurs on average in 20–30% of treatments.

The following steps may be considered for prevention of intradialytic hypotension. Blood volume monitoring (BVM) is strongly recommended in children. If relative blood volume (RBV) falls below 88% in the first hour of the treatment or below 84% at any time, UF should be discontinued until plasma refilling has occurred to adequately raise RBV. Some have advocated withholding antihypertensive medications on dialysis days. The half-life and proportion of antihypertensive drugs excreted by dialysis should be considered and this practice implemented on a situational basis. Other practices implemented to decrease the risk of hypotension include avoidance of food during dialysis or cooling the dialysate. Increasing the dialysate Na or ramping as described earlier and treating intradialytic hypocalcemia may also be of benefit. Mannitol 0.5–1.0 gm/kg or 25% albumin 1 gm/kg may be administered in the first hour of dialysis to prevent hypotension. In severe cases, midodrine 2.5–10 mg can be given 15–30 minutes before dialysis, and repeated at onset of hypotension during the first two hours of dialysis. It is important to remember hypotension occurs because vascular volume depletion exceeds the rate of refilling from the interstitium. Most dialysis machines have different UF profiles that can be adjusted to vary UF rates throughout the course of treatment. For a three-hour procedure it has been recommended that 50% of the planned total UF should occur in the first hour. Furthermore, traditional methods of iso-osmotic fluid removal (isolated UF) using sequential dialysis techniques (pure UF followed by dialysis) may achieve higher UF rates without inducing hemodynamic instability. UF only can be prescribed during the first or last hour or alternate with dialysis 30 minutes on–off. During isolated UF, the patient's temperature may fall because warmed dialysate is not flowing. For acute management for intradialytic hypotension, UF should be discontinued and normal saline bolus or 5% albumin 5 ml/kg/dose may be administered as an intravenous bolus. The patient should be placed in the Trendelenberg position. Finally, one should consider quotidian HD (increased time and/or frequency), such as short daily HD (SDHD) or nocturnal HD (NHD) prescribed 5–6 times per week to optimize hemodynamic stability.

Anticoagulation is usually provided during the HD treatment using unfractionated heparin. In some centers, a bolus dose of 10–15 u/kg of heparin (3–14.9 kg) or 15–20 u/kg of heparin (15–55 kg) is administered, followed by a continuous infusion of 10–20 u/kg/hr, which is stopped 30 minutes before the end of the dialysis treatment. A maximum amount of heparin 100 u/kg for a three-hour treatment and 130 u/kg for a four-hour treatment is recommended. Other centers may utilize interval boluses of heparin. Patients with a hypercoagulable state may require higher initial and maintenance doses of 25–30 u/kg of heparin. "Tight" heparin (ACT plus 140–180 seconds or 25% above initial baseline) is suggested for all children at risk of bleeding, and heparin free regimen is recommended in patients who have a risk of bleeding and weigh less than 10 kg. Furthermore, heparin may be held in children pre- or postoperatively to reduce the risk of surgical bleeding. Heparin Induced Thrombo-cytopenia (HIT) is uncommon in children. It is an antibody mediated activation of platelets (Platelet factor 4) which leads to thromboembolism. Heparin (including dialyzer prime) should not be used in the presence of HIT. Citrate anticoagulation of the extracorporeal circuit is possible without systemic effects, and is an option for patients with a bleeding risk. Poor hepatic metabolism can result in citrate toxicity. Citrate anticoagulation can also be complicated by hypocalcemia, hypernatremia, volume expansion, and metabolic alkalosis. Low molecular weight heparin has not been evaluated in pediatric HD.

Common Complications of Hemodialysis

Dialysis-related hypertension

Dialysis-related hypertension is predominantly caused by chronic volume overload. In a significant proportion of these patients, the blood pressure can be normalized with improved salt and fluid balance. Hypertension is defined as a mean of three casual blood pressure readings greater than the 95th percentile corrected for age, height, and gender. Additional parameters that influence the decision to treat include a wide pulse pressure, or if using 24-hour ambulatory BP, a blood pressure load (>40% of readings above 95th percentile of target values), or a sleep blood pressure decrease less than 10% of daytime baseline reading (nondipper). Treatment decisions will also be influenced by evidence of cardiovascular disease [e.g., left ventricular hypertrophy (LVH)].

Because elevated blood pressure is usually due to fluid retention, the treatment of hypertension should initially focus on accurate estimation and maintenance of dry weight. Also, the dialysis procedure can be prescribed to provide a lower sodium dialysate or adjustment of sodium profiles, or the frequency and duration of dialysis can be increased to facilitate fluid removal. Pharmacological treatment should consider drug pharmacokinetics during hemodialysis, including an estimate of drug half-life with end-stage renal function. For example, enalapril and captopril are cleared by HD but fosinopril is not. The beta-blockers atenolol and metoprolol are removed during HD, but clearance of propranolol is insignificant. Minoxidil is also cleared by HD but no data exists for doxazocin. Neither amlodipine, whose half-life is extended to about 50 hours in ESRD, nor angiotensin receptor blockers, such as losartan have significant clearance during HD.

Dialysis Dysequilibrium Syndrome (DDS)

DDS occurs as a result of cerebral edema swelling due to fluid shifts from the extracellular compartment to the intracellular compartment, which happens when plasma urea levels fall too rapidly during HD. This is most often associated with an initial HD treatment. Symptoms typically are progressive and include nausea, vomiting, headache, blurred vision, muscular twitching, disorientation, hypertension, tremors, seizures, and coma.

Patients at risk for developing DDS include children, those with preexisting neurologic disease; those with severe metabolic acidosis; new patients starting HD, particularly with a high predialysis urea; and patients with a high UF goal. Also at risk are those children who have a clinical situation associated with cerebral edema such as rapid rehydration therapy, hyponatremia, malignant hypertension, diabetes mellitus, or hypoglycemia.

Prevention of DDS can be achieved by adjusting the dialysis prescription to reduce the rate of plasma urea clearance, using a smaller dialyzer, decreasing the blood flow, or decreasing the dialysate flow rate. Intradialytic osmotic shifts can be minimized with the use of sodium profiles to provide high initial dialysate sodium concentrations, or treatment using sequential HD with an initial period of UF alone.

Mannitol is commonly used in pediatrics, both in a preventive and therapeutic role. A maximal intradialytic dose of 1 g/kg is recommended once a week in high-risk patients. If more frequent dosing is required, a smaller dose of 0.5 g/kg is advised. An alternative treatment is hypertonic sodium chloride infusion. Concurrent antiepileptic therapy is required if the patient is seizing.

Malnutrition, inflammation, and atherosclerosis

Malnutrition and inflammation have been reported to be strong predictors of mortality in dialysis patients; however, cardiovascular disease is the most commonly documented cause of mortality. Serum albumin levels are often low as both a marker of malnutrition as well as inflammation. C-reactive protein (CRP), an acute phase protein, is a recognized marker of inflammation and is often elevated in chronic HD patients. Attempts should be made at decreasing inflammation as much as possible. The dialysis prescription can be modified to become less inflammatory by using ultrapure dialysate and synthetic biocompatible membranes. Both ACE inhibitors and statins, more commonly recognized for their respective roles in treating hypertension and hypercholesterolemia, have also been reported to have anti-inflammatory actions.

Each patient receiving HD should be routinely followed by a renal dietitian at least monthly and malnutrition corrected. Many of these children will require supplemental enteric feeds (either orally or via gastrostomy tube) or intravenous intradialytic parenteral nutrition. Laboratory studies should be obtained at least monthly to assess nutritional stores, electrolytes, and clearances in HD patients.

Dialysis related carnitine disorder

A dialysis related carnitine disorder (DCD), usually manifests as anemia that is hyporesponsive to erythropoietin, intradialytic hypotension, cardiomyopathy, and weakness, asthenia, intradialytic muscle cramping, and reduced exercise tolerance. The aim of L-carnitine supplementation is to produce clinical improvement and restore the total body carnitine pool. Measurement of skeletal muscle L-carnitine concentrations is impractical in children. Therefore, deficiency is assessed from plasma-free carnitine levels, the ratio of acyl to free carnitine, and clinical evaluation. Treatment of carnitine deficiency is with intravenous L-carnitine at a dose of 20 mg/kg at the end of dialysis, with continuing treatment for 6–12 months. Oral carnitine supplementation is not recommended in ESRD due to concerns of toxicity from L-carnitine metabolites, which accumulate in renal failure.

Hyperhomocysteinemia

Plasma homocysteine elevations in CRF may be associated with atherosclerosis. Chronic inflammation may contribute to hyperhomocysteinemia. Folate, vitamin B12, and vitamin B6 therapy have the potential to improve cardiovascular morbidity both by lowering plasma homocysteine levels and by neutralizing elevated oxidative stress.

Assessment of Hemodialysis Adequacy

Dialysis adequacy should primarily be assessed by clinical evaluation of the patient with specific focus on energy level, nutritional state and appetite, growth, evidence of cardiovascular disease, and metabolic status (e.g., phosphate, parathyroid hormone levels).

Measurement of urea clearance by Kt/V_{urea} is also specifically recommended. The KDOQI recommendation for children on HD is a $spKt/V_{urea} > 1.4$ (based on a thrice weekly dialysis schedule). Single pool (sp) Kt/V_{urea} can be measured by kinetic modeling techniques which are available on a number of websites (e.g., www.Kt-V.net). An alternative is the formula

$$Kt/V = \text{Log n } (R - 0.008t) + (4\text{–}3.5\ R)\ UF/BW$$

In this formula R = post urea/pre urea, t = dialysis time in hours, UF is the fluid volume ultrafiltered in liters and BW is the estimated dry weight of the patient.

To minimize the effect of postdialysis rebound, blood for measurement of the postdialysis urea value should be drawn using the slow blood flow method:

1. At end of dialysis, turn off dialysate flow and decrease UF as much as possible
2. Decrease blood flow below 100 ml/min for 15 seconds
3. Obtain a blood sample

Or alternatively, using the stop dialysate method:

1. At end of dialysis, stop dialysate flow and decrease UF as much as possible
2. Maintain blood flow at normal rate for three minutes
3. Obtain a blood sample

Urea reduction ratio (URR) is a simplified estimate of the % urea removal during HD and is measured from the equation $(1 - R) \times 100$. URR is not recommended as the primary measure of dialysis adequacy because significant variations of Kt/V_{urea} may be obtained with each URR value depending on the amount of fluid removed.

The major advantage of kinetically modeled methods for estimating Kt/V_{urea} is that they also provide an estimate of urea generation rate, from which normalized protein catabolic rate (nPCR, an estimate of dietary protein intake in the clinically stable patient) can be estimated.

Summary

Hemodialysis is the mode of renal replacement in 36% of children with ESRD according to the NAPRTCS registry. The majority of these children have CVC as their mode of vascular access, and receive dialysis thrice weekly, each of which may be satisfactory provided transplantation is planned within a year. For those anticipating a longer time on HD, the central venous catheter should be replaced with AVF, and, especially for children without residual native renal function, more frequent HD sessions should be considered.

Suggested Reading

Chand DH, Valentini RP, Kamil ES. (2009) Hemodialysis vascular access options in pediatrics: considerations for patients and practitioners. *Pediatr Nephrol* 24(6): 1121–1128.

Fischbach M, Edefonti A, Schröder C, Watson A. (2005) Hemodialysis in children: general practical guidelines. *Pediatr Nephrol* **20**: 1054–1066.

Hothi DK, Geary DF. (2008) Pediatric hemodialysis prescription, efficacy, and outcome. In: Geary DF, Schaefer F. *Comprehensive Pediatric Nephrology*, Elsevier Saunders, Philadelphia, pp. 867–893.

KDOQI clinical practice guidelines and clinical practice recommendations 2006.

North America Pediatric Renal Trials and Collaborative Studies (NAPRTCS). (2008) *2008 Annual Report (Dialysis).*

Schröder CH, Geary DF. (2008) Dialysis modality choice and initiation in children. In: Geary DF, Schaefer F, *Comprehensive Pediatric Nephrology*, Elsevier Saunders, Philadelphia, pp. 817–822.

Sheth RD, Brandt ML, Brewer ED, Nuchtern JG, Kale AS, Goldstein SL. (2002) Permanent Hemodialysis vascular access survival in children and adolescents with end-stage renal disease. *Kidney Int* **62**: 1864–1869.

Valentini RP, Geary DF, Chand DH. (2008) Central venous lines for chronic hemodialysis: survey of the Midwest Pediatric Nephrology Consortium.

HYPERLINK"javascript:AL_get(this,%20'jour',%20'Pediatr%20Nephrol.');" *Pediatr Nephrol* **23**: 291–295.

Warady BA *et al.* (2004) *Pediatric Dialysis.*

Warady BA, Fischbach M, Geary DF, Goldstein S. (2007) Frequent Hemodialysis in Children. *Adv Chron Kidney Dis* **14**(3): 297–303.

39

Peritoneal Dialysis

Marcus R. Benz and Franz Schaefer

Introduction

The concept of peritoneal dialysis (PD) dates back to the late 19th and early 20th century when researchers demonstrated that the peritoneum constitutes a membrane with bidirectional permeability for small and middle molecules. The first chronic indwelling catheter for PD was placed in 1968 by Tenckhoff. In children, continuous ambulatory PD (CAPD) was first used in 1978 in Toronto, and soon practiced in many American and European centers. Nowadays, PD is the predominant initial dialytic modality in children with end-stage renal disease (ESRD), especially in children requiring renal replacement therapy (RRT) in the first decade of life. More than 60% of children with ESRD as their initial dialysis modality, mainly because PD is less restrictive socially and medically than hemodialysis (HD). Moreover, a permanent PD access can be accomplished at any age, whereas permanent vascular accesses are much more problematic in pediatric patients.

Key terms

The effectiveness of PD is influenced by three major components:

- *Peritoneal microcirculation*
    - Suggested peritoneal blood flow: 50–100 ml/min
- *Peritoneal membrane*
    - Capillary wall (mainly continuous type, less than 2% fenestrated)
    - Interstitium
    - Mesothelial cells

- *Dialysis fluid compartment*
  - Composition of solution
  - Modalities of delivery

For exchange of water and solute across the peritoneal membrane the following processes are involved:

- *Diffusion*
  - Solute exchange between blood and dialysis fluid separated by a semipermeable membrane following the concentration gradient
  - Spontaneous, based on free molecular movement, not energy consuming
  - Depending on height of concentration gradient, molecular weight, effective surface area and permeability of peritoneal membrane
- *Ultrafiltration (UF)*
  - Net removal of water from the blood in the dialysis fluid caused by the osmotic pressure of dialysis fluid (glucose or other osmotic agents in the dialysis fluid) as driving force
  - Hydrostatic pressure gradient due the dialysis fluid in the peritoneal cavity counteracts the osmotic pressure; this is less important for UF unless there are exceedingly high levels of intraperitoneal pressure (IPP)
  - UF reduced by lymphatic absorption (possible cause for reduced net UF in some children, as well significant absorption of macromolecules)
- *Convective solute transport*
  - Dissolved molecules dragged along (solvent drag) as water moves from blood to peritoneal cavity (even in the absence of a concentration gradient)
  - Depends on rate of UF and membrane permeability

Indications and Contraindications

The majority of pediatric patients can be managed with chronic peritoneal dialysis (CPD). Thus, the choice of CPD over chronic HD is most often based on patient/family preference, center philosophy, and modality availability.

Indications and predominant advantages for PD:

- Very small patients
- Lack of vascular access
- Contraindications to anticoagulation
- Cardiovascular instability
- Lack of proximity to a pediatric HD center

Absolute contraindications to PD:

- Omphalocele
- Gastroschisis
- Bladder exstrophy
- Diaphragmatic hernia
- Obliterated peritoneal cavity, and peritoneal membrane failure

Relative contraindications to PD:

- Impending abdominal surgery
- Recent major abdominal surgery
- Impending living/related renal transplantation
- Lack of an appropriate caregiver

The presence of a colostomy, gastrostomy (GT), ureterostomy, and/or pyelostomy does not preclude CPD. Patients with bladder augmentation and prune belly syndrome have also been successfully managed with CPD. Controversy exists as to whether the presence of a ventriculo-peritoneal cerebrospinal fluid shunt constitutes a contraindication to CPD. Limited experience suggests CPD is acceptable in this situation if no feasible alternative dialysis option exists, recognizing the risks of peritonitis in this patient population.

While PD is generally the preferred initial RRT in children, an individual decision needs to be made for every child. Besides the indications and contraindications given above, the following factors should be taken into consideration:

- *Patient age*: In infants, PD is the modality of choice due to the difficulty of creating a functioning arteriovenous fistula (AVF) for HD, the risks of infection, thrombosis, and malfunction of an indwelling venous catheter, and potential cardiovascular (CV) instability while undergoing HD.
- *Geographic location*: Whereas dialysis centers for adults are available ubiquitously, pediatric dialysis centers are not. If the pediatric dialysis center is a long distance from the patient's home, PD could suit the patient better than HD. For adolescents receiving HD, a boarding school near the center is an option in some countries.
- *Family composition and social support*: In general, home dialysis techniques are better compatible with social life and school attendance. However, this major advantage must be carefully weighed against the burden and responsibility of care imposed on the families by home dialysis. This burden may give rise to burnout, depression, and familial dysfunction. Thorough and careful evaluation of the family's social, psychological, and economic background, ideally by a multiprofessional team, including experienced physicians, dialysis nurses, psychologists, and social workers, is required to come to a fully informed decision. A home visit should be conducted by appropriate personnel prior to initiating PD. Due to the burden of PD at home, routine ongoing supervision by the multiprofessional team is necessary.
- *Patient compliance*: For home dialysis regimens, patient compliance is required. Devices such as individual smart media patient cards in modern cyclers could be an effective monitoring tool.
- *Residual renal function*: Native kidney urine output and residual function is better preserved in patient on PD compared with those on HD. The impact on quality of life can be tremendous.

PD Catheters

The ideal PD access provides high dialysate flow rates with no fluid leaks, minimal catheter movement at the skin exit-site (ES), has a low incidence of catheter-related infections, and placement of the catheter at a site that is both reachable and visible to the child or caregivers.

Catheter design

Key elements of catheter design are:

- *Material*: The catheters commonly used for chronic PD are constructed of biocompatible soft material, such as silicone rubber or polyurethane.
- *Intraperitoneal configuration (straight or curled)*: The straight internal portion of PD catheters has largely been replaced by coil

	N	%
Peritoneal Dialysis Courses	4352	100.0
Catheter		
Tenckhoff straight	1170	26.9
Tenckhoff curled	2677	61.5
Toronto western	26	0.6
Presternal	272	6.3
Other	88	2.0
Unknown/missing	119	2.7
Cuffs		
One	2263	52.0
Two	1951	44.8
Unknown/missing	138	3.2
Tunnel		
Swan neck/curved	1397	32.1
Straight	2801	64.4
Unknown/missing	154	3.5
Exit Site Orientation		
Up	535	12.3
Down	1425	32.7
Lateral	1735	39.9
Unknown/missing	657	15.1

Figure 1a.

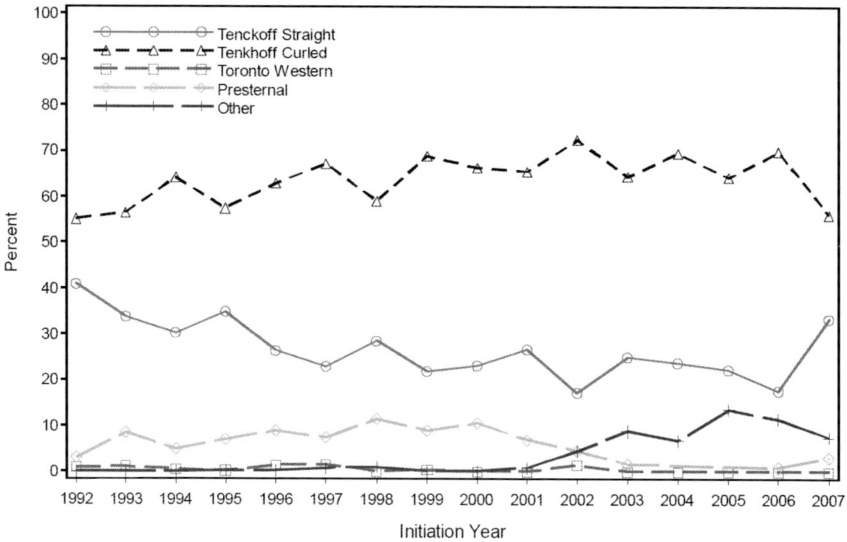

Figure 1b. Peritoneal dialysis catheter access type by initation year.

From NAPRTCS. (2009) *North American Pediatric Renal Trails and Collaborative Studies 2008 Annual Report*, EMMES Cooperation, Rockville.

catheters. The advantages of curled catheters include the reduced risk of blockade by omentum or bowel, reduced risk of migration out of the pelvis, less pain due to infusion or catheter tip pressure on the peritoneum, and better dialysate flow due to large number of side holes.

- *Number of Dacron cuffs (single or double)*: Retrospective studies and registry reports lend support to the use of double-cuff catheters. Lewis *et al.* showed that single-cuff catheters are associated with a higher incidence of ES infections and peritonitis. These data are supported by the NAPRTCS data registry, which also showed a longer time to first peritonitis episode in the double-cuff catheter group. In the International Pediatric Peritonitis Registry, the use of single-cuff catheters was independently associated with a poor outcome of gram-negative peritonitis. Hence, the use of single-cuff catheters should be restricted to neonates and young infants with short available tunnel distances for anatomical reasons, and to children with a high likelihood of a short PD duration (e.g., in acute kidney injury).

- *Positioning of single-cuff catheter*: The cuff of a single-cuff catheter should be positioned between the rectus sheaths and in the rectus muscle (not in superficial position).
- *Positioning of double-cuff catheter*: The outer cuff should be placed 1.5–2 cm from the exit-site to prevent cuff extrusion, and at least 1.5–2 cm from the inner cuff to form a decent subcutaneous tunnel. Any torsion should be avoided when placing the catheter. Advantages of double-cuff catheters include the prevention of organisms spreading from exit-site into the tunnel (reduced risk of exit-site infection and peritonitis).
- *Subcutaneous tunnel configuration (straight or swan-neck, i.e. inverted U-shape arc (170–180°) between cuffs)*: A swan-neck catheter was first described by Twardowski and was developed for the purpose of allowing the catheter to exit the skin in downward-pointing direction with a long subcutaneous tunnel (see below), and allowing the distal end of the catheter to enter the peritoneal cavity in an unstressed condition respectively without to much torque which reduces the risk of migration out of the pelvis. The swan-neck presternal catheter is a modification of this catheter type and may be useful in selected pediatric patients who are still in diapers, have gastrostomies, vesicostomies or ureterostomies, and are obese, crawling, or subject to recurrent ESI. Advantages of swan-neck catheters include the reduced risk of catheter displacement.
- *Exit-site orientation*: A PD catheter with a downward-pointing exit-site prevents the accumulation of dirt and debris at the exit site and/or catheter tunnel decreasing the risk of ESI or peritonitis. Furthermore, young children, who sometimes do not like to wear a face mask at the time of connection and/or dressing change, do not breathe on the notch of the catheter if it is placed in a downward-pointing position.
- Exit-site localization: The ES localization must be planned preoperatively and ideally discussed with the family beforehand. The ES should allow easy visual access and should not be compromised by bending movements of the patient. Leakage is minimal when the inner cuff is placed laterally from the midline with the tunnel passing vertically through the body of the rectus muscle. Midline catheter insertion should be avoided. In school children and adolescents, the exit-site localization should be either above or below the belt line

(adolescents mostly prefer below belt line). In infants, the exit-site is typically placed outside the diaper area to help prevent contamination. Also, proximity of the PD catheter exit-site to a GT/button exit-site, vesicostomy, ureterostomy, colostomy, or other stoma is a risk factor for infection. The exit-site should be located as remote as possible from such artificial orifices (e.g., contralateral side of abdomen). In difficult cases with multiple abdominal stomata, it may be necessary to extend the subcutaneous tunnel to the chest; the Twardowski swan-neck presternal catheter is an excellent option with low infection rates in such cases. The PD catheter should be positioned on the right-hand site of the abdomen, if the patient has the potential for having GT in the future. Otherwise, the PD catheter should be placed on the left-hand side to avoid interference with a future transplantation incision.

In summary, double-cuff swan-neck catheters with a downward-pointing ES configuration are associated with lowest infection rates and are generally recommended for children, but particular anatomical situations frequently necessitate modifications to this rule.

Catheter implantation

Preparation

Optimal timing for peritoneal catheter insertion is 2–6 weeks prior to use of the catheter. This is to ensure anchoring of internal and external cuffs and healing of the ES.

Preparation includes the decision where the ES of the catheter should be and what kind of catheter should be implanted. The catheter insertion site, exit-site and tunnel configuration should be determined well in advance of the surgical procedure, taking into account patient preference, scars from previous surgery, and the individual abdominal configuration, including skinfolds and belt line. It is helpful to draw the planned catheter trail on the skin (see Fig. 3).

Constipation is an independent risk factor for postplacement PD catheter migration. As constipation is common in patients with CKD, laxatives or enemas are often needed for preoperative preparation (avoid phosphorus containing enemas!).

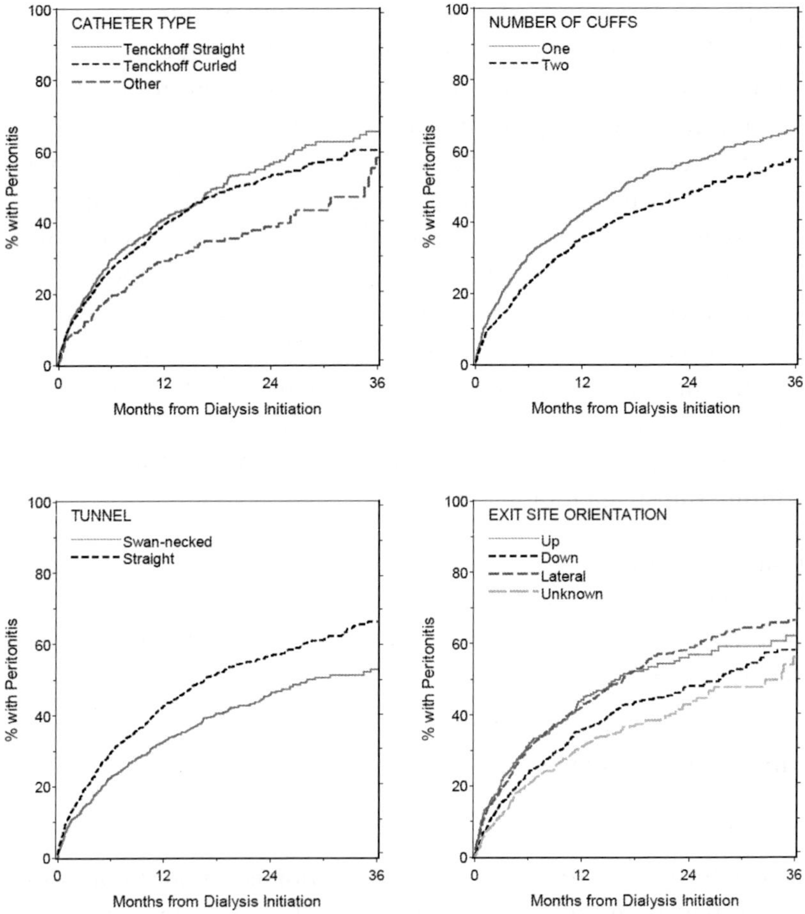

Figure 2. Time to first peritonitis infection by peritoneal dialysis access characteristics (PD index cases).

From NAPRTCS. (2009) *North American Pediatric Renal Trials and Collaborative Studies (NAPRTCS) 2008 Annual Report.* EMMES Cooperation, Rockville.

Small or latent hernias will inevitably be aggravated after start of PD. Therefore any known hernia should be repaired prior to or at the time of catheter placement. Most inguinal hernias manifest in young male infants with an open vaginal processus.

Perioperative antibiotic prophylaxis decreases the incidence of early peritonitis after PD catheter placement. Prophylaxis should be performed

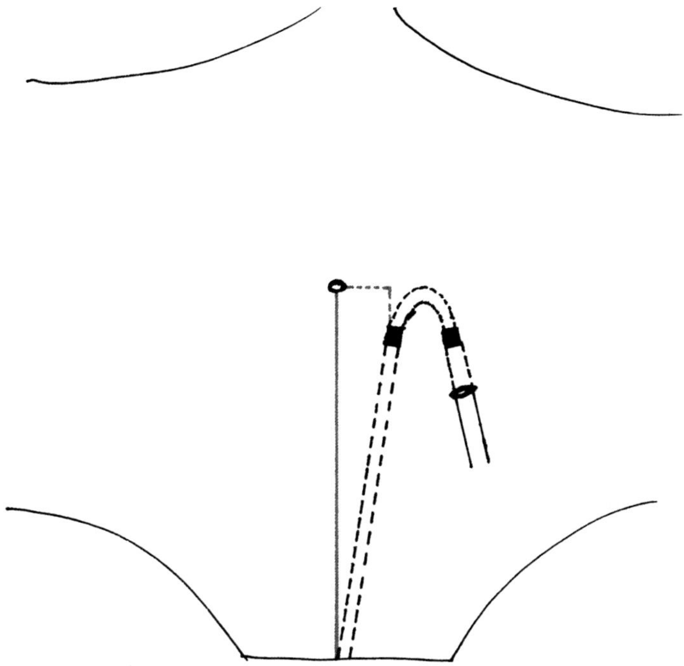

Figure 3. Determination of insertion site, exit-site and tunnel configuration prior to surgery.

with a first- or second-generation cephalosporin unless the patient is colonized with MRSA. Screening for nasal *Staphylococcus aureus* carriage may also be useful. If positive, caregivers should also be checked. A course of mupirocin 2% ointment applied to each nostril for five days, and reapplied every month for five days per month should be considered. Oral antifungal prophylaxis should be considered in a child with a gastrostomy tube.

Techniques

Open surgery or laparoscopic placement are possible.

Open technique

- Incision over the rectus muscle is mostly used (lateral/paramedial insertion of the rectus decreases risk of incisional hernias and leakage)

- Rectus muscle is split in parallel to fiber direction
- Posterior sheath is opened longitudinally
- Catheter is threaded over a stiffening wire to allow its placement deep in the pelvis (a few degrees to the right of midline but well within the pelvic brim, helps to prevent obstruction in case of a full rectum)
- Tip of catheter should be in the lowest part of pelvis *without* bending or kinking
- Posterior sheath is closed and inner cuff fixed to posterior sheath as part of its closure
- Inner cuff is positioned within the rectus muscle
- Anterior sheath is closed tightly around the catheter with a second purse-string suture around the cuff
- For tunneling, the catheter a lateral fascial opening is performed (as small as possible to prevent leakage)
- The catheter is then tunneled out to the skin with the outer cuff placed 1.5–2.0 cm from the catheter exit-site

    a. if <2 cm: risk for cuff extrusion
    b. if >2 cm: risk for formation of a deep sinus tract, granulation tissue formation, or tunnel infection

- Some centers use fibrin sealant around the outer cuff
- Exit-site should be as small as possible to prevent leakage and bacterial invasion
- Place catheter adapter and apply transfer set with cap
- Tape catheter securely to the abdomen
- Exit-site is dressed with nonocclusive absorbent dressing. Skin sutures should never be used to fixate the catheter!
- Apply antibiotic prophylaxis

The advantage of open technique is that it facilitates omentectomy. The disadvantages are that it requires significant incision in the peritoneum, and the need for extended rest period for healing.

Laparoscopic technique

First described in children in 2002, this technique is becoming increasingly popular.

- Vertical incision is made in the umbilicus and the umbilical fascia is sharply incised
- A 3 or 5 mm port is inserted via blunt dissection (size of the port is dependent on the size of the child)
- A corresponding 3 or 5 mm laparoscope is placed
- Peritoneum is carefully inspected for evidence of any hernias
- A sheath (20 French) is then inserted into the abdomen
- Using this sheath the PD catheter with a stiffener is inserted into the abdomen and placed in the pelvis under direct vision
- Using the peel-away sheath technique, the sheath is removed
- Control position of the catheter laparoscopically
- The inner cuff is fixed to the anterior rectus sheath with a purse-string suture
- Note that inner cuff is not visible in the peritoneal cavity
- Tunneling of catheter and creation of exit-site (see open technique)

The advantages of laparoscopic technique are the placement of PD catheter under direct vision, the need for a smaller peritoneal incision (lower risk for hernias and leakage), the fact that preexisting hernias can be detected easily, and that adhesions can be detected and unblocked. Disadvantages are that several peritoneal incisions are required, and the possible risk of hernias and leakage (e.g., third trocar required for omentectomy)

Omentectomy

Routine omentectomy remains controversial: omentectomy prevents PD catheter obstruction (reduces catheter occlusion rate from 10–23% to 5%) However, the incidence of catheter occlusion remains low. Overall, most pediatric surgeons recommend at least a partial omentectomy at the time of catheter placement. In infants and small children more extensive omentectomy may be required.

Careful attention to surgical technique and the experience of surgeon are probably more important than type of catheter used.

- Consider pediatric nephrologist or dialysis nurse presence in the operating room

- Check of catheter function in the operating room: free inflow and return of effluent should be verified and documented in the operating room.

Postplacement care and timing of catheter use

Placement should be timed to allow 2–6 weeks for healing prior to initiation of dialysis. This includes immobilization of catheter and minimizing exposure to bacterial colonization. A minimum dialysis-free period of at least two weeks is recommended. Some centers perform peritoneal flushing to check for catheter patency and function; however, other centers prefer to leave the catheter untouched until it is used for dialysis. If dialysis is required early, small volume exchanges in supine or recumbent position (low intra-abdominal pressure) may be performed with frequent checks for leakage.

Postoperative assessment and dressing changes should be performed weekly by experienced staff using aseptic technique with mask and gloves. Some oozing from the exit-site is common; therefore gauze dressing is recommended. The first dressing change should not be performed before day 5, unless there is evidence of bleeding, leaking, contamination, or infection.

Unnecessary palpation of the tunnel or mobilization of the catheter should be avoided. As much as possible, an increase of intra-abdominal pressure should be obviated (e.g., long crying in infants, heavy lifting, stair climbing, straining and constipation). Sufficient pain management should be provided.

At the initiation of dialysis:

- Nocturnal PD and other tasks to minimize increase in intra-abdominal pressure are recommended to avoid leakage
- PD should be started with low volume per exchange (10 ml/kg BW or 25–500 ml/m^2 BSA)
- Consider measurement of hydrostatic intraperitoneal pressure to assess patient tolerance of fill volume

During healing process (2–6 weeks) catheter and exit-site exposure to shower and bath water should be avoided — use occlusive dressing (Op-site). Training of patient and parents should be initiated early.

Chronic care of PD catheter

Long-term PD catheter management focuses on maintaining a healthy exit-site and catheter tract. This goal is achieved by:

- Assessment of exit-site (exit-site score)
- Early identification and treatment of exit-site problems
- Prevention of contamination
- Immobilization of the catheter (protection from trauma)

Dressings should be changed approximately three times per week. Some patients will elect not to wear a dressing after six weeks postplacement. Change dressing ahead of schedule in case of:

- Humidity penetration
- Pain
- Malfunctioning catheter
- Exit-site infection
- Unfixed dressing

Cleansing agent should be nonirritating, nontoxic, antibacterial and in liquid form (e.g., chlorhexidine). After drying the exit-site is covered with semipermeable dressing. Prophylactic use of mupirocin to *S. aureus* carriers (patient and caregivers) in both areas for five days (BID) per month. Alternatively, aminoglycoside cream can be administered to the exit-site with each dressing exchange.

Dressing recommendations

In case of an unremarkable exit-site score, change of dressing 2–3 times per week is sufficient. More frequent exist site care is associated with an increased risk of *Pseudomonas*-related peritonitis.

Cleansing should be done using a noncytotoxic and nonalcoholic agent in liquid form (e.g., poloxamer 188, ß-octenidine, chlorhexidine). The use of nonsterile agents (water/soap) increases the risk of *Pseudomonas*-related peritonitis. Additional dressing changes should be performed after taking a shower or bath and whenever the dressing becomes wet (e.g., intense sweating).

During dressing changes, doors and windows should be closed and every person in the room should wear a face mask:

- Disinfection of the hands is mandatory
- Crusts and scabs should be softened with sterile saline
- Exit-site should be kept dry
- Immobilization of catheter is recommended

PD and gastrostomy

Gastrostomy tubes are typically inserted via a percutaneous route using gastroscopy (PEG method). Gastrostomy is ideally undertaken together with PD catheter placement and PD initiation delayed for 2–6 weeks to allow gastrostomy healing.

In prevalent PD patients, PEG placement carries high risk of bacterial and fungal peritonitis, particularly in presence with severe malnutrition. Such patients should ideally receive a period of nasogastric feeding to improve their nutritional and immunological status prior to gastrostomy insertion. PD should be intensified prior to and, if possible, paused for three days following PEG placement.

Prescription

PD modality and prescription

Chronic peritoneal dialysis (CPD) can performed in different ways:

- Continuous ambulatory PD (CAPD) performed manually vs. automated PD (APD) performed with the help of a device (cycler).
- APD is administered as continuous cycling overnight.
  - Continuous cycling PD (CCPD): >50% fill volume instilled during daytime.
  - Nightly intermittent PD (NIPD): <50% fill volume instilled during daytime.
  - Tidal PD (TPD): Multiple short cycles with fixed partial drainage of dwell volume; full drainage every 4–5 cycles.

PD prescription should be individualized to meet ultrafiltration and clearance needs, as well as family lifestyle requirements.

CAPD

Prescription

- Inflow of dialysate solution and drainage is performed manually
- Double-bag PD solution container with Y set for infusion and drainage
- PD solution is warmed to body temperature prior to inflow
- 3–5 exchanges per day
- Initial fill volume 600–800 ml/m² BSA daytime, 800–1000 ml/m² BSA overnight

The advantages of CAPD is that it is sufficiently efficacious in children with residual function and there is no interference with evening activities. Disadvantages include the effort of manual daytime exchanges, the higher rate of peritonitis due to more frequent catheter access, and the increased risk of hernia and PD catheter leak.

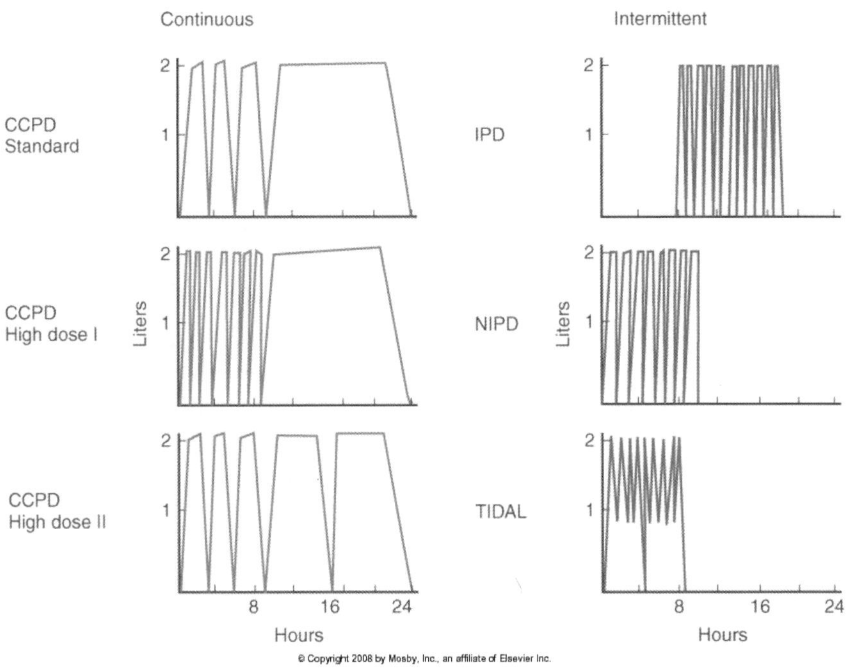

Figure 4. PC modalities.

From Verrina EE, Perfumo F. Pediatric dialysis prescription In: Geary DF, Schaefer F. *Comprehensive Pediatric Nephrology.*

APD techniques

Advantages of APD are that it does not interfere with daytime activities, and that compliance, lost dwell times, catheter flow rates can be checked easily. As well, because infants need high fluid intake for their calories, APD allows high UF due to short cycles, high dialysate flow, and high intraperitoneal volumes.

NIPD

Prescription

Should be guided by peritoneal transport characteristics as identified by peritoneal equilibration test [PET] (see below)

- Drain before fill reduces the risk of peritonitis
- 9–12 hours of total treatment time (to be balanced with schooling and social life requirements)
- 5–10 exchanges, dwell time of 45–120 min
- Fill volume: start with 800–1000 ml/m^2 BSA, increase to 1200–1400 ml/m^2 BSA maximum as required and tolerated.

The advantages of NIPD are that the recumbent position allows higher fill volumes than supine position in CAPD, there is decreased risk of glucose and fluid absorption during daytime, patient enjoys normal intraperitoneal pressure during day and improved body image, and the long-term preservation of the peritoneal membrane. The disadvantages include the risk of insufficient small molecule clearance in low/low–average transporters, and the fact that efficacy can be increased by increasing fill volume, number of exchanges/total treatment time, PD fluid glucose concentration.

CCPD

Prescription

- "Last bag" cycler option: Instillation of 50–100% of night-time fill volume before disconnection from cycler
- Drainage at time of reconnection in the evening

- If required for clearance and ultrafiltration, additional daytime exchanges can be provided, either manually or using latest cycler technologies (PD Plus™ Therapy, Fresenius; OCPD, Baxter)
- In case of poor return of daytime dwell, instillation of icodextrin based PD fluid is an excellent alternative to optimize ultrafiltration

The advantages of CCPD are that it is helpful in patients without residual renal function, the improved small- and middle-molecule clearance and the benefit for patients with low–average transport status. The disadvantages include glucose and potential net fluid resorption during daytime, high intraperitoneal pressure during daytime; increased risk of hernia, impaired appetite regulation by full abdomen and continuous glucose resorption, and impairment of body image.

Tidal PD

The optimum percentage of the fixed proportion of the fill volume which is drained at each cycle can be calculated by observing the drainage flow rate and using the point at which this declines. A combination with complete drainage from to time is possible. Patients with frequent cycler alarms due to poor drainage related to intra-abdominal adhesions or polyuria with net peritoneal fluid resorption, and patients with late outflow pain might benefit from a tidal regimen. Total small molecule clearances are not improved by tidal PD, but improved phosphate clearance has been reported.

PD devices and connectology

Transfer sets connecting the PD catheter with the PD fluid container are a potential source of bacterial contamination. Several technologies developed in recent years have reduced the risk of peritonitis. Catheter-to-transfer set connectors are Luer lock systems made from durable plastics or titanium. Transfer set-to container connection should be performed by Luer lock systems locked by pins. Spiking systems for connection carry a high risk of contamination and should be abandoned. Y sets comprising of a double-bag dialysate solution and an empty drainage bag have a rotating gear with a fixed position for any phase of the exchange/(Stay safe, Dianectan). These systems guarantee that the catheter has been automatically closed, and surrounded by a disinfectant when the cap is positioned.

Modern cycler devices for home-based therapy are of small size and lightweight, as well as intuitive and easy in handling (e.g., touch screen). They provide online warming of PD fluid and gravity-assisted roller or diaphragm pumps for dialysate drainage and infusion. Barcoded fluid bags and cassette receptacles for the tubing set minimize errors and infection risks. Pediatric tubing sets and software provide accurate delivery of small fluid volumes, low drainage flow rates, and minimal recirculating dead space volumes.

PD solutions

PD solutions contain an osmotic agent, an acid–base buffer and electrolytes in physiologic concentrations.

Osmotic agents

Glucose is the most widely used osmotic compound in PD solutions. Glucose induces the transport of water from the extracellular volume to the peritoneal cavity by way of crystalloid osmosis. Because water is transported through the system of ultrasmall pores (aquaporins), there is no direct transport of solutes. Glucose (molecular weight 180 Da) is continuously absorbed by the peritoneum, leading to rapid dissipation of the osmotic gradient, and rendering glucose unsuitable for maintenance of ultrafiltration during extended dwells. The transperitoneal glucose absorption rate varies widely between individuals but is relatively constant within subjects while on PD (see PET). Osmotic ultrafiltration can be adapted to patient needs by modulating glucose concentrations. Bags with low (1.4–1.5%), medium (2.3–2.4%), and high (3.9–4.5%) concentrations are available and can be mixed or alternated with modern cycler systems.

Problems of glucose-based PD solutions

- *Systemic metabolic effects*: Glucose absorption provides additional calorie supply to the patient. However, the continuous glucose load can aggravate hyperinsulinemia and dyslipidemia, contributing to cardiovascular risk.

- *Structural and functional effects on the peritoneum*: High glucose concentration may cause hyperosmolar stress and lead to formation of toxic glucose degradation products (GDPs) during heat sterilization. Mediated in part by GDP contaminants, glucose containing PD fluid affects mesothelial cell metabolism and induces glycation of peritoneal proteins and formation of advanced glycated end-products (AGEs), both locally and systemically. The mesothelial cell layer is gradually lost and the submesothelial space transformed to a thick layer of fibrous tissue. Moreover, glucose and GDPs induce peritoneal neoangiogenesis, leading to a gradual increase of vascular surface area and small-solute transport rates and ultrafiltration failure. In recent years, dual-chamber fluid bags have been introduced which allow sterilization of glucose at low pH, resulting in much reduced GDP formation. The use of such "biocompatible" PD fluids may help to preserve the peritoneal membrane. Icodextrin is a starch derivative consisting of glucose polymers that are too large to pass through the peritoneal membrane (MW around 20 kDa), but is absorbed into the lymphatic system. Icodextrin is hydrolyzed by amylase to maltose and a spectrum of oligosaccharides. Maltose levels reach steady state within two weeks and return to normal levels within two weeks of discontinuation. Maltose may be stored in tissues on continuous use. Except for exfoliative dermatitis and transient eczematoid rash, no related adverse clinical effects have yet been described, but long-term data in children are lacking. The ultrafiltration profile of icodextrin (available at 7.5% concentration) differs from that of glucose. Ultrafiltration occurs at a slower pace but continues to rise over 12–14 hours dwell time. At eight hours, net ultrafiltration is comparable to that achieved with 3.86% glucose. This profile makes icodextrin a suitable alternative to glucose for the daytime dwell) in children on automated PD and for the long night-time dwell in CAPD patients. Icodextrin is helpful in patients with type I ultrafiltration failure, as well as for transient ultrafiltration failure during a peritonitis episode.
- *Caveat*: Hyponatriemia can occur with icodextrin since sodium removal is relatively greater with icodextrin than with glucose containing PD solutions.

Amino acids can also be used as osmotic agents. A 1.1% amino acid PD solution produces similar ultrafiltration as 1.36% glucose. Amino acid PD fluid is highly biocompatible due to the lack of glucose and GDPs. Furthermore, they prevent amino acid loss into the dialysate and provide an additional source of nutrition. Downsides are the significant acid load, and their high cost, which preclude routine use.

Buffers

Metabolic acidosis is common in ESRD and can be offset by the provision of alkali in the PD fluid. Since bicarbonate precipitates with calcium and magnesium during heat sterilization, lactate, which is metabolized to bicarbonate after resorption, is used in conventional PD fluids. Such fluids areÿbuffered at acidic pH (around 5.5) to maintain glucose in solution. Although dialytic pH is neutralized within 30–60 min by transport of bicarbonate from the blood, fluids with acidic pH occasionally cause inflow pain and may cause mesothelial cell damage, particularly in patients with short cycles in whom peritoneal pH is never completely neutralized during PD treatment. The new generation of gas-tight dual-chamber PD fluids allows storing glucose at low pH, preventing GDP formation, and generating a neutral pH by mixing of the chambers at time of administration, thereby providing a more biocompatible solution (see Table 1).

Electrolytes

Sodium concentration in PD fluids is set to 132–134 mmol/L. Therefore, sodium mass transport is achieved mainly by convection rather than diffusion. In the initial phase of the dwell, inflow of free water via aquaporins results in diminished sodium concentrations (sodium sieving). The isotonic ultrafiltration achieved by convective mass transport constitutes a significant sodium loss in small infants, regularly resulting in a need for sodium supplementation (e.g. 300 ml daily UF = 40 mmol NaCl loss, i.e. 8 mmol/kg BW/day in child of 5-kg body weight).

PD solutions are available at reduced (1.0 mmol/L), normal (1.25–1.35 mmol/L) and high (1.75 mmol/L) ionized calcium concentrations, allowing to antagonize disorders of serum calcium. The higher

Table 1. PD solutions

	Acidic Lactate		Neutral pH/ Lactate	Neutral pH/ Bicarbonate	Neutral pH/ Bicarbonate/Lactate		Icodextrin
	e.g. Dianeal PD1 (Baxter)	e.g. Dianeal PD4 (Baxter)	e.g. Balance (Fresenius)	e.g. Bicavera (Fresenius)	e.g. Physioneal 35 (Baxter)	e.g. Physioneal 40 (Baxter)	e.g. Extraneal (Baxter)
Sodium [mmol/l]	132	132	134	134	132	132	133
Calcium [mmol/l]	1.75	1.25	1.25/1.75	1.75	1.75	1.25	1.75
Magnesium [mmol/l]	0.75	0.25	0.5	0.5	0.25	0.25	0.25
Chloride [mmol/l]	102	95	100.5/101.5	104.5	101	95	96
Bicarbonate [mmol/l]	—	—	—	34	25	25	—
Lactate [mmol/l]	35	40	35	—	10	15	40
Glucose [%]	1.36/ 2.27/ 3.86	1.36/ 2.27/ 3.86	1.5/ 2.3/ 4.25	1.5/ 2.3/ 4.25	1.36/ 2.27/ 3.86	1.36/ 2.27/ 3.86	Icodextrin 7.5%
pH	5.5	5.5	7–7.4	7.4	7.4	7.4	5–6

concentration results in diffusive calcium uptake exceeding convective calcium loss and resulting in positive calcium balance. The neutral dialysate calcium concentration reduces hypercalcemia (especially in children receiving high amount of phosphate binders), and accordingly avoids high calcium phosphate product.

Peritoneal equilibration test (PET)

Patient-specific peritoneal transport characteristics should be assessed soon after PD initiation and reassessed annually and whenever conditions with a suspected effect on peritoneal function occur (e.g., peritonitis). The Peritoneal Equilibration Test (PET) is the most widely used test for characterizing solute transport across the peritoneum. The PET allows for the measurement of low molecular weight solute transport and ultrafiltration capacity.

PET protocol

- Empty peritoneal cavity as completely as possible (initial drain).
- Instill 1000–1100 ml/m^2 BSA of 2.5% glucose PD fluid.
- Obtain dialysate samples at 0 (flush of peritoneal cavity), two and four hours, and blood sample at two hours dwell time. Alternative: *Short PET* — obtain two-hour blood and dialysate samples only.
- Measure creatinine, and glucose in dialysate effluent, creatinine in plasma.
- Calculate dialysate/plasma (D/P) ratios of solutes (creatinine, phosphate), and dialysate glucose concentration/initial glucose concentration (D/D_0). A shortened protocol takes only blood at the two-hour time point. A free online calculator of D/P, D/D_0 ratios and peritoneal transporter status assignment both for four-hour and two-hour PET is available at www.pedpd.org.
- Note: If dialysate creatinine is measured by the Jaffe method, correction for glucose in the PD fluid must be made.

PET Interpretation

- *High transporter status* implies rapid clearance of solutes from blood but also rapid glucose resorption, necessitating short cycle duration to achieve ultrafiltration. High transporters are at increased risk of fluid overload, hypertension, and left ventricular hypertrophy (LVH). They have higher dialytic protein and amino acid losses. Mortality and technique failure rate are increased in adult high transporters. NIPD with short cycles, CCPD with icodextrin daytime dwell or tidal APD are suitable treatment options.

- *Low transporter status* is associated with low small molecule clearances and high ultrafiltration. Use high fill volumes and long dwell times. Small molecule clearance is best achieved by CAPD or CCPD with 1–2 daytime dwells.

Increased intraperitoneal pressure (IPP)

In PD patients, increased intraperitoneal pressure (IPP) is a risk factor for hernias, hydrothorax, and fluid leaks resulting in abdominal wall or genital edema. IPP is mainly influenced by fill volume and body position, which is the greatest when sitting and lowest in recumbent position. Also, obese patients tend to have higher IPP. IPP can be measured in a standardized fashion to identify the optimal fill volume. During the procedure the fill volume should be increased in acceptable and realistic steps. In infants and children, IPP typically remains almost constant up to 1000–1200 ml/m^2 BSA dwell volume and increases exponentially at higher volumes.

IPP protocol

- Connect recumbent patient to CAPD twin bag system
- Attach outflow tube vertically to central venous pressure scale, with outflow bag in elevated position; point reference arrow (0 cm H_2O) to posterior axillary line with the patient in a supine position
- Instill PD fluid in incremental steps of 200 ml/m^2 BSA
- Switch to drain setting. Read water level at outflow tube in deep inspiration and expiration

IPP reference range

IPP is 0.5–2.2 cm H_2O in the empty abdominal cavity. IPP should not exceed 11–12 cm H_2O.

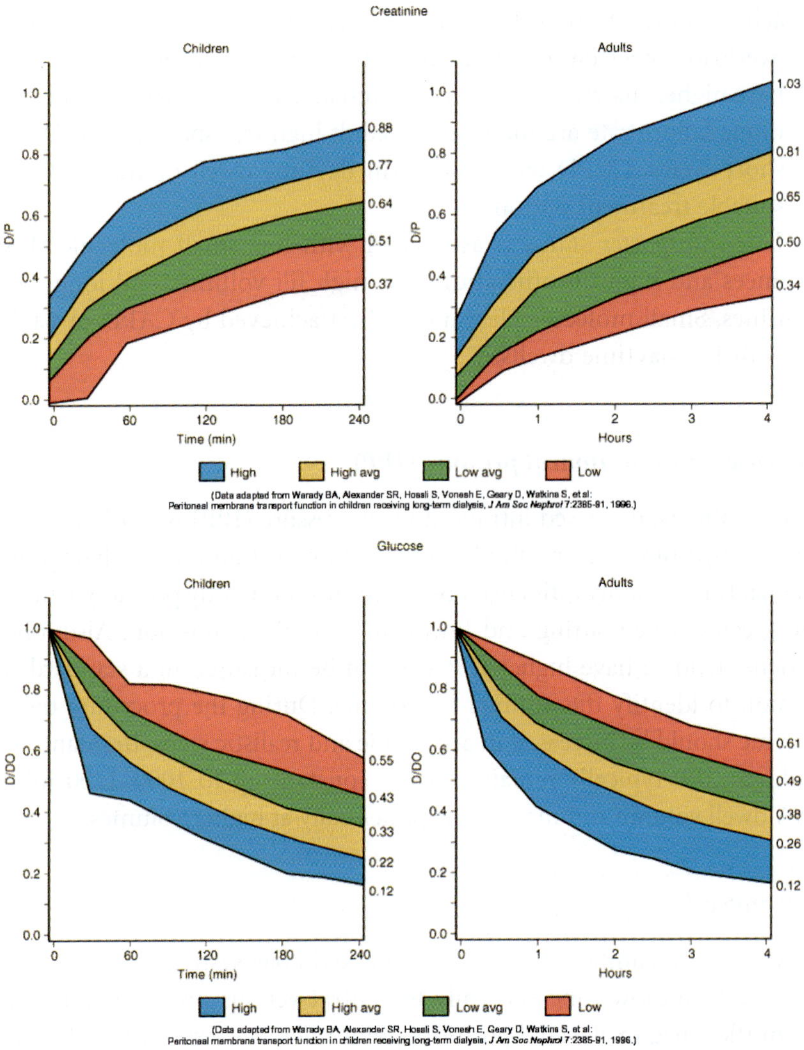

Figure 5. PET creatinine and glucose.

From Verrina EE, Perfumo F. Pediatric dialysis prescription. In Geary DF, Schaefer F. *Comprehensive Pediatric Nephrology*.

Mean IPP in children:

$$1000\text{–}1100\ \text{ml/m}^2\ \text{BSA} \rightarrow 8.2 \pm 3.8\ \text{cm}\ H_2O$$
$$1200\ \text{ml/m}^2\ \text{BSA} \rightarrow 9.5 \pm 2.9\ \text{cm}\ H_2O$$

Note: In the first few days after catheter implantation, IPP is higher, in part due to pain. Hence, patients should receive efficient analgestic medication and be kept supine for several days after catheter implantation in order to reduce the risk of fluid leaks.

Prescription targets

Prescription targets for children on CPD are not only PD adequacy measured by clearances and Kt/V urea, but also equally takes into account growth, nutrition, management of anemia, mineral homeostasis, and quality of life, as well as psychosocial adjustment of the child and family.

PD adequacy

Residual renal function is an important determinant of PD adequacy. Small molecule clearance from native kidneys is more closely related to clinical outcomes than dialytic clearance. Nephrotoxic drugs should be strictly avoided.

Clearance

Clearance describes the plasma volume from which a substance was removed in defined time and it is obtained from a collection of urine or dialysate normalized to 1.73 m^2 BSA.

Formula for creatinine clearance (CrCl) in dialysate:

$$\frac{\text{Cr in dialysate} \times \text{dialysis volume} \times 1.73}{\text{Collection period [min]} \times \text{Cr in serum} \times \text{BSA}}$$

In advanced renal failure, CrCl overestimates GFR because creatinine is secreted by the tubules. Therefore the average of creatinine and urea clearance is used to assess residual renal GFR. In PD, small molecule clearances

Table 2. Routine evaluation of children on chronic PD

Monthly	History • Daily fluid intake • Daily urine output • Daily ultrafiltration • Diet Anthropometry • Height (percentile or SDS) • Weight, BMI (for height age, percentile, or SDS) • Head circumference (in infants) • Blood pressure • Bioelectrical impedance (if available) Labs • Serum albumin • Hemoglobin, MCV, reticulocytes • Serum creatinine, urea, cystatin C • Serum electrolytes • Acid–base status • Intact parathyroid hormone
Every 3–6 months	Labs • Ferritin, transferrin saturation • 25-hydroxy vitamin D levels • serum IGF-I, IGFBP-3 (if on rhGH) Clearance: • 24-hour dialysate and urine collection o Creatinine clearance o Kt/V urea
Every 12 months	PET 24-hour ambulatory blood pressure monitoring ECG and echocardiography Hand and wrist X-ray for bone age, osteopathy Neurocognitive assessment (infants)

are calculated per week by convention. According to the KDOQI guidelines the following total (dialytic + renal) CrCl should be achieved:

- CAPD: >60 L/week × 1.73 m^2 BSA for high or high average transporters; >50 L/week × 1.73 m^2 BSA for low or low average transporters
- NIPD: >63 L/week × 1.73 m^2 BSA
- CCPD: >66 L/week × 1.73 m^2 BSA

Kt/V$_{urea}$

Urea clearance is expressed as Kt/V_{urea} and is normalized for urea distribution volume, which is assumed to be equal to total body water (TBW).

Anthropometric equations to calculate TBW in children

$$\text{Boys: TBW} = 0.1 \times (\text{Ht} \times \text{Wt})^{0.68} - 0.37 \times \text{weight}$$
$$\text{Girls: TBW} = 0.14 \times (\text{Ht} \times \text{Wt})^{0.68} - 0.35 \times \text{weight}$$

Weekly dialytic Kt/V_{urea} is calculated by the following formula from 24h dialysate collection.

Dialytic Kt/V urea:

$$\frac{\dfrac{\text{Urea in effluent} \times \text{Effluent volume} \times 7}{\text{Urea in serum}}}{\text{V}}$$

In patients with residual urine output, urinary urea clearance is added to peritoneal clearance in order to calculate the total urea clearance per week.

Total Kt/V urea:

$$\frac{\dfrac{[(\text{Effluent Urea} \times \text{Effluent volume}) + (\text{Urine Urea} \times \text{Urine Volume})] \times 7}{\text{Urea in serum}}}{\text{V}}$$

Total (dialytic + any residual renal) weekly Kt/V_{urea} should exceed 1.8.

Achieved small molecule clearances should be measured within 1 month of starting PD and monitored every 3–6 months thereafter.

Fluid and electrolyte balance

- In general, fluid, sodium, and potassium intake in the child on CPD needs slightly less restriction than in patients on hemodialysis. Fluid intake varies widely in children, depending mainly on residual urine output.

- Restriction of salt and fluid intake is usually necessary in oligo-anuric children and in patients with poor ultrafiltration due to membrane failure. Edema, hypertension, and LVH are unambiguous signs of fluid overload. Fluid-related hypertension is not easily corrected by antihypertensive medications. Fluid management should aim to normalize blood pressure without antihypertensive drugs.
- Infants with dysplasia commonly remain polyuric even when reaching ESRD. In these patients, ultrafiltration should be limited, and adequate salt and fluid intake ascertained in order to maintain residual urine output as long as possible.
- A peculiar aspect of CPD in neonates and young infants is their relatively greater electrolyte losses related to ultrafiltration. e.g., an anuric infant of 5 kg body weight requiring 250 ml of ultrafiltrate per day will lose approximately 35 mmol, i.e. 7 mmol/kg sodium and chloride per day. Failure to substitute these losses can lead to hypotonic or, more insidiously, isotonic dehydration. Arterial hypotension occurs in these children predominantly in the late night-time hours while on the cycler, and can lead to vascular events, such as sinus venous thromboses, and ischemic optical nerve atrophy.
- Hypokalemia sometimes occurs in neonates and young infants undergoing intensive PD, necessitating oral potassium supplementation. Hyperkalemia is a rare problem in children on CPD, seen occasionally in adolescents with suboptimal compliance to dietary potassium restrictions and/or missed dialysis cycles.

How to monitor fluid balance in children on PD?

- Body weight
- Blood pressure
- Bioelectrical impedance (if available)
- UF according to the report of the cycler in comparison to fluid intake
- Edema

How to manage fluid balance?

- Optimize PD prescription according to peritoneal transport characteristics (as identified by PET) and patient lifestyle needs.

- Dietary counseling: Assess amount of sodium intake, advise reduction.
- In patients with residual urine output: Consider loop diuretics
- Exclude malfunction of PD catheter
- Adherence? → individual education and training

Cardiovascular status

The vast majority of children with end-stage renal disease survive into adulthood. However, their long-term life expectancy is limited, mainly due to excessive cardiovascular comorbidity. Long-term dialysis predisposes to the development of a calcifying arteriopathy resembling accelerated atherosclerosis, combined with LVH and dysfunction. Hence, careful attention to cardiovascular risk factors should be a top priority in the clinical management of children on PD.

Dialyzed children are exposed to a large array of traditional, uremia- and dialysis-related cardiovascular risk factors. These may include:

- Hypertension (fluid-related)
- Left ventricular hypertrophy (volume and pressure overload)
- Dyslipidemia [increased triglycerides, LDL cholesterol, lipoprotein (a)]
- Obesity (dialytic glucose resorption, aggressive feeding protocols)
- Insulin resistance
- Lack of exercise
- Elevated serum calcium-phosphorus product (hyperphosphatemia, treatment with calcium containing phosphate binders, active vitamin D)

Table 3. Management of insufficient UF according to PET results in APD patients

High/high-average transporters: Short dwell time	Low/low-average transporters: Long dwell time
1) Stop daytime glucose dwell if daytime UF negative	1) Dwell volume↑
2) Number of cycles↑ (w/o change in dwell time per cycle)	2) Daytime icodextrine dwell
3) Dwell volume↑	3) Glucose concentration↑
4) Daytime icodextrin dwell	
5) Glucose concentration↑	

- Hyperparathyroidism
- Hyperhomocysteinemia
- Anemia
- Inflammation (PD-related and unrelated infections; uremic inflammatory state)
- Accumulation of advanced glycation end-products (resorption of glucose degradation products)

Clinical management should include regular monitoring of these risk factors, and aggressive prevention and treatment of modifiable conditions.

Nutrition

The goal of nutritional management of children on CPD is to optimize quantitative and qualitative nutrient intake and restore the physiological growth capacity, while minimizing the metabolic consequences of uremia.

Infants represent a unique subgroup within the ESRD population, with respect to the most severe anorexia and rapid growth failure observed in this age group but also in view of the unique option to provide an optimally balanced nutrition by way of enteral feeding. All children receiving PD should be followed at regular intervals by a renal dietitian.

Growth

In infants on CPD, growth failure can usually be avoided by consequent nutritional, electrolyte, and acid–base management. Most infants require aggressive nutritional support by nasogastric tube or PEG feeding. Ideally the PEG is placed prior to or simultaneously with the PD catheter and forced feeding is started as a preventive measure before significant malnutrition occurs. In addition, careful attention to correction of acidosis and electrolyte imbalance, treatment of renal osteodystrophy, and tailoring of CPD to achieve adequate dialysis will contibute to normal growth during this period.

Postinfantile growth is predominantly regulated by the somatotropic hormone axis, which is fundamentally altered in CKD. Circulating growth hormone levels are normal or elevated, but GH-dependent

IGF-1 production and bioactivity is impaired. Despite the resistance to endogenous GH, daily treatment with recombinant human growth hormone (rhGH) at pharmacological doses (0.05 mg/kg/day s.c.) increases IGF-I synthesis and bioactivity, and stimulates longitudinal growth in children with CKD. The growth response to rhGH correlated with residual renal function and is diminished in children on dialysis, most markedly so in anuric patients. Therefore, rhGH treatment should be started as early as possible in the course of CKD-associated growth failure.

Lifestyle compatibility

Children on PD have less social impairment, less depression, better adjustment, less behavioral disturbance, and fewer practical problems related to treatment than children on maintenance hemodialysis. Depression and anxiety are also less commonly observed in parents of children receiving PD, but this probably reflects the selection of families suitable for home dialysis. A potential for parental burn-out certainly exists in families managing extended CPD. The task to meet the medical, psychological and social needs of a child on CPD and still having sufficient time to meet the needs of other family members remains a continuous challenge to such families.

Beyond the period of infancy, short stature combined with alterations in body image related to the PD catheter may contribute to psychological maladjustment. Adolescents present a particular challenge with respect to diet and medication compliance, and the daily need for long hours of dialysis. In particular, acceptance of APD may be poor if dialysis prescription conflicts with evening social activities. Peer pressure, embarrassment about catheters, and fatigue may also result in failure to engage in physical activities with attendant health risks.

PD training

Standardized and empathic training by an expert is the key to successful PD performance. Apart from medical and technical contents, the training period should be used to develop a trustful relationship between family and medical staff.

The training should contain theoretical and practical issues:

- Theory (functions of the kidney, pathophysiology of renal failure, osmosis, diffusion, fluid balance)
- Practical/technical (aseptic technique, blood pressure monitoring, exit-site care, performance of PD exchanges, set-up and function of cycler, problem solving in case of alarms, NG/gastrostomy tube feeding (infants/small children))
- Peritonitis and ES/tunnel infection (recognition of signs and symptoms, initiating treatment, medicating bags for ongoing treatment; training may be limited to recognition of signs and symptoms due to low incidence of peritonitis in some centers)
- Noninfectious complications (hypotension/hypertension, catheter flow problems, hernias)

Complications

Infections (ES infection, tunnel infection, peritonitis) constitute the most common major complication limiting technique survival in pediatric PD. Mechanical complications are the second most common reason for catheter failure.

PD-related infections

ES infection/tunnel infection

Catheter ES/tunnel infections are a significant cause of catheter failure. Exit-site and tunnel infections tend to occur more frequently in pediatric than in adult CPD patients, possibly related to specific hygiene problems in young children ("diaper related") and/or the shorter length of the sinus tract with a higher risk of colonization of the subcutaneous cuff. *Staphylococcus aureus* is most common causative organism, accounting for 50% of infections, followed by *Pseudomonas aeruginosa.*

Prevention of exit-site infections is the primary goal of exit-site care which should encompass the following general principles:

- Regular monitoring using an objective ES scoring system (see Table 4 and/or photo documentation)

Table 4. Exit-site scoring system[a]

	0 Points	1 Point	2 Points
Swelling	No	Exit only (<0.5 cm)	Including part of or entire tunnel
Crust	No	<0.5 cm	>0.5 cm
Redness	No	<0.5 cm	>0.5 cm
Pain on pressure	No	Slight	Severe
Secretion	No	Serous	Purulent

[a] Infection should be assumed with a cumulative exit-site score of 4 or greater.

- Immobilization of the catheter
- Protection of the exit-site and tunnel from trauma
- Use of catheter dressing

Prophylactic use of antibiotics

The use of prophylactic antibiotic agents to decrease PD-associated *S. aureus* infections is supported by evidence in adults and children. Two approaches are currently used:

- Identification of patients and caregivers who are chronic nasal carriers of *S. aureus* by at least three nasal swabs; treatment of carriers with mupirocin b.i.d. for five consecutive days per month.
- Topical prophylaxis at the exit-site (mupirocin with each dressing exchange) in all patients.

The efficacy of topical prophylaxis may be jeopardized by emerging antibiotic resistance. Moreover, the routine topical use of mupirocin cream at the exit-site has been associated with increased *Pseudomonas* exit-site infection in adults and peritonitis in children. Gentamicin is an efficacious alternative to mupirocin, covering both the gram-positive and the gram-negative spectrum.

Treatment

Exit-site infections are routinely treated with oral antibiotics according to culture results. Intraperitoneal antibiotics are added only if improvement does not occur promptly. Refractory or recurrent infections suggest involvement of the subcutaneous cuff. In these cases surgical catheter replacement, usually performed as a one-stage intervention, is the standard procedure. Alternative approaches include surgical unroofing and peeling of the external cuff from the catheter, and selective replacement of the external infected portion by cutting right above the internal cuff. Repeated antibiotic therapies of recurrent infections should be avoided. Surgical intervention is indicated at the first relapse of an exit-site/tunnel infection.

Peritonitis

Background

The single most serious complication of CPD in children is peritonitis. More than 10% of peritonitis episodes in children lead to incomplete functional recovery or technique failure. Infectious agents can reach the peritoneum by one of several routes: transluminal (contamination), periluminal (exit-site/tunnel infection), enteric, hematogenous, and in rare cases ascending (through the vagina). Children are more prone to develop peritonitis than adults. *S. aureus* and *epidermidis*, and *Pseudomonas aeruginosa* are the most common causative bacteria. Their characteristic trait to adhere to the catheter (biofilm) makes eradication difficult and predisposes to recurrent peritonitis.

Reductions in peritonitis rates have been reported in both adults and children with technological advances, such as disconnect systems and flush-before-fill techniques, and improved prevention of exit-site infections by topical *Staphylococcus aureus* prophylaxis. Currently the mean peritonitis incidence in children on CPD is 1 infection every 18 patient-months. In a global pediatric peritonitis registry, gram-positive organisms were cultured in 44%, gram-negative organisms in 25%, and cultures remained sterile in 31% of cases. Gram-negative and specifically pseudomonas peritonitis were much more common in the United States, and associated with the use of mupirocin ES prophylaxis.

Fungal infections account for less than 2% of episodes. Prolonged use of antibiotics, malnutrition, and the presence of a percutaneous gastrostomy predispose to fungal peritonitis.

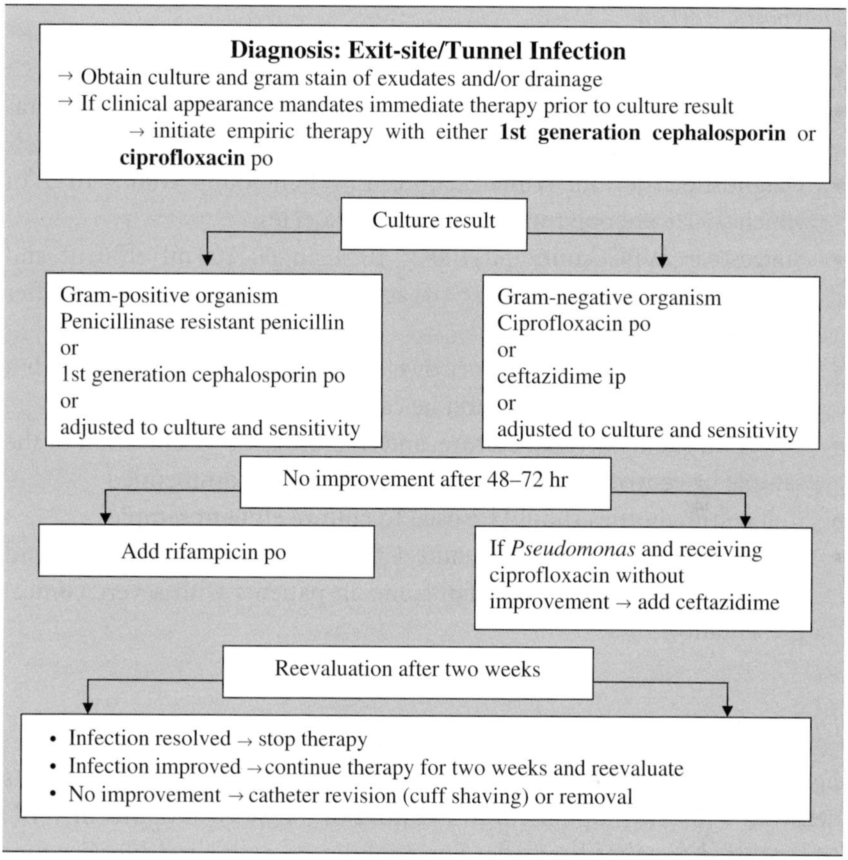

Figure 6.

From Warady BA, Schaefer F, Holloway M. (2000) International Society for Peritoneal Dialysis (ISPD) Advisory Committee on Peritonitis Management in Pediatric Patients. Consensus guidelines for the treatment of peritonitis in pediatric patients receiving peritoneal dialysis. *Perit Dial Int.* **20**: 610–624.

Clinical presentation

- Cloudy effluent
- Abdominal pain
- Fever
- Septic shock
- History of line contamination/damage

Diagnostic workup

- Sample should be obtained from first cloudy bag
- For immediate delivery (<60 min), transport sample at room temperature (otherwise store at 4°C)
- Diagnostic criterion: White blood cell (WBC) count $>100 \times 10^6$/L of which >50% are polymorphonuclear leukocytes
- Suggestive: WBC count $50–100 \times 10^6$/L in 50–100 ml effluent and typical signs and symptoms (if asymptomatic repeat testing after 4–6 hours)
- In patients on APD with short dwell times a second exchange with a dwell-time of 1–2 hours should be carried out
- For gram stain, bacterial culture, and microscopy concentration of the sample by centrifugation (15 min at 3000 g) is recommended
- Cell culture bottles should be used to culture effluent sample
- Do WBC and differential and Creactive protein in blood and perform blood culture in infants and in patients with severe clinical presentation

Differential diagnosis

Eosinophilic peritonitis should be considered if the culture remains negative. >100 eosinophils/ml in PD fluid or >10% eosinophils in WBC are required for the diagnosis. Eosinophilia in peripheral blood count may also be present. It is benign and usually resolves spontaneously over 2–6 weeks. Sometimes intraperitoneal hydrocortisone may be helpful.

Peritoneal hemorrhage

Children on CPD will occasionally experience bloody dialysate following minor trauma. Bleeding is probably due to catheter trauma in most cases. In postmenarchal girls, cloudy or bloody effluent can also be seen at times of ovulation and during menstruation. The correct diagnosis is established by effluent cell count. Conservative management is usually successful. The peritoneal cavity is flushed with PD fluid with the option of adding low-dose heparin to reduce the risk of clot obstructing the catheter.

Initial measures

- To reduce the severity of abdominal pain, several flushes may be performed prior to initiation of antibiotic therapy
- In patients who receive nocturnal automated peritoneal dialysis (APD) with short dwell times for routine therapy, continuous cycling with prolonged dwell times (3–6 hours) is recommended for 1–2 days until there is clearing of the peritoneal effluent; this does *not* apply to asymptomatic patients (in whom the routine prescription can be continued), patients requiring more frequent exchanges due to poor ultrafiltration, and patients receiving continuous ambulatory peritoneal dialysis (CAPD)
- The antibiotic loading dose should be administered during a standardized 3–6 hr dwell period
- Due to the prolonged half-life of glycopetides and cephalosporins (see empiric therapy), intermittent antibiotic loading is equally as effective as continuous application; when intermittent dosing is used, the antibiotic-containing dialysis solution must be allowed to dwell for at least six hours to allow adequate absorption of the antibiotic in systemic circulation
- The dwell which contains antibiotics should be a full exchange (approximately 1100 ml/m^2 BSA) as long as antibiotic treatment is continued

Empiric therapy

Empiric therapy antibiotic of peritonitis should be administered via the intraperitoneal route and provide coverage of gram-positive and gram-negative organisms, usually by a combination of a first-generation cephalosporin or vancomycin with a third-generation cephalosporin or an aminoglycoside (see Figs. 7 and 8). In view of the marked regional variation of antibiotic resistance patterns, the choice of empiric therapy should be guided by the local antibiotic resistance profile. The primary use of vancomycin, especially in the potentially oto- and nephrotoxic combination with aminoglycosides, should be restricted to centers with widespread methicillin resistance. Antibiotic therapy should be adapted as soon as culture results become available and continued for 10–21 days, depending on the causative organism.

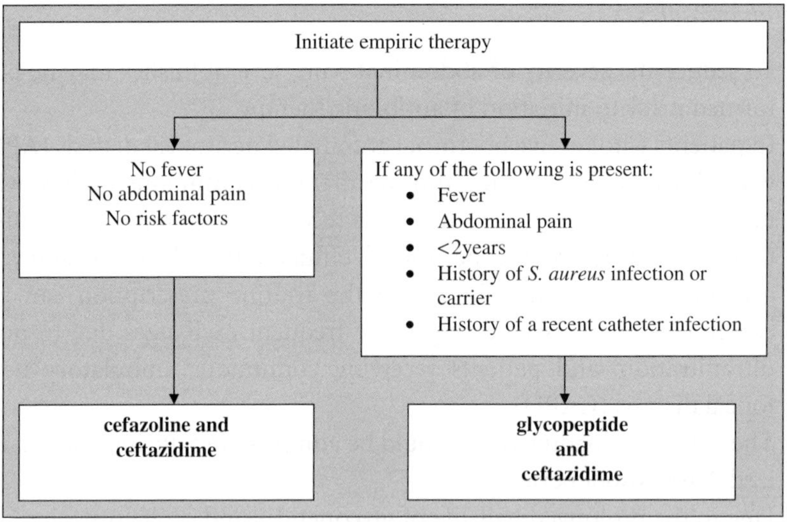

Figure 7. Empiric therapy of peritonitis.

Loading dose should be administered during a standardized 3–6 hour dwell period. Concentration-related loading doses assume usual patient specific fill volume (i.e. approx. 1100 ml/m² body surface area). If a smaller volume is instilled, the concentration must be increased to assure infusion of an equal mass of antibiotic. Intermittent antibiotic dosing should be applied in one bag per day for CAPD patients or during a full fill volume prolonged dwell for APD patients, unless otherwise specified.

Accelerated glycopeptide elimination may occur in patients with residual renal function. If intermittent therapy is used in this setting, the second dose of antibiotic should be time based on a blood level obtained 3–5 days after the initial dose. Redosing should occur when the blood level is <12 mg/L for vancomycin or 8 mg/L for teicoplanin. Intermittent therapy is not recommended for patients with residual renal function unless serum drug levels can be monitored in a timely manner.

Aminoglycosides and penicillins should not be mixed in dialysis fluid because of the potential for inactivation. Teicoplanin is not currently available in the United States. The therapeutic recommendations provided

	Loading Dose Continuous Therapy	Maintenance Dose Continuous Therapy	Intermittent Therapy (Once Daily)
Glycopeptide			
Vancomycin	1000 mg/L	25 mg/L	30 mg/kg q 5–7 days
Teicoplanin	400 mg/L	20 mg/L	15 mg/kg q 5–7 days
Cephalosporin			
Cefazolin/cefalothin	500 mg/L	125 mg/L	15 mg/kg q 24 hrs
Cefuroxime	200 mg/L	125 mg/L	15 mg/kg q 24 hrs
Cefotaxime	500 mg/L	250 mg/L	30 mg/kg q 24 hrs
Ceftazidime	250 mg/L	125 mg/L	15 mg/kg q 24 hrs
Ceftizoxime	250 mg/L	125 mg/L	–
Antifungal			
Amphotericin B	1 mg/kg IV	1 mg/kg/d IV	–
Fluconazole	–	–	3–6 mg/kg IP or po q 24–48 hrs
Flucytosine	50 mg/kg iv or po	25–37.5 mg/kg iv or po q 24 hrs	–
Aminoglycosides			
Amikacin	25 mg/L	12 mg/L	–
Gentamicin	8 mg/L	4 mg/L	–
Netilmicin	8 mg/L	4 mg/L	–
Tobramycin	8 mg/L	4 mg/L	–
Penicillin			
Azlocillin	500 mg/L	250 mg/L	–
Piperacillin	–	250 mg/L	150 mg/kg IV q 12 hrs
Ampicillin	–	125 mg/L	–
Oxacillin	–	125 mg/L	–
Nafcillin	–	125 mg/L	–
Amoxicillin	250–500 mg/L	50 mg/L	–
Quinolones			
Ciprofloxacin	50 mg/L	25 mg/L	–
Combinations			
Ampicillin/Sulbactam	1000 mg/L	100 mg/L	–
Imipenem/Cilistatin	500 mg/L	200 mg/L	–
Trimethoprim/ Sulfamethoxazole	320/1600 mg/L	80/400 mg/L	–
Others			
Clindamycin	300 mg/L	150 mg/L	–
Metronidazole	–	–	35–50 mg/kg/day po in 3 doses
Rifampin	–	–	20 mg/kg/day po (max dose 600 mg/day)
Aztreonam	1000 mg/L	250 mg/L	–

Figure 8. Antibiotic dosing recommendations; administration should be via intraperitoneal route unless specified otherwise.

above are those of the ISPD Advisory Committee on Peritonitis Management in Pediatric Patients and are, in large part, based upon adult experiences.

Once culture results and sensitivities are known, antibiotic therapy should be adjusted appropriately.

Culture negative peritonitis

- If culture remains negative and the patient's clinical condition is improving, combined therapy should be continued for two weeks
- In cases of no clinical improvement, repeat cell count, gram stain and culture
- Consider unusual pathogens

Fungal peritonitis

- If fungi are identified by gram stain or culture, treatment should be initiated with either intravenous amphotericin B, or a combination

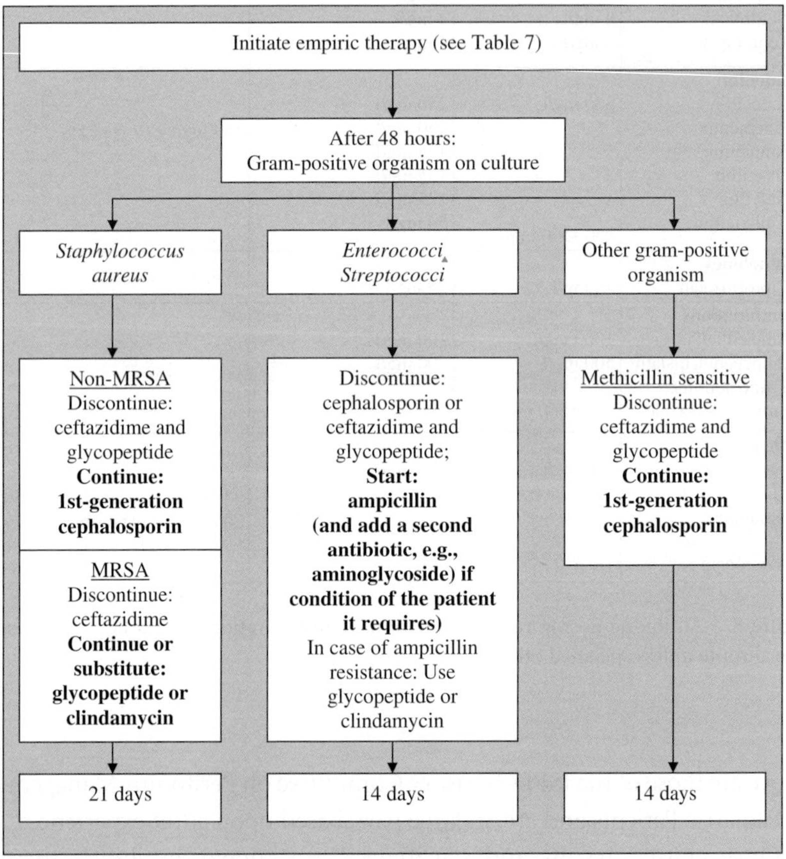

Figure 9. Gram-positive peritonitis.

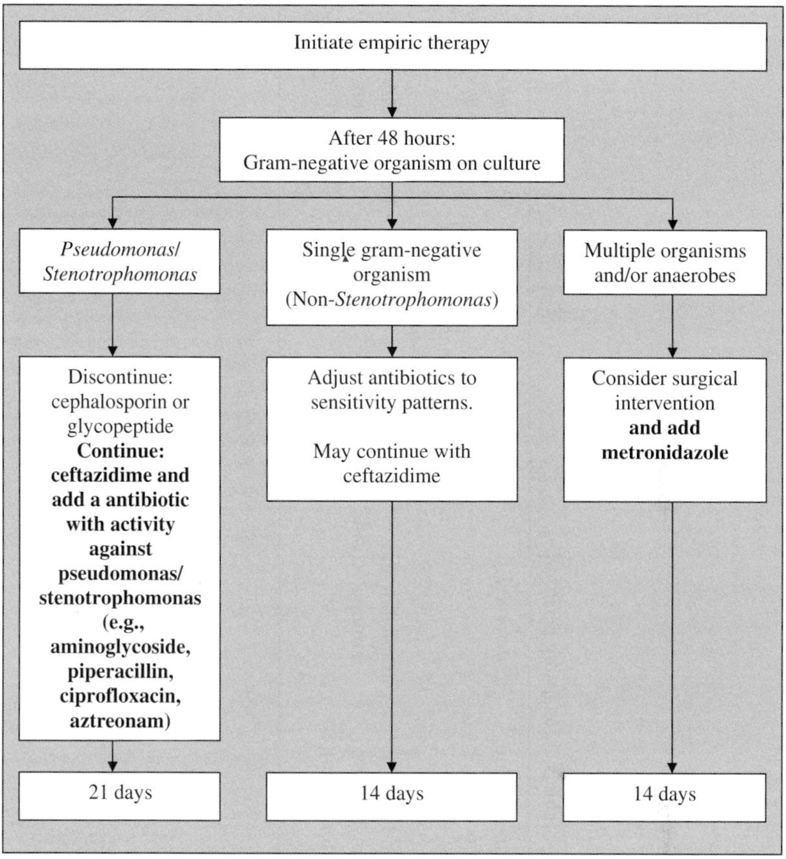

Figure 10. Gram-negative peritonitis.

of an imidazole/triazole (e.g., intravenous or oral fluconazole) and flucytosine.

- ○ amphotericin B 1 mg/kg BW IV
- ○ fluconazole 12 mg/kg PO/IP/IV once daily for 48 hours, then decreasing to 6 mg/kg once daily (maximum 200 mg PO/IP/IV)

- The PD catheter should be removed as soon as possible.
- In patients in whom the catheter is not removed initially, immediate catheter removal should take place if improvement does not occur within three days of treatment initiation.

Table 5. Relapsing peritonitis

Organism	Methicillin-sensitive *Staphylococci*	Methicillin-resistant *Staphylococci*	*Enterococci*	Gram-negative organism (other than *Pseudomonas/ Stenotrophomonas*)	*Pseudomonas/ Stenotrophomonas*
Treatment	First-generation cephalosporin and rifampin	glycopeptide or clindamycin with or without rifampin	ampicillin and aminoglycoside	ceftazidime	Remove Catheter plus ceftazidime and 2nd antibiotic
Duration (weeks)	3	3	3	3	≥2–3

- Treatment duration following catheter removal for all patients should be just under two weeks after complete resolution of the clinical symptoms of infection.
- Treatment duration without catheter removal should be 4–6 weeks.

Supportive therapy

- Intraperitoneal heparin inhibits fibrin clot formation and contributes to catheter patency in cases of severe peritonitis with massive protein exudation. It also has bacteriostatic and anti-inflammatory properties. The recommended dose of heparin is 200–1,000 U/L of dialysate until the effluent clears
- Intravenous immune globulin (IVIG) is recommended in patients with hypogammaglobulinemia
- Additional oral antifungal prophylaxis (e.g., nystatin) should be applied during administration of antibiotics

Catheter removal

The primary goal in managing peritonitis should always be the optimal treatment of the patient and protection of the peritoneum — and not saving the catheter. Indications for removal of the catheter include:

- Fungal peritonitis
- Sepsis or septicemic shock
- Exit-site or tunnel infection due to the same organism as that causing the peritonitis
- Relapsing peritonitis
- Persistently raised WBC after 3–4 days if infections is severe, or seven days if infection is mild
- Patient remains symptomatic after 3–4 days

After the catheter has been removed, a new catheter can be inserted after an interval of 2–3 weeks with at least two weeks of systemic antibiotic therapy during the intervening period.

Complications of peritonitis

- Catheter removal with subsequent need of HD
- Loss of UF leading to fluid overload

- Adhesions and failure for future PD
- Excessive loss of albumin and IgG resulting in malnutrition and secondary immunodeficiency
- Fungal peritonitis
- Ileus
- Pancreatitis

Prevention of peritonitis

- Use of double-cuffed swan-neck catheter type with downward directed exit-site reduces risk of peritonitis
- A single dose of an intravenous antibiotic given at the time of catheter placement decreases the risk of an early peritonitis episode; a first-generation cephalosporin is mostly used; however, vancomycin may be superior to a cephalosporin
- After catheter placement, dialysis initiation should be delayed for 1–2 weeks whenever possible
- During the period of wound healing, dressing changes should be reduced to minimum (not more than once per week)
- Careful training and education of parents and/or child

Sclerosing peritonitis

The peritoneum becomes thickened and fibrosed due to prolonged period on PD, prolonged use of bioincompatible PD fluid with high glucose concentrations, and recurrent peritonitis. This state leads to episodes of sterile peritonitis, poor ultrafiltration, and decreasing small solute clearance. Adhesions may cause gut obstruction (and malnutrition), as well as catheter obstruction and dislocation. Peritoneal biopsy is the gold standard diagnostic procedure; thickened bowel loops on the ultrasound or peritoneal calcifications are suspicious. Surgery is required in case of intestinal obstruction. Transfer to HD is often needed. Immunosuppressive medication has only limited evidence of efficacy.

Mechanical Complications

Hernias

The incidence of hernias detected after onset of PD in children is highly variable in the literature (17–81%). Multiple hernias are frequent and are likely to occur early in the course of CPD. Two types of hernias occur in children on PD due to increased intra-abdominal pressure: persistent congenital hernias that become apparent and hernias developing *de novo* in the abdominal wall (e.g., paraesophageal hernias).

The most commonly seen hernias are inguinal, umbilical and incisional. Incisional hernias occur more commonly when the PD catheter is placed through the midline instead of the paramedial approach through the rectus muscle. Enlargement of the herniation may occur as a result of increased abdominal wall pressure from dialysate in the cavity. Significant hernias left untreated increase the risk of further enlargement, pain, bowel entrapment, and subsequent discontinuation of PD. Risk factors for hernias include:

- Young age
- Prior abdominal surgery
- Glucocorticoid therapy
- Malnutrition, as well as obesity

Young male infants are at highest risk of inguinal hernias, since the obliteration of the *processus vaginalis* is frequently incomplete at time of PD initiation. The use of laparoscopy at the time of catheter placement can identify (congenital) hernias before they become symptomatic. If either inguinal, umbilical, or other significant abdominal wall hernias are identified by laparoscopy or clinical investigation, they should be repaired at the time the catheter is placed/prior to initiation of PD.

It has been proposed to monitor the intraabdominal pressure in children starting CPD in order to minimize the risk of hernia formation. At a given fluid volume normalized to body surface area, infants appear to develop a higher intraabdominal pressure than older children. The intraperitoneal pressure should not exceed 10 cm H_2O. APD with reduced exchange volumes and increased exchange frequency should be considered for patients felt to be at risk.

Leaks

Leakage of dialysate is uncommon and usually occurs in the immediate postoperative period (first month). Pericatheter and subcutaneous leaks are often related to:

- Poor implant]ation technique (inadequate closure of the layers of the abdominal wall, inappropriate large subcutaneous tunnel)

- Anatomical abnormalities
- Utilizing the catheter prior to healing
- Trauma

Dialysate can also leak from the peritoneal cavity into various tissue layers, most often into subcutaneous tissue around a previous surgical incision. In case of laparoscopic catheter placement, the trocar incision sites are possible locations of leakage to think of. The subcutaneous fluid expands because it is hypertonic and consequently absorbs water. A subcutaneous fluid leak into the genital area can be difficult to distinguish from an inguinal hernia. Aspiration of the subcutaneous fluid is not helpful and should be avoided. Ultrasound and MRI are helpful in establishing the diagnosis in case of doubt.

Conservative management, occasionally including temporary suspension of CPD, is usually sufficient to allow these leaks to resolve.

- Dialysis should be delayed as long as possible after catheter placement, because early high volume dialysis is associated with an increased risk of leakage
- In case of leakage, dialysis should be suspended for as long as possible in order to allow the site to heal; When dialysis is reinitiated, lower pressure is preferable by using low fill volumes

Hydrothorax

Hydrothorax is an uncommon complication of CPD in children and adults. It is usually right-sided. The prevalence of pleuroperitoneal connections in the general population is unknown, since they are not challenged with PD. It is believed that a tiny bleb arises on the surface of the diaphragm and then ruptures, forming a one-way valve leading to a tension hydrothorax. Alternatively, the potential pleuroperitoneal connection is present as a congenital defect in the diaphragm.

Differential diagnosis

- Congestive heart failure
- Fluid overload
- Hypoalbuminemia

MRI after intraperitoneal administration of dilute gadolinium contrast agent has been introduced as a noninvasive, radiation-free diagnostic. Transfer to hemodialysis will resolve the problem. For patients who need to return to CPD, sealing of the pleuroperitoneal connection with an intrathoracic sclerosing agent (i.e. tetracycline or autologous hemoglobin), or surgical patch-grafting have been reported.

Catheter obstruction

Inflow and outflow obstruction usually is an early complication but can also occur at later time points (especially during or following episodes of peritonitis). Catheter outflow occlusion is usually caused by omentum or adhesions to mesentery, ovarian tube fimbria in girls or other intra-abdominal structures. In case of catheter obstruction, laparoscopic exploration is the technique of choice.

To prevent early catheter obstruction, free return of effluent must be documented in the operating room immediate after catheter placement. For catheters that are functioning poorly but have not migrated out of the pelvis (see below), occlusion by fibrin, proteins, or blood is common. Tissue plasminogen activator (TPA) — urokinase or alteplase — instilled in the catheter for 30–60 min is effective in unblocking fibrin-clotted catheters.

Catheter migration

Catheter migration in the peritoneal cavity occurs in approximately 5–10% of catheters. This is usually a result of too much torque placed in the catheter at the time of surgical placement. In infants, catheter displacement is even more common due to shallow pelvis and proportional short abdomen. Occasionally, catheter migration may occur due to constipation and extensive bladder distension. Interventional radiology techniques or laparoscopy are used to reposition the catheter.

Cuff extrusion

Cuff extrusion may be caused by:

- Torque of the catheter
- Placement of the outer catheter cuff too close to exit-site
- Tunnel infection

The cuff may be peeled if there is no infection involving the tunnel and inner cuff. In case of deep infection, catheter replacement is obligate.

Miscellaneous

Hypogammaglobulinemia

Hypogammaglobulinemia is commonly present in infants and younger children on CPD. This may be particularly significant since mortality rates are highest in this age group of CPD children, and the majority of the deaths are from infection. This complication should be monitored and treatment with intravenous gammaglobulin considered especially in the setting of an active infection.

Bloody dialysate

Children on CPD will occasionally experience bloody dialysate following minor trauma. The bleeding is probably due to catheter trauma in most cases. Mild bleeding can mimic the cloudy fluid of peritonitis. Conservative management is usually successful. The peritoneal cavity is flushed with dialysate with the option of adding low-dose heparin to reduce the risk of catheter obstruction by clots. Patients, parents, teachers, and coaches often need reassurance that such episodes are of little consequence, and should not interfere with the normal physical or sporting activities.

Bloody dialysate can occur in postmenarcheal girls secondary to retrograde menstruation or at the time of ovulation.

PD in special conditions

Prune belly syndrome

Children with prune belly syndrome can be treated with CPD, despite their deficient abdominal musculature. To prevent leaks, the percutaneous catheter insertion technique can be helpful in achieving a watertight seal at the thin abdominal wall. A slow break-in period to permit healing is advised.

Ventriculoperitoneal shunt

Children with myelomeningocele typically have a neurogenic bladder which may lead to ESRD. In addition, these children often have hydrocephalus requiring ventriculoperitoneal (VP) shunting. When children with VP shunts require dialysis, the option of CPD is commonly entertained. The theoretical possibility of bacterial peritonitis episodes involving the VP shunt has led some to consider the presence of a VP shunt as a relative contraindication to CPD. However, uneventful PD with indwelling VP catheter has been reported.

Genitourinary surgery

Children with inadequate bladders are treated by a bladder augmentation procedure using bowel or dilated ureter. Creation of the augmented bladder requires extensive surgery with attendant risks for developing adhesions. In addition, the augmented bladder segment is attached to a vascular pedicle which resides in the peritoneal cavity. Despite the magnitude of the surgery and potential for complications, these children usually do well on CPD.

CPD can also be offered to children who require a vesicostomy or pyeloureterostomy. Many children on CPD require elective nephrectomy, usually for hypertension or to remove a potential focus of infection prior to renal transplantation. The posterior lumbotomy approach avoids invasion of the peritoneal cavity and allows continuing PD without interruption. For patients requiring nephroureterectomy via a transperitoneal approach, CPD must often be suspended for a brief period, relying on temporary HD.

Suggested Reading

[URL: www.kidney.org]

[URL: www.pedpd.org]

Chadha V, Schaefer FS, Warady BA. (2009) Dialysis-associated peritonitis in children. *Pediatr Nephrol* **25**(3): 425–440.

KDOQI Clinical Practice Guideline for Nutrition in Children with CKD. (2009) 2008 update. Executive summary. KDOQI Work Group. *Am J Kidney Dis* **53**(3 Suppl 2): S11–104.

Warady BA, Schaefer F, Holloway M, *et al.* (2000) International Society for Peritoneal Dialysis (ISPD) Advisory Committee on Peritonitis Management in Pediatric Patients. Consensus guidelines for the treatment of peritonitis in pediatric patients receiving peritoneal dialysis. *Perit Dial Int.* **20**: 610–624.

Warady BA, Alexander SR, Firanek C, *et al.* (2001) *Peritoneal Dialysis Catheter and Complications Management for Children.* Baxter Healthcare Corporation.

Warady BA, Feneberg R, Verrina E, *et al.* (2007) IPPR. Peritonitis in children who receive long-term peritoneal dialysis: a prospective evaluation of therapeutic guidelines. *J Am Soc Nephrol* **18**(7): 2172–2179.

40

Nutrition in ESRD

Natalie Lussier, Meredith Miller and Victoria Vitale

Introduction

The management of end-stage renal disease (ESRD) in children is complicated by the need to maintain normal patterns of growth and development in addition to the need to optimize medical care. The focus of nutritional care in patients with ESRD must include prevention of protein-energy malnutrition. In addition, patients require monitoring to avoid excessive weight for height while assuring adequate intake of micro- and macronutrients. Multiple factors often associated with ESRD including uremia, acidosis, abnormalities in the growth hormone axis, inadequate nutrient intake, metabolic bone disease, gastrointestinal reflux, delayed gastric emptying, and nausea may make achieving normal growth patterns challenging.

Growth delays during childhood, especially in the first two years of life, may impact normal brain development and final adult stature, and therefore, should be of great concern. Prevention of such delay should be a primary focus in the care of children with chronic kidney disease (CKD) with subsequent ESRD. The National Kidney Foundation's Kidney Disease Outcomes Quality Initiative (KDOQI) provides clinical practice guidelines, which serve as a useful reference for the care of children with ESRD receiving maintenance dialysis.

Evaluation of Nutritional Status and Growth

Multiple parameters must be considered in the evaluation of growth in children with ESRD. Thorough nutrition assessment and close monitoring by a registered dietitian (RD) experienced in pediatric kidney disease is warranted. Factors to be considered in assessment include:

- Review of dietary intake (3-day diet history or three 24-hour recalls)
- Length or height for age percentile or standard deviation score (SDS)
- Length or height velocity for age SDS (change over time)
- Estimated dry weight and weight for age percentile or SDS
- Body mass index (BMI), for-height–age percentile or SDS (using 2006 WHO growth standards for birth through two years and CDC growth charts >2 years)
- Head circumference-for-age or SDS (<3 years old only)
- Normalized protein catabolic rate (nPCR) in hemodialyzed adolescents
- Serum albumin

Online tools are available to assist in the assessment of growth and the calculation of SDS. Fluid overload is common in dialysis patients, especially anuric patients on hemodialysis (HD), so care must be taken in assessing dry weight by monitoring for hypertension, edema and jugular venous distention.

Disruption in the normal growth pattern is common in children with CKD. In the growth assessment, genetic height potential using the estimation of mid-parental height should be determined:

- Girls: 5 inches (13 cm) is subtracted from the father's height and averaged with the mother's height ± 8.5 cm
- Boys: 5 inches (13 cm) is added to the mother's height and averaged with the father's height ± 8.5 cm

Decreased growth velocity may not exclusively reflect nutritional status but may also be affected by growth hormone deficiency and warrants further evaluation. Prior to the initiation of growth hormone, factors to be considered and addressed include protein-energy malnutrition, salt wasting (common in polyuric infants), correction of serum bicarbonate levels, renal osteodystrophy, and corticosteroid use. Further discussion of growth hormone therapy is found in elsewhere in this manual.

Energy Requirements

Energy requirements should be considered 100% of the estimated energy requirement (EER) for chronological age using dietary reference intakes

Table 1. Equations to estimate energy requirements for children

Age	EER (kcal/d) = Total energy expenditure (TEE) + energy deposition
0–3 months	EER = [89 × weight (kg) – 100] + 175
4–6 months	EER = [89 × weight (kg) – 100] + 56
7–12 months	EER = [89 × weight (kg) – 100] + 22
13–35 months	EER = [89 × weight (kg) – 100] + 20
3–8 years	Boys: EER = 88.5 – 61.9 × age (yrs) + PA × [26.7 × weight (kg) + 903 × height (m) + 20
	Girls: EER = 135.3 – 30.8 × age (yrs) + PA × [10 × weight (kg) + 934 × height (m) + 20
9–18 years	Boys: EER = 88.5 – 61.9 × age (yrs) + PA × [26.7 × weight (kg) + 903 × height (m) + 25
	Girls: EER = 135.3 – 30.8 × age (yrs) + PA × [10 × weight (kg) + 934 × height (m) + 25
Overweight	Boys: TEE = 114 – [50.9 × age (yrs)] + PA × [19.5 × weight (kg) + 1161.4 × height (m)]
3–18 years	Girls: TEE = 389 – [41.2 × age (yrs)] + PA × [15 × weight (kg) + 701.6 × height (m)]

Adapted from KDOQI, September 2008.

Table 2. Physical activity coefficients (PA) for determination of energy requirements in children ages 3–18 years

Gender	Sedentary	Low active	Active	Very active
	Typical activities of daily living (ADL) only	ADL + 30–60 min if daily moderate activity (e.g. walking at 5–7 km/h)	ADL + ≥60 min of daily moderate activity	ADL + ≥60 min of daily moderate activity + an additional 60 min of vigorous activity *or* 120 min of moderate activity
BOYS	1.0	1.13	1.26	1.42
GIRLS	1.0	1.16	1.31	1.56

From Institute of Medicine. (2002) Dietary reference intakes for energy, carbohydrates, fiber, fat, protein, and amino acids (macronutrients). National Academy of Sciences, Washington DC.

(DRI) and adjusted for activity level and body weight (see Table 1). Modifications to caloric intake should be made based upon assessment of growth velocity and individual response (see Table 2).

When estimating energy needs in children receiving peritoneal dialysis (PD), consideration of glucose absorption from dialysate should be considered. The mean peritoneal glucose absorption rate of PD is estimated to be ~9 kcal/kg. The modification to estimated energy needs should only be considered when weight gain is excessive.

Supplemental nutrition should be considered when a child's usual intake does not meet energy requirements resulting in suboptimal growth. Modular products such as glucose polymers, liquid fat or a combination may be added to foods, formula or breast milk to limit renal solute load. Commercially available supplements can be used but consideration must be given to the product's nutrient composition and the child's specific dietary restrictions.

Oral supplementation is the preferred route of nutrition support; however, tube feeding should be considered when oral intake is inadequate. Selection and delivery of the tube feeding product must be tailored to the individual and may be affected by gastrointestinal tolerance, nutrient requirements, mineral and electrolyte imbalances, and actual oral intake. Special formulas designed for renal disease are available but are not always necessary for the dialyzed patient. When selecting method and timing of delivery, consideration should be given to maximizing oral intake. Infants may require boluses of the balance of their feeding after oral feeds, whereas some may require full nutrition via enteral supplementation. For older children, night-time tube feeds may be preferred to maximize oral intake during the day. In tube-fed children, oral aversion is not uncommon, thus care must be given to provide oral stimulation and encourage oral feeding as appropriate. In cases of significant aversion, consultation of a speech pathologist and/or an occupational therapist should be considered.

Hemodialysis treatments may provide an opportune time for nutrition supplementation; however, this remains controversial and requires close monitoring of vital signs. A list of oral and enteral products commonly used in the renal setting is presented in Table 3. In the event of a malnourished child who is unable to meet needs orally and/or enterally, intradialytic parenteral nutrition (IDPN) may be appropriate. The indication for IDPN needs to be evaluated on a case-by-case basis and is not discussed in-depth in this chapter.

Cardiovascular disease poses a significant risk for dialysis patients and dyslipidemia is common. The American Heart Association published a consensus statement endorsed by the American Academy of Pediatrics on dietary recommendations for children and adolescents. Diet prescription

Table 3. Enteral nutrition supplements and modular products

Product	Amount	kcal	CHO g	Pro g	Fat g	Na mg	K mg	P mg	Ca mg
Enlive (Abbott)	8 oz	250	52	9	0	45	45	280	50
Nepro Carb Steady (Abbott)	8 oz	425	37.9	19.1	22.7	250	250	170	250
NovaSource Renal (Nestle)	8 oz	475	47.3	17.4	24.1	210	192	154	308
Renalcal (Nestle)	8 oz	500	72.6	8.6	20.6	0	0	0	0
Resource Breeze (Nestle)	8 oz	250	54	9	0	<80	10	150	10
Suplena Carb Steady (Abbott)	8 oz	425	46.4	10.6	22.7	190	270	170	250
Similac PM 60/40 (Abbott)	8 oz	162	16.6	3.6	9.1	39	130	45	91
ProCel	1 scoop	28	<1	5	<0.5	10	35	27	40
ProMod (Abbott)	1 oz	100	14	10	0.6	55	20	95	—
ProStat Profile	1 oz	181	10	10	0	14.5	16	<6	—
ProStat 64	1 oz	72	3	15	0	14.5	18.4	<6	—
ProStat 101	1 oz	101	10	15	0	14.5	15.6	<6	—
ProStat AWC	1 oz	108	10	17	0	14.5	15.6	<6	—
ProStat RC	1 oz	72	3	15	0	14.5	18.4	6.7	—
Proteinex 15 (Llorens Pharmaceuticals)	1 oz	60	0	15	0	4	11	—	—
Proteinex 18 (Llorens Pharmaceuticals)	1 oz	72	0	18	0	5	13	—	—
Resource Beneprotein (Nestle)	1 scoop	25	0	6	0	10	35	15	30
Polycose Powder (Abbott)	1 Tbsp	23	5.6	—	—	<7	<1	<1	Neg
MCT Oil (Nestle)	1 mL	8	—	<1	—	—	—	—	—
Duocal (Nutricia)	10 grams (2 scoops)	49	7.3	0	2.2	<2	<0.5	<0.5	<0.5

Product information as at September 2010.

and supplementation should consider monitoring and treating hyperlipidemia to optimize cardiovascular health. The primary goal in the nutritional care for the pediatric ESRD patient remains providing adequate calories and nutrients for growth and development; however, when possible, diet modification for prevention or correction of dyslipidemia should be considered. With the epidemic of obesity posing an additional cardiac risk, dietary and lifestyle intervention in overweight and obese children with ESRD may be necessary.

Protein

The recommended protein intake for children with ESRD must take into consideration growth maintenance and adequate nutritional status as well as avoiding excess (see Table 4). The goal is to maintain dietary protein intake of 100% of the DRI for age plus an allowance for dialytic protein and amino acid losses. The calculation of protein requirement should utilize ideal body weight for overweight and obese children and dry weight in dialyzed children. In growth retarded children, protein needs should be based on DRI for height age to assure adequacy. It is also essential to provide adequate calories from fat and carbohydrates to prevent the utilization of protein as an energy source. Protein requirements may be increased in patients with proteinuria, catabolism, during peritonitis and in those on corticosteroids. As essential as adequate protein is to dialyzed patients, excess amounts of protein may be equally deleterious. Excess protein may exacerbate acidosis and make phosphorus control more challenging. Phosphorus content is naturally higher in protein rich foods and although animal proteins are the most digestible, they also provide the highest amount of phosphorus. A mixed intake of dietary protein from a variety of sources is optimal.

Calculation of nPCR reflects dietary protein intake but is affected by multiple other factors such as fluid overload. Similarly, although hypoalbuminemia is affected by multiple factors, it is consistently associated with increased morbidity and mortality. Routine monitoring of serum albumin has been a long-standing part of nutritional assessment of ESRD patients; however, factors such as systemic inflammation and volume overload can artificially depress the value.

Table 4. Recommended dietary protein intake in children with ESRD on maintenance dialysis

Age (years)	Healthy children (g/kg/day)	HD (g/kg/day)	PD (g/kg/day)
0–0.5	1.5	1.6	1.8
0.6–1.0	1.2	1.3	1.5
1–3	1.05	1.15	1.3
4–13	0.95	1.05	1.1
14–18	0.85	0.95	1.0

Other Nutrients

Patients receiving maintenance dialysis (HD and PD) are at significant risk for vitamin and trace-element deficiencies due to poor dietary intake, loss of nutrients through dialysis, abnormal renal metabolism, and poor absorption in the gastrointestinal tract. Growth and development are dependent upon meeting at least 100% of the DRI's for individual age groups (see Table 5).

Table 5. Recommended nutrient intake

Nutrient	Recommendation
Thiamin, riboflavin, pantothenic acid, pyridoxine (B6), biotin, cobalamin (B12), ascorbic acid (vitamin C), and folic acid	Supplementation of water-soluble vitamins is recommended, while all other vitamins should be obtained through diet to meet the DRIs for age
Zinc	Supplement required when deficiency is identified by serum laboratory values or symptoms of deficiency are present
Copper	Supplement required when deficiency is identified by serum laboratory values or symptoms of deficiency are present
Calcium	Diet should provide at least 100% of the DRI for age; in oligoanuric children, total oral and enteral intake along with phosphate binders should not exceed 150% of the DRI for age; monitor for hypercalcemia
Phosphorus	Diet should provide no more than 100% of the DRI/age when serum PTH is above target range and serum phosphorus is within the acceptable range for age; diet should provide no more than 80% of the DRI/age when serum PTH is above target range and serum phosphorus exceeds acceptable range for age
Vitamin D	Supplement with D2 or D3 when insufficiency or deficiency is present.
Sodium	Supplements should be considered for children with polyuria to avoid chronic intravascular depletion and to promote optimal growth; supplements should be considered for all infants on PD; restriction should be considered for children with prehypertension or hypertension (1,500–2,400 mg/day)

(*Continued*)

Table 5. (*Continued*)

Nutrient	Recommendation
Potassium	Limit dietary intake in children who have or are at risk of developing hyperkalemia (<30–40 mg/kg/day); a potassium binder may be required with oral and enteral supplements to reduce potassium content; children on PD rarely need a restriction
Fluids	Unrestricted unless warranted; replace insensible losses and urinary output

Suggested Reading

Byham-Gray L, Wiesen K. (eds.) (2004) *A Clinical Guide to Nutrition Care in Kidney Disease*, 1st ed., Renal Dietitians Dietetic Practice Group of the American Dietetic Association and the Council on Renal Nutrition of the National Kidney Foundation.

Centers for Disease Control and Prevention. (2009) *Clinical Growth Charts.* Atlanta, GA: [URL http://www.cdc.gov/growthcharts/clinical_charts.htm]

Edefonti A, Picca M, Damiani B, *et al.* (1999) Dietary prescription based on estimated nitrogen balance during peritoneal dialysis. *Pediatr Nephrol* **13**: 253–258.

McCann L. (ed.) (2009) *Pocket Guide to Nutrition Assessment of the Patient with Chronic Kidney Disease*, 4th ed., Chapters 1 and 11, National Kidney Foundation Council on Renal Nutrition, New York.

National Kidney Foundation. (2009) *KDOQI Clinical Practice Guidelines for Nutrition in Children with CKD: 2008 Update.* National Kidney Foundation, Inc., New York.

Otten JJ, Hellwig JP. (eds.) (2006) *Dietary Reference Intakes, the Essential Guide to Nutrient Requirements. Food and Nutrition Board.* The National Academies Press, Washington DC, pp. 69–166.

Solan P. (2008) Nutrition assessment and management of children with chronic kidney disease. *Pediatric Nutrition Practice Group of the American Dietetic Association*, **31**(2): 1–6.

World Health Organization. (2009) *Child growth standards.* Geneva, Switzerland [URL http://www.who.int/childgrowth/standards/height_for_age/en].

Part XV

Renal Transplantation

41

Pediatric Kidney Transplantation: Perioperative Management

Jens Goebel, William R. DeFoor and Curtis A. Sheldon

Medical Preparation

Preparing children for kidney transplantation is a multidisciplinary task shared by the nephrology care team in conjunction with other necessary services (e.g. pediatric urology, surgery, psychiatry, anesthesiology, and critical care). Treatment of children with CKD often includes antihypertensive and antiproteinuric therapy to delay progression to end-stage renal disease (ESRD) and to decrease cardiovascular (CV) morbidity. Kidney transplant is an elective procedure and patients should undergo the procedure in the healthiest state possible. CV fitness and absence of obesity reduce surgical and anaesthesiological risks and provide an advantage posttransplant. Appropriate renal management pretransplant, including prescription of phosphate binders and active vitamin D, and with regular monitoring of serum parathyroid hormone levels, also optimize posttransplant bone disease. Because transplanted children do not uniformly display catch-up growth, aggressive nutrition is required, and growth hormone therapy needs to be considered before, and possibly after, transplantation. Pretransplant, immunization status should be ascertained and all vaccinations administered, as live vaccines are avoided posttransplant, and response to inactivated vaccines may be blunted due to immunosuppression. Immunosuppressive therapy can exacerbate severe warts, and potential recipients should have warts treated prior to transplantation.

Individual issues need to be considered during recipient preparation. Patient and family psychosocial stability is tremendously important for posttransplant adherence to a relatively complex treatment regimen. Pretransplant, patients and families should be educated regarding the need for frequent and comprehensive follow-up especially for the first few months posttransplant. Logistical obstacles related to transportation and caregivers' time away from work should be planned for. As such, interventions may include counseling, intense psychological interventions, or involvement of authorities in complicated custodial situations. Appropriate financial coverage for posttransplant medications should be ensured and education on obtaining immunosuppressive drugs in the outpatient setting provided. Vascular and gastrointestinal (GI) tract access may need to be addressed: a central line may be needed posttransplant to facilitate frequent blood sampling, or in those necessitating peritransplant plasmapheresis for immunological reasons. A gastrostomy tube (GT) may benefit patients who require nutritional or fluid supplementation or are unable to take posttransplant medications orally. In the highly sensitized subgroup of patients (e.g. prior organ transplant, blood transfusions, pregnancy, etc.) at increased immunological risk may benefit from specialized immunological characterization and desensitization prior to transplantation.

Prior to transplant, the recipient's thrombosis risk should be assessed, as graft thrombosis can result in graft loss. Risk factors include hypercoagulopathy (e.g. chronic nephrotic states), antiphospholipid antibodies (30–50% of patients with systemic lupus erythematosus), prior postoperative venous thrombosis (e.g. a renal transplant vein) or thrombosis associated with vascular access (e.g. for dialysis). Hypercoagulability should be corrected before transplant whenever possible, and anticoagulation considered both perioperatively and postoperatively. Heparin use perioperatively remains controversial as a recent retrospective study showed that young recipient age, young donor age, and increased cold ischemia time were associated with graft thrombosis, but heparin administration did not decrease the incidence of early renal allograft thrombosis.

Surgical/Urological Preparation

The transplantation process, involving transplant surgeons and/or urologists, anesthesia, procurement teams and organ allocation personnel, is complex and potentially error-prone. However, when complications are averted or managed successfully, good long-term patient and allograft survival is achievable.

Preemptive transplantation, in which the patient receives a transplant prior to warranting dialysis, should be considered whenever feasible. Advantages of preemptive transplantation include minimization of CKD associated morbidity and dialysis related complications. Recent data from the North American Pediatric Renal Trials and Collaborative Studies (NAPRTCS) demonstrate a significant allograft survival advantage with preemptive transplantation, the reasons for which are likely several. Once accepted as a transplant candidate, the recipient undergoes careful preparation and critical concerns regarding the maximization of growth, nutrition, red blood cell mass, and acid-base, electrolyte, and CV and volume parameters.

Pediatric ESRD is often compounded by urinary tract disease, e.g. obstructive uropathy or high-grade vesicoureteral reflux (VUR). Consequently, optimization of urinary tract drainage including bladder management is key to transplant preparation (Tables 1 and 2). Because a dysfunctional bladder can adversely affect the allograft, surgical correction of urologic abnormalities is best performed before long-term immunosuppression. As such, transplantation should not preclude formal urological evaluation and preparation.

Table 1. Basic pretransplant evaluation of pediatric kidney transplant candidates

History/Physical Exam:
General history and physical examination
Immunization status
Serial anthropometric data (height, weight, and — as indicated, e.g. in very young children — head circumference)
Serial blood pressures
24-hour urine output (as indicated, e.g. in high-output CKD)
Hematological/Immunological Assessment:
Blood, Rh and HLA typing
Crossmatch with potential donors (if available)
Regular panel-reactive antibody (PRA) determination
Assessment for anti-HLA/donor-specific antibodies
Microbilogical/Virological Evaluation:
Urine culture
Rapid plasma reagent test
Mantoux test
Antiviral antibodies (cytomegalovirus, Epstein–Barr, herpes simplex, varicella, hepatitis B and C and human immunodeficiency viruses)

(*Continued*)

Table 1. (*Continued*)

Clinical Laboratory Evaluation:
Complete blood count, coagulation profile, kidney and liver function tests (including, calcium, phosphorus and albumin)
Quantification of urinary protein (as indicated)
Dental Evaluation (to assess for and remove potential sources of infection once chronic immunosuppression is needed)
Psychosocial Evaluation (to assess for nonadherence potential and other risk factors) and Intervention as indicated

Table 2. Staged urological pretransplant evaluation and interventions

History:
Primary diagnosis
Urinary tract infections
Bladder-related signs and symptoms (e.g. frequency, incontinence, poor stream, constipation)
Exam:
Genitalia, perineum and sacrum
Neurological exam of the lower extremities
First-line testing:
Urinalysis
Urine culture
Post void residual
Voiding cystourethrogram (VCUG, in selected cases, e.g. very young patients and patients with other evidence indicating lower urinary tract anomalies)
Second-line testing (as indicated):
Formal urodynamic evaluation
Cystourethroscopy
Non-surgical therapeutic interventions (as indicated):
Frequent/timed voiding
Bowel program
Anticholinergics
Clean intermittent catheterizations
Suppressive antibiotics
Surgical interventions (as indicated):
Native nephrectomy
Ureteral reimplantation
Bladder outlet reconstruction
Mitrofanoff/Malone antegrade continence enema (ACE) cecostomy
Bladder augmentation
Neobladder/conduit

All pediatric renal transplantation candidates undergo a urological history and physical examination. The presence of a urological cause of renal injury, a history of UTI, obstructive or irritative voiding symptoms, and an abnormal neurological or sacral examination are indications for evaluation with renal and bladder ultrasound (US), including postvoid residual measurement, radiographic voiding cystourethrography (VCUG), and formal urodynamic testing. Urine culture should be obtained. The presence of reflux, as well as detrusor or bladder outlet distortion on radiographic VCUG, is an indication for formal urodynamic testing, while otherwise unexplained functional or structural bladder abnormalities may require cystourethroscopy. In contrast, patients who have CKD secondary to a primary nephrological disorder and have no dysfunctional voiding symptoms or infection require neither VCUG nor urodynamic testing.

If a significant symptom complex or urodynamic abnormality is encountered, bladder control is attempted with a voiding regimen, anticholinergic therapy, and/or clean intermittent catheterization (CIC). Because dysfunctional defecation adversely affects voiding, aggressive bowel program may be indicated. Not uncommonly, voiding cannot be evaluated reliably because of urinary diversion or oliguria. In such instances, reversal of urinary diversion prior to transplant can be useful to ensure adequate bladder function and can be done without precipitating dialysis need. Rarely, oliguria precludes adequate assessment of structurally or urodynamically unsound bladder in which case bladder cycling via CIC can be helpful. If a continent, compliant, sterile, and evacuatable urinary tract cannot be ensured despite medical intervention, surgical reconstruction is indicated.

Table 3 outlines indications for pretransplantation native nephrectomy, including congenital nephrotic syndrome due to increased risk of vascular graft thrombosis and death from sepsis. Acquired renal cystic disease is a well-recognized entity in adults with ESRD with a definable malignancy risk, but is poorly established in children. Prophylactic native nephrectomy should be considered in conditions with an increased risk of renal malignancy.

Several strategic considerations regarding nephrectomy are relevant. While the chronic dialysis patient is awaiting transplantation, the presence of significant residual urine may obviate ultrafiltration facilitating

Table 3. Indications for pretransplant native nephrectomy

Chronic parenchymal infection, including infected reflux, hydronephrosis and urolithiasis
Persistent heavy proteinuria (associated with hypoalbuminemia and hypercoagulability or interfering with detection of FSGS recurrence posttransplant)
Cystic kidney disease causing complications (e.g. kidney size-related respiratory or gastrointestinal compromise)

fluid and blood pressure management. Hence, unilateral nephrectomy is done simultaneously with transplant, often through the same incision. If bilateral nephrectomies are required, differential function analysis by isotope imaging may identify the kidney with worse function which can be removed pretransplant and the remaining kidney removed at the time of transplant. Exceptions to this include the presence of renal-mediated intractable infection, hypertension, massively enlarged (e.g. polycystic) or significantly surgically altered kidneys (e.g. diversion), which may make nephrectomy at the time of transplantation unduly difficult. Nephrectomy incision should be positioned to maintain peritoneal integrity and not interfere with subsequent transplantation.

Management of VUR in native kidneys remains controversial. The current consensus is VUR associated with persistent/recurrent infection should be treated by ureteral reimplantation, or nephroureterectomy. Ureteral reimplantation is preferred in order to preserve the native ureter, facilitating the management of potential allograft ureteral complications. Additionally, high-grade dilating VUR is associated with sufficient morbidity to justify pretransplantation ureteral reimplantation. Additional considerations for reimplantation include dysfunctional bladder associated with persisting or recurring bacteriuria (symptomatic or asymptomatic) or requiring CIC.

Surgical reconstruction restoring continence pretransplant may be required in those with neurological [e.g. the VACTERL (vertebral abnormalities, anal atresia, cardiac abnormalities, tracheoesophageal fistula/esophageal atresia, renal agenesis or dysplasia, and limb defects)] association or structural (e.g. cloacal exstrophy) bladder impairment. Bladder outlet reconstruction and surgical establishment of a continent and easily catheterizable Mitrofanoff stoma are particularly successful and beneficial when indicated. Additionally, refractory fecal incontinence should be addressed. The Malone cecostomy as a continence enema has proved safe and effective.

Bladder augmentation may be necessary before transplantation to ensure continence and a urinary receptacle that operates at sufficiently low pressures to avoid allograft deterioration which has been demonstrated in bladders with high intravesical pressures [e.g. posterior urethral valves (PUV)]. That this is not simply a consequence of an irregular reservoir with inconsistent emptying is evidenced by transplantation into abnormal urinary bladders not associated with elevated intravesical pressures (e.g. prune belly syndrome). Several series, however, report excellent outcomes with transplantation into the nonsurgically altered PUV bladder. This conflicting experience can be explained by the large variability in urodynamic characteristics of the valve bladder, the limited number of patients reported in individual series, and improvement in valve bladder function with age in some patients.

These experiences have created controversy about augmentation in transplantation. As it can complicate recipient course, it should be performed only when definitive indication is demonstrable. Prior reports have included patients aged 6–20 years, with a primary diagnosis of PUV, followed by neurovesical dysfunction. Although ileocystoplasty is the most prevalent procedure, several other modalities have been successfully employed. The majority of patients (59%) received living related donor allografts; however, deceased donor allografts have been used with comparable success. Autoaugmentation and ureterocystoplasty can be performed extraperitoneally without interfering with peritoneal dialysis or intestinal function and without metabolic consequences. The clinical experience is quite limited, and applicability is low. Seromuscular augmentation is also without metabolic consequence, but clinical experience and applicability appear low in this relatively complex procedure. Ileocystoplasty and colocystoplasty are technically simple, extensively used procedures with good results, but often result in profound acidosis. Although ureteral or Mitrofanoff neourethral implantation can be successfully performed into the tinea of the colonic augmentation segment, reliable implantation is not possible with ileocystoplasty, autoaugmentation, and ureterocystoplasty. Both ileocystoplasty and colocystoplasty are associated with an increased incidence of bacteriuria, mucus production compromising catheter drainage, and bladder calculi. Gastrocystoplasty is applicable to the transplantation setting, avoids the risk of acidosis and calculi, and markedly reduces bacteriuria and mucus production. Ureteral and Mitrofanoff neourethral implantation are readily performed. The hematuria-dysuria complex is occasionally encountered, particularly during oliguric or anuric periods pretransplant. It is generally readily controlled by bladder cycling, histamine blockade, or proton pump inhibition.

Whenever possible, allograft ureteral implantation should be accomplished into the native component of the augmented bladder or into a gastrocystoplasty segment to reduce ureteral complications. If a nonreconstructable bladder is encountered, an intestinal conduit or continent diversion may be applicable. The risks of technical and infectious complications, however, are sufficiently high to obviate use unless native bladder rehabilitation is impossible. An isotopic neourethra and bladder provide an excellent alternative.

Obtaining a Donor Kidney

Approximately 3% of children waitlisted for deceased donor kidney die annually. Efforts focusing on optimizing organ donation rates from deceased donors and refining organ selection criteria are ongoing. The best kidney for a child is one from an otherwise healthy young adult donor, and a single kidney from a very young pediatric donor may not provide acceptable long-term function. However, consideration can be given to the transplantation of an *en bloc* pair of kidneys from a young donor into one recipient. Similarly, kidneys from expanded criteria deceased donors or non-heart-beating donors are used increasingly in adults; however, they are currently only indicated for children in extremely rare situations because they are unlikely to provide long graft survival. Historically, individuals who were being evaluated as potential deceased donors had suffered brain death, but donation after cardiac death (DCD) has more recently gained increasing acceptance.

The sequence of steps and diagnostic studies involved, including contraindications to the use of organs from any deceased donor, has been thoroughly mandated by the United Network for Organ Sharing (UNOS) and administered by the regional organ procurement organizations

(OPOs). Deceased donor management requires intensive, coordinated care by the intensive care unit and organ procurement team members. Hemodynamic stabilization is critical and generally involves central venous or pulmonary arterial pressure monitoring, volume and red blood cell expansion, replacement of coagulation components (for disseminated intravascular coagulopathy), correction of dysrhythmias, and the judicial use of vasopressors. Temperature regulation and respiratory support are also critical. Hormonal support is often indicated because of a precipitous decrease in levels after brain death and may include triiodothyronine, cortisol, and insulin. Arginine vasopressin is frequently indicated to reverse neurogenic diabetes insipidus.

Surgical organ retrieval is performed through a midline incision from the sternal notch to the pubis. The intestines are mobilized and the distal aorta and inferior vena cava isolated. Vascular anatomy of the liver, pancreas, and small intestine is defined and the aorta isolated at the diaphragmatic hiatus. The distal aorta is cannulated, supraceliac aorta clamped, venous drainage achieved (at the level of the right atrium), aorta flushed with cold preservation solution, and the abdomen packed with sterile saline ice slush. Organs are sequentially removed, beginning with the heart, followed by the lungs, liver, small intestine, pancreas, and finally, the kidneys. The kidneys are removed *en bloc* with the adjacent aorta and vena cava and the ureters divided at the level of the urinary bladder. Kidneys from the very young donor are not separated until a decision has been made about individual or en bloc transplantation. Otherwise, the kidneys are separated on the back table and cold stored in preservation fluid for distribution. Preservation fluid is designed to minimize the injury associated with hypothermia and hypoxia.

Although the short- and mid-term outcomes of deceased donor kidney transplantation in children approximate those of living donor transplantation, the latter is preferred, in part due to ease of timing. Once a transplant date is set, arrangements can be made to initiate immunosuppressive therapy pretransplant at those centers choosing this approach. While data supporting this practice as a means to improve outcome are not available, recent observations by several groups support the notion that exposure to mycophenolic acid, a commonly used antirejection agent, is insufficient in many patients early posttransplant if used at historically recommended doses. Accordingly, guidelines regarding the more aggressive use of this agent have recently been suggested. Live donor transplantation also makes pre-emptive transplant easier. When an adult kidney is placed into a small child, caution with pre-transplant immunosuppression should be exercised as these recipients can be quite uremic, and treatment with a calcineurin inhibitor (CI) for a number of days before transplantation may worsen this condition. Under these circumstances, a grafted adult kidney that functions immediately can remove uremic toxins at a staggering rate creating a clinical scenario similar to disequilibrium syndrome seen in hemodialysis.

As living related, and — increasingly — unrelated, donor renal allografts have become an integral component of pediatric renal transplantation, they are managed with additional precautions. Great care is required to ensure that the donor is acting on his or her own volition without coercion. Although the majority of allografts are obtained from direct relatives with a genetic advantage, suitable unrelated living donors are acceptable. Most centers require evidence of an ongoing emotional commitment (e.g. a step-parent) when entertaining unrelated directed donation, but unrelated, undirected (i.e. altruistic or "Good Samaritan") donation is now considered acceptable with adequate evaluation and allocation policies. UNOS strongly recommends an independent donor advocacy process purely focused on the assessment and support of the potential living organ donor as part of the evaluation.

The long-term outcome of transplantation favors the living donor (even unrelated) over well-matched deceased donor grafts, underscoring the critical impact of minimal cold ischemia time and the absence of pre and peri-procurement renal injury or disease. The decreased incidence of delayed graft function, fewer rejection episodes, and less cumulative exposure to immunosuppressant agents are important in children.

Morbidity associated with living related donor nephrectomy is small; however, systolic hypertension, proteinuria, and a reduced glomerular filtration rate have been documented decades after donation. Significant hypertension or symptomatic renal disease after nephrectomy is rare. General selection criteria and evaluation guidelines for potential living kidney donors have been established, but variability exists between individual centers, e.g. regarding acceptance of obese or hypertensive individuals. Donor evaluation or portions should be repeated as needed if transplant is postponed significantly.

Donor nephrectomy is performed simultaneously with surgical exposure of the recipient. Live donor nephrectomy has traditionally been performed through an extended flank incision, enabling excellent retroperitoneal exposure of renal hilar vessels and ureter. More recently, laparoscopic donor nephrectomy has increased because of improved safety and efficacy profile, specifically, less postoperative pain and a quicker return to normal activities. Consequently, the number of living renal donations has increased. Recent data suggesting small pediatric recipients of adult kidneys removed laparoscopically may be at risk for delayed graft function and early rejection has lowered the threshold for open donor nephrectomy in special situations.

The laparoscopic donor nephrectomy procedure has been well-described. Antiembolism sequential compression stockings are placed, and the patient is placed in a modified flank position. The abdomen is insufflated with carbon dioxide and four transperitoneal laparoscopic ports are placed. Access to the retroperitoneum is obtained by reflecting the colon after incising the line of Toldt. The kidney is gently mobilized taking care to avoid excessive dissection of the lower pole, which could interfere with ureteral blood supply, and the hilar vessels dissected to their junction with the aorta or vena cava. The ureter is mobilized with a generous cuff of retroperitoneal adipose tissue to maximize vascularity.

When the recipient is ready, the ureter is clipped and divided at the level of the iliac vessels, leaving the proximal end open. Good urine output is documented from both the divided ureter and the indwelling urethral catheter. The renal artery and vein are sequentially ligated, vessels divided, and the kidney is extracted from the Pfannenstiel incision. The kidney is immediately flushed with cold preservation solution, placed in saline ice slush and delivered to the recipient room. Hand-assisted laparoscopy has also been described for donor nephrectomy with similar outcomes.

Renal Transplantation

Establishment of compatibility

The first consideration regarding compatibility concerns the blood group antigen (ABO) system. Blood group polysaccharides are expressed on the endothelium of the allograft, and the presence of preformed antibodies results in hyperacute rejection if incompatible — similar to hemolytic blood transfusion reactions. As these antigens are not genetically linked to HLA, ABO incompatibility may occur in the presence of HLA identity. Because blood group O donors are "universal" donors, waitlisted patients with blood group O experience a comparably long wait. Live kidney donor ABO compatibility is also assessed analogous to blood transfusions. Blood group D (Rh) is not a relevant histocompatibility barrier to renal transplantation. Transplantation from a subset blood group A_2 donor to blood group B or O recipient can be successful in children; however, occasional accelerated acute rejections have been encountered, and anti-A immunoglobulin G (IgG) titers may influence both early and long-term graft survival, with a titer exceeding 1:8 indicating poor prognosis. Otherwise, ABO incompatibilities are avoided, although experience with ABO-incompatible live donor transplantation was reported in 1998, using aggressive recipient preparation consisting of plasmapheresis, immunoadsorption, and splenectomy at the time of transplantation, followed by allograft irradiation in the early posttransplantation period. This is not general practice in pediatric renal transplantation.

The clinical use of pretransplantation HLA cross-matching to avoid hyperacute and accelerated graft rejection has been extensively reviewed and center variability exists with respect to performance and interpretation. Traditionally, cross-matching is based on a complement-dependent lymphocytotoxic assay (using the serum of the potential recipient and tissue, e.g. lymphocytes, from the donor), which may be enhanced in sensitivity by the addition of antihuman globulin. Occasionally, a clinically insignificant positive cross-match is encountered related to presence of autoantibodies. Because these are often of the IgM isotype, incubation of the patient's sera with reagents such as dithiothreitol or dithioerythritol, which eliminate IgM isotype antibodies, is used to screen for autoantibodies. However, because not all autoantibodies are IgM and because not all IgM antibodies are insignificant, autoabsorption and retesting of the resultant autocrossmatch-negative serum for residual cytotoxic reactivity is more definitive. More recently, flow cytometry has been added to HLA cross-matching process as a complement-independent sensitive methodology. Most recently, bead technology provides identification and quantification of specific anti-HLA antibodies, allowing sensitized potential recipients to be studied in great detail, leading to the development of targeted approaches. The current listing process for potential deceased donor kidney transplant recipients in the United States now includes the bead technology-based calculation of a panel reactive antibody percentage (cPRA), replacing traditional determination of PRA using varying methodologies.

In the absence of autoantibodies, a positive serum complement-dependent cross-match is considered a contraindication to transplantation. Controversy exists about the significance of a positive flow cytometry cross-match in the presence of a negative complement-dependent crossmatch in primary transplants. In retransplantation, allosensitization from prior transplant, previous pregnancy, exposure to blood products, or a prior nonrenal organ transplant is problematic. Therapeutic options for allosensitized individuals include desensitization or paired kidney exchange. Either approach is labor-intensive and should be performed by centers with expertise and resources to maximize success. Paired kidney exchange is an option for ABO-incompatible donor–recipient pairs.

Matching of HLA antigens has been demonstrated to significantly impact allograft half-life, but such matching may be somewhat less important due to increased potency of newer immunosuppressive agents. Nonetheless, the matching process continues to play a role, especially in the allocation of deceased donor kidneys. Nationally, six-antigen–matched kidney sharing is mandated (5% of deceased donor transplants). In the absence of a six-antigen match, grafts are allocated locally based on HLA antigen matching in addition to the length of wait, the recipient allosensitization, recipient age, and other factors. Donor organs are matched and offered to centers for individual patients accordingly, based on allocation algorithms that undergo regular revisions and refinements. Because of additional neurodevelopmental advantages of kidney transplantation, waitlisted children receive an allocation advantage over adults.

Accepting the allograft

Once offered, kidney acceptance depends on many considerations, foremost the health of the recipient. Intercurrent illness is a contraindication to transplantation, especially if infectious in nature. Other considerations include recipient age, donor age, and the status of the kidney offered. The recipient's family is counseled regarding variables as indicated, allowing for an informed decision regarding the proposed allograft, especially when the donor meets "high-risk" criteria outlined by the Centers for Disease Control.

Very young recipient candidates may require a smaller graft if transperitoneal transplantation is obviated by peritoneal obliteration or if future obliteration is to be avoided. Published experience has demonstrated inferior outcomes when kidneys from very young donors (<6 years, and especially <2 years) are used in children. Such donor kidneys may fare better in adults and, in the very young donor, when used *en bloc*. Cold ischemia time is important. Donor age >50 years and death from CV disease are poor prognostic variables.

Transplantation process

Recipients entering the operating room for a kidney transplant should be in the best possible medical condition and dialysis dependent children should undergo dialysis treatment within 24hrs preceding transplant to optimize metabolic control (e.g. potassium or blood urea nitrogen), but should be relatively volume-loaded to ensure adequate allograft perfusion. Ultrafiltration should be adjusted pretransplant, possibly requiring an increase in antihypertensive drug therapy to compensate for this adjustment. If hemodialysis is required on the day of transplant, anticoagulation should be minimized or avoided to prevent excessive bleeding during surgery.

The transplant begins with general endotracheal anesthesia administration. The patient is positioned supine, a bladder catheter is placed, and the bladder is inflated under gravity flow with an antibacterial solution. Central venous access is obtained for monitoring and medication administration. A pulmonary arterial catheter is placed if indicated by primary pulmonary or cardiac disease. A second-generation cephalosporin is administered and intravenous hydration given. Red blood cell mass is expanded if indicated due to severe anemia.

The operation is performed through a "hockey-stick" incision, providing excellent retroperitoneal exposure. Younger recipients may require a transperitoneal approach due to limited retroperitoneal space. Retroperitoneal placement is preferred to preserve the peritoneal cavity for future dialysis if needed. General guidelines for allograft placement are shown in Table 4.

Table 4. General guidelines for allograft placement in children

Recipient weight	Graft placement (approach)
>20 kg	retroperitoneal (“hockey stick” incision, iliac fossa)
10–20 kg	retroperitoneal if possible
<10 kg	transabdominal (midline incision)

Blood volume is expanded to a central venous pressure (CVP) = 12–16 cm H_2O, with the expectation that vascularization of an adult allograft will result in acute blood sequestration of approximately 250–300 ml. Anastomotic sites are chosen, and venous and arterial trees are carefully mobilized with division of the overlying lymphatic vessels between ligatures. The anastomosis is placed at the level of the aorta or aortoiliac junction in infants and toddlers, in the common iliac artery in young children, and in the external iliac artery in adolescents and young adults. Vascular control is achieved with gentle application of vascular clamps or tapes, the venotomy placed, the recipient vein injected with a heparin-saline solution, and the venous anastomosis performed with 5–0 Prolene suture. The arteriotomy is then made, and arterial anastomosis is performed with 6–0 Prolene suture. The distal arterial tree is flushed with heparin-saline solution before the anastomosis. If the aorta is to be occluded, the patient is treated with heparin. Mannitol (0.5 mg/kg) and furosemide (0.5–1 mg/kg) are administered before completing the anastomoses. The vascular clamps are removed, with gentle finger pressure applied to the renal artery for three seconds to allow clearance of debris or air pockets before kidney revascularization. An intra-arterial injection of verapamil (0.1 mg/kg, maximum 5 mg) into the upstream artery with the distal artery still occluded may be performed at this time.

Attention is directed at ensuring that the kidney promptly attains good turgor. Studies have demonstrated the vascularization event to be associated with an abrupt fall in CVP by 4–7 cm H_2O in a small child. Mean aortic blood flow measurements reveal huge and sustained increases in aortic blood flow when a large graft is placed in a small recipient. Failure to achieve adequate turgor may necessitate additional volume expansion or addition of inotropic support, i.e. low-dose dopamine. Importantly, posttransplantation hypotension is a major risk factor for allograft loss and must be aggressively prevented.

Variations in vascular anatomy may obviate the use of a kidney from a prospective living donor or may create reconstructive challenges in deceased donor situations. Kidneys are removed *en bloc* from deceased donors with the adjacent vena cava and aorta, and are then visualized from a posterior perspective and the aorta opened in the midline, followed by midline division of the anterior aorta and vena cava. The kidney is thereby provided with an adjacent segment of both aorta and vena cava, enabling a significant degree of reconstructive flexibility. If a renal vessel is of good dimension, it may be simply divided, spatulated, and anastomosed. If the vessel is small, it may be prepared with a small patch of adjacent aorta or vena cava to facilitate anastomosis and minimize anastomotic stenosis or thrombosis. Multiple vessels entering the vena cava or aorta in a close cluster may be prepared on a single large cuff of aorta or vena cava). If multiple vessels entering the vena cava or aorta at sites remote from each other are encountered, reconstruction may be needed. If both vessels are small, two small patches may be anastomosed to create one larger cuff for anastomosis. If a dominant artery is present with a second smaller artery, an end-to-side anastomosis is undertaken. This type of vascular reconfiguration is tremendously enhanced by using an operating microscope. Occasionally, an extremely short renal vein is encountered, but mobilization of the venous tree is sufficient to enable a tension-free anastomosis. When this is insufficient, the renal vein may be extended by tubularizing adjacent flaps of vena cava.

Ureteral implantation into the bladder may be performed either transvesically (Paquin) or extravesically (detrusorrhaphy). Advantages of the extravesical approach include shortened operating time, very low incidence of anastomotic obstruction, and most importantly, dramatic reduction of postoperative hematuria and urinary extravasation. This is advantageous in the young recipient whose urethra may be easily occluded, even by a relatively small blood or fibrin clot. Ureteral implantation is considerably more critical in circumstances of dysfunctional voiding pathophysiology. An attempt is made to place the anastomosis somewhat lateral on the bladder where the bladder wall is less mobile, and a ureteral tunnel length: ureteral diameter ratio of 4:1 is sought. The detrusor is incised and a plane developed between it and the underlying bladder urothelium. A small defect is created distally in this mucosal trough, and spatulated anastomosis performed. The ureter is advanced distally with the first suture placed. As the remainder of the muscular defect is closed over the ureter to create a nonrefluxing implantation, a small bite of ureter is taken with every other or every third suture to prevent slippage of the ureteral anastomosis within the tunnel and erosion of the valvular mechanism over time. Because ureteral obstruction (e.g. from anastomotic edema) or extravasation represent potentially devastating complications, an internal indwelling stent is often placed temporarily during the early postoperative period.

Postoperative care

In addition to general perioperative care, which may require efforts at circulatory, respiratory, and nutritional support, postoperative care of the transplant recipient includes immunosuppression and fluid/electrolyte management. Generally, fluid management is approached by replacing insensible loss (calculated) and urine output on a volume basis. It is critical to recognize that hourly urine output may approach the patient's blood volume, particularly when an adult kidney is placed into an infant. This initial diuresis can cause major fluid and electrolyte disturbances, which must be anticipated and prevented.

Immunosuppressive therapy is in constant evolution to achieve the best possible antirejection prophylaxis without overimmunosuppression or induction of related toxicities. Immunosuppressive protocols cannot be administered in a "one size fits all" fashion: first-time Caucasian living donor recipients without presensitization require less antirejection prophylaxis than recipients of a repeat transplant, especially deceased donor, with evidence of presensitization, or African Americans. Genetic polymorphisms and related phenomena affecting drug metabolism and immunological responsiveness further reiterates individualization of immunosuppression. Therefore transplant programs generally adopt flexible immunosuppression protocols that are tailored to each recipient's risk profile. Additional guidance in the selection of pediatric immunosuppressive regimens is also derived from adult studies and from local practice and experience. A typical initial protocol in pediatric kidney transplantation consists of a CI, an antiproliferative agent, and steroids, possibly paired with a course of induction with a nondepleting anti-T cell antibody. The doses and target levels of these agents are geared towards the recipient's estimated risk for acute rejection, balanced against side effects and other potential disadvantages. Recent efforts by a variety of groups have further broadened the available choices for initial immunosuppression: complete steroid avoidance, induction with alternative antibody preparations, and introduction of a new class of maintenance immunosuppressants known as the inhibitors of the mammalian target of rapamycin (mTOR).

Hypertension frequently occurs or worsens in the immediate posttransplant setting for several reasons, including fluid liberalization and high-dose corticosteroid treatment. While mild blood pressure elevations may be temporarily desirable to enhance perfusion of the new allograft, more pronounced hypertension, especially if symptomatic, should be treated. Calcium channel antagonists are safe and effective, but may interfere with CI metabolism. Once transplant function has stabilized, the same group may be beneficial, although angiotensin-converting enzyme inhibitors (ACEIs) or angiotensin receptor blockers (ARBs) should be considered, especially if chronic allograft nephropathy is present.

Hypophosphatemia and hypomagnesemia can occur quickly posttransplant. The former is largely due to "hungry bones" and frequently requires phosphorus supplementation for several months. The latter is associated with CI, especially tacrolimus, therapy and may require supplementation, especially if clinical symptoms are present.

Prophylaxis against bacterial, viral, and fungal pathogens is essential posttransplant. Antibiotic coverage is provided perioperatively to prevent wound infections, then transitioned to a prophylactic regimen against UTIs and *Pneumocystis (carinii) jiroveci.* Specific guidelines have been developed for antiviral prophylaxis in the posttransplant setting, largely directed against cytomegalovirus (CMV) and prescribed based on risk profile, determined by recipient and donor CMV status and by the strength of immunosuppression used. Unfortunately, no effective prophylactic regimens for Epstein-Barr virus (EBV) infection are available. Since many pediatric transplant recipients are EBV-naïve and many adult donors carry EBV, primary EBV infection is a considerable problem, as EBV can drive the development of posttransplant lymphoproliferative disorder (PTLD). Antifungal prophylaxis is provided for the first several months posttransplant, when high immunosuppression doses are prescribed. Accordingly, a number of centers readminister infection prophylaxis during acute rejection episodes requiring aggressive immunosuppression.

Gastrointestinal prophylaxis includes either a histamine H2 receptor blocker or proton pump inhibitor, which are discontinued once all medicines are taken orally and if free of GI complaints.

Suggested Reading

Abraham EC, Wilson, AC, Goebel J. (2009) Current kidney allocation rules and their impact on a pediatric transplant center. *Am J Transpl* 9(2): 404–8.

Al-Akash SI, Ettenger RB. (2005) Kidney transplantation in children. In: Danovitch GM. (ed.) *Handbook of Kidney Transplantation*, 4th ed., Lippincott Williams and Wilkins, Philadelphia, p. 414.

Danovitch GM. (2005) Immunosuppressive medications and protocols for kidney transplantation. In: Danovitch GM (ed.) *Handbook of Kidney Transplantation*, 4th edition, Lippincott Williams and Wilkins: Philadelphia, pp. 72–134.

Davis CL. (2004) Evaluation of the living kidney donor: current perspectives. *Am J Kidney Dis* 43(3): 508–30.

Kidney Disease: Improving Global Outcomes (KDIGO) Transplant Work Group. (2009) KDIGO clinical practice guideline for the care of kidney transplant recipients. *Am J Transplant* 9(Suppl 3): S1–S157.

Neu AM, Fivush BA. (1998) Recommended immunization practices for pediatric renal transplant recipients. *Pediatr Transpl* 2(4): 263–269.

Ramos E, Kasiske BL, Danovitch G. (1998) Pre-transplant evaluation of the recipient. In: Norman DJ, Suki WN. (eds.), *Primer on Transplantation,* American Society of Transplant Physicians, Thorofare, p. 175.

Ryckman FC. (1997) Organ donation, procurement and preservation. In: Oldham KT *et al.* (eds.) *Surgery of Infants and Children: Scientific Principles and Practice,* Lippincott Raven Publishers. Philadelphia, p. 701.

Sheldon CA, Martin LW, Churchill BM. (1991) Surgical perspectives in pediatric renal transplantation. In: Gillenwater JY, *et al.* (eds.) *Adult and pediatric urology,* Mosby Year Book, St. Louis, p. 2301.

Sheldon CA, Snyder HM, et al. (1996) Principles of urinary tract reconstruction. In: Gillenwater JY, Grayhack JT, Howards SS (ed.) *Adult and Pediatric Urology,* Mosby Year Book, St. Louis, p. 2317.

42

Immunosuppressive Medications for Transplantation

Shefali Mahesh and Deepa H. Chand

Introduction

As immunosuppression is a requisite component of renal transplantation, knowledge of the various agents and combinations is critical to managing pediatric renal transplant recipients. Long-term, the goal is to preserve the allograft for as long as possible. Until recently the goals of transplantation focused on short-term survival, more specifically aimed at minimizing acute rejection episodes. Over the past few decades, great strides have been made in improving transplant immunosuppression regimens to achieve improved short-term survival. Consequently, emphasis has shifted to long-term allograft survival and decreasing the incidence of patient death with a functioning graft. As graft survival improves, the clinician is faced with the challenges of dealing with the adverse effects of prolonged immunosuppression and individual agent toxicity. Immunosuppression toxicity may manifest as chronic allograft nephropathy (CAN), one of the major causes of late allograft loss. Other factors contributing to CAN development include hypertension, hyperlipidemia, obesity, and diabetes. Thus, recently many different protocols have been put forth with a common aim of minimizing, withdrawing or avoiding immunosuppressive medications particularly corticosteroids and CNI.

Various immunsuppressant agents cause either lymphocyte depletion, diversion of lympocyte activity, or lymphocyte pathway blockade. The choice of immunosuppression regimen/combination is a paramount factor in renal transplant management. Specifically, the overall goal is to balance the risk of rejection to the complications associated with excessive immunosuppression, namely-malignancy, infection, and non-renal toxicity. This chapter provides a brief review of immunosuppressant medications currently being used in renal transplantation. It is important to remember that specific immunosuppressants and combinations of these will vary from institution to institution. This chapter will provide a general overview, however, specific guidance regarding combination therapy is deferred.

Induction

Induction therapy is defined as treatment with a biological agent begun before, at the time of, or immediately after transplantation. The purpose of induction is to deplete or modulate T cell responses at the time of antigen presentation. Traditionally, T cell depletion with the use of polyclonal antibodies was the mainstay. These agents induced depletion, however induced a cytokine release which produced significant side effects. These agents reduce early infection; but, the risk of post transplant lymphoproliferative disorder and infection preclude long-term use.

Antithymocyte antibodies

Polyclonal agents: ATGAM® and Thymoglobulin®

ATGAM® is an equine-anti-human polyclonal anti-thymocyte antibody preparation which is produced through the immunization of human T-lymphocytes into horses. A newer agent, Thymoglobulin® [anti-thymocyte globulin (rabbit)] is similar as it is a polyclonal anti-thymocyte preparation; however, it is a rabbit-anti-human product derived via injection of human T-lymphocytes into rabbits. Both preparations result in cytotoxic antibodies directed against human T-lymphocytes.

Mechanism of action

- Blocks T cell membrane proteins (CD2, CD3, CD45 etc.) to cause altered cellular function, cell lysis, and prolonged T cell depletion. These agents are not directed towards specific T cell subsets and hence, are very potent induction agents.

Adverse effects

- Systemic cytokine release syndrome resulting in fever, hypotension, shock, gastrointestinal (nausea, vomiting, diarrhea, dyspepsia)
- Serum sickness
- Leukopenia
- Thrombocytopenia
- Opportunistic infections (bacterial, candidal, etc.)
- Hypertension
- Headaches
- Hypertension
- Hyperkalemia

Monitoring

- CBC

Monoclonal antibodies

IL-2 Receptor Antagonists

These agents are more commonly used for patients who are at low or moderate risk of rejection. These agents are selective and therefore, have a favorable side effect profile as compared to polyclonal antibodies.

- Basiliximab: Chimeric mouse-human monoclonal antibody
- Daclizumab: Humanized monoclonal antibody (no longer available for kidney transplant rejection)

Mechanism of action

- Monoclonal antibodies do not deplete T lymphocytes, but rather reduce the responsiveness to lymphocyte actions.
- Chimeric monoclonal antibodies directed against the interleukin 2 (IL-2) receptor alpha chain (CD25) on activated T cells, inhibiting IL-2 induced T cell activation.
- Have limited efficacy but have low nonimmune toxicity because they do not trigger cytokine release
- Effects last for approximately 30 days.

Adverse effects

Hypersensivity reactions

- Hypertension
- Headaches
- Tremors
- Urinary system (urinary retention, dysuria)
- Opportunistic infection (bacterial, candidial, etc.)
- Gastrointestinal (abdominal pain, dyspepsia, nausea, vomiting, diarrhea, constipation).

Alemtuzumab (Campath)

This agent is not currently approved in the United States for renal transplantation, however has been used off label in renal transplantation induction.

Mechanism of action

- Recombinant humanized monoclonal antibody against CD52, causes severe depletion of lymphocytes.
- Binds specifically to antigen CD52, a glycoprotein expressed on the surface of B and T cells, monocytes, macrophages, natural killer (NK) cells, and granulocytes.
- Host immune response causes lysis of normal and leukemic cells, with presumed activity via complement-dependent cytotoxicity (CDC) and antibody-dependent cell-mediated cytotoxicity (ADCC).

Adverse effects

- First dose reaction
- Severe neutropenia, anemia, pancytopenia
- Autoimmunity (e.g. hemolytic anemia, thrombocytopenia, hyperthyroidism)
- Severe, life-threatening infections

Corticosteroids

Corticosteroids have been the cornerstone of transplant immunosuppression for decades. High dose methylprednisolone (2–10 mg/kg/dose to a maximum of 500 mg) is generally administered intravenously as an induction agent at the time of transplantation. Some centers include corticosteroids as part of a maintenance regimen as well.

Mechanism of action:

- At lower doses, corticosteroids inhibit DNA transcription factors. At higher doses, have receptor independent effects.
- Prevent T cell activation and proliferation
- Inhibit cytokine production (interleukin-1, interleukin-2, interleukin-6, interferon-gamma, and tumor necrosis factor (TNF)-alpha)
- Reduce MHC antigen expression
- Decrease neutrophil and monocyte activity

Adverse effects:

- Impaired linear growth
- Weight gain
- Cardiovascular: hypertension, hyperlipidemia, glucose intolerance
- Bone: Osteoporosis, avascular necrosis
- Cosmetic: cushingoid facies, acne, striae
- Easy bruising, poor wound healing
- Peptic ulcers
- Cataracts
- Mood changes

OKT3 (Muromonab)

This agent is a mouse-derived monoclonal antibody that has been used in the past for induction and treatment of rejection. This use of this agent has declined over time due to the availability of more efficacious and less toxic agents.

Mechanism of action

- Anti-CD3 antibody
- Binds to the delta chain of the T-cell receptor to inhibit nearly all T-cell functions leading to T-cell depletion

Adverse events

- Formation of anti-OKT3 antibodies, making it ineffective and limiting repeat use.
- Repeated use has been associated with and increase risk of PTLD
- First use reaction: fevers, chills, diarrhea, nausea, vomiting, hypotension, and pulmonary edema due to cytokine release.
- Acute kidney injury
- Central nervous system changes

Maintainance

Long-term immunosuppression to prevent rejection and deterioration of graft function. Agents with different mechanisms of action are used in combination to attain sufficient immunosuppression while minimizing the toxicities associated with individual agents. The aim is to prevent rejection and prolong graft survival while using the lowest possible immunosuppressive doses. In general, the longer the time from transplantation the lower the doses and levels of immunosuppression. This is based on the principle of development of "tolerance" to the grafted organ.

Calcineurin inhibitors

These medications are generally initiated within 1–2 days after transplantation. Some centers will initiate this agent 3–5 days pretransplant in living donor situations. It is important to postpone initiation in patients with delayed graft function due to nephrotoxic potential.

Cyclosporine

This agent has been used for nearly three decades as part of a maintenance therapy regimen in renal transplantation. It is an 11 amino acid peptide derived from *Tolypocladium inflatum.*

Mechanism of action

- Binds to cyclophilin and prevents activation of helper T cells, prevents production of IL-2, and other cytokines by calcineurin inhibition.

Adverse effects

- Nephrotoxicity due to afferent arteriolar vasoconstriction, and decrease in renal plasma flow.
- Hypertension due to fluid retention; stimulation of the sympathetic nervous system and renin angiotensin system; and inhibition of the action of nitric oxide; leading to intrarenal and systemic vasoconstriction.
- Central nervous system toxicity.
- Hyperkalemia, hypomagnesemia,
- Cosmetic side effects:
  - hirsutism, gingival hyperplasia
  - Metabolic disturbances: glucose intolerance, hyperkalemia, hypomagnesemia
  - Malignancy
  - Central nervous system changes
- Can induce hemolytic uremic syndrome.
- Increased risk of drug interactions due to metabolism via CP450 system.

Monitoring

- Because cyclosporine only partially blocks calcineurin, the clinical activity is proportional to tissue saturation, requiring diligent monitoring.
- Cyclosporine trough levels or two hours after dose (C2 level) should be obtained regularly.
- Generic forms are available and are not bioequivalent. Therefore, use of a consistent formulation is imperative.
- Monitor for drug interactions with agents affecting the cytochrome P450 system
- Hyperlipidemia is common and lipid panels should be monitored and intervention implemented accordingly.

Tacrolimus (FK506)

This agent is a macrolide antibiotic derived from *Streptomyces tsukubaensis*. This drug is more commonly used than cyclosporine; however, ultimately, the choice of calcineurin inhibitor used should be individualized.

Mechanism of action

- Binds to tacrolimus binding protein, and prevents activation of helper T cells, prevents production of IL-2 by calcineurin inhibition.

Adverse effects

- Malignancy: activation of Epstein-Barr virus in patients receiving tacrolimus has been associated with post-transplant lymphoproliferative disorder (PTLD).
- Neurotoxicity (tremors, weakness, paresthesias, seizures)
- Anemia
- Nephrotoxicity
- Metabolic disturbances:
    - diabetes mellitus,
    - hyperkalemia,
    - hypomagnesemia
- Cardiovascular:
    - hypertension, hyperlipidemia
- Infection
- Gastrointestinal (abdominal pain, constipation, diarrhea, vomiting, anorexia)
- Can reverse cosmetic side effects associated with cyclosporine.

Monitoring

- Tacrolimus trough levels
- Monitor for drug interactions with agents affecting the cytochrome P450
- Viral monitoring
- Routine blood counts to evaluate anemia, leukopenia

Antimetabolites

These agents are inosine monophospate dehydrogenase inhibitors. When used in conjunction with calcineurin inhibitors for maintenance therapy, they have been shown to improve allograft and patient survival. They can be used with other agents, do not require monitoring and do not increase cardiovascular or other organ toxicity.

Adverse effects

- Bone marrow suppression (leukopenia, megaloblastic anemia, thrombocytopenia)
- Liver toxicity (cholestasis, hepatitis, portal vein obstruction, elevation in transaminases)
- Malignancy
- Gastrointestinal (aphthous stomatitis, anorexia, nausea, vomiting, diarrhea)
- Alopecia

Monitoring

- Complete blood count (CBC)
- Pancreatic and liver enzymes

Mycophenolate Mofetil

Has largely replaced azathioprine as an antiproliferative agent due to superior efficacy. It is a prodrug that is metabolized to mycophenolic acid.

Azathioprine

Mechanism of action

- Releases 6-mercaptopurine and converts 6-MP to tissue inhibitor of metalloproteinases which is converted to thioguanine nucleotides that decreases DNA and RNA synthesis; The exact mechanism of immunosuppressive activity is unknown, but is believed to be dependent on several factors.
- Incorporates into nucleic acids resulting in chromosome breaks, disintegration of nucleic acids, or synthesis of abnormal proteins; It may also inhibit coenzyme formation and functioning, interfering with cellular metabolism and inhibiting mitosis.

- Suppresses cell-mediated immunity and causes alterations in antibody production, in renal transplant.
- Has mostly been replaced by mycophenolate mofetil.
- Remains an option for patients who are unable to tolerate mycophenolate mofetil due to side effects.

Mechanism of action

- Inhibits synthesis of guanosine monophosphate nucleotides that block purine synthesis to impair B and T cell proliferation.

Adverse effects

- Bone marrow suppression (leukopenia, megaloblastic anemia, thrombocytopenia)
- Hypertension
- Infection (may induce cytomegalovirus activation)
- Malignancy
- Gastrointestinal (abdominal pain, dyspepsia, anorexia, nausea, vomiting, diarrhea)

Monitoring

- CBC

mTOR Inhibitors

This class of agents was initially designed to be used in conjunction with calcineurin inhibitors. However, this combination has resulted in increased nephrotoxicity, hemolytic uremic syndrome and hypertension. These agents must be used cautiously as part of combination therapy.

Rapamycin (Sirolimus)

Mechanism of action

- Binds to FKBP12. This complex inhibits target of rapamycin ("TOR") Inhibits IL-2 driven cell proliferation.

Adverse effects

- Impaired wound healing
- Worsening of delayed graft function
- Metabolic (hyperlipidemia, hypertriglyceridemia)
- Pulmonary (pneumonitis, insterstitial lung disease)
- Oral stomatitis
- Joint pain
- Hematologic (thrombocytopenia)
- May enhance calcineurin inhibitor nephrotoxicity.

Monitoring

- Serum trough levels
- Lipid monitoring required.

Everolimus

Everolimus, an inhibitor of mammalian target of rapamycin (mTOR), is under consideration for use in renal transplantation. Everolimus binds with high affinity to the intracellular protein FK506 binding protein-12 (FKBP-12) to form a complex, inhibiting activation of mTOR. Inhibition of mTOR by everolimus has been shown to reduce cell proliferation, angiogenesis, and glucose uptake *in vitro* and/or *in vivo*. It is currently used as an antineoplastic agent, but it remains a newer agent on the horizon.

Rituximab

This chimeric monoclonal antibody is specific against CD20. Due to anti-neoplastic properties, it is sometimes used for the treatment of some forms of PTLD. Although it is not FDA approved for transplant immunosuppression, it has been used successfully to mitigate antibody mediated rejection in transplant patients.

Mechanism of Action

This agent binds to CD20 on B lymphocytes to induce B cell lysis.

Adverse Effects

- Infusion reactions
- Pulmonary fibrosis has been reported

Monitoring

- CD 20 and CD 19 levels

Emerging Concepts

The ultimate goal in kidney transplantation is to avoid the use of immunosuppression completely. However, this goal is not eminently consistently possible. Therefore, the current goal is to minimize toxicities while optimizing allograft survival.

In pediatric renal transplantation, great focus has been placed on steroid avoidance or minimization. Until recently, steroids have been the mainstay of immunosuppressive protocols for transplantation. The well established toxicities of long-term corticosteroids have prompted minimization in transplant immunosuppressive regimens. The goal has been to minimize steroid exposure and side effects, with no change in rejection rate or graft survival.

There is accumulating evidence that there is a place for steroid minimizing regimens, but there is limited evidence in high-risk patients and long-term outcomes still need to be defined. Many terms have been utilized such as steroid avoidance, steroid sparing, steroid withdrawal, steroid minimizing, steroid-free, etc. When assessing or utilizing these protocols, the reader must define the terminology and determine the risk associated with each. Generally speaking, steroid-free implies the complete absence of steroid use, for either induction or maintenance; steroid minimization refers to a rapid steroid taper spanning from weeks to months from time of transplant; and there are many variations of terminology in between.

Benefits of steroid reduction include improved cardiovascular health, improved linear growth, and a decreased risk of hypertension, metabolic syndrome, and diabetes mellitus In children, improved growth and bone health are additional considerations supporting steroid minimization.

Numerous studies have failed to demonstrate an increase in acute rejection episodes or early graft failure with rapid taper schedules. However, it should be noted that these protocols have usually been limited to the low-risk population, typically first transplant recipients. Reports of successful minimization in high-risk populations, such as those with retransplants, African Americans, children, recipients with potentially recurring diseases, are increasing.

There have been concerns that late steroid withdrawal may set the stage for acute rejection and graft failure. This was attributed to the fact that even though steroids inhibit T cell proliferation by suppressing cytokine production they up-regulate the expression of cytokine receptors. Therefore, when steroids are discontinued, the overactive pro-inflammatory cytokines increase T cell proliferation and may trigger rejection.

Many of the adverse effects related to steroids are observed with higher doses. Whether or not low doses of steroids that are commonly used for maintenance immunosuppression have the same adverse effect profile is unclear. Overall there is moderate evidence for trade-offs between steroid avoidance compared to steroid maintenance, with increased incidence of acute rejections but prevention of steroid related adverse effects.

In conclusion, a variety of agents and protocols are available. Most commonly used regimens include prednisone, calcineurin inhibitors and mycophenolate mofetil for maintenance therapy. Most immunosuppression protocols are decided on a case to case basis by the transplant team.

Suggested Reading

Halloran PF. (2004) Immunosuppressive drugs for kidney transplantation. *New Eng J Med* **351** (26): 2715–2729.

Matas AJ. (2008) Steroid elimination — who, when, how?. *Transplant Proc* **40** (10, Suppl): S52–S56.

NAPRTCS 2008 Annual Report.

43

Transplant Outcomes

Corina Nailescu

Transplant Outcomes

Graft survival

The past two decades have brought a significant improvement in graft survival rates in pediatric kidney transplantation. According to the North American Pediatric Renal Trials and Collaborative Studies (NAPRTCS), the cumulative distribution of kidney graft survival has improved with each ten-year cohort for both living donor (LD) and deceased donor (DD) transplants. For LD recipients the estimated graft survival probabilities at one year and seven years, respectively, improved from 91.2 ± 0.59% and 72.2 ± 1.05% in transplants performed between 1987 and 1995 to 95.3 ± 0.41% and 78.9 ± 1.40% for transplant performed between 1996 and 2007 ($p < 0.001$). Likewise, corresponding estimates for recipients of DD kidney transplants showed an improvement from 80.7 ± 0.81% and 56.2 ± 1.16% at one year and seven years, respectively to 93.4 ± 0.57 and 65.3 ± 2.05% ($p < 0.001$). Notice in Fig. 1 that more recent DD source transplants (1996–2007) have a graft survival experience very similar to that of LD transplants from the earlier (1987–1995) era.

Determining factors for graft survival

Recipient age

If estimated survival rates are categorized by age groups, the improvement has been particularly dramatic in the youngest patients. In fact, according to the 2007 Annual Report of the US Organ Procurement and Transplantation Network and the Scientific Registry of Transplant Recipients (OPTN/SRTR), as shown in Table 1, graft survival rates in

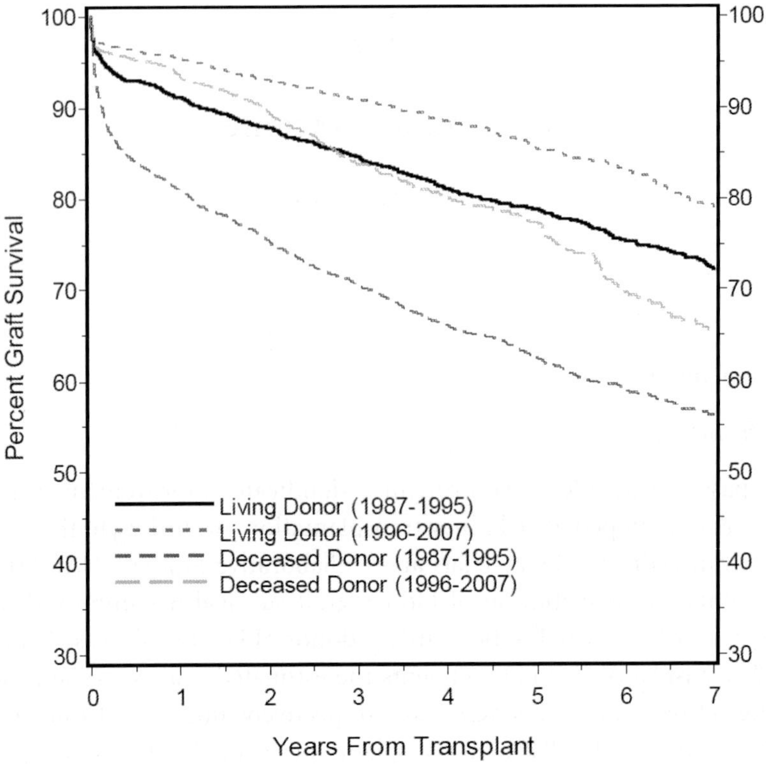

Figure 1. Percentage of living donor and deceased donor graft survival among pediatric kidney transplants in NAPRTCS by cohort year (NAPRTCS 2008 Annual Report).

Table 1. Adjusted graft survival for all LD kidney transplants at five years based on age groups (OPTN/SRTR Data as at May 1, 2007).

		5 Years Adjusted Graft Survival (Transplanted between 2000–2005)		
		N	%	SE
Total	All	37,369	80.3%	0.3%
Age	<1 year	19	89.6%	6.8%
	1–5 years	575	88.5%	1.8%
	6–10 years	460	84.6%	2.5%
	11–17 years	1,406	74.4%	1.8%
	18–34 years	8,213	79.2%	0.7%
	35–49 years	12,125	82.7%	0.5%
	50–64 years	11,633	80.7%	0.6%
	65+ years	2,938	73.1%	1.3%

young pediatric patients with LD kidney transplants aged 1–5 years are the best of all age groups (88.5 ± 1.8%). Unfortunately, adolescent kidney transplant recipients do not reflect the same outcome. For recipients of LD grafts aged 11–17 years, the five-year estimated graft survival is only 74.4 ± 1.8% compared with the overall all age survival rate of 80.3 ± 0.3%. Therefore, adolescents are only second to recipients aged older than 65 years in terms of poor graft survival. The reason for this disappointing outcome in adolescents is not exactly known, although there are speculations about the role of nonadherence and the relatively high incidence of focal segmental glomerulosclerosis (FSGS).

Recipient race

The risk for graft failure is increased by a factor of 1.5–2.0 in African American children, as well as in adults. The reason for this finding is not entirely understood, but is was speculated that it might have to do with socioeconomic factors.

Donor type

The LD grafts have overall a better survival rate compared with DD ones. However, as can be noted in Fig. 1, the difference in graft survival between LD and DD grafts had a tendency to diminish in the recent years. The use of unrelated LD has become more and more popular. The survival rates for the unrelated LD transplants are certainly better than the DD ones, but not as good as the related LD. The data in children come from the previous decade via a study done through NAPRTCS, which showed that unrelated LD transplants have a low rate of acute tubular necrosis (ATN) that is similar to that of related LD transplants. However, unrelated LD transplants have a high incidence of acute rejection, and the graft survival at 12 and 24 months posttransplantation was inferior to related LD transplants. For example, estimated primary graft survival probabilities (+/– SE) at 12 months posttransplant were 0.825 +/– 0.071 for unrelated LD, compared to 0.911 +/– 0.006 for related LD, and 0.815 +/– 0.009 for DD.

Ischemia time

Cold ischemia damage has a detrimental effect on graft function and survival. The longer the cold ischemia time, the more severe the permanent damage is. Once the cold ischemia time exceeds 24 hours, the effect is even more prominent. The relative hazard (RH) for cold ischemia time longer than 24 hours as an individual prognostic factor for graft survival was 1.15 ($p = 0.0251$) compared with cold ischemia time less than 24 hours.

Human leukocyte antigens (HLA) mismatch

In light of the better immunosuppression protocols that became available over time, HLA mismatch tends to have less influence on graft survival. However, there are still significant differences in graft survival observed with HLA-B mismatch in both LD and DD transplants. According to the most recent NAPRTCS report, the RH of HLA-B mismatch as an individual prognostic factor for graft survival was 1.39 ($p = 0.0056$) in LD and 1.16 ($p = 0.0133$) in DD when comparing the 1–2 mismatch group with the 0 mismatch group.

Pretransplant blood transfusions

Multiple blood transfusions have been associated with a higher risk for graft loss and it is now common practice to avoid them pretransplantation. This is particularly true for DD patients, in which the RH for more than five blood transfusions as an individual prognostic factor for graft survival was 1.28, ($p = 0.0002$). In LD, the effect of multiple blood transfusions is still present, but less pronounced ($RH = 1.24$, $p = 0.0122$). While having more than five blood transfusions is a well recognized risk factor for poor graft survival, interestingly a study from the previous decade suggested that a history of fewer than five blood transfusions might actually be associated with a decreased risk of acute rejection.

Pretransplant dialysis status

Preemptive transplantation, which is the "gold standard" in the world of pediatric kidney transplantation, provides better graft survival, in addition to a better quality of life. This is true for both LD ($RH = 1.16$, $p = 0.0444$) and DD ($RH = 1.21$, $p = 0.0520$) transplants when comparing patients who had preemptive transplantation with those who were on dialysis pretransplant, regardless of dialysis modality. When comparing peritoneal dialysis (PD) with hemodialysis (HD), there was no difference in long-term graft survival. However, short-term, the use of PD prior to transplant reduced the risk of delayed graft function when compared with HD.

Nonadherence

Graft survival may be affected by nonadherence with medications and medical follow-up. According to the United States Renal Data System (USRDS), noncompliance as the cause of graft loss is highest in patients 13–17 years of age, as shown in Fig. 2b. Therefore, the poor graft outcome in adolescents is thought to be largely due to nonadherence.

Other

A multitude of other factors have a significant impact upon graft survival, including delayed graft function, graft vascular thrombosis, hypertension, recurrence of the primary disease on the graft, acute rejection episodes, infections, cancers, chronic allograft nephropathy (CAN), and cardiovascular disorders (see Fig. 2a).

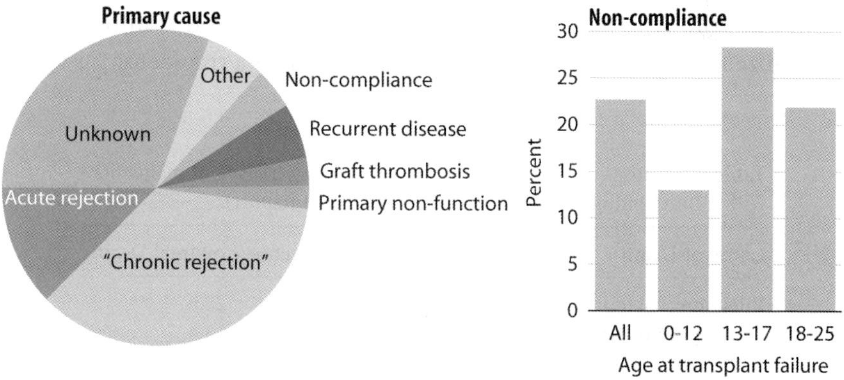

(a) (b)

Figure 2. **(a)** Primary cause of graft loss in pediatric kidney transplant recipients age 0–17 at transplant, age 0–25 at death-censored graft failure and whose grafts failed during 2002–2006 (N = 1,801) (b) Percentage of non-compliance as the cause of graft loss in the same population (USRDS 2008 Annual Report).

Patient survival

According to NAPRTCS, the most common three causes of death in pediatric kidney transplant recipients with a functioning graft are infections, cardiopulmonary diseases, and malignancy, as shown in Table 2. There is some concern that infection rates are increasing, which is thought to be a result of more efficient and potent immunosuppression medications. A recent NAPRTCS analysis revealed that the risk for hospitalizations due to infections exceeded the risk resulting from acute rejection.

Immediate Postoperative Period

Short-term graft survival has improved dramatically in the last decade due to multiple factors, including the use of newer immunosuppressive drugs, improved pre and posttransplant care and better donor selection. The recent 1-year graft survival was 95.3 ± 0.41 and 93.4 ± 0.57 for LD and DD pediatric kidney transplants, respectively. However, a still fairly common scenario is acute allograft dysfunction (AAD), which is broadly defined as a sudden deterioration of the graft function within the first six months posttransplant. AAD can occur in the immediate postoperative period, in which case the term used is delayed graft function (DGF). In the situations where the graft never gains adequate function, the terminology used is primary graft nonfunction, which causes 2.3% of the graft losses. AAD is seen more commonly in DD transplants compared with LD. It is important to minimize the occurrence of AAD, as by itself AAD is a risk factor for CAN,

Table 2. Causes of death among pediatric kidney transplant recipients with a functioning graft (NAPRTCS 2008 Annual Report).

Cause of Death	Percentage of Total Deaths
Infection (bacterial and viral)	28.6
Cardiopulmonary	15.4
Malignancy	10.6
Hemorrhage	6.0
Dialysis-related complications	2.9
Recurrence of the primary disease	1.8
Other	24.9
Unknown	9.7

Table 3. Causes of acute allograft dysfunction

Prerenal	Renal	Postrenal	Vascular
Poor fluid intake	Rejection:	Blocked catheter	Thrombosis
Excessive fluid loss	— Hyperacute	Ureteric stenosis	Stenosis
Hypotension	— Acute		
	Infections:	Functional:	
	— Bacterial (UTI)	— Morphine-induced urinary retention	
	— Viral (BKV, CMV)	— Incomplete bladder emptying	
	Tubulointerstitial Diseases:		
	— Acute tubular necrosis		
	*Hypoperfusion		
	*Medications		
	— Acute interstitial nephritis		
	*Medications		
	Glomerular diseases:		
	— Recurrence		
	— *De novo*		

the number one cause of graft failure in children. The different causes of AAD are delineated in Table 3.

Hyperacute rejection

Hyperacute rejection occurs as a result of preformed antibodies to donor antigens. The reaction between the recipient antibodies and HLA class I or II antigens on donor endothelial cells leads to arteriolonecrosis and occlusion of vascular lumina within minutes to hours. Clinically, it is easily identified when the graft becomes blue prior to closure of the abdomen and should always be considered in cases of primary nonfunction. The diagnosis can be confirmed by using a Doppler ultrasound which shows no flow to the kidney, or by using a nuclear scan that would show no uptake. The presence of preformed antibodies can be detected pretransplant by using the cross-matching test, which is performed routinely. The techniques available for cross-matching have improved over time and their use contributed to dramatic reduction in hyperacute rejection. The most commonly currently used techniques are the complement-dependent cytotoxicity cross-matching, flow cytometric cross-matching and ELISA. However, despite the array of tests available, a minority of patients still develop hyperacute rejection after having a negative cross-match. NAPRTCS data reported hyperacute rejection as responsible for 0.7% of graft losses. Unfortunately the only treatment for hyperacute rejection is allograft nephrectomy.

Delayed graft function

DGF is defined as the need for dialysis in the first week posttransplantation. DGF is mainly due to ischemia-reperfusion injury, and the most common histologic finding is ATN. DGF occurs more frequently in DD transplants due to the higher incidence of ATN, which is worse with longer cold ischemia times. DGF is much more frequent in the adult population where extended-donor criteria are used. It is important to minimize its occurrence, as DGF is an independent poor prognostic factor for graft survival. In the LD group, 5-year graft survival rates are 84.8% for grafts without ATN and 64.6% for grafts with ATN ($p < 0.001$). Among DD grafts, 73.4% of subjects without ATN are estimated to be functioning at 5 years as opposed to 55.9% of those with ATN ($p < 0.001$). The most significant risk factors for DGF are African-American ethnicity, cold-ischemia time longer than 24 hours, previous transplant, history of >5 blood transfusions pretransplant, previous native nephrectomies and panel reactive antibody (PRA) >50%. The diagnosis of DGF is suspected when there is no urine production postoperatively. If anuria occurs, the fluid status of the patient should be assessed, preferably using central venous pressure monitoring, and the position and patency of the Foley catheter should be checked. If the patient is well-hydrated and there is no technical problem related to urine drainage, a Doppler ultrasound, and a nuclear scan should be obtained. If there is good perfusion and radiotracer uptake to the graft, respectively, the most likely diagnosis is DGF, although some practitioners would recommend a kidney biopsy to rule out hyperacute rejection. The usual treatment of DGF is dialysis; either HD or PD can be used, depending on what type of access is present. If the patient had a preemptive transplantation, the most commonly used dialysis modality for DGF is HD. Approximately 50% of posttransplant patients with DGF recover enough renal function to stay off dialysis by the tenth postoperative day. It is common practice to avoid the use of calcineurin inhibitors (CNIs) and other nephrotoxic medications until renal function recovers.

Graft vascular complications

Vascular thrombosis is responsible for approximately 10% of graft loss in pediatric kidney transplant recipients. The percentage of vascular thrombosis as a cause of graft loss has decreased over time probably as a result of a better pretransplantation screening for prothrombotic states. However, the risk for graft vascular thrombosis remains particularly elevated in children less than two years of age due to a discrepancy between donor and recipient blood vessels, in recipients of DD kidneys from donors <5 years, in recipients of a second kidney transplant, when cold ischemia time was longer than 24 hours, and in children who were undergoing PD before transplant. Several thrombophilic disorders have been identified as risk factors for allograft loss resulting from thrombosis, including protein C deficiency, protein S deficiency, factor V Leiden mutation, antiphospholipid antibodies and prothrombin gene abnormalities. If oliguria occurs after good urine output has been established, graft thrombosis should be suspected. The diagnosis is made by Doppler ultrasound of the graft, which shows absence of arterial flow; or by nuclear scan, which shows no graft uptake of the radiotracer. The treatment involves surgical exploration with thrombectomy. In addition, there are options of anticoagulation with heparin or of thrombolysis with streptokinase or urokinase, but the use of these agents is very controversial. When a prothrombotic state is diagnosed pretransplantation, prophylactic treatment with heparin, warfarin, low-molecular weight heparin or aspirin can be used after the immediate postoperative period.

Renovascular stenosis can be another surgical complication in the immediate postoperative period. The diagnosis is suspected when there is a sudden onset of renin-mediated hypertension with or without graft dysfunction. The diagnosis can sometimes be made by Doppler ultrasound, although the gold standard for diagnosis is conventional arteriogram with possible balloon angioplasty and/or stent placement of vascular reconstruction, depending on the particular situation.

Other surgical complications

Urine leak is a very rare, but serious surgical complication due to ureteral necrosis at the anastomosis site. A risk factor for this particular surgical complication in adults has been found to be the use of sirolimus, which is associated with poor wound healing. The diagnosis is made by testing the fluid obtained from the abdominal drain for BUN and creatinine which are found to be similar to urine levels. The treatment is prompt surgical intervention, but the prognosis is fairly poor.

Obstruction can be secondary to ureter kinking, ureteral wall edema, or lymphocele related compression. A very rare cause of obstruction is polyoma BK virus infection, but does not usually occur in the immediate postoperative period. The diagnosis is made by graft ultrasound revealing hydronephrosis. The treatment usually involves surgical reintervention, stent placement, or drainage of the lymphocele, depending on the etiology.

Acute rejection

Introduction/importance

Acute rejection (AR) is defined by an AAD due to activation of immunological mechanisms that try to reject the graft which is sensed as a "nonself." AR most commonly occurs in the first three months after transplantation, but can essentially occur at any time. When AR occurs within one week posttransplantation, it is referred to as accelerated AR. The incidence of AR has decreased over time due to advances in immunosuppression medications, but still 46.9% of transplants had at least one rejection episode (42% in LD and 53% in DD) and the number of rejections per transplant ranged from 0–12. AR is still a major concern for two main reasons. First, AR is second only to CAN as a cause of graft loss, accounting for 13.1% of losses. Secondly, the occurrence of one or more episodes of AR increases the risk for CAN by threefold. Therefore, prevention and prompt treatment of AR are essential for good long-term outcome of the graft. Although the pathophysiological mechanisms are intertwined, AR has been traditionally classified into acute cellular rejection (ACR), when the mechanisms of injury are primarily T cells mediated, and acute humoral rejection (AHR), which is antibody mediated. The two types of AR have differences in terms of histological characteristics, treatment and prognosis.

Pathogenesis

The transplanted organ is perceived by the recipient as "nonself" and leads to immune system activation which then attacks and attempts to destroy the graft. Donor antigens are recognized as foreign by the recipient, primarily the so-called major histocompatibility complex (MHC). The MHC antigens are encoded by a cluster of genes on human chromosome 6 that encode for two types of HLA: class I and class II. HLA class I antigens are constitutively expressed by most nucleated cells and are subclassified into HLA-A, B and C, with HLA-A and HLA-B being the most antigenic. The HLA class II are constitutively expressed by a relatively small number of cell types (B lymphocytes, macrophages, dendritic cells), but they can be induced by interferon and other agents on several other cell types, including endothelial cells and T lymphocytes. They are subclassified into HLA-DR, HLA-DP and HLA-DQ, with the HLA-DR being the strongest inducers of the immunologic response to "nonself." In addition to the MHC, there are also minor transplantation antigens, as evidenced by AR episodes that occur when an organ is transplanted from an HLA-identical donor. However, the main mechanism in ACR is common. The donor's HLA class II antigen is recognized by the recipient's CD4+ T helper cells via the T cell receptor (TCR). Stimulation of the TCR activates certain signaling pathways that ultimately promote interleukin-2 (IL-2) gene transcription. IL-2 is a potent inducer of lymphocyte proliferation, as well as upregulator of IL-2 receptors on the T cell surface, thus leading to autocrine stimulation. In general, as a result of the interaction with the foreign antigen, the naïve CD4+ T helper cells differentiate into two different subpopulations, Th1 and Th2. Th1 cells are mainly involved in ACR by producing cytokines that promote T cell proliferation and differentiation and induce cytotoxicity in macrophages, natural killer cells, and cytotoxic T cells. Cytotoxic T cells contribute to graft destruction either by enzymatic cytolysis mediated by perforin and granzyme B, or by inducing apoptosis. Natural killer (NK) cells, macrophages, eosinophils, and granulocytes also respond to factors made by Th1 cells and contribute to graft dysfunction and rejection. Th2 cells are mainly involved in AHR by inducing B cells to differentiate into plasma cells and produce large amounts of specific antibodies. Antibodies act on the endothelium where they fix complement and lead to subsequent cytolysis.

Clinical presentation

The most common clinical scenario is a patient who is found to have an acute rise in creatinine, possibly also hematuria and proteinuria, with no clinical symptoms. Less often, a patient can present with vague symptoms of graft tenderness, fever and fatigue. There are certain transplant centers where "surveillance" graft biopsies are performed, where mild rejection can be diagnosed before any clinical signs or laboratory abnormalities are apparent. However, the use of surveillance biopsies is generally not common practice.

Diagnosis

The gold standard for the diagnosis of AR is a kidney biopsy. The sample is generally considered adequate if it contains cortex with at least ten glomeruli and at least two arteries. The diagnosis is made based on light microscopy only, which offers the advantage of obtaining the results quickly, usually the same day, which is crucial for initiating prompt treatment. The diagnosis of acute rejection is reported according to the Banff 97 Diagnostic Categories (see Table 4). Figure 3 shows a typical histological image of ACR. In addition to the histological criteria described in Table 4, the diagnosis of AHR is based on two other important features that prove the antibody-mediated disease. One is the deposition of C4d, which is a terminal component after an antigen-antibody complex fixes complement, in the peritubular capillaries. The other diagnostic element is serologic evidence of antidonor anti bodies. Because a kidney biopsy is an invasive procedure that can potentially be complicated by infection, bleeding and even graft loss, there has been a lot of interest in finding less invasive techniques to diagnose AR based on blood or urine samples. These potential markers of rejection are still in the experimental stage and are not clinically used. The most promising blood markers are perforin and FasL, which can be measured by RT-PCR in peripheral blood lymphocytes. Other peripheral blood lymphocyte markers have been described, such as granulysin, granzyme B, IL-13 and 15 and 18 taken together, IL-4 and tumor necrosis factor-alfa (TNF-α), but their expression has been also found in the setting of infection, which makes their clinical utility less likely. As far as urine markers, increased levels of

Table 4. The Banff 97 diagnostic categories for renal allograft biopsies

1. Normal
2. Antibody-mediated rejection
   - I. ATN-like: C4d+, minimal inflammation
   - II. Capillary: Margination and/or thromboses, C4d+
   - III. Arterial: Transmural inflammation/fibrinoid changes, C4d+
3. Borderline changes: Suspicious for acute rejection, with foci of mild tubulitis (≤4 mononuclear cells/tubular cross section), but no intimal arteritis
4. Acute cellular rejection
   - IA. Significant interstitial infiltration (>25% of parenchyma) and foci of moderate tubulitis (>4 mononuclear cells/tubular cross section or group of ten tubular cells)
   - IB. Significant interstitial infiltration (>25% of parenchyma) and severe tubulitis (>10 mononuclear cells/tubular cross section or group of ten tubular cells)
   - IIA. Mild to moderate intimal arteritis affecting ≤25% of the luminal area.
   - IIB. Severe intimal arteritis affecting >25% of the luminal area.
   - III. Transmural arteritis and/or arterial fibrinoid change and necrosis of medial smooth muscle cells with accompanying lymphocytic inflammation
5. Chronic/sclerosing allograft nephropathy
   - I. Mild interstitial fibrosis and tubular atrophy
   - II. Moderate interstitial fibrosis and tubular atrophy
   - III. Severe interstitial fibrosis, tubular atrophy and tubular loss
6. Other changes not considered to be due to rejection

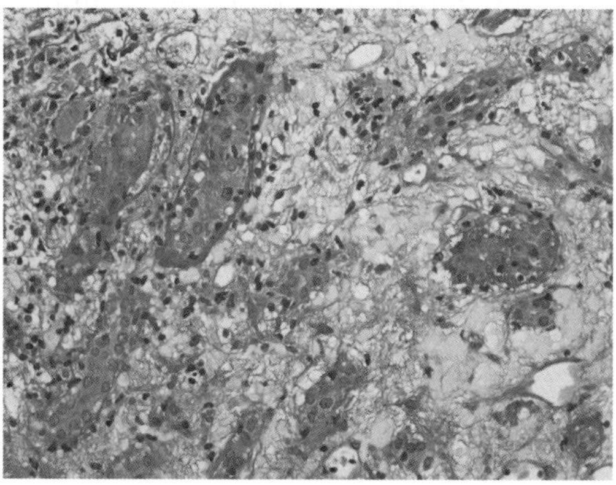

Figure 3. Severe tubulitis (Banff 1B) and interstitial edema seen in a case of acute cellular rejection (PAS staining, x400) (Photograph courtesy of Dr. Carrie Phillips, Department of Pathology, Indiana University, Indianapolis, IN).

granzyme B, perforin, interferon-γ-inducible chemokine IP-10, the chemokine receptor CXCR3 and FOXP3 have been found to be associated with AR. In the future, DNA microarray technology and urine proteomics might offer solutions to finding useful biomarkers for AR from either blood or urine samples.

Treatment and prognosis

For Banff IA and IB ACR, high dose intravenous "pulse" steroids are the first line of treatment, regardless of whether the patient was receiving steroids. Usual doses used are 3–10 mg/kg/day intravenously daily for 3–5 days, followed by an oral steroid taper. Steroids can reverse an episode of ACR in 60–70% of cases and are fairly well tolerated. For Banff IIA, IIB and III ACR and also in cases of Banff IA and IB ACR with no response to steroids, antibodies against lymphocyte cell surface antigens can be used. Today the most commonly used is antithymocyte globulin, which is a polyclonal antibody, while OKT3, a monoclonal antibody, is less commonly used. These anti-T cell antibodies can reverse ACR in 50–90% of cases, but are associated with significant side effects, including severe infections and malignancies. During treatment with anti-T cell antibodies, antiviral and antifungal prophylaxis should be prescribed. Episodes of ACR that are resistant to anti-T cell antibodies have been treated with other unconventional agents. The most promising appears to be alemtuzumab (Campath-1H), a humanized anti-CD52 panlymphocytic (both B and T cells) monoclonal antibody that is approved for the treatment of chronic lymphocytic leukemia. However, one should be very careful when considering the risks of using such medications, particularly malignancy and infections, against the benefits. AHR should be treated with plasmapheresis until there is clinical improvement, which has been reported to require up to six sessions. In addition, intravenous immunoglobulins (ivIg) can be used with doses ranging from 0.4–2.0 g/kg. The most promising results with ivIg have been obtained with the high-dose ivIg protocol developed at Cedars–Sinai Medical Center in Los Angeles, CA, which used 2 g/kg as a single dose. Recently, rituximab, an anti-CD20 monoclonal antibody, has been used in treating AHR with some positive results.

Long-Term Complications

Chronic allograft nephropathy

Introduction/importance

While short-term graft survival has improved significantly in the last two decades, long-term graft survival has not shown such a dramatic improvement. CAN, also known as chronic allograft dysfunction, refers to a gradual and progressive deterioration of the transplanted kidney and has specific histological findings. It is thought that CAN is a common final pathway in response to various types of kidney insults, of which some are immunologic (this component is referred to as chronic rejection) and others are nonimmunologic (see Table 5). CAN is the number one cause of graft loss in pediatric kidney transplant recipients.

Pathogenesis

As expected by the multitude of contributing factors, the pathophysiology of CAN involves multiple mechanisms. The immunological mechanisms are due to low-grade inflammation caused by chronic rejection. The nonimmunologic mechanisms involve ischemic damage to the tubules, afferent arteriole vasoconstriction and injury to the endothelium from CNI toxicity and infection-mediated inflammatory reaction. Once chronic changes have occurred, proteinuria and subsequent hyperfiltration, possibly associated with hypertension, will manifest. These conditions will cause further nonspecific fibrosis mediated by the profibrotic transforming growth factor-beta (TGF-β), endothelin-1, reactive oxygen species and angiotensin II. Special consideration is given here to the use of CNIs. It is clear that CNIs cause nephrotoxicity as shown by the number of patients who develop chronic kidney disease (CKD) after using CNIs for nonkidney transplant related reasons, such as other solid organ transplants, stem cell transplants and autoimmune diseases. Acutely, CNIs can cause dose-dependent reversible afferent arteriole vasoconstriction, which can decrease glomerular filtration rate (GFR). The pathophysiology of chronic CNIs toxicity, however, is poorly understood. From animal models, it is thought to be related to activation of the renin-angiotensin system activation inhibition of nitric oxide.

Table 5. Etiological factors for CAN and possible interventions for prevention and treatment

Etiological Factors	Intervention
Immunologic	Prevention and prompt treatment of AR
Acute rejection episodes, mainly:	
Repeated episodes	
AHR	
Steroid-resistant AR	
Late AR episodes	
HLA-disparity	Good matching
Higher preformed antibody level before transplantation	Strategies to minimize panel of reactive antibodies
Nonimmunologic	
Donor factors:	
Advanced donor age	Avoidance of older/marginal donors
DD kidney versus LD	Promote LD transplantation when possible
Cold ischemia time >24 hours and subsequent DGF	Minimize cold ischemia time
Recipient factors:	
Hypertension	Maintain blood pressure in normal range
Hyperlipidemia	Control hyperlipidemia
Recurrence of the original kidney disease	Specific treatment
Dysfunctional lower urinary tract	Good collaboration with Pediatric Urology
Exogenous factors:	
CNIs toxicity	Reduce, avoid or stop CNIs
Infections (CMV, Polyoma BK virus)	Screen for and treat infections

Clinical presentation

Typically there is a gradual and progressive deterioration of kidney function noticed clinically as early as three months posttransplantation, although on protocol biopsies it has been described as early as one month after transplant. Proteinuria and increases in blood pressure are often seen. Due to the decrease in kidney function, the patient might encounter complications of CKD, including anemia, secondary hyperparathyroidism, metabolic acidosis, etc.

Diagnosis

In the vast majority of cases, the diagnosis is solely made on clinical grounds, as described above. Most patients presenting with clinical evidence of CAN are not biopsied solely for diagnostic purposes, although the definitive diagnosis of CAN is indeed based on biopsy. There are two situations when a patient is subjected to a biopsy that would show evidence of CAN. One would be a situation when there is another indication for a graft biopsy, such as an acute rise in creatinine. The other situation is if the patient was transplanted at one of the few centers where protocol biopsies are done. Protocol or "surveillance" biopsies are performed at some centers at certain interval posttransplantation; changes of CAN may be evident upon biopsy long before there is any clinical indication of a problem. The incidence of CAN in pediatric protocol biopsy cohorts ranged from 30–100% at two years posttransplant, with changes of CAN present as early as one month posttransplantation. Biopsy results for CAN are reported according to the Banff 97 classification (see Table 4). The glomerular lesions of CAN are referred to as transplant glomerulopathy and consist of varying degrees of glomerulosclerosis with an increase in mesangial matrix, mesangial interposition, and irregular thickening of the basement membrane. The tubulointerstitial space in CAN is characterized by tubular atrophy and interstitial fibrosis. In chronic CNIs toxicity, striped fibrosis with tubular atrophy, due to arteriolar spasm, is seen in the interstitium. The typical vascular changes seen with CAN are arterial and arteriolar narrowing due to myointimal proliferation and medial hypertrophy (see Fig. 4). Arteriolar hyaline changes, especially if they are nodular, and arteriolar myocyte vacuolization are suggestive of CNIs toxicity. Immunofluorescence may show the presence of granular mesangial IgM and to a lesser degree C3 deposition. Glomerular and peritubular capillaries staining for C4d has been reported. By electron microscopy, there is separation of the endothelial cells from the basement membrane with the accumulation of a granular material in the subendothelial space.

Treatment

As the pathophysiology of CAN is multifactorial, its prevention and treatment consists of addressing all the possible modifiable factors involved (see Table 5). The few studies on protocol biopsies in pediatric kidney transplant recipients suggested that treatment of subclinical rejection found on protocol biopsies in patients with stable graft function has been associated with a better outcome (better GFR and less fibrosis on further

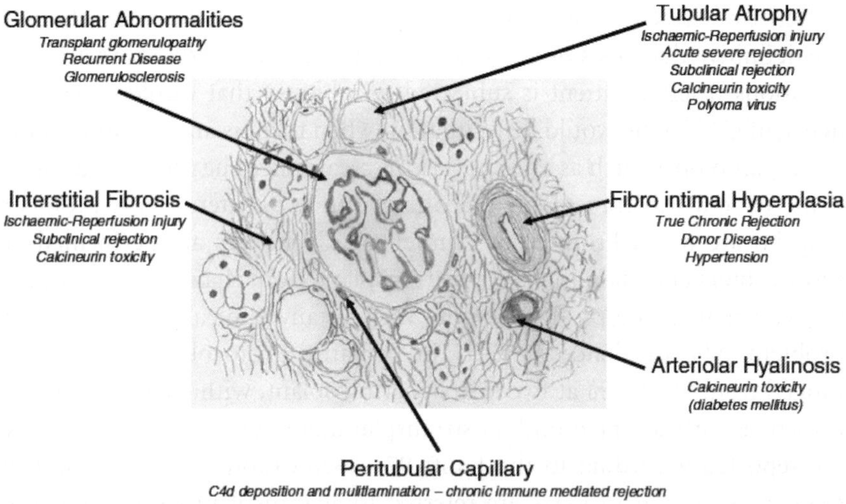

Figure 4. Schematic illustration of biopsy features of a renal allograft showing histopathological features characteristic of CAN. Italicized words indicate potential precipitating factors for CAN associated with the areas they specifically target. [Reproduced with permission from Fletcher *et al.* (2009) *Pediatr Nephrol* **24**: 1465–1471.]

biopsies). However, since treating subclinical rejection means using methylprednisolone and augmenting the maintenance immunosupression, the benefits of treating subclinical rejection needs to be weighed against the risk of infections and malignancy caused by enhancing immunosuppression. In addition, in an effort to prevent CAN, several studies have examined the effects of early (3–4 months posttransplantation) withdrawal of CNIs. In one study, patients received sirolimus, cyclosporine, and prednisone for three months, followed by the randomization to either withdrawal or continuation of cyclosporine. Patients who underwent cyclosporine withdrawal had better GFR and less CAN compared with the ones who continued with cyclosporine, with no increase in the incidence of AR episodes. Furthermore, recently there are some CNIs-free protocols, but they are still in the experimental phase.

Infectious complications

Improvements in graft survival have resulted from the availability of more potent immunosuppression medications. However, as a result, the problem of posttransplant infections has become of a higher magnitude, to the point that infections are currently the number one cause of death and of hospitalization posttransplantation. Pediatric kidney transplant recipients are more susceptible for infections due to multiple reasons: the immunosuppressive medications currently in use are all nonselective, thus suppressing not only responses to allograft, but also to infectious organisms; CKDs stage IV or V that the patients suffer from before transplantation are also a cause of reduced immunity; and the surgical stress associated with transplant procedure. In addition to the infections that can be a cause of concern in any pediatric patient who underwent a major surgery, or in any immunosuppressed patient, three types of viral infections deserve special consideration in the pediatric population: cytomegalovirus (CMV), Epstein–Barr virus (EBV), and polyoma BK virus. As these viral infections are usually more clinically significant when they manifest as a primary infection, children are clearly at risk as many of them are naïve to these viruses prior to transplantation and acquire the infections via the transplanted organ from an adult donor.

Cytomegalovirus

Introduction

CMV is a DNA virus of the herpes virus family that tends to be acquired during childhood followed by a dormant state of the virus in the reticuloendothelial system. There are three patterns of CMV infection posttransplantation: primary infection, reactivation, and superinfection. Primary infection, which is the most clinically significant, occurs when a recipient is seronegative prior to transplantation and acquires the infection most likely from a seropositive donor. Reactivation occurs when a recipient is seropositive pretransplant, receives a graft from a seronegative donor and becomes ill due to the immunosuppression state causing the dormant CMV to replicate. Superinfection occurs when a seropositive recipient receives a kidney transplant from a seropositive donor. Both CMV reactivation and superinfection tend to be clinically milder than primary infection.

Clinical presentation

In the absence of preventive therapy, symptomatic CMV infection usually presents within 1–3 months posttransplantation. However, with the use of preventive therapy, symptomatic CMV infection may present within 1–3 months after the prophylaxis is discontinued. CMV infection can present as either CMV syndrome or CMV disease. CMV syndrome is characterized by nonspecific symptoms, such as fever, malaise, and myalgias associated with leukopenia and thrombocytopenia. CMV disease is characterized by clinical evidence of specific organ involvement. The most common sites of CMV disease are lungs (pneumonitis), liver (hepatitis), and gastrointestinal tract. Unlike patients with the acquired immunodeficiency syndrome, CMV chorioretinitis is rare in solid organ transplant recipients.

Diagnosis

In addition to the clinical presentation, one should have evidence of active viral replication of CMV as reflected by CMV DNA PCR or CMV pp65 antigenemia assay. Because these tests can be positive in asymptomatic patients, whenever the diagnosis of organ invasive CMV disease is considered, a biopsy of the involved organ should be considered. Viral cultures of urine or bronchoalveolar lavage are not useful, as patients can shed CMV asymptomatically in these secretions.

Prevention and treatment

CMV prevention protocols vary widely between different transplant centers, consisting of universal prophylaxis or preemptive treatment. However, most centers recommend universal prophylaxis (consisting of intravenous ganciclovir followed by oral ganciclovir or valganciclovir, which has better bioavailability) for high-risk patients (seronegative recipients of seropositive organs and seropositive recipients of seropositive organs) and some centers even for intermediate-risk (seropositive recipients of seronegative organs) patients. The standard duration of therapy is 100 days (approximately three months), although some centers have extended it to six months based on some data suggesting a significant reduction in late CMV infections by using this approach. For low-risk patients (seronegative recipients of seronegative organs), the most widely used approach is preemptive therapy with intravenous ganciclovir at the first sign of CMV infection. For the treatment of CMV syndrome or disease, intravenous ganciclovir is the first-line agent, although recent data suggest that high doses of oral valganciclovir may also be used. Additionally, a reduction in immunosuppression is recommended. Clinical response usually occurs within 5–7 days of treatment. However, the patients should be treated until there is no more evidence of active viral replication as measured by the CMV DNA PCR or CMV pp65 antigenemia assay. Patients who show evidence of resistance to ganciclovir should be treated with alternative agents, such as foscarnet and cedofovir. In severe cases, CMV immune globulin can be used in conjunction with the antiviral agent.

Prognosis

Without preventive therapy, the incidence of symptomatic CMV infection is over 50%. Prior to the availability of ganciclovir, fatal disseminated CMV infection occurred in 4% of CMV infected children after kidney transplantation. Fortunately, since the appearance of ganciclovir, mortality resulting from CMV infection has become an extraordinary event. As a prognostic factor, CMV infection is a risk factor for EBV-associated post-transplant lymphoproliferative disorder (PTLD) and for AR.

Epstein–Barr virus

Introduction

EBV is another herpes virus that can be acquired during childhood followed by a dormant state of the virus in the reticuloendothelial system. There are also three different patterns of EBV infection: primary infection, reactivation and superinfection, of which the primary infection is the most clinically significant.

Clinical presentation

EBV infection can be asymptomatic or can present as a nonspecific viral syndrome, similar to CMV, usually in the first year after transplantation. While the initial clinical presentation of EBV infection can go unnoticed, its real importance stays in the fact that it can trigger PTLD that tends to occur later.

Diagnosis

In addition to the clinical presentation, one should have evidence of active viral replication of EBV as reflected by a positive EBV DNA PCR. If possible, the PCR technique should be quantitative, providing a baseline estimate for future monitoring of treatment. In addition, serologic evidence of seroconversion can be useful (EBV antiviral capsid IgM positive or a significant rise in EBV antiviral capsid IgG titer). By contrast, anti-nuclear antigen antibodies tend to become positive 1–2 months after the acute infection, indicating a past EBV infection. While there is no data in pediatrics, the adult literature suggests monitoring EBV PCR every three months for the first year posttransplant in seronegative recipients of seropositive donors.

Prevention and treatment

Oral ganciclovir and valganciclovir are also sometimes used for prevention of EBV associated disease. An EBV vaccine, directed against an EBV glycoprotein, is under testing in the United Kingdom.

Polyoma BK virus

Introduction

BK virus is a member of the polyoma group of viruses that is usually acquired during childhood and tends to remain dormant in the uroepithelium.

Clinical presentation

Clinically, BK virus-associated nephritis (BKVAN) closely resembles acute rejection. While in general the onset of the disease occurs at a mean period of 10–13 months posttransplantation, it can present as early as six days posttransplantation or as late as five years. The incidence of BKVAN in pediatric kidney transplant recipients is 3–8%.

Diagnosis

Findings of significant BK active viral replication (plasma DNA PCR load >10,000 copies/mL), plus kidney dysfunction defines presumptive

BKVAN. However, the gold standard is a graft biopsy with special immunostaining. BKVAN is an interstitial nephritis, so the following findings are characteristic: tubular injury (apoptosis, desquamation), tubulitis (lymphocyte permeation of the tubular basement membrane), interstitial mononuclear, or polymorphonuclear cell infiltrates in the areas of tubular damage (see Fig. 5a). In addition, there are characteristic cytopathic changes, such as intranuclear basophilic viral inclusions without a surrounding halo and anisonucleosis, hyperchromasia, and chromatin clumping of infected cells. With electron microscopy, intranuclear viral inclusions can be seen. In addition, immunohistochemistry tests using antibodies directed specifically against BK or against the cross-reacting SV40 large-T antigen are available and when positive are pathognomonic (see Fig. 5b).

Prevention and treatment

Preventive strategies have suggested serial urine BK PCR monitoring and preemptive reduction in immunosuppression upon first positive result. However, there is no consensus in this matter. Once BKVAN occurs, treatment includes reduction of immunosuppression and antiviral therapy.

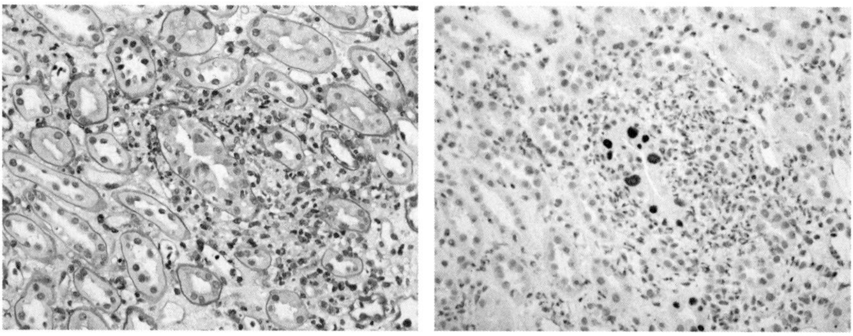

(a) (b)

Figure 5. (a) BK virus infection characterized by disrupted epithelium associated with invading lymphocytes (tubulitis) and pleomorphic nuclei with amphophilic inclusions (PAS staining, ×400). (b) BK virus is confirmed by immunohistochemical staining for the large T antigen of SV40 seen here in tubular cells (anti-SV40 immunoperoxidase, ×400) (Photograph courtesy of Dr. Carrie Phillips, Department of Pathology, Indiana University, Indianapolis, IN).

The agents that have been used are cidofovir and leflunomide, which is an agent that has both antimetabolite and antiviral properties.

Malignancy

Although not such as significant problem compared with the adult population, malignancy post-kidney transplant in children has been an increasing problem largely due to the recent use of more potent immunosuppressive medications. Malignancy is the third most common cause of death with a functioning graft as well as a significant cause of graft loss. According to NAPRTCS, 2.4% of pediatric kidney transplants are complicated by malignancy. The risk seems to be independent of gender or in LD versus DD, but when age group is factored, patients age 2–5 years old are affected almost twice as often as the pediatric group overall. Approximately 85% of all post-kidney transplant malignancies are PTLD and this is why we will give special consideration to this entity. Among the other malignancies, nonmelanoma skin cancers are the second most common, followed by melanoma. Table 6 describes the most common risk factors for malignancy after kidney transplantation in children.

Posttransplant lymphoproliferative disorder

Introduction

PTLD consists of a group of abnormal proliferation, generally of B cells but not always, and generally thought to be induced by EBV infection. PTLD seems to be a biphasic disease that has two peaks of occurrence. The highest rates are seen in the first 12 months posttransplantation, with a mean at six months. There is a second peak that occurs 5–10 years after transplant.

Pathogenesis

Primary EBV infection usually occurs during childhood, so 90% of the adult population has serologic evidence of past infection. During the primary infection, the virus enters the B-lymphocytes following an

Table 6. Risk factors for malignancy after kidney transplantation in children

Pretransplantation
ESRD is associated with an impairment of the immune system
Immunosuppressive drugs formerly used for the primary kidney disease
Genetic conditions:
— Denys–Drash syndrome predisposes to Wilm's tumor due to a mutation of the Wilm's' tumor suppressor gene WT1
—Frasier syndrome predisposes to dysgerminomas
Bladder augmentation by enterocystoplasty can lead to adenocarcinomas, transitional cell carcinomas and squamous cell carcinomas
Posttransplantation
Immunosuppressive therapy, mainly:
— Antithymocyte globulin
— OKT3
— Calcineurin inhibitors
Viral infections:
— EBV: PTLD and renal leiomyosarcoma
— HHV8: Kaposi's sarcoma
— HPV: cervical cancer and other vulvar and vaginal malignancies
— HTLV-1: leukemia
— BK virus: brain tumors and renal carcinoma

HHV8: human herpesvirus 8, HPV: human papillomavirus, HTLV-1: human T-lymphotropic virus.

interaction with the CD21 surface molecules. Subsequently the virus remains in the B-lymphocyte nuclei in a dormant state for a lifetime. Intermittently there is low-grade viral replication, but in a healthy person, this is kept under control by a cytotoxic T cell (CD8+) EBV-specific immune response. Impairment of the EBV-specific cytotoxic T cell response induced by immunosuppressive medications is thought to lead to uncontrolled viral replication in transplant patients.

Clinical presentation

The most common scenarios are unexplained fever, malaise and weight loss, cervical adenopathy, enlarged tonsils, and allograft dysfunction with graft tenderness.

Diagnosis

The diagnostic work up is prompted either by symptoms or as a result of the EBV surveillance posttransplantation, which some centers perform at regular intervals posttransplantation for the first year in seronegative recipients of seropositive donors and consists of EBV PCR (see Fig. 6). EBV PCR is of most value in detecting early-onset PTLD. Late-onset PTLD may present in the absence of a positive EBV PCR. The latest World Health Organization classification divides PTLD into four classes (see Table 7).

Prevention and treatment

Until vaccination becomes available, prevention of PTLD consists of EBV surveillance and reduction of immunosuppression in case of primary EBV infection. Treatment options for patients with proven PTLD are described in Table 8.

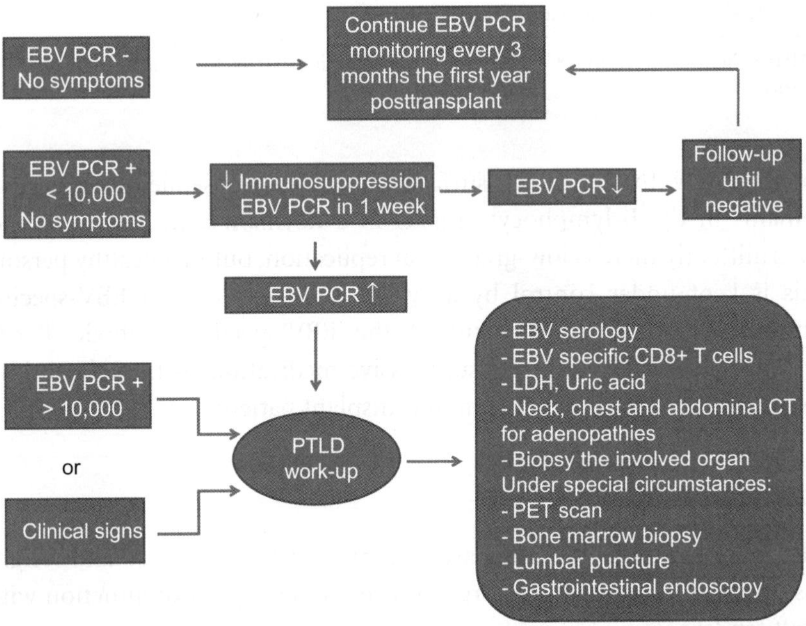

Figure 6. EBV surveillance and diagnostic work up in case of suspected PTLD.

Table 7. World Health Organization (WHO) classification of PTLD

Early lesions:
—Plasmacytic hyperplasia
—Infectious mononucleosis-like lesion
Polymorphic PTLD
Monomorphic PTLD (classify according to the lymphoma they resemble)
—B-cell lymphomas
Diffuse large B-cell lymphoma
Burkitt lymphoma
Plasma cell myeloma
Plasmacytoma-like lesion
Other
—T-cell lymphomas
Peripheral T-cell lymphoma
Hepatosplenic T-cell lymphoma
Other
Classical Hodgkin lymphoma-type PTLD

Table 8. Treatment options for patients with proven PTLD

Therapy	Comments
Reduction of immunosuppression	Usually enough for early lesions and polymorphic PTLD
Anti-EBV therapy with ganciclovir	Widely used, but the benefit is unproven
Rituximab (monoclonal antibody to CD-20 antigen on the surface of B-cells)	Promising results for polymorphic PTLD non-responsive to reduction of immuno-suppression; multicenter trials in progress
Surgery	For localized disease, excisional biopsies, bowel obstruction
Chemotherapy	For monomorphic PTLD and Hodgkin lymphoma

Prognosis

There is a very wide range, with various studies reporting 0–80% mortality. Worse prognosis is seen in late-onset PTLD, T-cell lymphomas and Burkitt-like lymphomas.

Recurrence of disease posttransplantation

In the 2008 NAPRTCS report, recurrence of the original kidney disease was responsible for 6.8% of all graft failures. For index grafts, recurrence of the original disease represented 6.4% of the causes of graft failure, while for subsequent grafts it represented 9.7% of the graft failures.

In general, the diseases that tend to recur on the graft are glomerular in origin and recurrence can occur at any time posttransplantation. However, certain diseases tend to recur early after transplantation, such as FSGS, hemolytic uremic syndrome (HUS), membranoproliferative glomerulonephritis (MPGN), IgA nephropathy, and Henoch–Schönlein purpura (HSP) (see Table 9). On the other hand, other diseases tend to be late recurring, such as membranous nephropathy (MN), and systemic lupus erythematosus (SLE). MN can be found in a graft biopsy in three situations: In a patient known to have had MN as the primary kidney disease (recurrent MN), in a patient who had an alternative disease as the cause of ESRD (*de novo* MN), or in a patient whose cause of ESRD remains unknown (in which case it is not possible to determine whether this represents recurrent or de novo disease). In adults, where MN is much more common than in children, the rate of recurrence is 5–10%, but it usually does not cause significant graft damage. There are no studies reporting on the prevalence and risk factors for recurrence of MN in children. The only large pediatric series looking at the outcome of kidney transplantation in children with SLE nephritis reported only one case of graft loss in 94 children who underwent 100 kidney transplants.

In addition to glomerular diseases, certain metabolic diseases can recur on the graft. The classical one is primary hyperoxaluria type I (oxalosis), for which the standard of care previously was kidney-only transplantation, in which case the enzyme deficiency persisted after the transplantation leading to continuous deposition of calcium oxalate crystals and subsequent graft function deterioration. This has led to the change in standard of care, so that patients with oxalosis now receive combined liver and kidney transplantation.

Growth retardation

Despite the fact that kidney transplantation offers a better quality of life compared with dialysis, growth retardation continues to be a concern for

Table 9. Recurrence of disease post-transplantation

Disease	Risk factors for recurrence	Frequency of recurrence	Frequency of graft loss	Treatment	Comments
FSGS	— Aggressive primary FSGS; — Onset before age 6 years; — Previous recurrence predicts recurrence in 75–100% of subsequent grafts; — Diffuse mesangial proliferation on biopsy	15–60% index 80% subsequent	50%	Plasmapheresis	The most common cause of graft loss due to disease recurrence
MPGN type I	Not known	10–70%	15–35%	As the primary disease	
MPGN type II	Not known	90–100%	25%	High dose steroids Plasmapheresis	
HUS	— CNIS — Factor H deficiency	1–50%	80%	Stop CNIs Plasmapheresis	Recurrence more frequent in atypical HUS compared with typical
IgA nephropathy	LD transplants	15–80%	5%	As the primary disease	Recurrence rate significantly higher in LD transplants compared with DD
HSP	LD transplants	30–50%	10–25%	As the primary disease	Recurrence rate significantly higher in LD transplants compared with DD

both patients and parents. The majority of patients will already have a height deficit due to their CKD at the time of transplantation. In the 2008 NAPRTCS Report, at the time of transplantation, the mean height deficits for all pediatric kidney transplant recipients is −1.78 standard deviations. This deficit is greater for males (−1.82) than females (−1.72).

After transplantation, there is usually accelerated growth for up to three years, which seems to be more prominent for younger patients, particularly less than six years old. Between age 6 and 12 years, there is still some minimal catch up growth, but beyond age 12 there is no benefit from kidney transplantation in relationship to growth. The growth impairment is thought to be in part related to the use of steroids. There is data showing that patients receiving alternate-day steroids had better growth with no adverse effects on the graft survival, compared with patients receiving every day steroids. More recently, steroid-free immunosuppression was also associated with significantly greater linear growth in pediatric kidney transplant recipients than was observed in historical controls receiving steroid-based therapy. Despite the advantages of transplantation, many pediatric transplant patients still do not reach normal adult height. In cases where growth is still not satisfactory after transplantation, growth hormone therapy has been used. In one study conducted by NAPRTCS, growth velocity in the group administered growth hormone posttransplantation was significantly increased during the first year of treatment, but the effect became limited with time. No significant adverse effects on five-year graft survival or function were observed.

Metabolic syndrome

Hypertension is fairly common in children with kidney transplants. Older data reported up to 70% of the children with kidney transplant requiring antihypertensive medications. Major contributing factors to the development of hypertension are obesity, high renin release from the native kidneys, the use of steroids and CNIs, AR and CAN, and recurrent or de novo glomerulonephritis. Recently, steroid-free immunosuppression regimens have been found to be associated with significantly lower incidences of hypertension (14.3%) compared with steroid-treated patients (57%) at 20 months posttransplantation. Development of hypertension creates a vicious cycle, as it was shown to be independently associated with a subsequent deterioration of renal function, and graft failure. In addition, hypertension also exacerbates proteinuria, which is a known independent risk factor for the progression of renal disease.

A recent multicenter retrospective review of demographic, clinical, laboratory, and echocardiographic parameters at time of and at one-year posttransplant was conducted in 234 pediatric recipients in order to estimate the prevalence of metabolic syndrome and its association with cardiac abnormalities in children with kidney transplants. 37.6% met criteria for metabolic syndrome. Among the overweight patients, 40% had metabolic syndrome. Among obese patients, 74.5% had metabolic syndrome. The prevalence of metabolic syndrome at time of transplant was 18.8%, compared with 37.0% at one-year posttransplant ($p < 0.0001$). Among patients without metabolic syndrome at time of transplant, 27.9% had developed metabolic syndrome by one-year posttransplant.

Suggested Reading

Cochat P, Hébert D. (2008) Demographics of pediatric renal transplantation. In: Geary DF, Schaefer F. (eds) Comprehensive Pediatric Nephrology. Mosby Elsevier, Philadelphia.

Fletcher JT, Nankivell BJ, Alexander SI. (2009) Chronic allograft nephropathy. *Pediatr Nephrol* 24(8): 1465–1471.

Health Resources and Services Administration, Healthcare Systems Bureau, Division of Transplantation, Rockville, MD. *2007 Annual Report of the U.S. Organ Procurement and Transplantation Network and the Scientific Registry of Transplant Recipients: Transplant Data 1997–2006.* [URL: http://optn.transplant.hrsa.gov]

Neu AM, DV, (2008) Prevention and treatment of infectious complications in pediatric renal allograft recipients. In: Geary DF, Schaefer F. (eds) Comprehensive Pediatric Nephrology, Mosby Elsevier, Philadelphia.

Neu AM, Fivush BA. (2007) Outcomes and risk factors. In: Fine RN, Webber SA, Olthoff KM, Kelly DA, Harmon WE (eds) *Pediatric Solid Organ Transplantation*, 2nd ed., Blackwell Publishing, Malden.

North American Pediatric Renal Trials and Collaborative Studies (NAPRTCS). (2008) *Annual report 2008* [URL: https://web.emmes.com/study/ped/annlrept/annlrept.html]

Smith JM, McDonald R. (2007) Posttransplant management. In: Fine RN, Webber SA, Olthoff KM, Kelly DA, Harmon WE. (eds) *Pediatric Solid Organ Transplantation*, 2nd ed., Blackwell Publishing, Malden.

Swerdlow SH, Webber SA, Chadburn A, Ferry JA. (2008) Posttransplant lymphoproliferative disorders. *WHO Classification of Tumours of Haematopoietic and Lymphoid Tissues.* International Agency for Reasearch on Cancer (IARC), Lyon.

United States Renal Data System (USRDS). *2008 Annual Data Report.* [URL: http://www.usrds.org]

Wilson AC, Greenbaum LA, Barletta GM, *et al.* (2010) High prevalence of the metabolic syndrome and associated left ventricular hypertrophy in pediatric renal transplant recipients. *Pediatr Transplant* **14**(1): 52–60.

Part XVI

Cardiovascular Disease

44

Cardiovascular Disease in Pediatric Chronic Kidney Disease

Amy C. Wilson and Mark M. Mitsnefes

Introduction

Despite significant advances in the care of children and adolescents with chronic kidney disease (CKD), long-term survival of children with CKD in the United States remains far lower than for the general population. For children on dialysis, the anticipated lifespan is reduced by 40–60 years and for transplant patients by 20–25 years, when compared to an age- and race-matched population. The most likely cause of this reduction in survival is an excessive burden of cardiovascular mortality, related to both accelerated ischemic heart disease and premature development of dilated cardiomyopathy in young adult survivors of childhood onset CKD.

Risk Factors for Cardiovascular Disease

As in adults, the risk factors thought to be responsible for accelerated cardiovascular disease (CVD) in children with CKD can be divided into two primary groups:

1. Traditional risk factors for atherosclerotic disease (e.g. dyslipidemia, diabetes, hypertension, smoking) which are common in the general adult population as well
2. Uremia-related risk factors which are unique to or far more prevalent among patients with CKD

A majority of adults who develop end-stage renal disease (ESRD) do so as a complication of diabetes or generalized atherosclerosis. The frequency of both traditional and uremia-related risk factors for CVD is high, and

Table 1. Key risk factors for CVD in pediatric CKD and relevance after renal transplant

Risk Factor (RF)	Prevalence	Impact of Renal Transplant (RT)
Hypertension	48–87%	Prevalence increases significantly after RT, to ~80–90% at one year
Dyslipidemia	50–90%	Highest rates occur after RT, largely iatrogenic
Obesity	10–30%	Rates double in first year after RT
Abnormal glucose metabolism	Up to 30%	Studied almost exclusively in RT; minimal data in children with CKD or ESRD
Sedentary lifestyle/ poor overall fitness	Near 100%	Contrary to expectations, does not improve significantly after RT
Coexistence of multiple RF	Up to 66%	Emerging data indicates prevalence rises sharply after RT
Anemia	18–86%	Previously thought less common after RT; new data shows prevalence up to 86% after RT
Hyperparathyroidism	30–60%	Improves after RT

cardiac disease is already well established at the onset of ESRD in these patients. Although children have neither diabetes nor symptomatic atherosclerosis at the time of starting maintenance dialysis, they unfortunately share similarly high rates of CVD risk factors (see Table 1).

In addition to traditional risk factors, there are a host of uremia-related risk factors that uniquely increase risk for atherosclerotic CVD in patients with CKD. These are primarily evident in patients on maintenance dialysis rather than in those with early CKD or following successful transplantation. Although maintenance dialysis is typically a temporary state prior to transplantation in children, the consequences of even relatively short-term dialysis persist well beyond successful transplant into adulthood.

Volume overload among patients on maintenance dialysis is frequent. This is primarily related to failure to achieve and maintain a true dry weight, and is a primary mechanism for the development and persistence of hypertension in the maintenance dialysis population, particularly for patients treated with intermittent hemodialysis (HD) rather than peritoneal dialysis (PD). Furthermore, chronic volume overload in children is associated with higher rates of cardiac structural, and functional abnormalities.

Anemia is another highly prevalent uremia-related CV risk factor in children and adolescents with advanced CKD. Unlike other major uremia-related risk factors, it appears relatively early in the course of CKD. Despite wide use of recombinant erythropoiesis stimulating agents (ESAs), it remains common, affecting up to 70% of patients with ESRD. Dialyzed children with anemia are 55% more likely to be hospitalized than those with normal hemoglobin and are at increased risk for both cardiac morbidity and mortality. In addition, anemia is associated with left ventricular hypertrophy (LVH), a known CV risk. Until recently, posttransplant anemia has been underappreciated. However, with introduction of more potent immunosuppression therapy, recently reported posttransplant anemia rates are similar to those in ESRD.

Abnormalities in calcium-phosphorus metabolism are universal among patients with advanced CKD, and they appear to be among the most important drivers of cardiac and vascular disease progression in this population. Secondary hyperparathyroidism affects approximately 30–45% of children with CKD stage 2–4 and nearly 60% of children on dialysis. Associations between abnormal mineral metabolism and changes in vascular structure in children with CKD have also been documented. Although activated vitamin D supplementation in ESRD is an established therapy for control of secondary hyperparathyroidism, there is evidence that such supplementation may enhance vascular calcium deposition. Nutritional vitamin D deficiency is also quite common in children with CKD and is associated with secondary hyperparathyroidism even among those patients with normal activated vitamin D levels.

Malnutrition and inflammation appear to be intimately related to the development of vascular disease in adults with CKD. The same inflammatory markers have been identified at high levels in children on maintenance dialysis. However, there is no strong evidence to guide inflammation-related risk-modification in children with CKD.

Spectrum of Cardiovascular Findings in Pediatric CKD

Clinically evident cardiovascular lesions (symptomatic coronary artery disease, myocardial infarction, cerebrovascular accident) are fortunately rare in children and adolescents with CKD. However, there is increasing evidence demonstrating significant subclinical cardiovascular abnormalities in this population, all of which are independent predictors of CVD morbidity and mortality in the general population, and in adults with CKD.

Left ventricular structure and function

As in adults, LVH develops relatively early in the course of CKD in children, and becomes more common as renal function declines. Although some small retrospective studies demonstrate regression of LVH with better BP and volume control while on dialysis, others have demonstrated advancement of LVH. Unfortunately, LVH remains common after pediatric renal transplant. Overall, reported prevalence ranges from 20–85%, with most studies finding that 30–50% of children with CKD, ESRD, or renal transplant have LVH, which is often severe. LVH is also frequent in adult survivors of ESRD in childhood (4–50%), as is diastolic dysfunction (13%).

Diastolic dysfunction is thought to be the initial functional LV abnormality evident in children with CKD. Recent studies utilizing tissue Doppler imaging substantiated that diastolic dysfunction is common in this population. Overall, children on maintenance dialysis have worse diastolic dysfunction than those with either CKD stage 2–4 or functioning renal transplants. Functionally, although diastolic dysfunction is generally asymptomatic, it is independently associated with reduced maximal aerobic capacity in children with CKD.

Systolic function has classically been thought of as preserved in children with CKD. While that appears to be true of overt systolic function abnormalities as assessed by LV contractility or endocardial shortening fraction (eSF), recent studies have demonstrated that subclinical systolic dysfunction, as assessed by abnormal midwall shortening fraction, is common in children with CKD, affecting up to 40% of HD patients.

Large vessel disease

Large vessel disease occurs at disturbingly early ages among children with CKD. Known abnormalities range from early changes in endothelial function, as assessed by flow mediated dilatation of the brachial artery, to increased carotid intimal media thickness (cIMT), coronary artery calcification (CAC), and frank atherosclerosis. Major risk factors for early vascular disease include longer duration of dialysis dependence, higher calcium-phosphorous product, cumulative dose of calcium-based phosphate binders, and cumulative dose of activated vitamin D (specifically calcitriol).

Importantly, although multiple studies have demonstrated increased cIMT in children with CKD, ESRD, and transplant, recent work has shown that exceptional blood pressure control can result in stabilization of cIMT in renal transplant recipients. With respect to CAC, cross-sectional studies have demonstrated substantial rates of CAC (as measured by computed tomography) in children with ESRD. Investigation of the etiology of vascular calcium accumulation indicates that accumulation begins well in advance of initiation of maintenance dialysis, but accelerates and leads to overt changes in vascular structure only following initiation of dialysis. Unfortunately, noninvasive studies (including carotid ultrasound and computed tomography) have not proven to be sensitive early indicators of increased calcium load.

Evaluation and Management of CV Risk in Pediatric CKD

The most significant change in paradigm regarding management of CV risk in children with CKD came with the 2006 release of the American Heart Association guidelines for CV risk reduction in high risk pediatric patients. There, for the first time, pediatric CKD patients were stratified as "high risk" for the development of CVD, with associated "pathological and/or clinical evidence for manifest coronary disease before 30 years of age." This group is otherwise limited to patients with homozygous familial hypercholesterolemia, type 1 diabetes, heart transplant recipients, and Kawasaki disease patients with current coronary aneurysms. The panel's treatment recommendations for children with CKD refer the reader to several National Kidney Foundation Kidney/Dialysis Outcomes and Quality Initiative (NKF K/DOQI) clinical practice guidelines.

The avoidance of long-term dialysis, with preference for preemptive transplantation when feasible, significantly reduces cardiovascular risk. Although far from perfect with regard to CV risk, successful transplantation eliminates or significantly improves uremia-related risk factors and increases predicted life expectancy by 20–30 years as compared to long-term dialysis. Otherwise, management strategies are specific to the stage of CKD (predialysis, dialysis, or transplant) as each has a unique subset of common risk factors. Current recommendations for management of the most common risk factors are summarized in Table 2.

Table 2. Summary of treatment goals for CVD risk factors in pediatric CKD

Risk factor	Treatment Goal
Hypertension	Blood pressure <90th percentile for age, sex, and height, or <120/80 mmHg, whichever is lower.
Dyslipidemia	Maintenance of total cholesterol, LDL, HDL, and triglycerides in age-appropriate ranges for high CVD risk patients.
Obesity and physical inactivity	Maintenance of normal body habitus (BMI between 5–85th percentile for age, sex).
Hyperinsulinemia/ hyperglycemia	Maintenance of normoglycemia and normal insulin sensitivity.
Abnormal mineral metabolism	Phosphorus, Ca x P, and intact PTH goals vary by age and CKD stage.
Anemia	Maintenance of hemoglobin in the range of 11.0–12.0 gm/dL in patients receiving erythropoeisis stimulating agent (ESA) therapy, along with maintenance of adequate iron stores.
LVH	Maintenance of normal LV mass and function; in those patients with preexisting LVH, normalization of echocardiographic findings.

Hypertension

Hypertension therapy is determined by CKD stage. Angiotensin-converting enzyme inhibition (ACEi) and/or angiotensin-receptor blockade (ARB) is preferred in stage 2–4 CKD. Among patients on maintenance dialysis, meticulous attention to management of volume overload is essential, which may necessitate more frequent or intense dialysis than a standard thrice-weekly regimen. Significant improvements in volume control, hypertension, and regression in LVH can be achieved via use of intensive dialysis regimens in children. Following transplant, in addition to judicious use of antihypertensive agents, minimization/avoidance of iatrogenic causes of hypertension (calcineurin inhibitors, corticosteroids) should be considered.

Guidelines suggest that ambulatory blood pressure monitoring (ABPM) be considered to assess for nocturnal hypertension but stop short of recommending its routine use. However, newer literature suggests that use of annual ABPM leads to improved attainment of goal BP compared to standard therapy following renal transplant. Moreover, masked hypertension (ambulatory hypertension in the presence of casual BP <95th percentile) is known to be common among children with CKD of all stages and is associated with a two-fold increase in frequency of LVH. Therefore, routine use of ABPM in children with CKD (beginning in early CKD and continuing thereafter) may significantly improve ascertainment and management of hypertension.

Dyslipidemia

The most recent guidelines for lipid screening and treatment in childhood state that for children eight years and older with diabetes, statin therapy should be considered for those with LDL ≥130 mg/dL. Although these guidelines do not specifically address children with CKD, given that the 2006 guidelines from the American Heart Association clearly place patients with CKD in the same high CV risk group as those with diabetes and heart transplant, it could be argued that statin therapy be standard of care for patients with CKD who are eight years and older with LDL ≥130 mg/dL. No data exist regarding changes in long-term outcome related to tight lipid control in children with CKD; however, emerging data suggest a survival benefit associated with statin use in adult renal transplant recipients. Statins are also considered standard of care in all patients >1 year of age following pediatric heart transplantation (with the goal of reducing LDL to below 100 mg/dL), due to the associated reduction in incidence of transplant vasculopathy. Emerging evidence in adults suggests potential for similar improvements in renal transplant. Although it remains unclear what, if any, benefit such treatment would have on long-term graft or patient survival, one might speculate that strategies improving graft survival could improve cardiovascular outcomes over decades.

Obesity and physical inactivity

Evidence from adult maintenance dialysis populations suggests a survival advantage conferred by higher body mass index (BMI); however, this appears to be limited to those with low body fat and high muscle mass. No large studies have evaluated the safety and efficacy of weight loss in overweight dialysis patients; as such, recommendations suggest that weight loss programs in ESRD patients be approached only with supervision from appropriate physicians and registered dietitians. However, increased physical activity is encouraged for most children with CKD. After pediatric renal transplantation obesity is associated with higher rates of graft loss and graft dysfunction. Obesity also reduces efficacy of antihypertensive therapy in children.

Hyperinsulinemia/hyperglycemia

No formal recommendations exist for frequency or type of glucose monitoring or assessment of insulin resistance in children with CKD without preexisting diabetes. For those children with known type I diabetes and CKD of any cause, K/DOQI guidelines defer to the American Diabetes Association standards of care for children and adolescents. Following transplantation, serum glucose should be monitored routinely given the high incidence of posttransplantation diabetes. There are no formal guidelines for assessments of insulin resistance in these patients. However, there may be a role for regular assessments even in patients with earlier stages of CKD.

Abnormal mineral metabolism

Although there is evidence suggesting that calcium and phosphorous load are associated with significant increase in risk for early CV disease, there is little evidence supporting improved CV outcomes associated with achievement of these treatment goals. More research is needed regarding optimal management of calcium-phosphorous metabolism, including that regarding the role of noncalcium containing phosphorous binders, and calcimimetics in children with ESRD.

Anemia

Notably, anemia in renal transplant recipients may be more difficult to treat successfully secondary to relative ESA-resistance due to multiple factors (immunosuppression-related bone marrow suppression, infections, malignancy, inflammation related to rejection, etc.). Also of note, patients in the early pretransplant period are at somewhat higher risk for iron deficiency than at other stages of disease, related to low pretransplant iron stores in the face of increased iron utilization following resumption of erythropoiesis after successful transplant.

Left ventricular hypertrophy

Guidelines recommend screening echocardiography within three months of beginning dialysis, with follow-up examinations every six months for those with abnormal studies or annually if normal. As noted previously, meticulous attention to volume control is the treatment strategy most likely to result in improvement of LVH in the maintenance dialysis patient, although there is certainly a role for antihypertensive therapy (specifically ACEi/ARB) as well. Following transplant, antihypertensive therapy and ACEi/ARB become the main therapeutic approach. Given the high frequency of LVH in renal transplant recipients, our center continues with routine echocardiography following transplantation as well, with studies at one year posttransplant and then every two years thereafter if normal, or annually (at a minimum frequency) if abnormal. There is not enough evidence to recommend a routine evaluation for other intermediate CV outcomes (e.g. IMT or CAC) in children with CKD.

Summary

Cardiovascular disease is the most common cause of death in young adults with childhood onset of CKD. The likely reason for increased CVD in these patients is high prevalence of traditional and uremia-related CVD risk factors. Early markers of cardiomyopathy, such as left ventricular hypertrophy (LVH) and LV dysfunction, and early markers of atherosclerosis, such as increased carotid artery intima-media thickness (IMT), carotid arterial wall stiffness and coronary artery calcification (CAC) are frequently found in this patient population. Aggressive treatment of modifiable CV risk factors early in the course of childhood CKD is important for prevention of development and progression of future CVD.

Suggested Reading

Daniels SR, Greer FR, and the Committee on Nutrition. (2008) Lipid Screening and Cardiovascular Health in Childhood. *Pediatr* **122**: 198–208.

Gruppen MP, Groothoff JW, Prins M, *et al.* (2003) Cardiac disease in young adult patients with end-stage renal disease since childhood: a Dutch cohort study. *Kidney Int* **63**: 1058–1063.

Kasiske B, Cosio FG, Beto J, *et al.* (2004) Clinical practice guidelines for managing dyslipidemias in kidney transplant patients: a report from the Managing Dyslipidemias in Chronic Kidney Disease Work Group of the National Kidney Foundation Kidney Disease Outcomes Quality Initiative. *Am J Transplant* **4**(Suppl. 7): 13–53.

Kavey RE, Allada V, Daniels SR, *et al.* (2006) Cardiovascular risk reduction in high-risk pediatric patients: a scientific statement from the American Heart Association Expert Panel on Population and Prevention Science. *Circulation* **114**: 2710–2738.

National High Blood Pressure Education Program Working Group on High Blood Pressure in Children and Adolescents. (2004) The fourth report on the diagnosis, evaluation, and treatment of high blood pressure in children and adolescents. *Pediatr* **114**(Suppl 2): 555–576.

National Kidney Foundation Task Force on Cardiovascular Disease. (1998) Controlling the epidemic of cardiovascular disease in chronic renal disease: What do we know? What do we need to know? Special report from the National Kidney Foundation Task Force on Cardiovascular Disease. *Am J Kidney Dis* **32**(Suppl. 3): 1–121.

National Kidney Foundation. (2003) K/DOQI Clinical Practice Guidelines for Managing Dyslipidemias in Chronic Kidney Disease. *Am J Kidney Dis* **41**(Suppl 3): S61–S70.

National Kidney Foundation. (2004) K/DOQI Clinical Practice Guidelines on Hypertension and Antihypertensive Agents in Chronic Kidney Disease. *Am J Kidney Dis* **43**(Suppl 1): S223–S229.

National Kidney Foundation. (2005) Section III. State of the Science: Novel and controversial topics in cardiovascular diseases, in K/DOQI Clinical Practice Guidelines for Cardiovascular Disease in Dialysis Patients. *Am J Kidney Dis* **45(Suppl. 3)**: S76–S114.

US Renal Data System. *USRDS 2003 Annual Report.* Bethesda, The National Institute of Diabetes and Digestive and Kidney Diseases. [URL: http://www.usrds.org] Accessed January 21, 2009.

Part XVII

Neonatal Nephrology

45

Neonatal Renal Physiology

Abiodun A. Omoloja

Introduction

Understanding newborn renal physiology is of cardinal importance in appreciating the unique conditions peculiar to this subset of the pediatric population. It becomes very important considering how alerted renal physiology at such young age can contribute to ill health, and renal disease as children or adults. Such an example is the association of very low birth weight and prematurity with focal segmental glomerulosclerosis (FSGS). Much of what is known about human fetal and newborn renal physiology is based on animal models. Despite these limitations, better understanding of fetal and newborn renal physiology continues to occur resulting in improved clinical care, reduced short and long term morbidity and mortality. Finally, it is important to note that division of this segment into fetal and newborn renal physiology is artificial. In reality, it is a continuum. Expression and activity of the renal transporter Na^+/K^+-ATPase for example commences *in utero*, continues throughout infancy and childhood and reaches maximal activity in adulthood.

Fetal Renal Physiology

Kidney development commences early in gestation with two transient but functional units, the pronephros and mesonephros that appear at the third and fifth week of gestation, respectively. Involution of these units occurs with formation of the metanephros, the definitive kidney, occurring at around the fifth week (Fig. 1). Urine production starts at about

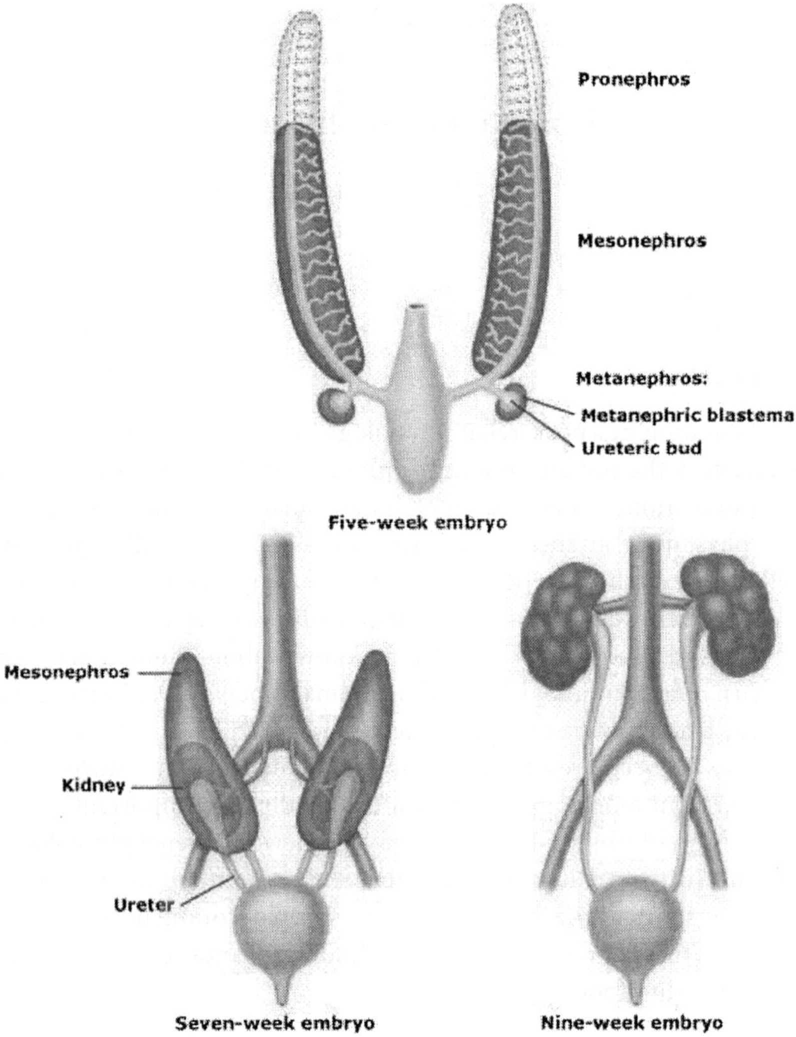

Figure 1.

the tenth week of gestation. The metanephros is formed when the ureteric bud and metanephric blastema meet, and a host of signaling occurs that triggers normal renal development. Significant increase in size occurs thereafter, with ultrasound (US) visualization of the kidney by the 18th week of gestation. Nephrogenesis is concluded by the 36th week of gestation.

Glomerular filtration rate

Renal function in the fetus is characterized by low glomerular hydrostatic pressure resulting in low glomerular filtration rate (GFR). This is due to combined low systemic blood pressure (SBP), low renal blood flow (RBF), and high renal vascular resistance (RVR) in the renal arteriolar and efferent vascular circulation. Indeed, RBF accounts for only 2–4% of cardiac output in the fetus as compared to 10% and 25% in one–week-old full-term infants and adults, respectively. This is achieved by a delicate balance between the overriding renin angiotensin system (RAS), renal sympathetic nervous system and other regulatory mechanisms. Low glomerular filtration surface, intraglomerular pressure, and hydrostatic pressure ensure a physiologically low fetal GFR. Fetal fluid and electrolyte balance are maintained entirely by the placenta throughout gestation; hence, GFR remains minimal and unchanged relative to fetal size during prenatal period.

Accurate evaluation of fetal GFR is difficult from the both ethical and medical standpoints. Plasma creatinine (Cr), a commonly used surrogate to evaluate GFR is freely filtered across the placenta. So fetal Cr is a reflection of the mother's Cr throughout gestation and for the first couple of weeks after delivery. Amniotic fluid volume estimation, which estimates fetal urine production, is an indirect method of evaluating GFR. Several other factors determine amniotic volume thus making this method less reliable. Filling and emptying of the bladder with urine, known as bladder cycling, is another noninvasive method used to evaluate GFR. Using US, filling and emptying of the bladder which occurs every 40 minutes near term is monitored. It is estimated that fetal urine flow rate increases from about 22–40 weeks gestation in a linear fashion from 5 ml/hour to 30 ml/hour. This can be increased dramatically by the administration of intravenous furosemide to a pregnant woman, thus knowledge and effects of maternal medication on fetal renal function is important when evaluating GFR. By the 34th week of gestation, GFR is about 14 ml/min per 1.73 m^2 and increases to 21 ml/min per 1.73 m^2 at term.

Despite the above limitations in evaluating fetal renal function, important facts to remember are that low fetal GFR parallels change in renal mass and increasing gestational age. So a preterm or small for gestational age (SGA) infant will have a reduced GFR compared to a full term or appropriate for gestational age (AGA) infant. It must also be remembered that a low fetal GFR permits conservation of much needed energy for growth and development, as reabsorption of fluid, electrolytes and several other tubular functions are energy dependent processes. Hence energy expenditure is focused on growth and development of the fetus. However, the low fetal GFR, perfect for growth and development under normal circumstances, prevents and retards rapid postnatal renal adaptation to intra and extrauterine stressors like sepsis, perinatal asphyxia, use of angiotensin converting enzyme (ACE) inhibitors, and nonsteroidal anti-inflammatory drugs (NSAIDS). NSAIDS which freely cross the placenta are potent cyclooxygenase inhibitors with adverse renal effects especially in the term and preterm infant. Significant renal anomalies have been reported with exposure to NSAIDS in utero. While benefits of antenally administered glucocorticoids for pulmonary maturation is without doubt in preterm infants, the same cannot be said about renal maturation and function.

Tubular function

Similar to low GFR, fetal tubular renal function is minimal when compared to postnatal life. Tubular function commences in the second trimester and continues well into postnatal life.

Tubular reabsorption of sodium is low resulting in a high fractional excretion of sodium (FENa) estimated at about 10% or more. Distribution and activity of the tubular active transport systems, Na^+/K^+-ATPase and Na^+/H^+ exchanger increase as gestation progresses. Other mediators of improved tubular function include expression of receptors to atrial natriuretic factor (ANF), thyroid hormones, and catecholamines. Increased expression, distribution and maturation of receptors facilitate improved fetal ability to conserve sodium along the nephron as term approaches. The ability to secrete potassium from the distal tubule is low, although this improves as term approaches due to increase in Na^+/K^+-ATPase activity and increased tubular surface area. Overall, low tubular potassium secreting ability maintains fetal serum potassium higher than a full term. Proximal tubular glucose reabsorption during fetal life increases *pari passu* with GFR — due mainly to increase in cell membrane and basolateral membrane surface area; hence, glucosuria is more common in the preterm as compared to term infants.

Calcium homeostasis is maintained by production of $1,25(OH)_2D_3$ by the maternal fetal unit and fetal kidney especially for rapid growth and development that characterizes the last trimester. It is estimated that mean intrauterine accumulation of calcium is 130 mg/kg each day. A positive fetal phosphate balance in the third trimester is also observed that continues well into postnatal life. Plasma phosphate concentration is higher than adults mainly due to the rapid growth of the fetus that occurs in the third trimester.

Placental maintenance of acid-base balance leaves minimal role for fetal kidney. However with increasing gestational age, there is an increasing participation of the fetal kidney in maintaining acid–base balance by reabsorbing filtered bicarbonate and secretion of hydrogen ions. In severe or prolonged acidotic conditions, such as prenatal asphyxia, the fetal kidney is able to secrete hydrogen ions to alleviate acidosis. The ability to concentrate urine remains poor for reasons mentioned earlier, hence fetal urine is always hypotonic (despite a relatively large amount of sodium), throughout gestation. Low sodium and water reabsorptive ability of the fetal kidney is considered by some to be an adaptive mechanism to conserve for much needed growth.

Premature and Term Renal Physiology

A host of well-coordinated events occur at the time of transition from intra to extrauterine life. Successful transition depends on gestational age and other prevailing maternal and fetal conditions, such as maternal fever, intrauterine medications exposure, preeclampsia and presence of congenital anomalies to mention a few. Alterations to the normal sequence of adaptive measures can result in immediate or long term consequences. For example, reduced renal mass due to prematurity has been associated with increased incidence of hypertension, hyperlipidemia, and diabetes in adulthood.

Glomerular filtration

At birth, there is a rapid and significant reduction in RVR and increase RBF and GFR. GFR in newborn term infants, estimated at about 20 mls/minute/1.73 m^2, doubles in the first 2 weeks of life, an increase that continues until about the age of 3 years when adult GFR of 120 ml/min/1.73 m^2 is attained (see Fig. 2). This increase is due to a host of vasodilatory mediators that counteract the predominant *in utero* vasoconstrictive mediators (Table 1). Recruitment of new and growth of existing glomeruli with increased filtration surface area are additional mechanisms that result in increased GFR in infancy.

A high plasma level of vasodilatory prostaglandins permit arteriolar dilation thus increasing glomerular hydrostatic pressure with resulting increased GFR. Nitrous oxide generated from local endothelium is another essential intrarenal vasodilator in the developing kidney opposing the vasoconstrictor mechanisms. Adrenomedullin, a vasodilator peptide is

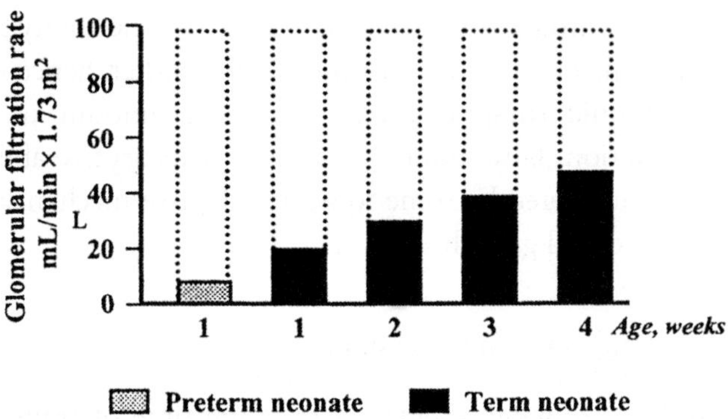

Figure 2. Glomerular filtration rate during the first month of life of preterm and term neonates, compared with adult values (*open columns*). (Adapted from Guignard JP, Torrado A, Da Cunha O, (1975) *et al.* Glomerular filtration rate in the first three weeks of life. *J Pediatr* 87: 268.)

Table 1.

Vasoconstrictive Mediators	Vasodilatory Mediators
Adenosine	Nitric Oxide
Angiotensin II	Norepinephrine
Atrial naturetic peptide	PGE_1
Bradykinin	PGE_2
Dopamine	Thromboxane A_2
Endothelin	Vasopressin
Epinephrine	

known to decrease RVR and increase RBF in animals, though its role in humans remains unknown. These vasodilators increase RBF by as much as 10% of cardiac output within one week of postnatal life. Most of the increased flow supplies the cortex with about 10% perfusing the medulla. Other vasodilator mediators include the diuretic peptide bradykinin (BK) produced by killikrein in the connecting tubules. Expression of B2 receptors through which BK exerts its effects, is higher in the neonatal kidney as compared to the adult kidney, suggesting a role in the transition from intra- to extrauterine life. ANF is another mediator that may have a dual role as a vasodilator and diuresis mediator. Its level, which is initially high at birth, gradually decreases by the second week of life. A dramatic increase in SBP also occurs. Renal autoregulation of RBF, an important mechanism designed to maintain renal perfusion when SBP is low, is present in newborns but set at a much lower threshold than adults or children.

Despite the role of vasodilatory mediators in increasing GFR, the RAS is still an important mediator in maintaining appropriate GFR. Plasma renin activity, presence of angiotensin II receptors and expression of the renin gene are all higher in neonatal renal tissue compared to adults. Angiotensin II increases GFR by preferentially constricting the efferent arteriole thereby maintaining glomerular capillary pressure. The sympathetic nervous system also contributes significantly to vasoconstrictor activity directly via stimulating release of renin. Endothelin (ET), a potent vasoconstrictor peptide is elevated in both term and preterm neonates, as higher concentrations are needed in newborns as compared to adults to maintain the same renal vasoconstriction effect. The newborn kidney is especially sensitive to medication effects that can alter concentrations of these vasoactive mediators (see Fig. 3).

Standardized evaluation of GFR is rarely performed in the newborn; instead Cr is used to estimate renal function as in children and adults. This is fraught with multiple limitations. At birth, Cr is a reflection of maternal Cr because it freely filtered across the placenta. In term infants, the Cr decreases by 1–2 weeks of age to a level adequately reflecting the infant's renal function. This drop is much slower and prolonged for very preterm infants, lasting up to 4 weeks (Fig. 4). Also in the very preterm, a transient increase in Cr occurs within the first week life before gradual decrease is observed. Passive reabsorption or back diffusion of Cr across

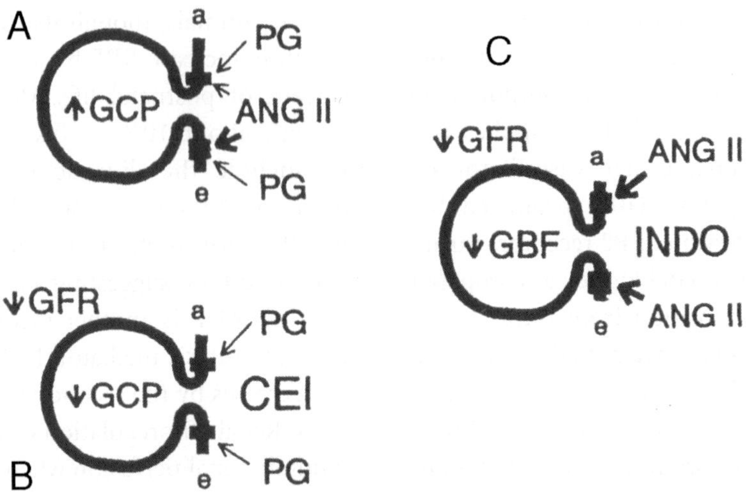

Figure 3. Control of glomerular filtration rate (*GFR*) in neonate. *A*, glomerular capillary pressure (*GCP*) is maintained by greater angiotensin II (*ANGII*) vasoconstriction at efferent (e) than afferent (α) arteriole but effects are attenuated by concurrent vasodilation mediated by prostaglandins (*PG*). *B*, angiotensin converting enzyme inhibitors (*ACE-i*), such as captopril, allow unopposed vasodilation by prostaglandins, reducing glomerular capillary pressure and glomerular filtration rate. *C*, indomethacin (*INDO*) reduces prostaglandin synthesis, allowing unopposed angiotensin II mediated vasoconstriction, resulting in reduced glomerular blood flow (*GBF*) and decreased glomerular filtration rate.

the immature tubules is thought to be the reason. Due to these limitations of utilizing Cr to evaluate GFR, cystatin C, has been touted as a viable alternative. Cystatin C is a low molecular weight protein produced constantly by all nucleated cells and cleared from circulation almost exclusively by glomerular filtration and has shown some promise in evaluating GFR in newborns; larger studies are still needed to verify its accuracy.

Important facts to remember are that GFR is lower in the very preterm infant due to incomplete nephrogenesis and a much slower improvement in renal function occurs over time as compared to a full term infant. Also, using Cr in the newborn to monitor GFR should depend on serial readings of Cr. Regardless of gestational age, all newborns should void within 24 hours of life, with preterms usually voiding earlier than full terms. Other factors that may affect time of first void include breast milk or formula fed and intercurrent illness.

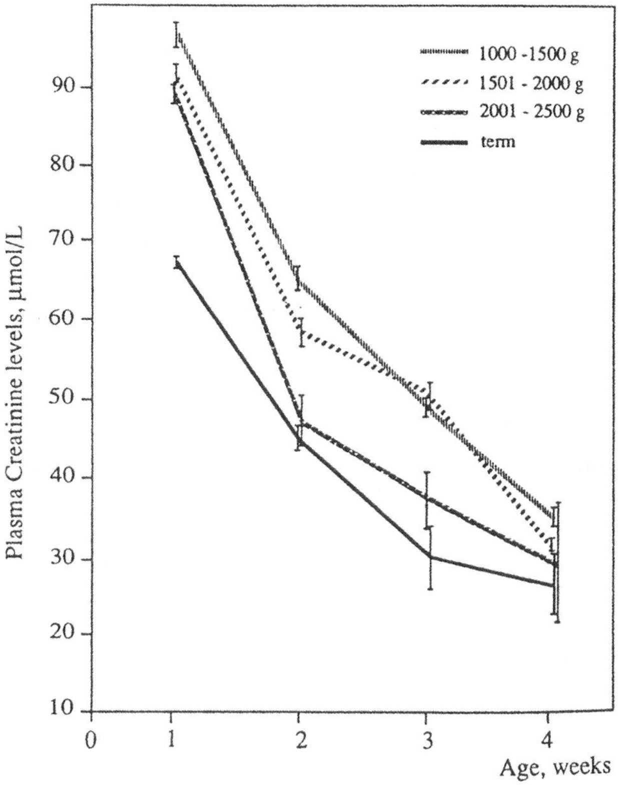

Figure 4. Plasma creatinine in term and low-birth-weight infants during the first 4 weeks of life. (From Bueva A, Guignard JP: Renal function in preterm neonates. *Pediatr Res* **36**: 572, 1994.)

Tubular function

At birth, the newborn kidney begins a brisk period of diuresis that lasts for about two weeks leading to a 10–15% loss of extracellular fluid. The physiologic drop in birth weight observed in newborns irrespective of gestational age is attributed to this diuretic phase.

Diuresis occurs with sodium loss in the urine. The fractional excretion of sodium (FENa) can be as high as 5% compared to 1% in a mature adult. FENa eventually drops with subsequent positive sodium balance and accompanying water retention. High ANF levels are observed, especially in preterms during this time of natriuresis and diuresis. In preterm infants, the reduction in FENa is delayed with more sodium losses, resulting in early hyponatremia within the first few weeks of life. Gallini *et al.* demonstrated an inverse relationship between gestational age and FENa in a cohort of preterms. Unlike early hyponatremia, late hyponatremia occurs after resolution of diuresis and natriuresis noted in the first two weeks of life. This is observed in rapidly growing low birth-weight babies at about six weeks of age due to increased need of sodium for normal growth. Low activity of tubular Na^+/K^+-ATPase results in decreased sodium absorption in the loop of Henle so greater amount of filtered sodium is delivered to the distal tubule. Irrespective of postnatal age, a persistent negative sodium balance in newborns markedly prevents growth and underscores importance for sodium supplementation of between 2–4 mEq/kg/day depending on gestational age. Al-Dahhan *et al.* demonstrated that sodium supplementation in the second week of life promoted weight gain that continued even after discontinuation of supplementation.

Neonatal intracellular potassium is higher than adults and remains so for up to four months, mainly because of the rapid growth that characterizes this period. Proximal tubular reabsorption of potassium, unresponsiveness to aldosterone by the distal tubule, limited excretory capacity of the collecting tubule and intestinal absorption permit potassium retention which is instrumental in maintaining a positive balance. Newborns with adequate potassium stores eliminate excess ingested potassium mainly via the intestinal tract with the rest taking place in the urine.

A positive phosphate balance is critical to support the rapid skeletal growth in newborns and similar to potassium, serum phosphate is higher in neonates compared to adults due to efficient reabsorption in the proximal tubule and intestinal tract. Phosphate conservation is important since human breast milk contains much less phosphorus relative to infant formulas. Karlen *et al.* showed that preterm breastfed infants had higher urinary losses of phosphate in the first week of life compared to term breastfed infants. But by the second week of life, tubular reabsorption was similar to full terms at about 95%. Due to renal phosphate retaining ability, urinary phosphate is closely tied to dietary phosphate. A low-phosphate diet results in high tubular reabsorption and vice versa. Thus, a preterm with phosphate-free urine is likely receiving inadequate dietary phosphate and is at risk for neonatal hypo-phosphatemic rickets. Intestinal absorption and renal phosphate retention are also promoted by growth hormone. Production of 1,25-dihydroxyvitamin D by newborn proximal renal tubules which began *in utero* is increased rapidly after birth.

Bicarbonate reabsorption in the proximal tubule is low during early postnatal life due to weak expression and maturation of transporters and enzymes such as Na^+/H^+ exchanger and carbonic anhydrase. This leads to a reduced renal threshold for bicarbonate reabsorption in the proximal renal tubule, manifesting as a plasma bicarbonate concentration of about 19–21 mmol/L in full term neonates and 16–21 mmol/L in extreme preterm infants. Another speculated reason for relatively low bicarbonate levels in the newborn is expanded extracellular fluid volume. Distal as compared to proximal tubular function is more mature and functional in newborns. This feature permits a term neonate to reduce urine pH to values similar to adults in the presence of acidosis. It is however important to note that this is dependent on the ability to generate urinary buffers (ammonium and phosphate), which is in turn dependent on diet and health status. An ill and catabolic infant can easily develop metabolic acidosis, more so if premature.

Several factors limit maximal concentrating ability in a newborn, namely reduced responsiveness of collecting ducts to vasopressin, anatomic immaturity of the renal medulla and low concentration of urea and sodium within medullary tissue. Also, in the premature (unlike term) newborns, the threshold for the release of vasopressin is higher, resulting in significant dehydration and or hypernatremia before concentration of urine begins. Maximal urine concentrating ability within the first three weeks of life due to dehydration and vasopressin is below 430 mOsm/kg H_2O and 630 mOsm/kg H_2O, respectively, in 4 and 6 week old infants (Fig. 5).

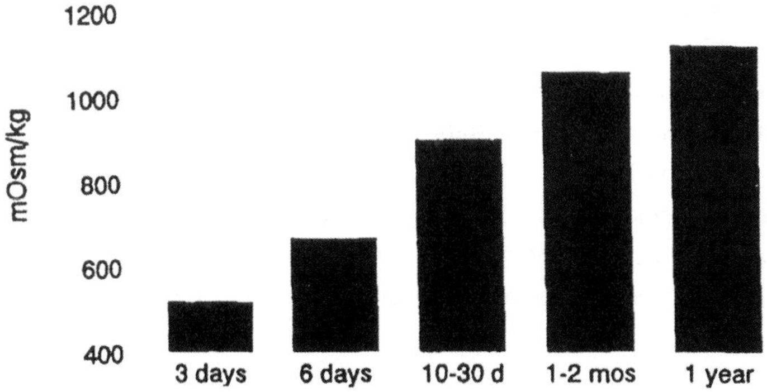

Figure 5. Increase in renal concentrating capacity in term neonate with most adult concentrating capacity achieved within first month of life.

The renal effects of prenatal glucocorticoids administered to enhance lung maturity remain unknown and controversial. Transient improvement of renal function in preterms, higher mean arterial blood pressure within the first 3 days of postnatal life, altered renal development and higher BP as adults, have been described. Unfortunately there are no large and long-term robust studies performed investigating this relationship. Most studies to date are either animal data or case series with no standardization of type of glucocorticoids administered, stage of gestation/nephrogenesis or dose and frequency of glucocorticoids administration.

Suggested Reading

Al-Dahhan J, Haycock GB, Nichol B, *et al.* (1984) Sodium homeostasis in term and preterm neonates. III. Effect of salt supplementation. *Arch Dis Child* **59**(10): 945–950.

Armangil D, Yurdakok M, Canpolat FE, *et al.* (2008) Determination of reference values for plasma cystatin C and comparison with creatinine in premature infants. *Pediatr Nephrol* **23**(11): 2081–2083.

Benini D, Fanos V, Cuzzolin L, Tato L. (2004) In utero exposure to nonsteroidal anti-inflammatory drugs: neonatal renal failure. *Pediatr Nephrol* **19**(2): 232–234.

Bueva A, Guignard JP. (1994) Renal function in preterm neonates. *Pediatr Res* **36**(5): 572–577.

Figueroa JP, Rose JC, Massmann GA, *et al.* (2005) Alterations in fetal kidney development and elevations in arterial blood pressure in young adult sheep after clinical doses of antenatal glucocorticoids. *Pediatr Res* **58**(3): 510–515.

Gallini F, Maggio L, Romagnoli C, *et al.* (2000) Progression of renal function in preterm neonates with gestational age < or = 32 weeks. *Pediatr Nephrol* **15**(1–2): 119–124.

Guignard JP, Drukker A. (1999) Why do newborn infants have a high plasma creatinine? *Pediatr* **103**(4): e49.

Rodriguez SJ. (20002) Renal tubular acidosis: the clinical entity. *J Am Soc Nephrol* **13**(8): 2160–2170.

Senterre J, Salle B. (1988) Renal aspects of calcium and phosphorus metabolism in preterm infants. *Biol Neonate* **53**(4): 220–229.

van den Anker JN, Hop WC, de Groot R, *et al.* (1994) Effects of prenatal exposure to betamethasone and indomethacin on the glomerular filtration rate in the preterm infant. *Pediatr Res* **36**(5): 578–581.

46

Neonatal Disorders

Deepa H. Chand, Heather Stewart and Maria E. de Ferris

Introduction

There is no consensus in the definition of neonatal acute kidney injury (NAKI), but most accepted definitions incorporate the acute reduction of renal function leading to concurrent solute and fluid retention. NAKI can be defined as an absolute increase in serum creatinine of more than or equal to 0.3 mg/dL, a percentage increase in serum creatinine of more than or equal to 50% (1.5-fold from baseline), or a reduction in urine output (documented oliguria of less than 0.5 mL/kg/h for more than six hours.

Neonatal Acute Kidney Injury (NAKI)

Incidence of NAKI

Depending on the series and study design, the incidence of NAKI ranges from 1–24% of neonatal ICU admissions and can be classified as prerenal (75%), intrinsic renal (10%) or postrenal (5%) or oliguric and nonoliguric (better prognosis). If the insult persists, both pre- and postrenal failure may become intrinsic renal failure.

Etiology and diagnosis of NAKI

Because nephrogenesis is not complete until 36 weeks gestation and the renal maturation process extends into the infant period, neonates, especially those born prematurely, are at increased risk of developing NAKI. Further, a complicated prenatal, perinatal, and postnatal course can predispose the infant to NAKI. Many children suffer from comorbidities, both congenital and acquired, which can impair renal function. Common

Table 1. Etiology (based on location) of neonatal acute kidney injury and diagnostic tests

Prerenal	Sepsis and multiorgan system failure
	Hypovolemia due to dehydration, patent ductus arteriosus or cardiac surgery
	Urine Na <20; FENa ≤1; RFI <1; increased beta 2-microglobulins and NAG
	Acute tubular necrosis secondary to perinatal asphyxia or neonatal hypoxia
Renal (Intrinsic)	*In utero* exposure to nephrotoxic agents (e.g. ACEi)
	Vascular thrombosis
	Postnatal exposure to nephrotoxic agents (e.g. indomethacin, aminoglycosides)
	Congenital conditions (e.g. renal agenesis, dysplasia)
	Hereditary renal disease (ARPKD)
	Full-term babies: Urine Na >50; FENa >2.5–3%; RFI >4
	Preterm babies (<32 weeks): FENa >6%; RFI >8
	Urinalysis: blood, protein, RBCs, casts (granular or hyaline)
Postrenal	Congenital urinary tract anomalies (i.e. Cloaca)
	Congenital urinary tract obstruction (PUV, UPJ or UVJ Obstruction)
	Diagnostic test: Renal ultrasound

ACEi = angiotensin-converting enzyme inhibitor; PUV = posterior urethral valves; UPJ = uretero-pelvic junction; UVJ = uretero-vesical junction; FENa = fractional excretion of sodium; RFI = renal failure index; NAG = N-acetyl-beta-D-glucosaminidase

conditions include hypovolemia, administration of nephrotoxic agents, and sepsis, all of which can adversely affect renal function. The etiology of NAKI can be summarized based on its classification as shown in Table 1.

Diagnosis of NAKI

Elevated serum creatinine

In full-term neonates, a serum creatinine >1.3 mg/dL for at least two days (if maternal renal function is normal); or increasing by 0.3 mg/dL/day or fails to fall below maternal plasma creatinine within 5–7 days. In preterms, the physiological decline of serum creatinine can extend over two weeks.

Evaluation of NAKI should include a detailed history and physical exam. Prenatal events, postnatal course, medications, family history, and maternal history should be recorded. Physical examination should focus on the major organ systems, but one should also note any dysmorphic features, sacral abnormalities, ear deformities, and abnormal skin findings.

Quantity of urine output should be noted in addition to the presence or absence of gross hematuria. Acute presentation of gross hematuria, especially in the presence of umbilical catheters, may be indicative of thrombosis. Serum electrolytes, BUN, creatinine, and complete blood count should be obtained. Urinary electrolytes may be obtained to assess imbalances, specifically to determine if renal losses are excessive. Renal ultrasound is helpful in as it can rule out obstructive uropathy, renal vein thrombosis, and renal parenchyma disease. Genetics consultation should be obtained if congenital syndrome is suspected. Although early markers of NAKI such as serum and urine endothelin-1 have been described, these tests are not widely available nor have they been validated in large cohorts.

Management of NAKI

The management of NAKI should be supportive. First, nephrotoxic agents should be avoided and discontinued if possible. Necessary nephrotoxic medications should be dosed according to estimated renal function.

As oliguric NAKI has a poorer prognosis than nonoliguric NAKI, accurate urine output is essential. This may require the placement of a bladder catheter in many instances. Weight measurements are often helpful; however, this may be difficult in the neonatal intensive care (NICU) setting. Similarly, an accurate record of intake should be documented. If hypovolemia is present, the patient's volume status should be repleted. This can be accomplished by using crystalloid solutions; however, in some instances (i.e. acute blood loss) colloid may be preferred. Fluid resuscitation should be performed cautiously so as to avoid volume overload if possible. This may be challenging in certain situations if capillary leak is present, as the patient may have total body volume overload despite intravascular hypovolemia. In a patient with volume overload, fluid intake should be restricted to urine output (when present), plus insensible losses.

The use of diuretic therapy is controversial; however, if used, the patient's serum electrolytes should be monitored closely. Furthermore, if loop diuretics are used for a prolonged period of time, follow-up renal ultrasound is warranted to monitor for nephrocalcinosis. It is important to remember that high doses of diuretics may be necessary to allow delivery of the medication to the renal tubules.

Electrolyte management should include monitoring of serum potassium (K^+) and avoiding excessive intake based on serum levels. Blood is often drawn via heel stick in infants, and as such, results should be interpreted with caution as hemolysis secondary to technique can falsely elevate the serum K^+. Hence, blood draws from a central line or venous draw are advisable. When initiating feedings in these neonates, breast milk contains the lowest K^+ load, however, if commercial formulas are necessary, consultation with a renal dietitian may provide options. Similarly, many infants with NAKI may also have sodium, calcium, and phosphorus abnormalities. These should be evaluated using serum and urine studies to determine if supplementation or restriction is required. Supplementation of electrolytes due to excess urinary excretion can be provided by enteral route, if functional. If necessary, supplementation can be given intravenously. If continued supplementation is necessary, total parenteral nutrition should be adjusted accordingly to compensate for these losses.

Many neonates with NAKI may develop hypertension. Hydralazine and propranolol are often effective in the treatment of NAKI associated hypertension.

Renal replacement therapy (RRT)

Indications for RRT in the neonate are similar to those in older children. However, nuances to the infant population include difficulty in establishing large bore vascular access due to small vessel size and difficulty in placing a peritoneal dialysis catheter due to lack of subcutaneous fat, predisposing to catheter leak. In the cases of premature infants, consultation with the surgeon is imperative to determine if access can be placed. Parents should be strongly advised of the potential risks of RRT in this population as the risk of mortality is significant.

Renal Vein Thrombosis (RVT)

Epidemiology

The incidence of RVT is not clear. Risk factors for RVT in neonates include hypervolemia, polycythemia, hypercoagulable states, and dehydration. Maternal diabetes may predispose the infant to develop an osmotic diuresis with associated dehydration, decreased perfusion pressure, and thrombosis. Other risk factors include umbilical vein catheterization, sepsis, dehydration, birth asphyxia, or thrombocytopenia. Intrauterine cases have been reported. Maternal history of systemic lupus erythematosus may be a risk factor for antiphospholipid antibodies, predisposing to RVT.

Clinical presentation

The clinical presentation of RVT includes acute development of gross hematuria, hypertension, enlarged kidney, shock, thrombocytopenia, lower extremity edema, and abdominal distention.

Diagnosis

Diagnostic evaluation includes complete blood count with emphasis on platelet count, coagulation studies, and renal ultrasound (US) with Doppler. A renal US confirms the diagnosis with an enlarged hyperechoic kidney and thrombi on the renal vein that can even extend to the inferior vena cava noted by Doppler. Other diagnostic tests to determine hypercoagulability may be indicated.

Treatment

The treatment of RVT should be aimed at stabilization of the intravascular volume while correcting electrolyte abnormalities. The use of heparin is controversial, but if there is a bilateral involvement, a loading dose of 50–100 units per kg is followed by continuous infusion of 25–50 units per kg to maintain a PTT of 1.5 times normal. There is limited experience with tissue plasminogen activator at a dose of 0.02 to 0.03 mg/kg with the same goals for the PTT followed by low molecular weight heparin. If bleeding occurs, e-caproic acid should be at the bedside.

Neonatal Hypertension

Incidence and diagnosis

Neonatal hypertension has an incidence of approximately 3% in the NICU. Renovascular etiologies, such as RVT and renal artery stenosis secondary to vascular thrombosis, occur as a complication of umbilical catheterization. Neonatal hypertension is diagnosed by the presence of blood pressures (systolic and/or diastolic) ≥95th percentile (or more than two standard deviations above the mean values).

Although renovascular hypertension is the most common etiology, other causes of neonatal hypertension that are important to consider and evaluate include coarctation of the aorta, mid-aorta syndrome, polycystic kidney disease, renal parenchymal disorders, and acute kidney injury (AKI). Specific etiologies of AKI include acute tubular necrosis (ATN) from hypovolemia and tubulointerstitial nephritis (TIN) often secondary to medications. Nonrenal etiologies include bronchopulmonary dysplasia (BPD), hyperthyroidism, congenital adrenal hyperplasia, increased intracranial pressure, and maternal illicit drug use (cocaine). Iatrogenic causes include pain (especially postoperative), medications, and fluid/electrolyte abnormalities.

Evaluation

A thorough history should be obtained and detailed physical examination performed. Prenatal history including maternal drug use (prescribed or illicit), perinatal history including presence of oligo- or polyhydramnios, and postnatal course including umbilical catheter use should be noted. Particular attention should be given to femoral pulses and four limb blood pressures obtained to evaluate for coarctation. The mid-aorta syndrome, considered by some to be an extension of coarctation is a segmental narrowing of the distal thoracic or abdominal aorta, and may present with abdominal bruit. Renal and bladder US should be obtained to evaluate for renal parenchymal disorders, cystic kidney disease, or obstructive uropathy. Laboratories, including serum electrolytes, blood urea nitrogen, creatinine, and complete blood count, should be obtained. Echocardiogram should be obtained to evaluate for structural abnormalities, as well as to assess cardiac function. Urine output should be quantified as should total intake. Urinalysis should be obtained to evaluate for hematuria and proteinuria.

Further testing should be conducted based on index of suspicion and may include thyroid function tests, adrenal testing, and tests to detect infectious, neurologic, drug, endocrine, or metabolic causes of neonatal hypertension.

Most neonates with hypertension are asymptomatic, however, symptoms, if present can vary. These are often nonspecific and include feeding intolerance, irritability, lethargy, tachypnea, cyanosis, apnea, and seizures. Renal manifestations may include hyponatremia, polyuria, or proteinuria. Sometimes, heart failure may be present.

Treatment

The blood pressure at which treatment should be initiated is not clear as no published guidelines exist. Most practitioners will initiate medication when the SBP >99th percentile or if end-organ damage is present. The goal of therapy is to normalize blood pressures, while minimizing morbidity. Choice of medication should be based on cause of hypertension. For example, correction of hyperthyroidism will result in resolution of hypertension as will treatment of congenital adrenal hyperplasia with glucocorticoids. Urinary obstruction should be relieved if present. If pain is present, this should be addressed adequately.

In the presence of thrombosis, patients should be monitored by ultrasound. In general, the benefits of thrombolytic therapy should be weighed against the risk of bleeding and mortality. The use of anticoagulants and/or thrombolytic agents is limited to severe thromboembolic events that compromise the viability of a vital organ or extremity.

Many classes of medications have been used in neonates, including diuretics, angiotensin converting enzyme (ACE) inhibitors, beta blockers, calcium channel blockers, and direct peripheral vasodilators. The etiology of the hypertension should be considered when choosing appropriate therapy. As a general principle, shorter acting agents should be used to allow titration as needed.

Most often, ACE inhibitors are used; however, they are contraindicated in patients with bilateral renovascular disease or renovascular disease in a solitary kidney. In these scenarios, AKI can occur as a result of loss of the angiotensin II-mediated maintenance of glomerular capillary pressure. Controversy exists regarding the use of ACE inhibitors in severely premature infants due to potential impact on nephrogenesis. Enalaprilat offers an intravenous alternative. The beta-blocker propranolol has been efficacious and well-tolerated in neonates. Labetalol is another agent, often used in central and catecholamine induced hypertension due to alpha-1 and beta-blockade. Beta-blockers are contraindicated in infants with BPD due to risk of bronchoconstriction. Dihydropyridine calcium channel blockers, such as nicardipine and amlodipine, are peripheral vasodilators and useful in neonatal hypertension in most circumstances. Peripheral vasodilators such as hydralazine can be given either orally or intravenously and act very rapidly to lower blood pressure. Intravenous nitroprusside is a potent vasodilator used solely in cases of severe hypertension. It has a very rapid onset of action and short duration of action, making it very useful acutely. However, its major complication is thiocyanate toxicity, which occurs with prolonged administration (>72 hr).

Regardless of which agent is used, the onset of action, duration of action, and potential side effects should be known. Therapy should be initiated with low dosages initially and titrated to desired effect. Whenever possible, one agent should be used and dosing maximized before addition of a second agent. Development of potential side effects should be monitored. Duration of treatment will vary and as such, these patients need to be monitored very closely, both in the NICU setting and after hospital discharge. Close outpatient follow-up is warranted.

Nephrocalcinosis

Nephrocalcinosis is common in preterm infants, with reported incidence of up to 64% in extremely low birth-weight infants. This is often multifactorial in nature, affected by postnatal course, and occurs as a result a of complicated NICU course. As loop diuretics induce hypercalciuria, children treated for conditions such as BPD, cardiac conditions, and volume overload are at increased risk. Other predisposing factors include prolonged parenteral nutrition which increases urinary oxalate excretion and administration of nephrotoxic agents which impair tubular function. Nephrocalcinosis commonly occurs in congenital syndromes such as William's syndrome, distal renal tubular acidosis, Bartter syndrome, and neonatal hyperparathyroidism. Neonates suspected to have these disorders should be screened for nephrocalcinosis.

Diagnosis is made by renal US with shows medullary calcification. Urinary studies including calcium: creatinine should be obtained. Serum laboratory studies should be obtained to evaluate electrolytes, with special attention to serum calcium, phosphorus, and bicarbonate levels. Measurement of serum parathyroid hormone levels should be considered.

Treatment and outcomes

Prevention remains the mainstay of treatment. If diuretics are necessary, consideration should be given to use of a thiazide diuretic, especially if long-term use is required. Combined or alternating therapy may also provide synergistic benefits, as well as possibly decrease the risk of nephrocalcinosis. Offending agents should be minimized or discontinued if possible. Renal US should be obtained at regular intervals to follow renal growth and progression of nephrocalcinosis.

Long-term nephrocalcinosis may resolve spontaneously over one to two years. However, lower GFR, hypercalciuria, and impaired tubular function (concentrating ability, acidification impairment, etc.) have all been reported long-term.

Suggested Reading

Andreoli SP. (2004) Acute renal failure in the newborn. *Semin Perinatol* **8**: 112–123.

Askenazi D, Ambalavanan N, Goldstein S. (2009) Acute kidney injury in critically ill newborns: What do we know? What do we need to learn? *Pediatr Nephrol* **24**: 265–274.

Chua A, Sarwal M. (2005) Acute renal failure management in the neonate. *Neoreviews* **6**: e369–e376.

Gouyon JB, Guignard JP. (2000) Management of acute renal failure in newborns. *Pediatr Nephrol* **14**: 1037–1044.

Lee M, Chua A, Yorgin P. (2005) Neonatal peritoneal dialysis. *Neoreviews* **6**: e384–e391.

Nafday SM, *et al.* (2005) Renal Disease. In: MacDonald MG. (ed.), *Neonatology: Pathophysiology and Management of Newborn* (6th ed.), Lippincott Williams and Wilkins. 981–1065.

Reznik VM, Griswold WR, Peterson BM, *et al.* (1991) Peritoneal dialysis for acute renal failure in children. *Pediatr Nephrol* 5(6): 715.

Subramanian S, Agarwal R, Deorari A, *et al.* (2008) Acute renal failure in neonates. *Indian J Pediatr* 75(4): 385–391.

Symons JM, Chua AN, Somers MJ, *et al.* (2007) Demographic characteristics of pediatric continuous renal replacement therapy: a report of the prospective pediatric continuous renal replacement therapy registry. *J Am Soc Nephrol* 2(4): 732–738.

Yorgin P, Lee M. (2005) Neonatal hemodialysis and continuous renal replacement therapy. *Neoreviews* **6**: e377–e383.

Part XVIII

Congenital Renal Diseases

47

Hydronephrosis, Obstructive Uropathy, and Multicystic Dysplastic Kidney

Eric Z. Massanyi and Daniel R. McMahon

Hydronephrosis

Hydronephrosis, the most common prenatally detected ultrasonographic abnormality, is found in approximately 1% of pregnancies and it is a clinical sign, not a specific diagnosis. Prenatal hydronephrosis warrants additional radiographic imaging postnatally. Etiologies are numerous (e.g. vesicoureteral reflux (VUR) and obstruction) and specific diagnosis determines treatment course. VUR is the most common cause (up to 40%).

The degree and laterality of hydronephrosis depends on the stage of pregnancy as well as the underlying etiology. Ultrasonography (US) can detect the bladder and kidneys at 15 weeks of gestation and distinguish a renal sinus by 18–20 weeks. After 20 weeks, the fetus is larger, and anomalies are easier to define. In many cases, prenatal hydronephrosis may not be associated with any postnatal pathology, and premature diagnosis of hydronephrosis may cause significant parental anxiety for the pregnancy duration. Caution should be exercised in making specific recommendations as the postnatal prognosis may differ significantly from the prenatal appearance.

Pathogenesis

The ureteral bud arises from the mesonephric duct during the fifth week of gestation. It joins and interacts with the metanephric blastema and induces differentiation and growth of the renal parenchyma. Most nephrons are present by the middle of the second trimester, and maturation is complete by 36 weeks of gestation. The ureteral bud undergoes multiple generations of division to complete the collecting system from the proximal tubules to the distal hemitrigone of the bladder.

Embryologically, the ureter develops as a solid cord of tissue that lengthens and canalizes during development. Distal to the ureter, the urogenital sinus undergoes differentiation to form the bladder and urethra at 10 and 12 weeks of gestation, respectively.

The placenta maintains salt and water homeostasis for the developing fetus; however, the fetal kidney begins producing hypotonic urine between the fifth and ninth weeks of gestation with output increasing throughout gestation. An anomaly at any point in the urinary tract can cause partial or complete obstruction of urine flow, causing proximal collecting system dilation manifesting as hydronephrosis. Anomalies produced include ureteropelvic junction (UPJ) obstruction, obstructing megaureter, ectopic ureter, ureterocele, and posterior urethral valves (PUV). If the process is partial or transient, it may not be pathologic, but rather may be a normal part of development in some fetuses, leaving no pathology postnatally. However, if significant obstruction persists, renal tissue maturation can be affected, resulting in nephropathy.

Hydronephrosis can be associated with nonobstructive collecting system distension secondary to VUR, in association with nonrefluxing, nonobstructing megaureters, or in Eagle–Barrett (prune belly) syndrome. Obstructive lesions are generally more harmful to developing kidneys and can lead to oligohydramnios, impairing lung development, which may be incompatible with life.

Clinical presentation

Typically, prenatal hydronephrosis is a radiographic finding of which the presentation varies widely and depends on severity and etiology. In the modern era, most cases are discovered prenatally, and most infants are asymptomatic and otherwise healthy. Less often, hydronephrosis is associated with palpable mass, respiratory distress, failure to thrive or urinary tract infection (UTI). Older children presenting with UTI or abdominal pain may be detected incidentally.

Diagnosis

Hydronephrosis is most often brought to medical attention via prenatal US. If an abnormality is detected, a dedicated US of the genitourinary system should be performed to evaluate the collecting system architecture, renal architecture and size, parenchymal echogenicity, bladder appearance, and amniotic fluid volume. The differential diagnosis of hydronephrosis is broad; however, many clues can be obtained from initial US. Hydronephrosis severity is a significant factor that can herald an obstructive process and various grading systems exist, including subjective numerical grading and objective measurement of the anterior-posterior diameter of the renal pelvis. Most commonly, hydronephrosis is described as mild, moderate, or severe based on degree of dilation and appearance of the ureter, pelvis, calicies, and surrounding parenchyma. Dilated calices or caliectasis with thinning renal parenchyma are suggestive of severe hydronephrosis with higher intrarenal pressures. Another widely used system for grading, developed by the Society for Fetal Urology, is graded from I–IV (see Fig. 1). Some type of intervention will likely be necessary with grade III–IV hydronephrosis. Renal anterior-posterior (AP) pelvic diameter is also used to evaluate the significance of dilation. In one study, >90% of fetuses with an AP diameter of >2 cm ultimately required surgical intervention while <5% of fetuses with an AP diameter <1 cm did so. More conservatively, a renal AP pelvic diameter of at least 4 mm before 33 weeks of gestation and at least 7 mm after 33 weeks of gestation is considered significant.

Renal architecture, renal size, and echogenicity of the renal parenchyma are important in developing a differential diagnosis and predicting potential renal function. Increased echogenicity may be associated with renal dysplasia but this finding is not as reliable in the perinatal period as it is later in life. Differentiation between hydronephrosis and polycystic kidneys or cystic dysplastic kidneys can be difficult. Hydronephrosis tends to be an orderly process with visible connections between the dilated calyces and pelvis. Cystic kidneys do not appear as orderly, and cystic connections are unidentifiable.

The presence of a distended bladder without functional emptying is also important in developing a differential diagnosis. A filled bladder should be visualized, with functional emptying observed. A system that does not empty properly, with significantly dilated bladder and upper tract, may suggest the presence of PUV, prune belly syndrome, or urethral atresia. A keyhole sign is usually indicative of PUV. Bladder visualization may also reveal ureterocele.

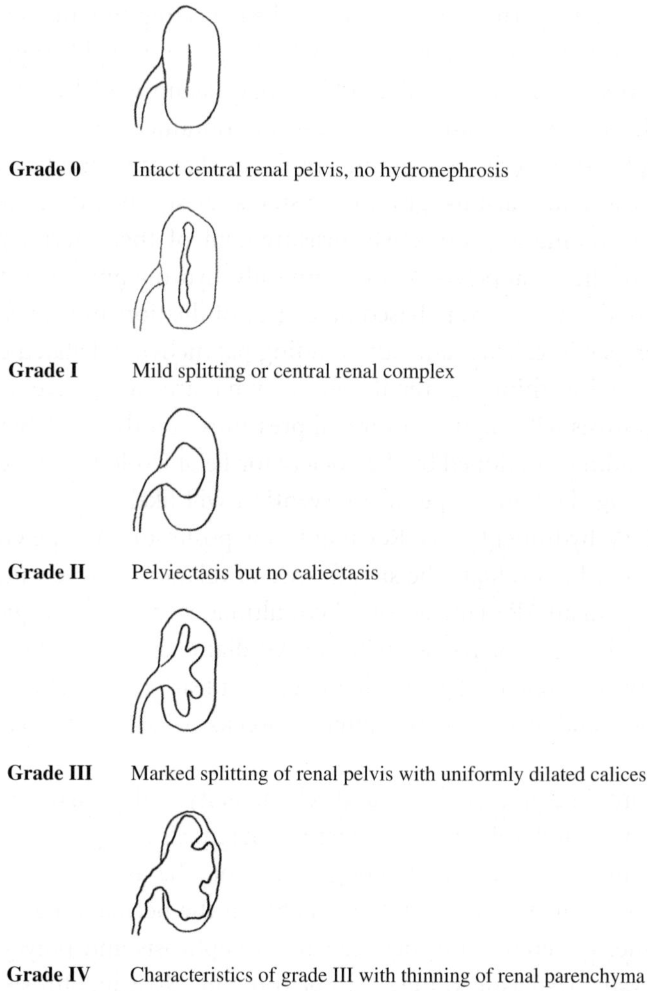

Figure 1. SFU grading system of hydronephrosis.

Amniotic fluid volume should also be assessed if hydronephrosis is identified as its presence is vital to normal fetal development. Oligohydramnios can cause pulmonary hypoplasia and compression deformities of the head, thorax, and limbs. A normal amniotic fluid index (AFI) is 5–25 cm. If an AFI shows fluid level <5 centimeters (or <5th percentile), the absence of a fluid pocket 2–3 cm in depth, or a fluid volume <500 mL at 32–36 weeks gestation, then oligohydramnios should be suspected.

Treatment

Treatment and prognosis of hydronephrosis is directed at the underlying etiology. Rarely, prenatal intervention may be indicated if life-threatening; however, most management occurs postnatally. Bilateral hydronephrosis and AP diameter >10 mm are concerning and require diligent prenatal monitoring. The frequency of prenatal follow-up evaluation should be based on severity of hydronephrosis, unilateral, or bilateral presence, and amniotic fluid volume. In general, for mild to moderate hydronephrosis with normal amniotic fluid, the fetus can be reevaluated in 4–6 weeks with a repeat US to rule out progression. Rarely, patients with severe obstructive uropathy that is life-threatening (usually due to oligohydramnios and pulmonary hypoplasia) may be candidates for prenatal treatment. This combination is most often due to PUV and *in utero* vesico-amniotic shunting has been advocated; unfortunately, the results have been disappointing as the intervention occurs too late to avoid renal dysplasia. It is important to identify other congenital abnormalities and assess renal function via fetal urine sampling before proceeding with this potentially fatal procedure. *In utero* intervention should only be performed by centers with significant experience. Urinary electrolyte assessment is based on 2–3 serial bladder aspiration. Since fetal urine should be dilute in comparison to post-natal values, favorable fetal urinary electrolytes would include sodium <100 mEq/l, chloride <90 mEq/l, osmolarity <210 mOsm/l and β-2 microglobulin <10–20. If age is >28–30 weeks, little will be gained from *in utero* intervention, and preterm delivery considered.

It is reasonable to obtain a renal US with or without voiding cystourethrography (VCUG) at 1–2 months of postnatal age to reevaluate mild or unilateral prenatal hydronephrosis. Significant bilateral or severe hydronephrosis should be evaluated shortly after birth with US. Noteworthy, US may underestimate the degree of hydronephrosis immediately postnatally secondary to fetal dehydration and transitional nephrology. Further testing may be necessary to guide further management. VCUG will assist in identifying VUR, PUV, and occasionally ureteroceles. Diuretic renographic scintigraphy with the use of mercaptoacetyltriglycine (MAG3) should generally be reserved for infants with grade 3–4 hydronephrosis at significant risk for

Table 1. Postnatal management for hydronephrosis

Prenatal Findings	Antibiotics	Imaging	Timing	Surgery
Mild hydronephrosis	+/−	US, +/− VCUG	2–3 Months	Unlikely
Modeste/severe hydronephrosis	Yes	US, VCUG, +/− MAG3	1–2 Months 2–3 Months	Unlikely
Severe unilateral hydronephrosis	Yes	US, VCUG, +/− MAG3	1 Month 1–3 Months	Possible
Severe bilateral hydronephrosis	Yes	US, VCUG, probable MAG3	<1 Week 3–5 Weeks	Probable
Hydronephrosis with duplication + intravesical defect	Yes	US, VCUG, MAG3	<1 Month 3–5 Weeks	Probable
Unilateral cystic kidney	Yes	US, VCUG, DMSA	<1 Month	Unlikely

obstructive pathology. Table 1 highlights current recommendations regarding additional imaging and surgery. Often antimicrobial prophylaxis (i.e. amoxicillin 10 mg/kg/day) is continued until the evaluation is complete.

Prognosis

The prognosis is largely dependent on the underlying etiology of the dilated collecting system. Obstructive lesions and lesions with bilateral renal involvement are uniformly more threatening than nonobstructive and unilateral lesions. The survival rate with unilateral renal obstruction approaches 100%, with only 15–25% of patients requiring surgery. In the presence of bilateral obstruction, oligohydramnios correlates with adverse outcome as associated pulmonary hypoplasia, and compression deformities of the skeletal system can impair quality of life and survival. The timing of oligohydramnios is an important determinant of fetal outcome. The earlier a lesion develops, the more likely it is to have an effect on the fetal kidney, lungs, and overall outcome of the fetus. Many fetuses have an excellent prognosis, and this should be communicated to the parents. If a fetus has US findings suggestive of an adverse outcome, discussing the implications and consultation with pediatric urologists and/or pediatric nephrologists is important.

Obstructive Uropathy

Obstructive uropathy, the leading cause of renal dysfunction during infancy, often requires renal transplantation long-term. Obstruction adversely affects normal renal development, and may inhibit renal function even after the obstruction is relieved. Obstructive uropathies can be congenital or acquired, vary in severity, and can occur at any level from the kidney to the urethra (see Table 2).

The vast etiologic spectrum and variability of obstructive changes pose major challenges in diagnosing, and managing these conditions. Management of obstruction must be tailored individually with the goal

Table 2. Causes of urinary tract obstruction

Upper tract obstruction
• UPJ obstruction
• Intermittent hydronephrosis
• Multicystic kidney
• Obstructive megaureter
• Ureteral valves, kinks, and stenosis
• Prune belly syndrome
Nonobstructive hydroureteronephrosis
• Nonobstructive, nonrefluxing hydroureteronephrosis
• Refluxing megaureter
• Prune belly syndrome
• Residual hydroureteronephrosis
Bladder outlet and urethral obstruction
• PUV
• Anterior urethral valves
• Polyp of verumontanum
• Prune belly syndrome
• Hydrometrocolpos/cloacal anomaly
• Primary bladder neck obstruction
• Urethral atresia and stenosis
• Prostatic rhabdomysocarcoma
Nonobstructive vesicoretention
• Neurogenic bladder
• Megaureter, megacystis syndrome (reflux)
• Vesicourethral dysenergia
• Prune belly syndrome
• Congenital idiopathic megacystis
• Urinary tract dilation associated with imperforate anus

of preserving renal function to prevent chronic kidney disease (CKD) with minimal intervention.

Pathogenesis

Fetal genitourinary obstruction system may affect the upper urinary tract, unilaterally, or bilaterally, or may involve the bladder outlet and urethra. The most common upper urinary tract obstruction is UPJ obstruction, while PUV are the most common cause of lower tract obstruction. Hydronephrosis, urinary stasis, and residual urine may occur without considerable narrowing of the urinary tracts or increased pressure. These nonobstructive conditions may lead to infection and renal damage. Conversely, obstruction can result in damage without intervening infection.

Congenital obstruction affects renal development. Obstruction during fetal renal development can cause dysplasia, fibrosis, and abnormally increased interstitial tissue. Intercellular communication and renal architecture may become distorted, leading to diminished renal function. Acquired obstruction can still lead to renal deterioration from increased intrarenal pressure, pyelonephritic damage, and hyperperfusion.

Clinical presentation

Prenatal US has radically altered the clinical manifestations of obstructive conditions. Most individuals are detected incidentally, with many asymptomatic infants at birth. Clinical manifestations correlate with severe obstructive conditions, such as PUV or massive hydronephrosis and include straining to void, poor urinary stream, or palpable/enlarged bladder. Infants and younger children may present with UTIs or failure to thrive. Older patients may report abdominal pain. Metabolic findings include reduced filtration with an elevation in serum creatinine indicating glomerular injury, acidosis from tubular injury, and nephrogenic diabetes insipidus from collecting duct abnormalities. Hypertension may be seen due to elevated renin activity. Concomitant genitourinary abnormalities, such as hypospadias, and genital or anal anomalies may accompany congenital urinary obstruction. Occasionally, anal dimples may be found on physical examination signifying neural tube defects, such as spina bifida or tethered cord. Abnormal ears, single umbilical arteries, and limb abnormalities may also be present.

Patients with UPJ obstruction clinically present with episodic abdominal pain, flank pain, emesis or UTI; however, many are now incidentally diagnosed due to prenatal hydronephrosis. UPJ obstruction is characterized radiographically by unilateral pelvicaliectasis without ureteral dilation. Functional dilation may occur as a consequence of elevated bladder pressures, especially in males.

Ureterovesical junction (UVJ) obstruction, characterized by hydroureteronephrosis can present with pain or infection with variable degree of dilation. Greater ureteral dilation is seen near the level of the bladder. Causes of obstruction include primary ureter obstruction, ectopic ureter, or ureterocele. VUR may also produce similar findings, which are indistinguishable by US.

The presentation of PUV is highly variable. More severe cases are typically found on prenatal US, but less severe lesions may present as new onset incontinence in late childhood. In more severe cases, the bladder is thickened and distended and bilateral hydroureteronephrosis with increased renal parenchymal echogenecity is seen. Occasionally, the bladder may take up much of the fetal abdomen as urinary ascites may be present. Often times, amniotic fluid volume decreases by mid-second trimester due to fetal urinary obstruction. Prenatal US may reveal a dilated posterior urethra.

In the female fetus, bladder outlet obstruction with bilateral hydroureteronephrosis and dilated bladder may suggest cloacal anomaly or urogenital sinus causing vaginal distention and urinary obstruction. There is usually a retrovesical cystic structure representing the fluid-filled vagina.

Ureterocele can be diagnosed more definitively in the neonatal period. Patients are prone to febrile UTI. Presence of upper pole hydronephrosis in a duplicated system and a dilated ureter that can be traced to the bladder is suggestive. The bladder often demonstrates a thin-walled cystic structure associated with the base of the bladder away from the midline. Although upper tract dilation may not be seen in a poorly functioning kidney or upper pole, ureteroceles typically present with upper pole dilation due to system duplication in females, whereas single system ureteroceles are more common in males. Upper pole hydronephrosis may also represent ectopic ureter in the absence of an intravesical cystic structure. The appearance of bilateral single system ectopic ureters is distinct from that of the more common duplex ectopic ureters. Bilateral single ectopic ureters are usually associated with significant renal abnormalities and hypoplasia of the bladder.

Diagnosis

Actual diagnosis of obstructive uropathy by imaging studies is key in determining if intervention is appropriate. US, VCUG, and nuclear scans are employed. Ultrasonographic evaluation and chemistries will determine if urgent urinary drainage is required. VCUG, indicated in cases of suspected upper and lower urinary tract obstruction, provides information regarding the bladder outlet, and determines presence of associated VUR.

Differential function of each kidney can also be determined by obtaining a MAG3 scan to assess upper tract function and drainage. Detection of functioning renal tissue and renal scarring is best performed by ^{99m}Tc dimercaptosuccinic acid (DMSA) renal scintigraphy.

Treatment

Renal deterioration associated with obstructed urinary tracts is due to elevated intrarenal pressure, pyelonephritic damage, and hyperperfusion. Hence, relief from obstruction, prevention and treatment of infection, and stabilization of renal function are treatment goals. Prenatal diagnosis allows for evaluation of degree of obstruction present and prevention of infection before emergencies arise. When renal and bladder pressures are low and the child appears well, antimicrobials can prevent infections while the need and type of permanent intervention is further evaluated. When azotemia and sepsis are present, temporary drainage may be required to stabilize electrolyte imbalance, eliminate infection, and restore renal function prior to surgical intervention. Relief of obstruction is achieved by permanent or temporary drainage of urine. CIC is generally preferable to indwelling urethral catheter due to lower infection risk; however, in patients suspected of PUV with a tenuous urethra, an indwelling feeding tube is a safer short-term solution. If necessary, needle aspiration of the bladder or dilated upper urinary tract can be diagnostic and therapeutic, and an angio-cath left as a drainage tube.

Most infants with PUV are treated with cystoscopic valve ablation; however, management should be individualized. At times, the degree of obstruction, the level of renal function, the presence and severity of VUR, patient age, and urethral size may necessitate short-term vesicostomy with subsequent valve ablation.

Diuretic urography is considered the gold standard for evaluation of UPJ obstruction. In reality, there is no modality that is completely reliable in distinguishing obstructive from nonobstructive hydronephrosis. Many now view diminished function as the only indication for intervention in an asymptomatic patient. Others base the decision to intervene on a combination of grade of hydronephrosis, drainage times on sequential studies, patient age and differential renal function. Pyeloplasty has a success rate of approximately 95%.

In cases of ureteroceles and ectopic ureteroceles, endoscopic incision provides drainage, but can also cause VUR. Alternative management includes partial nephrectomy, uretero-ureterostomy, uretero-pyelostomy, or ureterocele excision with ureteral reimplantation.

Ectopic ureters are amenable to ureteral reimplatation or uretero-ureterostomy. Rarely, cutaneous pyelostomy or ureterostomy may be indicated. Nephrectomy is reserved for units with minimal function (i.e. <15%).

Prognosis

It is difficult to predict which patients will progress to end-stage renal disease (ESRD). Even in patients who undergo surgical intervention, further renal deterioration may occur. Serum creatinine remains the best indicator of further renal deterioration after obstruction is corrected. Patients who achieve a nadir creatinine less than 0.8 mg/dl tend to have adequate long term renal function, but renal function should be monitored intermittently.

Multicystic Dysplastic Kidney

Multicystic dysplastic kidney (MCDK), the most common cause of newborn abdominal mass, is the most common cystic malformation of the kidney. MCDK, a form of unilateral renal dysplasia characterized by the presence of multiple renal cysts of varying size without a normal pelvocaliceal system, is associated with ureteral atresia.

Importantly, the affected kidney is nonfunctional, is not reniform in shape, and lacks an organized calyceal drainage system. Minimal stroma separates multiple cysts and is often described as having "a bunch of grapes" appearance. Kidney size is variable, ranging from small to filling most of the abdomen. Less frequently, two other variations of MCDK are found. Solid cystic dysplasia is found with small or microscopic cysts with stromal predominance. If renal pelvis can be identified, the kidney is referred to as a hydronephrotic multicystic kidney.

MCDK should not be confused with polycystic kidney disease or other renal cystic diseases. The Urology Section of the American Academy of Pediatrics established the National Multicystic Kidney Registry, a large, multicenter, longitudinal database that helped clarify the appropriate management of MCDK.

Pathogenesis

Etiology and pathogenesis of MCDK is poorly understood with multiple postulated theories over the last century. Generally, most believe MCDK is caused by obstruction or metanephric differentiation abnormality. A combination of increased and decreased gene expression involving nephrogenesis and antiapoptosis is thought to be involved. Some have suggested that stability of growth and transcription factors determines whether the MCDK will dilate, shrink, or persist unchanged. Several anecdotal cases of Wilm's tumors that have developed from MCDK implicate gene overamplification. Others suggest that MCDK is a severe form of gestational hydronephrosis occurring secondary to collecting system or ureter atresia or obstruction. The left kidney is more frequently involved, similar to primary obstructive megaureter and UPJ obstruction. In animal models, several attempts have been made to induce MCDK by creating obstruction have been unsuccessfully made, despite successful induction of renal dysplasia.

The metanephric blastema forms the proximal portion of the nephron from the glomerulus to the distal convoluted tubule. The ureteral bud, arising from the mesonephros, forms the distal portion of the nephron, including the collecting duct, renal pelvis, and ureter. Failure of the ureteric bud to fuse with the metanephric blastema has been implicated. The cysts may also be secondary to premature termination of tubule division at the ureteric bud ampullae with subsequent failure of metanephric differentiation.

Typically, MCDK is sporadic and rarely inherited; however a few autosomal dominant cases have been reported. Other reported causes include chromosomal abnormalities, teratogen exposure, and maternal cocaine use during pregnancy.

Clinical presentation

MCDK often presents as abdominal mass in infants; however, identification has increased substantially due to improved prenatal US. In asymptomatic patients, incidental diagnosis is made during unrelated imaging evaluation.

The incidence of MCDK is 1:2400 to 1:4300. Males are more likely to unilateral disease (2.4:1); however, bilateral disease (more properly termed cystic dysplasia) occurs more frequently in females (2:1). Bilateral disease is more likely associated with chromosomal and congenital anomalies. When the diagnosis is made *in utero*, it is bilateral in 19–34%, and presentation often includes oliogohydramnios and Potter's syndrome, which are incompatible with life.

Unilateral disease suggests normal life expectancy, however, up to 50% of patients with MCDK have other genitourinary anomalies. UPJ obstruction occurs contralateral to the MCDK in 3–12%, and 15–43% will have VUR in the contralateral kidney.

Periodic US should be obtained and has demonstrated 60–70% of MCDK involute prenatally or postnatally. Later in life, the renal finding may be referred to as a "nubbin" or "renal aplasia/agenesis." The contralateral kidney should undergo compensatory hypertrophy with normal function. If the kidney enlarges, compressive effects may compromise pulmonary or gastrointestinal function. Hypertension has been reported in association with MCDK.

Diagnosis

Since most patients with MCDK are asymptomatic, incidental diagnosis is common. In an infant with abdominal mass, US is recommended. In MCDK, the affected kidney will contain multiple randomly arranged cysts of variable size separated by little to no echogenic parenchyma without a larger central or medial cyst. On US or CT, the cysts do not appear to communicate; however, when injecting contrast, cysts are visibly connected by a network of tubular ducts. A single ostium can be seen opening into a set of channels from each cyst, suggesting the cysts originate from the ureteric bud rather than the blastema.

If US findings are not classic for MCDK or obstruction is questioned, DMSA scan will help determine presence of functional renal tissue and diagnose MCDK as MCDK lacks function. Since this results in a solitary functioning kidney, VCUG should be obtained upon diagnosis to rule out VUR (see Fig. 2).

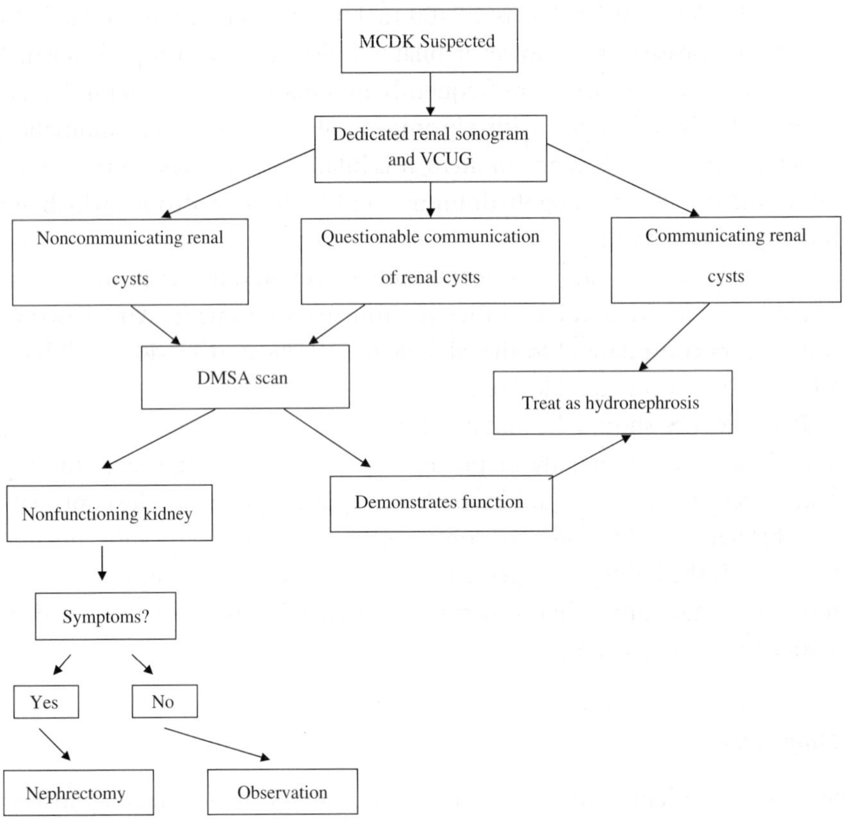

Figure 2.

Treatment and prognosis

MCDK may persist without any change in size, may also grow, spontaneously involute, or rarely, calcify. Most cases of unilateral MCDK undergo spontaneous involution, due to presumed resorption of cystic fluid. Some cases demonstrate increasing size before involution. The Multicystic Kidney Registry reported 260 patients whose cases were conservatively followed with US, showing 54% were undetectable at the end of 5 years.

The vast majority of MCDK require no treatment, and nephrectomy is reserved for those with symptoms from mass effect, hypertension, pain, malignancy, or recurrent infection. Neonates with compromised respiratory function may require percutaneous aspiration of cystic fluid to postpone nephrectomy.

Potential for malignant degeneration of MCDK is concerning. Many cases of Wilm's tumor and other renal tumors have cystic components, while some preknown MCDK undergo malignant transformation. It is therefore difficult to ascertain if a kidney with malignancy was truly a MCDK at birth, therefore further testing should be considered in situations not classic for MCDK. No patient in the Multicystic Kidney Disease Registry has developed a malignancy. Some have estimated Wilm's tumor is 4 times more likely to occur in MCDK than in the general population. Even with this increase, the incidence of Wilm's tumor among MCDK is 1 in 2000; therefore, prophylactic nephrectomy is not recommended. Furthermore, if Wilm's tumor does develop, survival is greater than 90%.

Hypertension has been reported in <1% of patients in the AAP Registry; however, blood pressure should be monitored closely and complete evaluation conducted hypertension develops before considering nephrectomy. The etiology is questionable in most and blood pressure will remain elevated in up to 50% of those that undergo nephrectomy. If a patient with MCDK is found to have contralateral VUR, the patient should receive prophylactic antibiotics until resolution or definitive management.

Many MCDK will remain the same size or involute as the person grows older. The most common risk of a MCDK left in situ is pain from growth, amenable to nephrectomy. MCDK should be followed using US at regular intervals until the kidney involutes. Current recommendations are to obtain renal US every three months during first year of life, followed by every six month US until the patient is five years of age. Alternatively, many practitioners obtain quarterly US during the first year of life followed by annual US.

Suggested Reading

Colodny AH. (1995) The management of multicystic dysplastic kidney in infancy. *Urology* **45**: 1084–1045.

Crombie WJ, Lee K, Houde K, Holmes L. (2001) Implications of prenatal ultrasound screening in the incidence of major genitourinary malformations. *J Urol* **165**: 1677–1680.

Fernbach SK, Maizels M, Conway JJ. (1993) Ultrasound grading of hydronephrosis: introduction to the system used by the Society for Fetal Urology. *Pediatr Radiol* **23**: 478–480.

Glassberg KI, Stephens FD, Lebowitz RL, *et al.* (1987) Renal dysgenesis and cystic disease of the kidney: a report of the committee on terminology, nomenclature and classification, section on urology, American Academy of Pediatrics. *J Urol* **138**: 1085–1092.

Herndon CD, Ferrer FA, Freedman A, McKenna PH. (2000) Consensus on the prenatal management of antenatally detected urologic abnormalities. *J Urol* **164**: 1052–1056.

Herndon CDA, Cain MP. (2009) Prenatal diagnosis of urological disease. *AUA Update Series* **28**: 21–33.

McKenna P, Ferrer F. (2002) Prenatal and postnatal urologic emergencies. In: Belman B, King L, Kramer S. (eds.) *Clinical Pediatric Urology* (4th ed.) Taylor & Francis, London pp. 170–172.

McLean RH, Gearhart JP, Jeffs R. (1988) Neonatal obstructive uropathy. *Pediatr Nephrol* **2**: 48–55.

Peters CA. (2007) Perinatal urology. In: Wein AJ, Kavoussi LR, Novick AC, Partin AW, Peters CA (eds.) *Campbell-Walsh Urology*, (9th ed.) Saunders, Philadelphia: Saunders pp. 3176–3197.

Peters CA, Chevalier RL. (2007) Congenital urinary obstruction: pathophysiology. In: Wein AJ, Kavoussi LR, Novick AC, Partin AW, Peters CA. (eds) *Campbell-Walsh Urology*, (9th ed.) Saunders, Philadelphia pp. 3163–3175.

48

Polycystic Kidney Disease

John J. Bissler

Introduction

Renal cystic diseases have a wide spectrum of presentation with variablility in age of onset, severity during childhood, and presence of comorbidities such as retinal disease, abnormal olfaction, and *situs inversus.* Recent insights into the pathogenesis of polycystic kidney diseases (PKD) have helped not only explain these associations, but also identify novel therapeutic targets. More than 20 different genes causing PKD have been cloned using over the last 15 years. The common factor that unifies PKD is dysfunction of a cellular organelle called the primary cilium and the associated basil body. Continued research toward understanding the etiology and pathogenesis of PKD has already begun to result in targeted clinical trials. This chapter focuses on renal cystic disease from the genetic and cell biology standpoint in order to create a cogent clinical discussion.

Pathogenesis

Polycystic kidney disease anatomically describes the renal phenotype associated with diseases, such as autosomal dominant and recessive polycystic kidney disease, maturity onset diabetes in the young, oral facial digital syndrome, Bardet Biedl syndrome, tuberous sclerosis complex (TSC), and nephronophthisis (NPHP) (Table 1). These are all syndromic cystic renal diseases linked to genes whose protein products localize to renal tubular cell primary cilia or centrosomes. This is much more than "guilt by association," because animal models that disrupt the structure of function of the primary cilia lead to PKD.

Table 1.

Syndrome	OMIM	Mutated gene
Autosomal dominant polycystic kidney disease	173900	PKD1, PKD2
Autosomal recessive polycystic kidney disease	263200	PKHD1
Jeune	208500	IFT80
Orofaciodigital (type 1)	311200	OFD1
Meckel–Gruber		MKS1
	249000	MSK3
Nephronophthisis		NPHP1
	266900	NPHP2 (inversin)
		NPHP3
		NPHP4
		NPHP5
		NPHP6
		NPHP7
		NPHP8(RPGRIP1L)
		NPHP9 (NEK8)
Bardet–Biedl	20990	BBS1
		BBS2
		BBS3/ARL6
		BBS4
		BBS5
		BBS6/MKKS
		BBS7
		BBS8
		BBS9
		BBS10
		BBS11/TRIM32
		BBS12
Joubert	213300	AHI1
Tuberous Sclerosis	191100	TSC1
Complex		TSC2
Von Hippel–Lindau	193300	VHL

Primary cilia originate from the mother centriole in a variety of cells throughout the body. Cilia function as specialized sensors capable of detecting and measuring mechanical, chemical, and peptide cell signaling stimuli. A recent comparative analysis of genomic and proteomic data suggested that the vertebrate cilium may have over 1,000 different polypeptides. In addition to renal cystic disease, ciliary and basal body proteins are also strongly linked to cancer. Renal cystic disease and cancer both exhibit abnormal cell proliferation and changes in ciliary cell signal molecules, including the polycystins and trp channels, Wnt, hedgehog, as well as mitogen and growth factor pathways. Mouse models disrupting cilia develop a cystic renal phenotype. Cilia are also critical for vision, auditory and olfactory reception as well as embryonic development. This developmental link to primary cilia helps to explain the association of some renal cystic disease with retinal abnormalities, anosmia, and *situs inversus.* The developmental role of cilia and timing and extent of mutations also influence the phenotypic expression of renal cystic disease.

Clinical Presentations

Autosomal dominant polycystic kidney disease

Autosomal dominant polycystic kidney disease (ADPKD) has an incidence of 1:400 to 1000, making it one of the most common monogenic disorders (see Fig. 1). Approximately 4.4% of patients requiring renal replacement therapy (RRT) for end-stage renal disease (ESRD) in the United States have ADPKD. This disease process has phenotypic variety, as well as variable expressivity. Cysts develop not only in the kidney but also in the liver, pancreas, seminal vesicles, and arachnoid. ADPKD also is associated with abnormal vasculature, including intracranial aneurysms. These berry aneurysms are about five times more common than in the general population and are a significant cause of morbidity and mortality in ADPKD.

The *PKD1* (16p13.3) and *PKD2* (4q21) genes are linked to ADPKD. Mutations in the *PKD1* gene account for approximately 85% of familial disease, and mutations in the *PKD2* gene account for the remainder. The average age of onset of ESRD for patients with *PKD1* gene mutations is 54.3 years of age, while *PKD2* is 74 years. A developmental component for ADPKD has been revealed in murine models. Heterozygous mice for either *PKD1* or *PKD2* develop a few cysts, mainly in the liver, at older ages; however, studies using conditional knockouts of the *PKD1* gene have demonstrated that inactivation of this gene prior to postnatal day 13 has a very severe phenotype with progressive cystic disease, whereas inactivation at a later time point is phenotypically vastly different. These results

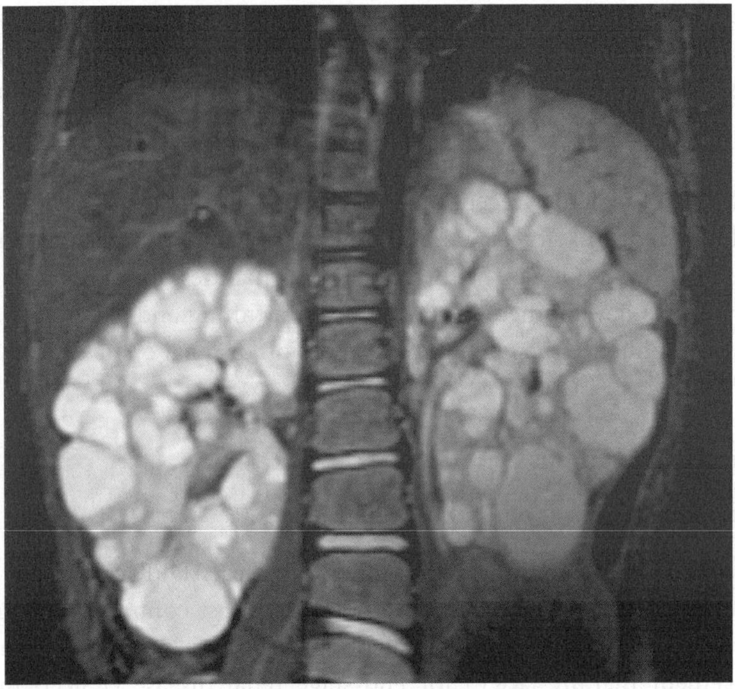

Figure 1. MRI of a child with severe ADPKD.

Note: The numerous cysts (white) in the kidneys bilaterally in this coronal view; MRI (without gadolinium) using the fast spin echo inversion recovery (FSEIR) technique.

indicate an important developmental switch that may be associated with non-regulation of polycystin during renal development. The development of cystic disease has also been associated with a second somatic mutation leading to the loss of a functional *PKD1* gene. Haploinsufficiency can also lead to ADPKD if the *PKD1* hypomorphs produce only small amounts of polycystin 1.

Autosomal recessive polycystic kidney disease

Autosomal recessive polycystic kidney disease (ARPKD) has an estimated incidence of 1 in 20,000 and most commonly presents *in utero* or in the neonatal period with enlarged, echogenic kidneys (Fig. 2). The ARPKD phenotype can extend from Potter sequence with pulmonary hypoplasia,

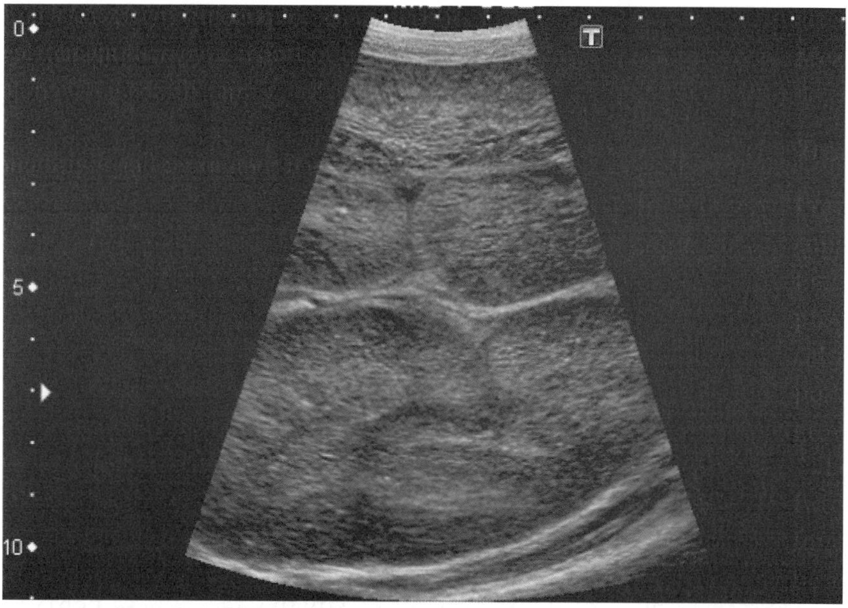

Figure 2. Ultrasound of markedly enlarged kidneys in a patient with severe ARPKD.
Note: The kidneys meet in the midline, and the top kidney is the left, the bottom kidney is the right in this interpolar region view.

characteristic facies, spine, and liver abnormalities to much less renal involvement, such as Caroli disease, which includes congenital hepatic fibrosis, plus intrahepatic bile duct dilatation. Approximately 30% of children with ARPKD die in the neonatal period, primarily from respiratory insufficiency. In those that survive, hypertension and chronic kidney disease (CKD) are frequent. Caroli disease can occur in infants as well as in adolescent and adult patients. The classic renal pathology of ARPKD is fusiform dilatation of the collecting duct as associated with mutations in the polycystic kidney and hepatic disease 1 (*PKHD1*) gene (6q21).

Tuberous sclerosis complex

Renal cystic disease occurs in approximately 45% of patients with TSC. TSC is caused by mutations in either the *TSC1* or the *TSC2* gene. The cystic disease varies from microcystic disease undetectable by imaging studies, to a devastating polycystic phenotype. This latter severe, very early onset phenotype is associated with mutations involving the adjacent *TSC2* and *PKD1* genes on chromosome 16p13 and account for about 2% of TSC patients. Such patients frequently exhibit new mutations, mosaicism for genomic rearrangements, and often develop significant renal dysfunction as teenagers. However, extrapolating older studies regarding progression of CKD to current patients may be inaccurate because patients are now routinely treated with long-acting angiotensin converting enzyme (ACE) inhibitors, and angiotensin receptor blockers (ARB), which may alter the cystic phenotype. TSC-related renal cystic disease also seems to have a cilial association similar to other forms of PKD including other tumor suppressor associated cystic disease.

Nephronophthisis

The incidence of NPHP varies depending on geographic location, occurring at a rate of approximately 1 in 50,000 live births in Canada and about one case per million in the United States. NPHP progresses to ESRD in approximately 10% to 15% of children and accounts for approximately 5% of patients with ESRD in the United States. NPHP is classified based on the age of onset of disease, including the infantile, juvenile and adolescent forms. Like other cystic diseases, NPHP is characterized by a significant urinary concentrating defect resulting in polyuria, polydipsia, and nocturia, as well as secondary enuresis; but, unlike other diseases, it is associated with significant anemia disproportionate to the degree of renal dysfunction. Renal ultrasound (US) often reveals kidneys of small to normal size; late in the disease process, medullary cysts can develop. Edema is rare until the development of ESRD. Depending on the genetic mutation, additional findings can occur with NPHP. Senior–Löken syndrome, accounting for approximately 10% of NPHP, manifests with development of coarse nystagmus and/or blindness at birth or within the first 2 years of life in early-onset disease. Late-onset Senior–Löken syndrome typically presents with night blindness, progressing to overt blindness by school age.

Nephronophthisis manifesting with a specific constellation of extrarenal manifestations constitutes Joubert syndrome. These include coloboma of the eye with or without retinal degeneration, cerebellar vermis aplasia or hypoplasia leading to ataxia, developmental delay, polydactyly, cleft lip/palate, and episodic tachypnea and dyspnea. Magnetic resonance imaging (MRI) of the brainstem reveals the "molar tooth" sign, a pathognomonic finding for Joubert syndrome. In the first two years of life, patients can also develop a failure in initiating fast eye movements resulting in ocular motor apraxia, sometimes referred to as Cogan's ocular motor apraxia or saccadic initiation failure, resulting in impaired horizontal eye movement. Patients also may develop hepatomegaly with portal fibrosis and mild bile duct proliferation. This phenotype may be differentiated from classic congenital hepatic fibrosis by less prominent bile duct proliferation. Using positional cloning, ten genes associated with NHP have been identified with some loci associated with specific phenotypes (see Table 1).

Medullary cystic kidney disease

Medullary cystic kidney disease (MCKD) has very similar histopathology to NPHP, but it is much less prevalent, manifests in adulthood, and is inherited in an autosomal dominant fashion. There are two loci linked to MCKD: one on chromosome 1q21 and the other on chromosome 16p12 that encodes Tamm Horsfall protein (uromodulin). The PKD that develops has renal pathologic findings virtually identical to NPHP, though it manifests in adults and may be associated with hyperuricemia.

Bardet–Biedl syndrome

Estimates of the prevalence of Bardet–Biedl syndrome range from approximately 1 in 18,000 for Newfoundland, 1 out of 13,000 for the Bedouin of Kuwait, and in the United Kingdom approximately 1 out of 125,000. Patients with Bardet–Biedl syndrome demonstrate an array of renal findings, including renal fetal lobulation with calyceal cysts and diverticula, microcysts, diffuse cortical loss, focal scarring, and progression to ESRD in 5% to 30% of patients. First-degree relatives of patients with Bardet–Biedl syndrome also have a higher incidence of renal cell carcinoma. The extrarenal manifestations of Bardet–Biedl syndrome, include polydactyly, central obesity related to hyperphagia, developmental delay, and hypogenitalism in males. In addition, approximately one half of patients exhibit anosmia.

Diagnosis

The diagnosis of PKD is most often made by imaging. If cysts are large, US demonstrates hypoechoic cysts, but if cysts are numerous and small, US may reveal increased echogenicity. Computed tomography (CT) and MRI have increased sensitivity for detecting small cysts. Because cysts develop over time in all patients, an imaging study free of cysts must be interpreted cautiously especially in ARPKD. However, in ADPKD, the patient must be free of cysts after the age of 30 to be confident that the patient has not inherited the disease-causing allele. Cysts can be distributed throughout the kidney parenchyma, focused in the cortical region, as with glomerulocystic disease, or in the medulla, as with diseases like medullary cystic kidney disease or NPHP. Determination of the specific type of PKD depends on the patient and family medical history, as well as the patient's physical exam.

Treatments

While pediatric PKD represents a wide array of phenotypes, they all exhibit several common features that make an initial approach rather straightforward. All forms of PKD are associated with a urinary concentrating defect. While older, neurologically intact, patients can generally maintain their intravascular volume status because they can obtain access to water; infants and developmentally delayed patients can develop significant hypovolemia if they develop increased volume output, decreased intake, or both. A typical example of this latter situation occurs with gastroenteritis. Because urine output is often used in children to assess hydration status, and patients with PKD can have urinary concentration defects, practical advice for families can involve the purchase and use of a scale appropriate for the child's size in order to assess hydration. Parents often sense a change in behavior of the child, even before the onset of significant symptoms, such as diarrhea or vomiting. In this circumstance, parents should be instructed to weigh the child when they are first concerned about the possibility of illness. If additional symptoms develop or worsen, they should reweigh the child to allow the pediatrician to accurately assess the actual percent of dehydration. Animal studies also reveal that suppression of antidiuretic hormone by increased water intake reduced the cystic burden in PKD rats.

Although not all forms of PKD are associated with hypertension, blood pressure control is of critical importance. Hypertension is the second leading cause of ESRD in the United States, and accelerates loss of renal function in other renal diseases. Animal studies suggest that suppression of the renin-angiotensin axis may slow the progression of renal cystic disease, and these preclinical studies have resulted in a clinical trial called HALT. While it is not definitively clear if ACE inhibitors, ARB, or both, decrease the rate of renal reserve loss in pediatric patients with PKD, these agents are very well-tolerated, and are very effective to control blood pressure.

Patients with large cysts, such as occur in ADPKD, TSC, or Bardet–Biedl syndrome, can develop gross hematuria. This hematuria can be caused by nephrolithiasis due to hypocitraturia or trauma. Large cysts can exert such hydraulic force with blunt trauma that the renal parenchyma can be disrupted leading to significant hemorrhage. In this latter case, it is critical to determine the rate of blood loss. Hemorrhages need immediate attention.

Prognosis

The prognosis of each of the different PKD is unique, both to the specific disease as well as to the individual patient. Both types of PKD, ADPKD, and ARPKD have a variable phenotype making it necessary to individualize follow-up and treatment. Beyond excellent blood pressure control and assuring a healthy lifestyle that includes adequate exercise, there is a great deal of promise surrounding possible pharmacologic therapies that are currently being trialed. Given the apparent unifying ciliary hypothesis of PKD, it is possible that these clinical trials may bode well for all PKD. Animal studies have demonstrated beneficial affects of ACE inhibitors with or without ARB. Such a preclinical success is related to the HALT trial. Likewise, research for the vasopressin-2 receptor blocker called tolvaptan has led to phase 2 and 3 trials. Clinical trials with pravastatin, octreotide and lanreotide likewise are underway. Finally, the mammalian target of rapamycin (mTORC) signaling pathway has also been shown to be upregulated and inhibitors of this pathway have shown benefit in animal studies, and in some human reports have been suggested that they may reduce cyst size leading to trials using mTOR inhibitors such as sirolimus or everolimus. End points for these trials include safety, renal volume, and glomerular filtration rate. These trials will be finishing in the upcoming years and hopefully will yield crucial insight about the pharmacologic modulation of the different PKD forms.

Suggested Reading

Adeva M, El-Youssef M, Rossetti S, *et al.* (2006) Clinical and molecular characterization defines a broadened spectrum of autosomal recessive polycystic kidney disease (ARPKD). *Med (Baltimore)* **85**: 1–21.

Bissler JJ, Dixon BP. (2005) A mechanistic approach to inherited polycystic kidney disease. *Pediatr Nephrol* **20**: 558–566.

Bissler JJ, Siroky BJ, Yin H. (2009) Glomerulocystic disease. *Pediatric Nephrology* (In Press).

Guay-Woodford LM, Desmond RA. (2003) Autosomal recessive polycystic kidney disease: the clinical experience in North America, *Pediatr* **111**: 1072–1080.

Hildebrandt F, Attanasio M, Otto E. (2009) Nephronophthisis: disease mechanisms of a ciliopathy. *J Am Soc Nephrol* **20**: 23–35.

Onuchic LF, Furu L, Nagasawa Y, *et al.* (2002) PKHD1, the polycystic kidney and hepatic disease 1 gene, encodes a novel large protein containing multiple immunoglobulin-like plexin-transcription-factor domains and parallel beta-helix 1 repeats. *Am J Human Genet* **70**: 5.

Rakowski SK, Winterkorn EB, Paul E, *et al.* (2006) Renal manifestations of tuberous sclerosis complex: incidence, prognosis, and predictive factors. *Kidney Int* **70**: 1777–1782.

Romio L, Wright V, Price K, *et al.* (2003) OFD1, the gene mutated in oral-facial-digital syndrome type 1, is expressed in the metanephros and in human embryonic renal mesenchymal cells. *J Am Soc Nephrol* **14**: 680–689.

Siroky BJ, Czyzyk-Krzeska MF, Bissler JJ. (2009) Renal involvement in tuberous sclerosis complex and von Hippel-Lindau disease: shared disease mechanisms? *Nat Clin Pract Nephrol* **5**: 143–156.

Torres VE, Harris PC, Pirson Y. (2007) Autosomal dominant polycystic kidney disease. *Lancet* **369**: 1287–1301.

Ward CJ, Hogan MC, Rossetti S, *et al.* (2002) The gene mutated in autosomal recessive polycystic kidney disease encodes a large, receptor-like protein. *Nat Genet* **30**: 259–269.

Yoder B.K. (2007) Role of primary cilia in the pathogenesis of polycystic kidney disease. *J Am Soc Nephrol* **18**: 1381–1388.

49

Nephronophthisis

Rene G. Van De Voorde III

Introduction

Nephronophthisis and medullary cystic kidney disease are two heritable disorders which are often grouped together and termed the nephronophthisis-medullary cystic disease complex. These diseases share many clinical and histopathologic features as well as being equally difficult to diagnose. They are, however, distinct disorders with dissimilar inheritance patterns, extrarenal manifestations, and timing of the onset of renal failure. Medullary cystic kidney diseases, which have autosomal-dominant inheritance patterns, typically present with adult-onset renal failure so they are less likely to present in childhood and will be covered only briefly. Nephronophthisis (NPH) is a genetically heterogenous group of autosomal-recessive renal cystic disorders that often present with subtle symptoms in children, often unrecognized for a long time, but have serious consequences, as they contribute to a large percentage of pediatric patients with end-stage renal disease (ESRD).

The term "familial juvenile nephronophthisis" was first coined by Fanconi in 1951, though the disorder was initially described six years earlier by Smith and Graham. Over the years, three clinical variants of the disease have been described based on the age of onset of ESRD (juvenile, adolescent, and infantile) with juvenile NPH by far the most common form. Its incidence has been estimated as almost 1 per million in the United States, but as high as 1 per 50,000 live births in Canada. Despite this low overall incidence, NPH is one of the most common genetic causes of ESRD in the first two decades of life. It is the attributable cause of ESRD in 2–2.8% of all pediatric patients in North America (NAPRTCS data, 2007), but comprises an even higher fraction (estimated at 15%) of pediatric cases in Europe.

Pathogenesis

The histologic appearance of NPH is a characteristic triad of findings consisting of tubular basement membrane disruption, tubulointerstitial nephropathy, and corticomedullary cysts. However, the pathogenetic mechanisms of NPH had long been elusive. The mutated gene product in juvenile NPH, nephrocystin or nephrocystin-1, was originally localized to the adherens junctions and focal adhesions of renal epithelial cells so these mutations were thought to primarily affect cell–cell and cell–matrix signaling. However, with the advances in positional cloning of genes and the increased ability to characterize encoded proteins over the past decade, greater insight into the pathogenesis of NPH was revealed.

In 2003, the protein products in classic juvenile NPH (nephrocystin) and infantile NPH (inversin) were localized to the primary cilia of renal tubular cells. Primary cilia are highly conserved structures which sense a wide variety of extracellular cues, and act as mechanosensors to fluid movement in the tubule which then elicit transduction pathways within the tubular cell which regulate the cell cycle, proliferation, and apoptosis. Defects in these proteins, termed cystoproteins, can lead to changes in cell polarity, a disruption of the longitudinal orientation of tubular cells, and, ultimately, dilation of the tubules and cyst formation. Thus, the current thinking is that the different diseases of NPH are actually disorders of the cilia, or ciliopathies.

This theory of pathogenesis also helps explain the variety of extrarenal findings (retinal changes, cerebellar malformations, situs inversus) associated with NPH. Retinal photoreceptor cells have connecting cilia, similar to the primary cilia of renal epithelial cells. Neuronal growth and distribution in the brain are assisted by similarly structured microtubules, while left–right orientation of the body (heterotaxy) is a primary function of cilia.

Nine NPH genes and their protein products have been identified to date (see Table 1) with this number steadily increasing over the past five years. However, the causative gene is still unknown for nearly 70% of all worldwide cases of NPH, so new genes will likely be identified in the near future.

Table 1. NPH genetics and extrarenal findings

NPHP gene (disease)	Chromosome	Other organs involved (% of time)	Syndrome or additional physical findings
NPHP1	2q13	Eye (6%)	Senior Loken Syndrome, oculomotor apraxia Cogan
(Juvenile NPH)		Cerebellum (1%)	Joubert Syndrome Type 4
NPHP2	9q31	Eye (10%)	
(Infantile NPH)		Heart (10%)	— situs inversus
NPHP3	3q22	Eye (13%)	
(Adolescent NPH)		Liver (3%)	Boichis Syndrome- hepatomegaly, portal fibrosis
NPHP4	1p36	Eye (33%)	Senior Loken Syndrome, oculomotor apraxia Cogan
NPHP5/IQCB1	3q21	Eye (100%)	Senior Loken Syndrome (early onset)
NPHP6/CEP290	12q21	Eye (100%)	Early retinitis, rarely microophthalmos or coloboma
		Cerebellum (90%)	Joubert Syndrome Type 5
		Brain (90%)	— mental retardation
		Liver (10%)	— bile duct proliferation
		Bone (10%)	— polydactyly
NPHP7/GLIS2	16p	None	
NPHP8/RPGRIP1L	16p	Eye (100%)	— coloboma
		Cerebellum (100%-missense)	Joubert syndrome
		Brain (100%- truncating)	— occipital encephalocele
		Liver (100%- truncating)	
NPHP9	17q11	Eye (30%)	
Unidentified	—	Bone, Eye (50%), Cerebellum (25%)	Mainzer-Saldino syndrome- cone-shaped phalangeal epiphyses, retinal changes, ataxia
	15q13, 3q24	Bone	Jeune syndrome- short ribs (asphyxiating thoracic dysplasia)
	—	Bone, Hair/Nails	Sensenbrenner syndrome- cranioectodermal dysplasia
	4p16	Bone	Ellis van Creveld syndrome- chondroectodermal dysplasia
	—	Eye, Ear, Endocrine	Alstrom syndrome- retinitis, deafness, obesity, diabetes
	—	Eye, Endocrine	RHYNS syndrome- retinitis, hypopituitarism, skeletal dysplasia

Clinical Presentation

The typical presenting symptoms of juvenile NPH are the manifestations of diminished tubular capacity to concentrate the urine. Polyuria, polydipsia, hyposthenuria, and secondary enuresis occur in more than 80% of patients. These symptoms are initially mild, so that patients are often able to maintain volume balance, but are susceptible to dehydration if fluid intake is limited. Increased nocturnal fluid intake, to maintain euvolemia, typically presents by early school age (6–10). However, these patients typically lack other symptoms of renal disease (edema, hypertension, urinalysis findings) so that the diagnosis may be easily missed for several years. Estimates are that symptoms often begin around age five or six, while a slight increase in creatinine does not occur until age nine. Eventually, signs and symptoms of chronic kidney disease (CKD) develop, such as nausea, growth retardation, and aminoaciduria, but typically late in the disease process and many patients are diagnosed at or near the time of ESRD.

Pallor is another very characteristic finding of juvenile NPH. Unlike other renal disorders where anemia often reflects the degree of renal impairment, the anemia seen in NPH is disproportionate to the degree of renal impairment and may occur before any elevation in serum creatinine, such that its association with renal disease may be missed. The etiology of the severe anemia in NPH is abnormally decreased erythropoietin production by the peritubular cells of the kidney, which is not surprising given the histopathologic picture of NPH.

Often the diagnosis of NPH is made at the time of ESRD development, which varies by type of NPH. Infantile NPH has ESRD onset at a median age of less than three years, adolescent NPH (type 3) is age 19 years, and juvenile NPH (predominantly types 1 and 4) by age 13 years. If someone has findings suggestive of NPH but has not developed ESRD by age 25, then medullary cystic kidney disease should be considered.

Although NPH is considered a renal cystic disease, radiologic evidence of cysts is not a hallmark finding. Except in infantile NPH, a renal ultrasound will normally reveal normal to small kidneys with normal contours, increased echogenicity, and loss of corticomedullary differentiation. Corticomedullary cysts may be seen on ultrasound, but are more sensitively detected by thin section (1–2 mm) CT scan, and can be diagnostic.

However, corticomedullary cyst development is a late finding and may not always be present. Unlike the cysts in polycystic kidney disease (PKD), the cysts of juvenile NPH develop from a loss of normal tissue, not a proliferation of abnormal tissue, and are not evenly distributed throughout the kidney, so they are less evident. The exception is infantile NPH, which has radiologic findings similar to polycystic kidney disease (PKD), with enlarged kidneys and cortical cysts. Not surprisingly, the clinical features of infantile NPH are more similar to PKD, as proteinuria and hypertension are typically present.

Although the clinical findings of juvenile NPH may be overlooked, a unique finding of NPH is its pleiotropic nature with the potential involvement of multiple other organ systems outside of the kidney. Up to 10% of patients with NPH, and 100% of patients with some NPH types, will have extrarenal findings (see Table 1). Retinal involvement, termed Senior Loken syndrome, has been found in up to 10% of families with juvenile NPH with no obvious correlation to genotype. Retinitis pigmentosa is most commonly seen with progressive development of night blindness and loss of visual fields. However, an early onset of retinitis may also be present with profound loss of vision in the first years of life. Abnormal brain development can also be seen in some forms of NPH. Cerebellar vermis aplasia has been associated with NPH, referred to as Joubert syndrome. It may be symptomatic with ataxia, hypotonia, or neonatal dyspnea and have classic head MRI findings ("molar tooth sign"). Oculomotor apraxia type Cogan, which is the transient inability of horizontal eye movement, may be noted in infants and toddlers with NPH who jerk their head about to compensate for their ocular restriction. Liver fibrosis has been associated with adolescent NPH, while situs inversus has been seen in the infantile form. Additionally, several other rarer anomalies have also been associated with NPH.

Diagnosis

When there are no extrarenal findings, the diagnosis of NPH requires a high index of suspicion for the disorder, because it lacks early hallmark findings. Patients will have a low urine osmolality (<400 mOsm) on first morning voids, but this may also be seen in other renal concentrating defects. Previously, the diagnosis of NPH would be delayed until the late stages of CKD when a renal biopsy was often indicated and would reveal the characteristic findings of tubular basement membrane thickening and disruption, dilated and atrophic tubules, and corticomedullary cysts. Additionally, thickening and splitting of Bowman's capsule may also be seen with only rare glomerular changes such as segmental sclerosis.

However, with advances in genetic testing, earlier, and more definitive, diagnosis is possible and may be done before the glomerular filtration rate decreases. In patients with a clinical and radiographic picture suggestive of juvenile NPH, molecular genetic analysis for NPHP1 (and NPHP4) gene mutations is commercially available. DNA may be extracted from blood or saliva and tested for the homozygous deletion in NPHP1, which is seen in 60% of patients with juvenile NPH. Heterozygous gene deletion testing is also available by fluorescence *in situ* hybridization (FISH). Negative results do not rule out NPH as there are additional loci and genes for NPH, but a positive result can confirm the diagnosis, with the possible avoidance of renal biopsy. An algorithmic approach (see Algorithm 1) to juvenile NPH has been previously suggested. Incidentally, genetic testing for mutations to NPHP2 and NPHP5 are also available.

The differential diagnosis for NPH includes other disorders which may cause CKD with negative urinalysis findings, including chronic pyelonephritis, obstructive uropathy, cystic renal dysplasia, PKD, medullary sponge kidney, and drug injury. A renal ultrasound may reveal other findings such as renal scarring, hydronephrosis, cortical cysts and enlarged kidneys, or calcifications and ductal ectasia that are consistent with alternate diagnoses.

Treatment/Prognosis

The management of NPH includes correction of specific sequelae of the disorder, as well as the manifestations of CKD. Since tubular fluid and sodium losses are often present, some patients may require an initial correction of water and electrolyte imbalances through enteral or parenteral supplementation. Anemia, particularly severe in NPH, merits early treatment with recombinant human erythropoietin and iron supplementation, often before the later stages of CKD. Additionally, growth hormone should be used for those patients with impaired linear growth. There is no other intervention to slow disease progression as hypertension and proteinuria are not common. In animal models, an experimental vasopressin receptor agonist has been shown to mitigate the mouse equivalent of adolescent NPH but there have been no human studies to date.

In all variants of NPH, there is gradual progression to ESRD such that all patients will ultimately require renal replacement therapy. Preemptive transplantation should be considered; however, potential related donors should be carefully screened for NPH since they, and other relatives, could be at risk for having the disorder as well. Fortunately, disease recurrence has never been reported in transplanted patients.

Suggested Reading

Hildebrandt F, Rensing C, Betz RC, *et al.* (2001) Establishing an algorithm for molecular genetic diagnostics in 127 families with juvenile nephronophthisis. *Kidney Int* **59**: 434–45.

Hildebrandt F, Zhou W. (2007) Nephronophthisis-associated ciliopathies. *J Am Soc Nephrol* **18**: 1855–1871.

Hildebrandt F, Attanasio M, Otto E. (2009) Nephronophthisis: disease mechanisms of a ciliopathy. *J Am Soc Nephrol* **20**: 23–35.

Omran H, Ermisch-Omran B. (2008) Nephronophthisis and medullary cystic kidney disease. In: Geary DF, Schaefer F (eds.) *Comprehensive Pediatric Nephrology*, 1st ed., pp. 143–152, Mosby, Philadelphia.

Salomon R, Saunier S, Niaudet P. (2008) Nephronophthisis. *Pediatr Nephrol*, published online July 8, 2008.

[URL http://www.renalgenes.org/nephronophthisis.html].

[URL: http://emedicine.medscape.com/article/982359-overview] Accessed June 6, 2009.

50

Rare Genetic Disorders

Rene G. Van De Voorde III

Introduction

Since renal diseases are already uncommon among children, many are considered rare disorders. The heritable disorders discussed in this chapter are infrequently encountered in pediatric nephrology practice (Table 1). Despite being "zebras," they are important to recognize because of either their distinctive features or the potential for early treatment, and reduction of morbidity.

Cystinosis

Nephropathic cystinosis is an autosomal recessive, lysosomal storage disorder which affects the kidney and other tissues. It is the most common heritable cause of Fanconi syndrome, yet its incidence is 1 in 200,000 live births. Early identification of the disorder is essential as it presents during infancy and prompt treatment may delay organ dysfunction.

Cystinosis is caused by mutations to the gene encoding cystinosin, the lysosomal exporter of cystine, mapped to chromosome 17. In the lysosome, the amino acid cysteine is oxidized into its disulfide, cystine. With defective cystinosin, cystine cannot be transported out of the lysosome, and accumulates into intracellular crystals. The exact mechanisms of tissue injury are unclear, but it is thought that lysosomal cystine directly increases apoptosis, though extent of crystal content does not correlate with tissue injury.

The initial clinical findings of cystinosis are related to Fanconi syndrome presenting during infancy. Presenting symptoms are polyuria [with dilute (< 300 mOsm/L) urine output of at least 2 liters daily] and polydipsia- with

Table 1. Rare genetic disorders

Disease	Gene (chromosome)	Distinctive features
Cystinosis	CTNS (17p13)	Fanconi syndrome; photophobia, corneal cystine crystals; hypothyroidism; decreased sweating, tearing, and salivation; blond hair, fair complexion
Dent Disease	CLCN5 (Xp11) OCRL1 (Xq26)	Significant low molecular weight proteinuria; hypercalciuria, nephrocalcinosis
Lowe Syndrome	OCRL1 (Xq26)	Fanconi syndrome; congenital cataracts, glaucoma; mental retardation, delayed speech and ambulation; stereotypical behaviors, temper tantrums; elongated face, deep-set eyes; scoliosis, arthritis
Nail Patella Syndrome	LMXB1 (9q34)	Absent or dystrophic nails; patellar aplasia/hypoplasia or dislocations; limited elbow pronation/supination, radial head hypoplasia; iliac horns; glomerulonephritis-like findings
Primary Hyperoxaluria, type 1	AGXT (2q37)	Recurrent urolithiasis (renal colic, hematuria), nephrocalcinosis; late oxalosis with bone pain and spontaneous fractures

an increased susceptibility to dehydration as an infant. Other classic urinary findings include glucosuria, proteinuria, phosphaturia, and bicarbonaturia. Linear growth retardation, secondary to acidosis, and profound electrolyte losses, often presents by age one year as does hypophosphatemic rickets. Decreasing glomerular filtration rate (GFR) often does not begin until late childhood with serum creatinine being normal initially. Photophobia, from cystine crystal formation within the cornea, presents in early childhood while hypothyroidism, from thyroid crystal accumulation, develops by age ten. Other features of the disorder include fair complexion (blond hair, blue eyes) and decreased tearing, salivation, and sweat production.

Early diagnosis, to prompt preventive therapy, is crucial. Chemical evaluation of the serum and urine may reveal hypokalemia, hypophosphatemia, and renal tubular acidosis, which helps differentiate from Bartter syndrome and diabetes insipidus. Confirmation of cystinosis is made by measuring leukocyte cystine content on serum assay, with subjects having cystine levels >2 nmol/mg protein and normal individuals <0.2. The presence of corneal cystine crystals on slit lamp examination is also diagnostic, but may not be present before 15 months of age. Neonatal testing of the placenta and prenatal diagnostic amniocentesis may also be performed.

Treatment consists of symptomatic therapy of fluid, electrolyte, and mineral imbalances of Fanconi syndrome with water, potassium, phosphate, and alkaline replacement. Growth hormone is frequently required at an early age, whereas thyroxine is also eventually needed. However, prompt diagnosis is most important because of the ability to potentially delay tissue injury with cystine-depleting therapy with cysteamine. Cysteamine crosses into the lysosome and has an exchange reaction producing cysteine and cysteine-cysteamine, both of which may exit the lysosome via a lysine transporter. Oral administration of cysteamine every 6 hours may deplete intracellular cystine by 90% and delay renal and other tissue damage. Corneal crystals need to be treated with topical cysteamine eye drops, 6–12 times daily, to ameliorate ophthalmic symptoms.

Before the use of cysteamine, end-stage renal disease (ESRD) would often occur by age 12 years, but now may be delayed until age 30 in treated patients. Dialysis may be performed effectively, but transplant is still preferable, with heterozygous relatives acceptable as donors. Renal transplantation does not correct the metabolic defect of the disease, as it can affect all tissues; therefore continued cysteamine therapy is necessary. With cystinosis patients living longer, other disease complications have become more prevalent, such as myopathy, gastrointestinal (GI) dysmotility, pancreatic insufficiency, and diabetes mellitus.

Lowe Syndrome

Lowe syndrome, or the oculo-cerebro-renal syndrome of Lowe, is a X-linked recessive (XLR) disorder, with a prevalence of 1 in 500,000. It has a classic triad of diagnostic findings — congenital cataracts, neonatal or infantile hypotonia proceeded by developmental delay, and Fanconi syndrome — which often leads to early diagnosis in most patients.

Lowe syndrome has been linked to several described mutations to the OCRL1 gene, located on the long arm of the X chromosome. Its gene product, inositol polyphosphate 5-phosphatase, localizes to the Golgi apparatus and its impairment alters intracellular protein sorting of the renal epithelium and optic lens, resulting in altered endocytosis.

Boys with Lowe syndrome typically present as neonates with bilateral cataracts, hypotonia, and areflexia. Dense cataracts form in utero, from altered migration of crystalline embryonic epithelium of the lens, and are often apparent on initial red reflex exam. Fanconi syndrome typically presents after three months of age with failure to thrive from persistent renal tubular acidosis and salt/water wasting. Low molecular weight (LMW) proteinuria is often present early and is the most sensitive marker of renal dysfunction.

Initial renal symptoms include fluid and electrolyte disorders as renal function remains stable during the first decade of life. Dehydration episodes are common and aggressive fluid and caloric replenishment is often needed to maintain normal growth. Patients also have significant phosphaturia, causing hypophosphatemia and growth impairment. Rickets, with classic radiographic findings, often develops. Hypercalciuria, from high urinary sodium and parathyroid hormone (PTH) levels, is often present and nephrocalcinosis may be seen on renal ultrasound.

While renal findings develop, there is persistence of both ocular and developmental abnormalities. Bilateral glaucoma develops in 50–60% of subjects, typically in the first year of life, while corneal keloids develop 25% of the time. Delayed development of language and motor milestones is nearly universal. Unassisted ambulation is delayed past the third birthday in nearly all boys and often past the sixth birthday. Only 10% of Lowe patients have borderline intelligence with greater than one-third having profound mental retardation. Additionally, behavioral changes with stereotypical behaviors in infancy, temper tantrums in childhood, and aggressiveness in adolescence are seen in more than 80% of patients.

The diagnosis of Lowe syndrome is suspected by clinical findings. However, the diagnostic standard is decreased (<10%) activity of inositol polyphosphate 5-phosphatase in cultured skin fibroblasts. This testing is available commercially and is abnormal in >99% of affected males. Sequence analysis of the OCRL1 gene can be performed for confirmation of the diagnosis, as mutations will be found in 95% of subjects. Unaffected carriers of the disease can also be identified by the presence of punctuate white-grey opacities in their lenticular cortex as seen on slit-lamp examination.

The treatment of Lowe syndrome includes aggressive treatment of proximal tubulopathy. Citrate or bicarbonate replacement is needed to maintain a serum HCO3 >20 mEq/L. Potassium citrate is preferred as it may replace concurrent potassium deficits. Sodium and fluid supplementation may be necessary, depending on the extent of renal losses, and replacement via nasogastric or gastrostomy tube should be considered. Phosphorus and vitamin D replacement is also needed to treat rickets, with a goal of maintaining normal serum calcium and PTH. LMW proteinuria does not typically cause protein malnutrition, but carnitine supplementation is needed in one-third of individuals with low serum levels. Extrarenal therapies include early rehabilitative services such as behavioral modification planning, speech, and physical therapy. Ophthalmologic interventions include early cataract removal, use of corrective glasses to promote visual development, and ongoing monitoring for glaucoma and corneal scars.

In the first years of life, there is moderate morbidity and mortality risk from metabolic derangements and respiratory illnesses, because of poor cough clearance secondary to hypotonia. Impaired renal function does not typically develop until the second or third decade. In these older patients, interstitial fibrosis and tubular atrophy gradually progress, leading to secondary glomerulosclerosis and decreasing GFR. ESRD inevitably develops, typically by age 30, without many options to delay progression. Dialysis and renal transplantation have been performed successfully in patients, but may require greater discussion because of the potential ethical and complexity issues regarding long-term care.

Dent Disease

Dent disease is an XLR disorder of the proximal tubule, characterized by LMW proteinuria and hypercalciuria. Similar disorders such as XLR nephrolithiasis, XLR hypophosphatemic rickets, and LMW proteinuria of Japanese children, share some, but not all, disease characteristics with Dent disease. However, with advancing genetic analysis, it was discovered that these were all varied mutations of the same gene and, hence, were grouped together as Dent disease type 1. Dent disease type 2 is clinically similar, but involves mutations to a different gene on the X chromosome. Because of this variability in terminology, overall prevalence of the disorder has not been reported and may be underestimated.

The mutation isolated in 60% of all Dent disease is to the CLCN5 gene located on chromosome X. This gene encodes a voltage-gated chloride channel found primarily, but not exclusively, in the proximal tubule, thick ascending limb, and collecting duct. This channel permits acidification of proximal tubular endosomes by counterbalancing chloride entry. Loss of this channel does not allow for endocytosis of LMW proteins in the proximal tubule. Additionally, proximal tubular reabsorption of PTH is also reduced and leads to activation of distal receptors and increased urinary calcium excretion, though the direct mechanism is less apparent. The mutation identified in 15% of Dent disease (type 2) is in OCRL1, the same gene in Lowe syndrome. Though it is unclear why the full spectrum of Lowe syndrome is not seen, changes to the encoded phosphatase is thought to affect endosomal tracking via direct action on the endosomal protein clathrin.

Patients with Dent disease typically present in childhood with polyuria, microscopic hematuria, and proteinuria. Nocturia and polyuria are seen in early childhood though impaired urinary concentration is not as prominent as in other Fanconi syndromes. Similarly, glucosuria and phosphaturia are variably present. However, LMW proteinuria is often significant (1–2 grams daily) and present in early childhood, though not necessarily symptomatic. Significant hypercalciuria (8–10 mg/kg/d) may also be present in younger children with the development of nephrocalcinosis in 75% of patients, often in childhood, and urolithiasis in 50% of patients. Though serum calcium and PTH are normal, rickets has been seen in 25% of patients, predominately reported in Europe. Renal dysfunction develops in two-thirds of patients, often starting in late childhood.

The diagnosis should be suspected in children with significant hypercalciuria or nephrocalcinosis, and proteinuria. Vastly elevated urinary retinol binding protein is a sensitive and specific disease marker, but not diagnostic. Female carriers often also have LMW proteinuria and may be tested. Commercial genetic tests for CLCN5 and OCRL1 mutational analysis are available, but only account for 75% of the known mutations.

Primary treatment focuses on the reduction of hypercalciuria to prevent nephrocalcinosis, and nephrolithiasis. Dietary sodium intake should be restricted while dietary calcium should be normalized, as to not worsen any bone disease. Additionally, thiazides are recommended to decrease calcium excretion. Phosphate and vitamin D supplementation are recommended if bone disease is present, with doses adjusted to normalize serum alkaline phosphatase levels, while closely monitoring urinary calcium. Mouse studies have shown benefit of increased dietary citrate and may be beneficial, while angiotensin converting enzyme (ACE) inhibitors may have some antifibrotic effects but are unlikely to improve proteinuria.

Advancing tubular atrophy and interstitial fibrosis eventually lead to glomerulosclerosis and renal dysfunction. ESRD typically develops by age 30–40 and thought to be associated with nephrocalcinosis, but not always. Patients with Dent disease do well with dialysis and are excellent transplant candidates.

Hyperoxaluria

Primary hyperoxaluria is an autosomal recessive disorder affecting hepatic peroxisomes, with primary effects on the kidney from oxalate accumulation. It occurs in two forms, more commonly type 1 (PH1), which occurs in 1 in 120,000 European births with higher rates in areas of the world with increased consanguinity. PH1 occurs due to defective alanine:glyoxalate aminotransferase (AGT), an enzyme which normally converts glyoxalate to glycine in the liver peroxisome. The gene encoding AGT has been mapped to chromosome 2 and different mutations may cause either complete absence of AGT, nonfunctional enzyme, or reduced AGT activity. Decreased glyoxalate conversion to glycine leads to increased conversion to oxalate, via an alternate pathway, and oxalate accumulation within the body. PH2 also leads to oxalate accumulation by decreased glyoxalate conversion to glycolate.

Oxalate overproduction leads to massive amounts in the urine and subsequent risk of urinary complications. Typically, patients have recurrent urolithiasis starting in early childhood, with 50% having symptoms before age five. Nephrocalcinosis on ultrasound or bilateral radio-opaque stones on X-ray should raise suspicion for PH1. An infantile form of PH1 is seen with early nephrocalcinosis and rapid GFR decline, with half of patients having ESRD diagnosed simultaneously with their PH1. Less aggressive forms of PH1 may not be diagnosed promptly, with up to five years from initial symptoms to diagnosis; therefore, a high index of suspicion is warranted.

The diagnosis of PH1 is first suspected by markedly elevated urinary oxalate excretion. Normal urine oxalate levels are <0.5 mMol/1.73m^2/day, where levels exceeding 1 mMol/1.73 m^2/day are suggestive of the disorder. However, a definitive diagnosis is made by liver biopsy and testing both AGT levels and activity. Genetic analysis is not routinely performed for diagnostic purposes but may be considered for genotyping, as certain mutations are more responsive to pyridoxine therapy.

The initial treatment goal in PH1 is to minimize renal oxalate deposition and risk of urolithiasis. Dietary avoidance of foods high in oxalate (tea, chocolate, spinach) has a very limited effect. Increasing fluid intake to maintain high urine output (2–3 liters/day) is recommended and the use of thiazides may also reduce urine calcium levels. Potassium citrate, orthophosphate, and magnesium supplementation may be used to increase the urinary solubility of calcium oxalate. Urologic involvement in the presence of stones should be prompt to avoid obstructions and minimize long-term risk factors.

Pyridoxine, a co-enzyme to AGT, can reduce urine oxalate concentrations by one-third, but only 10–30% of patients are pyridoxine-responsive. Pyridoxamine, which chelates oxalate precursors, has encouraging results in animal studies, but is not yet approved for humans.

The bacteria *Oxalobacter formigenes* has been shown to reduce urine and plasma oxalate in PH1 patients when given enterally.

Eventually, PH1 patients will have a gradual decline in GFR and ESRD is typically reached by age 25–40, but much more rapidly (by age five) in the infantile form. As GFR declines below 30–50 ml/min, plasma oxalate levels increase and deposition into other tissues occurs, primarily bone, heart, and vasculature. Standard dialysis is unable to remove oxalate chronically, and alternate dialysis plans are needed. Isolated renal transplant may be considered, but this is only temporizing, as graft function will ultimately be lost with oxalate reaccumulation. Combined liver–kidney transplant or preemptive liver transplant are the only permanent treatments as the liver graft should have normal AGT activity and act as enzyme replacement.

Nail Patella Syndrome

Nail Patella syndrome (NPS), also referred to as hereditary osteo-onychodysplasia, is characterized by the clinical tetrad of nail, knee, and elbow anomalies with the presence of iliac horns. It is an autosomal dominant disorder occurring once every 50,000 births but, because of its inheritance pattern and classic findings, it's not difficult to diagnose. Renal involvement is variable.

NPS is associated with mutations to the LMXB1 gene, located on chromosome 9. This gene encodes a transcription factor for multiple other genes, including those for normal development of dorsal limb structures, and the coordinated expression of type IV collagen in the glomerulus.

NPS typically presents with nail and joint findings, as renal involvement, if present at all, develops later. Nail changes are present in >90%, often at birth. Nails may be split, dystrophic, or absent. Triangular nail lunules are a characteristic finding of NPS. Nail involvement is typically bilateral and symmetric, with fingers involved more than toes and radial (thumb, index) more than ulnar nails. Nearly all patients have either knee (75%) or elbow (70%) abnormalities, and often both. Patellar aplasia or hypoplasia may be found either by palpation or radiography. Subjects often suffer from recurrent patellar dislocation from abnormal condylar or muscle development, with contractures and arthritis developing with time. Elbow abnormalities include radial head hypoplasia or limited pronation, and supination. Iliac horns, bony processes projecting posteriorly, and laterally from the iliac crests, are found in 30–70% of subjects. Iliac horns are considered pathognomonic for the disorder, but are asymptomatic so they must be sought by radiography as they are typically not palpable.

Renal involvement is seen in only 30–45% of NPS patients with variation even within families. It presents as a mild glomerulonephritis, with proteinuria but hematuria and hypertension may also develop. Nephrotic syndrome has been seen with NPS, including the infantile form, while other nephropathies have also been associated. Renal biopsy may show basement membrane thickening with negative immunofluorescence. Electron microscopy reveals increased lucencies of the basement membrane, classically described as appearing moth-eaten. This appearance is secondary to the disordered array of type IV collagen, much like Alport's syndrome, causing irregular thickening of the membrane. There is no correlation between the ultrastructural appearance and disease severity, so biopsies are not necessarily prognostic.

The diagnosis of NPS is made from clinical nail findings and radiologic abnormalities of the knees, elbows, or pelvis. Diagnostic confirmation may be made by genetic analysis, which is commercially available and reveals mutations in 85% of subjects.

Primary treatment surrounds the orthopedic issues associated with the disorder including early physiotherapy, splinting, and bracing to avoid joint degeneration and future surgeries. In the 30–40% with renal involvement, prevention of disease progression with ACE inhibition, hypertension control, and treatment of chronic kidney disease sequelae is indicated. In those patients developing nephrotic syndrome, corticosteroids may induce remission while diuretics minimize edema. Additionally, regular screening for glaucoma should be performed in all NPS patients, as it is more prevalent and occurs earlier than in the general population. One third of NPS patients with nephropathy (5% overall) will progress to ESRD, at a mean age of 33 years. Renal transplantation in these patients have good outcomes; however, circumspect screening of related donor candidates should be performed because of the heritable nature of the disorder.

Congenital Nephrotic Syndrome

Congenital nephrotic syndrome has been defined as heavy proteinuria occurring before three months of age; this is in contrast to heavy proteinuria later during the first year termed infantile nephrotic syndrome. However, the diseases causing nephrosis in the first year of life are mainly genetic disorders affecting glomerular structure, with overlapping times of onset and histologic pictures. Therefore, there is no diagnostic rationale for making the distinction between congenital and infantile presentations and these disorders are grouped together here under the term congenital nephrotic syndrome (CNS).

Most cases of CNS are from genetic mutations which encode for either structural components or regulatory proteins of the glomerular filtration barrier (see Table 2). The most prevalent form of CNS is the Finnish type (CNF), which is seen in 1 in 10,000 births in Finland, but much less commonly elsewhere. It is caused by mutations to the NPHS1 gene encoding nephrin, a critical protein of the slit diaphragm. The absence of nephrin causes a loss of effective charge- and size-selectivity, allowing plasma proteins to leak across into the luminal space. Mutations to the NPHS2 gene encoding podocin, a podocyte protein which targets and anchors nephrin, have also been associated with up to half of CNS cases in Europe and are found in 95% of identified causes of CNS. Less common mutations may occur to genes encoding for laminin β-2 (primary component of the glomerular basement membrane), WT1 (transcription factor for embryonic development of the kidney and genitalia), and PLCE1 (enzyme which generates second messengers for cell growth and differentiation). Secondary causes of CNS have also been associated with congenital infections (syphilis, toxoplasmosis, hepatitis B, HIV) and maternal lupus.

CNS may be suspected antenatally, as proteinuria occurs before birth and elevates alpha-fetoprotein (AFP) levels. In the absence of anencephaly or neural tube defects, amniotic AFP levels ten-fold greater than normal are indicative of CNS. At delivery, the placenta is often very large, >25% of the newborn weight. Postnatally, the first sign is often generalized edema, but this may not be noted until infancy. The evaluation reveals edema, massive proteinuria (>2000 mg/dL) and hypoalbuminemia (<1.5 g/dL), making the diagnosis of CNS. In CNF, renal function is often normal for several months and declines late in infancy or early

Table 2. Congenital nephrotic syndrome (CNS)

Disorder	Protein (chromosome)	Distinctive features
CNS- Finnish type (CNF)	Nephrin (19q13)	No extrarenal manifestations except for minor flexion deformities from large placenta; Large echogenic kidneys on US late in infancy
	Podocin (1q25-31)	No extrarenal findings; often FSGS on biopsy, lack of podocin staining
Denys Drash syndrome	WT1 protein (11p13)	Male pseudohermaphroditism (46 XY), abnormal gonadal development (US), Wilms tumor risk- often bilateral nephrectomies needed
Galloway Mowat syndrome	Unknown	CNS anomalies (microcephaly, structural anomalies), mental retardation, hiatal hernia, diaphragmatic abnormalities
Isolated diffuse mesangial sclerosis	Phospholipase C epsilon (10q23)	Isolated diffuse mesangial sclerosis on biopsy, may respond to immunosuppression
Pierson syndrome	Laminin β-2 (3p21)	Ocular findings (pinpoint pupils, cataracts, retinal changes), developmental delay

childhood. Other etiologies of CNS, particularly those with extrarenal findings, often have more rapid decline in GFR. Although the CNS disorders having extrarenal findings are less common, a complete physical examination looking for these findings is indicated. Thorough examination of the genitalia (male pseuodohermaphroditism), eyes (microcoria), and head (microcephaly) should be performed at a minimum while karyotyping, head and abdominal ultrasound, and ophthalmologic examination should be considered.

The diagnosis of CNS is made by clinical findings of severe proteinuria and hypoalbuminemia. The specific CNS etiology is not typically made by renal biopsy, as the findings of minimal change, focal sclerosis, or diffuse mesangial sclerosis may overlap with different entities. Immunohistochemistry for nephrin, podocin, or laminin β-2 may be performed. However, genetic analysis is the preferred method of diagnosis as testing for NPHS1, NPHS2, WT1, and LAMB2 mutations are clinically available.

The treatment of CNS is very different from other forms of nephrosis as steroids and immunosuppressants do not cause remission. Therefore, the goals of therapy are to control edema, prevent complications of severe proteinuria, and optimize nutrition. Reduction of proteinuria is only accomplished by reducing renal blood flow. Angiotensin converting enzyme inhibitors and indomethacin are frequently used together and, when medical therapy is insufficient, unilateral nephrectomy should be considered. Parenteral albumin infusions via central venous catheters are often necessary to limit swelling. The main complications of such severe proteinuria are infectious risk, and hypercoagulability. IVIG infusions and prophylactic antibiotics may be considered but seem to have limited efficacy. Increased suspicion of septicemia with prompt therapy is warranted. Aspirin and dipyridamole have also been used to reduce thrombotic risk. Loss of thyroid-binding globulin often causes hypothyroidism so thyroxine substitution is also required for appropriate growth. Lastly, a low-sodium, high-calorie, high-protein diet is indicated for adequate growth and may need to be given via nasogastric or gastrostomy tube.

CNS patients historically had very poor prognoses, often succumbing early to infectious complications. More recently, with more aggressive CNS therapy and better outcomes with infant dialysis, patients may do well and grow enough to allow for renal transplant, the only curative treatment. Renal transplant outcomes are similar to other disorders with transplant at younger ages. There has been a noted (25%) risk of recurrence of disease in CNF, but was seen only with the homozygous Fin-major genotype.

Suggested Reading

Cochat P, Liutkus A, Fargue S, *et al.* (2006) Primary hyperoxaluria type 1: still challenging! *Pediatr Nephrol* **21**: 1075–1081.

Gahl WA, Thoene JG, Schneider JA. (2002) Cystinosis. *N Engl J Med* **347**: 111–121.

Jalanko H. (2007) Congenital nephrotic syndrome. *Pediatr Nephrol* [Online].

Ludwig M, Utsch B, Monnens LAH. (2006) Recent advances in understanding the clinical and genetic heterogeneity of Dent's disease. *Nephrol Dial Transplant* **21**: 2708–2717.

[URL: http://www.ncbi.nlm.nih.gov/bookshelf/br.fcgi?book=gene&part=lowe] (Gene Reviews website for Lowe Syndrome)

[URL: http://emedicine.medscape.com/article/1106294-overview] (e-Medicine website for Nail-Patella Syndrome)

[URL: http://www.uptodate.com/patients/content/search.do?search=Lowe%20 syndrome&source=RELATED_SEARCH] (UpToDate search on Lowe syndrome)

Index